# Principles and Practice of Dental Care

# Principles and Practice of Dental Care

Editor: Dave Clark

FOSTER ACADEMICS

www.fosteracademics.com

www.fosteracademics.com

FOSTER ACADEMICS

**Cataloging-in-Publication Data**

Principles and practice of dental care / edited by Dave Clark.
p. cm.
Includes bibliographical references and index.
ISBN 978-1-63242-499-0
1. Dental care. 2. Dentistry--Practice. I. Clark, Dave.
RK61 .P74 2017
617.6--dc23



Foster Academics,
118-35 Queens Blvd., Suite 400,
Forest Hills, NY 11375, USA

ISBN 978-1-63242-499-0 (Hardback)



Printed and bound in China.

# Contents

# Preface

Every book is initially just a concept; it takes months of research and hard work to give it the final shape in which the readers receive it. In its early stages, this book also went through rigorous reviewing. The notable contributions made by experts from across the globe were first molded into patterned chapters and then arranged in a sensibly sequential manner to bring out the best results.

Dental care involves the prevention and management of chronic mouth and facial pain and other diseases and disorders that affect the oral cavity. It is a sub-discipline of dentistry which deals with the study, diagnosis and treatment of diseases related to oral cavity. This book outlines the different techniques through which dental disorders could be treated. This book is compiled in such a manner, that it will provide in-depth knowledge about the theory and practice of dental care and dentistry. It is a resource guide for experts as well as students. Coherent flow of topics, student-friendly language and extensive use of examples make this book an invaluable source of knowledge.

It has been my immense pleasure to be a part of this project and to contribute my years of learning in such a meaningful form. I would like to take this opportunity to thank all the people who have been associated with the completion of this book at any step.

**Editor**

# 1

# Liquid-Supported Dentures: A Soft Option—A Case Report

**Anoop Jain,[1] Shivakumar Puranik,[1] M. S. Jagadeesh,[2] Puttaraj Kattimani,[3] Savita Akki,[4] Pawan Kumar,[5] and Vijaya laxmi'[6]**

[1] *Department of Prosthodontics, HKE'S S N Institute of Dental Sciences & Research, Gulbarga, Karnataka 585105, India*
[2] *Department of Prosthodontics, Farooqia Dental College and Hospital, Mysore, Karnataka 570015, India*
[3] *Department of Prosthodontics, Pandit Deendayal Upadhyay Dental College Hospital & Research Centre, Solapur, Maharastra 413255, India*
[4] *Department of Prosthodontics, SB Patil Dental College & Hospital, Bidar, Karnataka 585401, India*
[5] *Department of Prosthodontics, Al-Badar Dental College & Hospital, Gulbarga, Karnataka 585105, India*
[6] *Department of Prosthodontics, G. Pulla Reddy Dental College, Andhra Pradesh 518002, India*

Correspondence should be addressed to Anoop Jain; dranoopjn@gmail.com

Academic Editors: L. Junquera, A. Kasaj, C. Ledesma-Montes, and A. Markopoulos

Liquid-supported denture technique allows continued adaptation of denture to the mucosa both at resting and functional state. A complete denture prosthesis is unacceptable if it violates the foundation on which it rests. In this case, a technique for fabrication of a complete denture prosthesis that eliminates the disadvantages of tissue conditioners and soft liners (i.e., poor bond strength to acrylic, candidal colonization, etc.) and preserves the remaining tissues is described. Liquid-supported denture can be a permanent solution to some patients with problematic conditions like diabetes, xerostomia, atrophied ridge, and so forth.

## 1. Introduction

Flabby ridge is a superficial area of mobile soft tissue affecting the maxillary or mandibular alveolar ridges. It can be developed when soft tissue replaces the alveolar bone and it is a common finding, particularly in long term denture wearers [1]. These soft tissue changes and bone resorption occurs because of muscle dynamics or tissue irritation, which ultimately affects the residual ridge dimensions [2]. Thus, complete denture seldom remain in close adaptation to the adjacent mucosa. However, it also has to support the teeth during function and thus should be rigid. An ideal denture base should be flexible, as it has to continuously adapt to the mucosa. However, it also has to be rigid so as to support the teeth during function. These properties cannot be combined in one material, but are possible by using combination of materials [3].

Several techniques have been tried on the tissue surface of the dentures. In 1961, Chase introduced the use of elastic impression material to relieve traumatized tissue. But this can be only a temporary provision. Moreover, it might easily derive candidal growth. Since then a variety of tissue conditioning materials has been introduced. Another group of materials called soft liners has been used to relieve "denture sore mouth" problems. But soft liners are also only temporary provisions because due to loss of plasticizer over a period of time, they lose their plastic properties. In a flabby ridge condition, an ideal denture should be able to withstand masticatory forces and have flexible tissue surface to reduce stress concentration and trauma on the underlying tissues [4]. A Liquid-supported denture can hence be a solution for this problem. This paper describes the fabrication of a mandibular complete denture with its base covered with a preshaped, close fitting, and flexible sheet containing a thin film of viscous liquid, which fulfills the aforementioned requirements.

## 2. Case Report

A 56-year-old male patient reported to HKE'S S N Institute of Dental sciences & Research, Gulbarga, Karnataka, India, for replacement of missing teeth. The patient had a history

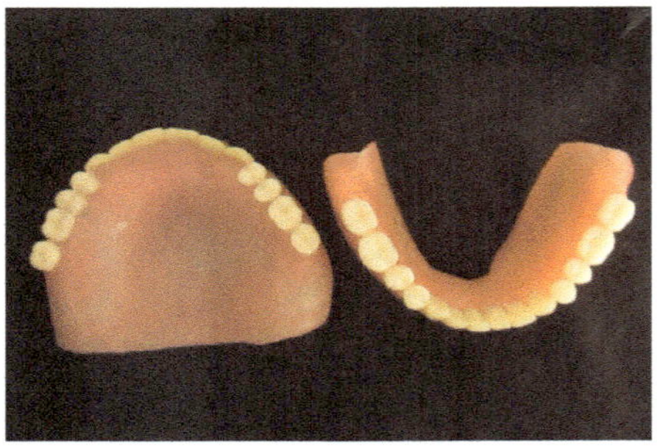

FIGURE 1: Patient's old denture.

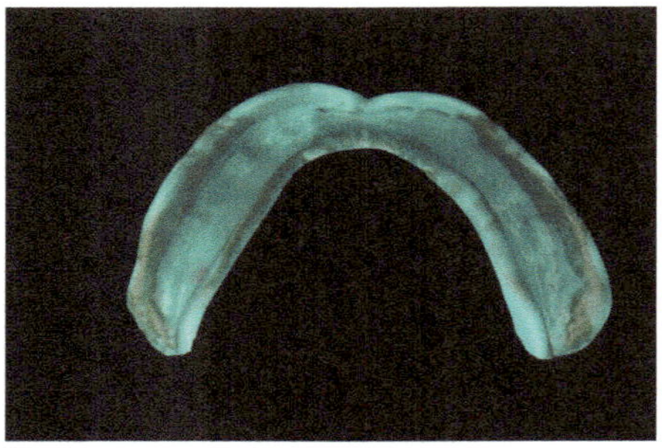

FIGURE 2: Final impression made with elastomeric impression material.

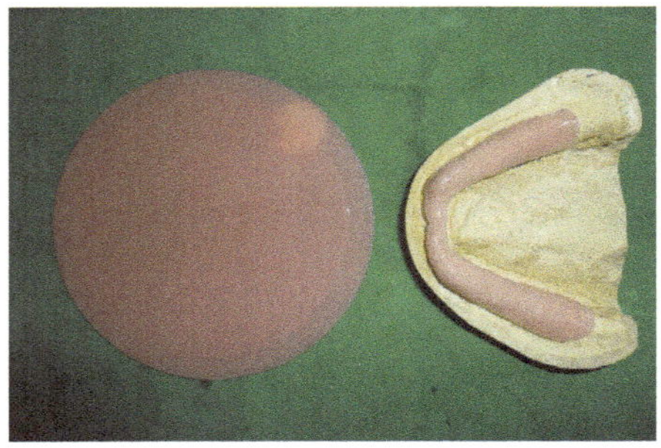

FIGURE 3: Vacuum heat-pressed polyethylene sheet (1.5 mm thick).

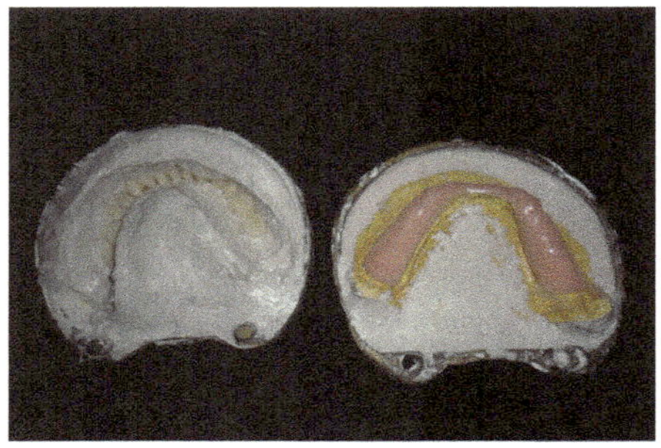

FIGURE 4: Vacuum heat-pressed polyethylene sheet (1.5 mm thick) incorporated at the time of packing.

of wearing maxillary and mandibular complete dentures since the past 6 years (Figure 1). His chief complaint was the poor fit of the denture, and it felt loose while eating. Patient had a history of diabetes and hypertension since last 9 years. The patient was wearing complete dentures even at the night. He was also using denture adhesive. By intraoral examination, a completely edentulous mandibular arch with flabby tissue existing in the mandibular anterior region was observed. It was decided to give a conventional maxillary complete denture opposing a Liquid-supported mandibular complete denture because of flabby soft tissues in anterior mandibular region. Primary impressions were made with alginate (Prime Dental products pvt. Ltd., Mumbai, India). Full complete double spacer was applied in the mandibular anterior region because of flabby soft tissues in the anterior region. Border molding was performed by using low fusing impression compound (DPI pinnacle tracing sticks, Dental products of India), and final impression was made with light body additional silicone impression material (Aquasil, Dentsply/caulk) (Figure 2). Denture base of 3 mm thickness was fabricated for mandibular denture base and 2mm for maxillary 3 denture base. Jaw relations record and trial of waxed up denture was done by conventional method. The mandibular denture design was modified to make a Liquid-supported denture. Maxillary complete denture was acrylised using conventional procedure.

Steps in fabricating a Liquid-supported denture.

(1) Vacuum heat-pressed polyethylene sheet (Biostar vacuum forming machine, Scheu-dental, Germany) of 1.5 mm thickness was adapted on the mandibular master cast. The sheet acted as a temporary spacer, and it was made 2 mm short of the sulcus (Figure 3).

(2) After dewaxing, 1.5mm temporary polyethylene sheet was adapted on the mandibular cast, and vaseline was applied over it so that this temporary sheet can be retrieved easily (Figure 4). Now, the denture was acrylised using heat cure resin along with the sheet. The mandibular denture with this 1.5 mm thick temporary polyethylene sheet was then finished and polished in conventional manner (Figure 5).

(3) The mandibular denture was inserted in to the patient's mouth to check for retention, support, stability, and border extension. The patient was asked to wear the denture for two weeks to get adjusted to it (Figure 6).

(4) After two weeks, the patient was recalled to convert the mandibular denture into a Liquid-supported one. Temporary polyethylene 1.5 mm thick spacer sheet was removed from the mandibular denture.

(5) An additional silicone putty impression was made of the tissue surface of the denture, and the cast was made of it. This was done to record the exact junction of the sheet to the denture. The impression was poured with dental stone, which will form negative replica of the ridge. Now, again the cast was poured upon the negative replica to produce positive replica of the ridge. On this cast, a 0.5 mm thick final polyethylene sheet was vacuum heat pressed which

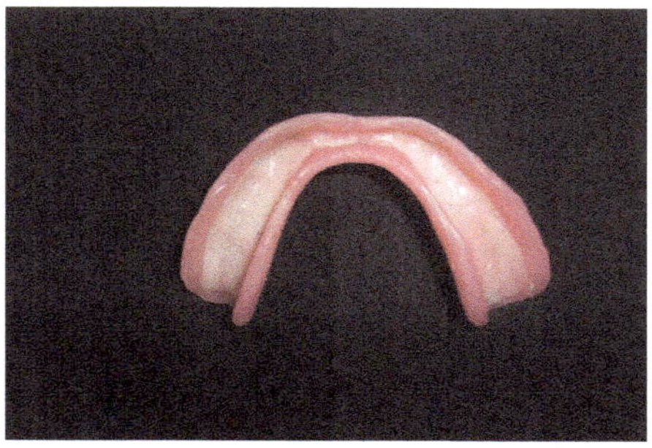

FIGURE 5: Polished denture with 1.5 mm thick temporary polyethylene sheet.

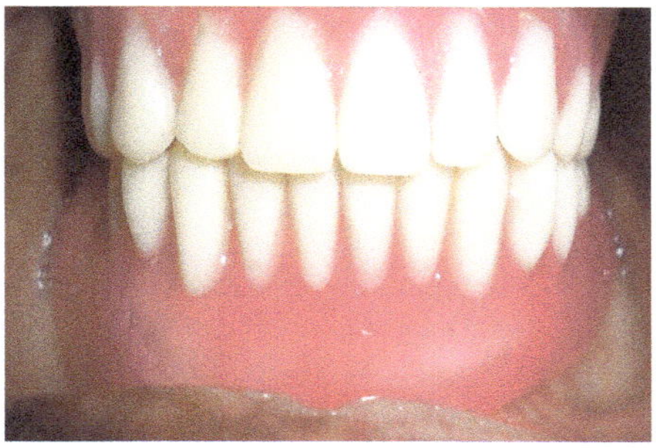

FIGURE 6: Intraoral view of maxillary and mandibular complete dentures.

was used in place of 1.5 mm thick sheet creating a 1 mm space between tissue surface of the denture and permanent polyethylene sheet (Figure 7).

(6) The polyethylene sheet was cut using the putty index as guide. The borders of the 0.5 mm thick sheet were placed in the crevice formed due to removal of 1.5 mm thick sheet. Cyanoacrylate adhesive and autopolymerizing acrylic resin were used to seal the borders and prevent escape of liquid (Figure 8).

(7) The space created due to the replacement of a 1.5 mm thick sheet with a 0.5 mm thick sheet was filled with viscous liquid, that is, glycerine. This was done by making two holes drilled on the buccal flange in the molar area of the denture by round bur and injecting viscous liquid, that is, glycerine through these holes, and one hole was sealed with autopolymerizing cure acrylic resin.

(8) The occlusal vertical dimension was adjusted by fitting the denture in the patient's mouth, and the other hole was sealed using the autopolymerizing cure acrylic resin. Then, the mandibular Liquid-supported denture was delivered (Figure 9).

(9) Denture care instructions were given to the patient. The patient was told to clean the tissue surface using cotton. The patient was recalled for followup.

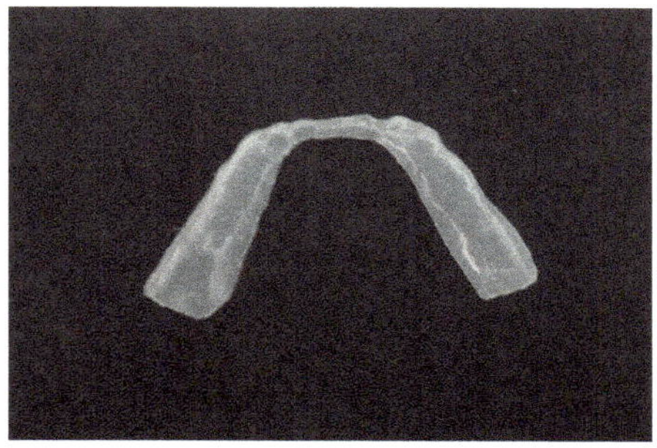

FIGURE 7: Vacuum heat-pressed 0.5 thick final polyethylene sheet.

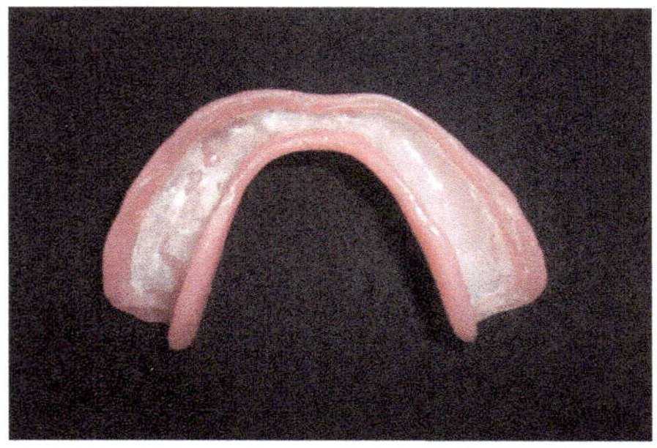

FIGURE 8: Liquid-supported mandibular denture with 0.5 mm thick final polyethylene sheet filled with glycerine (tissue surface).

## 3. Discussion

In this case where the presence of flabby tissue in mandibular arch (anterior portion) was treated by a modified design, that is, Liquid-supported denture. The principle of this design was that a Liquid-supported denture is flexible and continuously adapts itself to the mucosa. However, it is also rigid enough to support the teeth during actual use. Thus, the denture base is covered with a close-fitting flexible foil to keep a thin film of liquid in its place. This design will act as a continuous reliner for the denture and thus has an advantage over the existing denture designs. When no forces are applied, the foil remains in the resting position and act as a soft liner, and when the dentures are in use, vertically directed loads are distributed in all directions by the liquid resulting in optimal stress distribution (Figure 10). Thus, Liquid-supported denture provides benefits of both tissue conditioners and soft liners. This helps in long-term the preservation of bone and soft tissues. Apart from the combined benefits of tissue conditioners and soft liners, the load from biting forces and even bruxism will be distributed over a larger surface [5].

*The Precautions are as follows (see [6]):*

(i) thickness of denture base should be at least 3 mm;

(ii) The seal should be perfect and should be checked for microleakage;

(iii) denture care instructions should be given to the patient;

(iv) in case the liquid leaks out, the patient should inform the dentist, and the denture should be refilled;

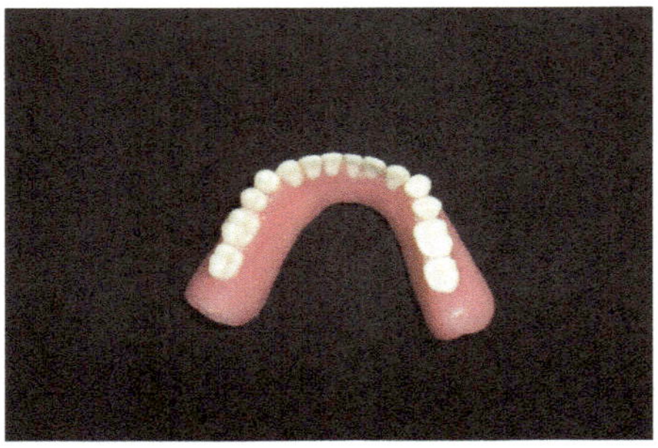

FIGURE 9: Final mandibular denture (Polished surface).

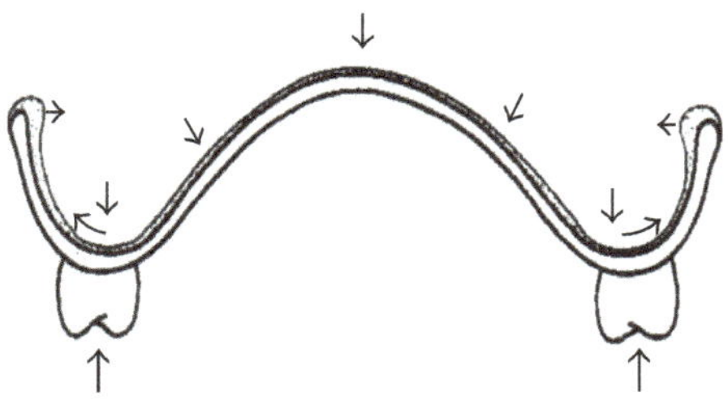

FIGURE 10: Unidirectional loading of denture resulting in multidirectional distribution of hydrodynamic pressure throughout fluid and clasping pressure at border of denture.

(v) repair is possible if the sheet gets ruptured and can be replaced over preserved stone cast.

For a liquid cushion, glycerine was used, which is clear, colorless, and odourless with a good pharmaceutical action. To prevent the liquid from leakage, a dense foil must be used [7]. The problem faced in fabrication of complete denture is the difficulty in a achieving complete seal at the junction of polyethylene sheet and denture base. The main drawback of liquid-supported denture is the relining procedure, which is not possible with this liquid supported denture [8].

## 4. Conclusion

Days and nights change, men, tissues, so do our treatments. Ultimately, Devan's dictum holds true "Our objective should be perpetual preservation of what remains, rather than meticulous reconstruction of what is lost." The seeds of success or failure of the prosthesis lies in the hands of the dentist. Liquid-supported denture by acting as a continuous reline provides solution to some problematic prosthodontic situations like patients with bruxism or clenching habits, in xerostomia patients, or those patients with atrophic ridge, superficial mental nerve, and so forth. Liquid-supported denture with its shock absorbing effect thus fulfills a valuable role in prosthetic dentistry.

## References


[1] R. W. I. Crawford and A. D. Walmsley, "A review of prosthodontic management of fibrous ridges," *British Dental Journal*, vol. 199, no. 11, pp. 715–719, 2005.

[2] D. A. Atwood, "Post extraction changes in the adult mandible as illustrated by microradiographs of midsagittal sections and serial cephalometric roentgenograms," *The Journal of Prosthetic Dentistry*, vol. 13, no. 5, pp. 810–824, 1963.

[3] C. L. Davidson and G. Boere, "Liquid-supported dentures, part I: theoretical and technical considerations," *The Journal of Prosthetic Dentistry*, vol. 63, no. 3, pp. 303–306, 1990.

[4] D. Kakade, S. Athavale, S. Shingote, and B. Dammani, "Liquid-supported denture: a gentle option," *Journal of Indian Prosthodontist Society*, vol. 7, no. 1, pp. 35–39, 2007.

[5] W. W. Chase, "Tissue conditioning utilizing dynamic adaptive stress," *The Journal of Prosthetic Dentistry*, vol. 11, no. 5, pp. 804–815, 1961.

[6] G. Boere, H. de Koomen, and C. L. Davidson, "Liquid-supported dentures, part II: clinical study, a preliminary report," *The Journal of Prosthetic Dentistry*, vol. 63, no. 4, pp. 434–436, 1990.

[7] M. K. A. Razek and Z. M. Mohamed, "Influence of tissue-conditioning materials on the oral bacteriologic status of complete denture wearers," *The Journal of Prosthetic Dentistry*, vol. 44, no. 2, pp. 137–142, 1980.

[8] S. Narula, K. Meenakshi, M. Handa, D. Garg, B. Singh, and D. Lakhani, "Fluid retained denture: a case report," *Indian Journal of Stomatol*, vol. 3, no. 3, pp. 84–86, 2012.

# 2

# Implant Prosthetic Rehabilitation with Bone Regenerative Techniques after Fracture of the Upper Central Incisors

**Massimo Amato,[1] Vincenzo Bruno,[2] Giuseppe Pantaleo,[2] Antonio Cerutti,[3] Gianrico Spagnuolo,[2] and Gilberto Sammartino[2]**

[1] *Department of Medicine and Surgery, University of Salerno, Fisciano, 84084 Salerno, Italy*
[2] *Department of Neurosciences, Reproductive and Odontostomatological Sciences, University of Naples Federico II, 80131 Naples, Italy*
[3] *School of Dentistry, University of Brescia, 25121 Brescia, Italy*

Correspondence should be addressed to Gianrico Spagnuolo; gspagnuo@unina.it

Academic Editors: G. Danesh and M. A. de A. M. Machado

A case of implant-bone prosthetic rehabilitation, after the fracture of the maxillary central incisors, which had been treated with grafting of a bone substitute, is reported. This case was followed by the normal procedures of implantology within the traditional timeframe for bone regeneration. However, a barrier membrane was not used which shows that even along with the use of graft material a sufficient amount of bone could be achieved for a subsequent rehabilitation. Therefore, after a five-year follow-up period, osseointegration was maintained with no marginal bone loss.

## 1. Introduction

Dental trauma could be the most common uncomfortable distress of the facial region. Dental coronal fractures and dislocations occur frequently, and because of their position, the teeth of the anterior maxillary area are therefore more usually subjected to this type of injury [1]. Following dental trauma, psychological stress along with the physical pain has been suggested as the main causes of discomfort for the patient, in particular if there is an extensive loss of coronal structure. The restoration of the anterior maxillary teeth and especially of fractured central incisors represents a key intervention for the dentist which could be challenging [2].

## 2. Case Presentation

A 39-year-old caucasian man was referred to the Dental School of the University Federico II of Naples in 2008. His main complaint was localized pain in region 1.1 and 2.1 during the function, the clinical examination showed that either the two fixed prosthesis elements where of ceramic metal as well as the presence of a secreting fistula in correspondence of the mucosa in the apical area of 1.1. A periapical radiograph was performed and the medical history was documented which has no relevance with regard to the disease in question. Dental history reports that prior treatments and retreatments on these teeth have been completed before the prosthesis.

The clinical and radiographic findings showed a probable root vertical fracture of the tooth 1.1 as well as a possible vertical fracture of the tooth 2.1 (Figure 1).

For aesthetic reasons, an alginate impression was taken and a plaster cast was made to construct an interim prosthesis.

Therefore, a decision was made to place two commercial teeth in a row on a steel wire to construct a prosthesis similar to the Maryland Bridge.

Probable causes were an inadequate apical seal and/or one or more vertical root fractures that were not captured via periapical radiograph.

The periapical radiograph from 1.1 revealed an osteolytic area in the middle third of the root. This osteolytic area also enveloped apical third of the root.

A beta-lactam antibiotic (Amoxicillin) was given orally 2 gr one hour before the surgery, and a diagnostic flap surgery was planned, which allowed to establish the correct treatment plan.

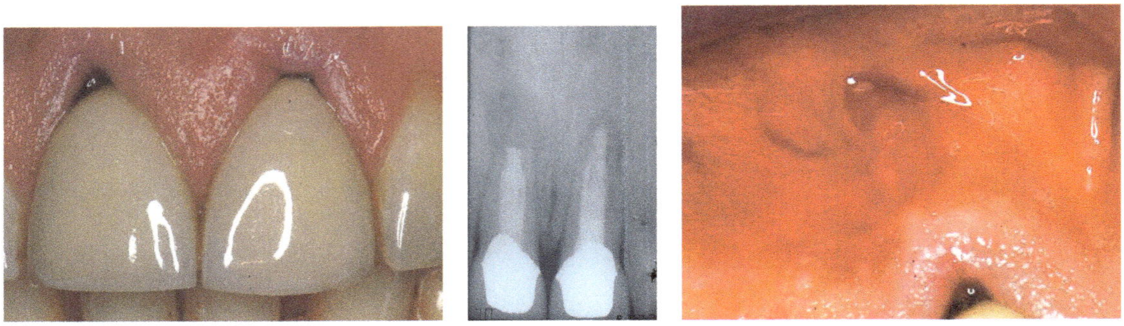

(a) (b) (c)

FIGURE 1: Radiographic (a) and clinical control (b) with the presence of a secreting fistula in correspondence with the mucosa in the apical area of 1.1 (c).

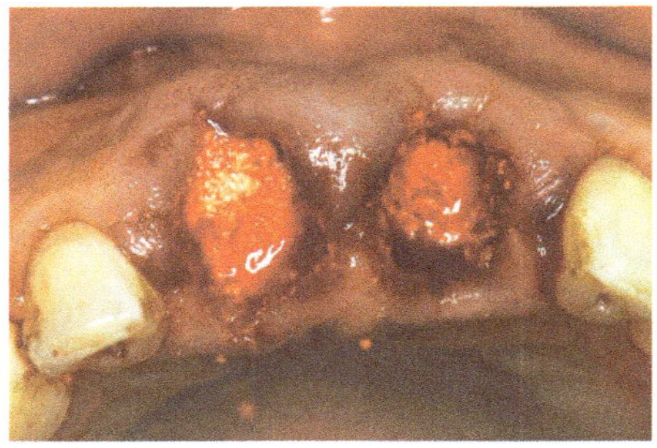

FIGURE 2: Filling of granules of bone substitute (Bio-Oss spongiosa) into the socket.

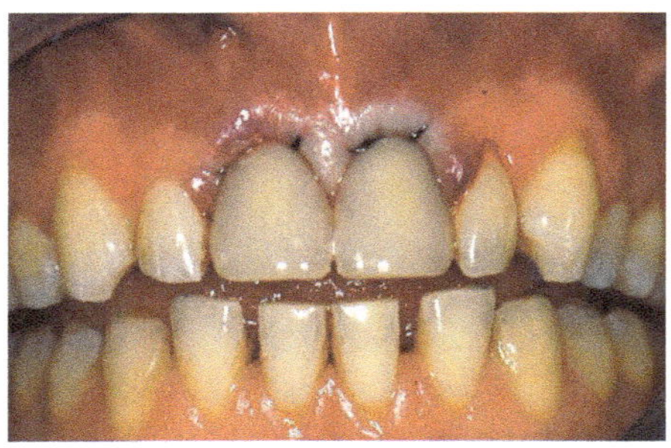

FIGURE 3: Temporary adhesive system attached to the adjacent teeth.

Previous to local anesthesia, a diagnostic flap was opened, respecting marginal soft tissues. The root's vertical fracture of 1.1 was immediately evident, while curettage of the exposed portion of the root of 2.1 also revealed a further fracture in the apical mesial portion of the root. The teeth were gently extracted with particular attention to the preservation of the hard and soft tissues at the sites. The extraction sockets were debrided using piezosurgery devices and alveolar surgical curettes to remove the granulation tissue [3]. The socket walls were then carefully probed to assess the presence of any fenestration or dehiscence defects [2]. Atraumatic avulsion was required to maintain the integrity of the vestibular bone, which specifically in the frontal region is as usual particularly thin. The preservation of the buccal bone is extremely important to obtain a good esthetic outcome in the frontal area and medium- and long-term maintenance [4]. If any trauma were to occur to the buccal bone crest, it would hinder the recovery and cause additional damage. The extraoral view of the roots confirmed the diagnosis. The alveolar bone review showed a defect of 8 mm. According to the conclusion of Darby et al., 2009, a decision was made to adopt a technique for ridge preservation [1, 5]. In particular, the circumferential gap was filled with granules of bone substitute (Bio-Oss, spongiosa, 0.5 mm). This material has exceptional biological and mechanical properties as well as biocompatibility. Its high porosity provides all the necessary space for angio- and osteogenesis. The microstructure of the Bio-Oss surface promotes optimal proliferation of osteoblasts and particles integrate with the newly formed bone. The slow rate of conversion of Bio-Oss in autologous bone (remodeling) stabilizes the structure of the newly formed to maintain a good long-term bone volume increased (Figure 2) [6, 7].

The Vicryl polyglactin (91, 3/0) absorbable suture was used to close the flap. The interim prosthesis was delivered by using an adhesive system to attach to the adjacent teeth. This prosthesis allows to achieve an acceptable esthetic outcome, as well as a good phonatory function and an initial tissue conditioning for the pontic areas (Figure 3) [8].

The postoperative therapy requires good oral hygiene, rinsing with mouthwash containing 0.2% chlorhexidine solution twice a day, and an evening application of the same product in gel form, as well as the administration of a nonsteroidal anti-inflammatory aid (Ketoprofen 80 mg) for three consecutive days.

The patient was asked to be seen for regular followups for the next three months.

At the end of the 3 months, the patient showed remarkable healing of the soft tissues, and the gingiva appeared with an excellent color and texture of the tissue too. It also began to outline the proper and harmonious design of the facial mucosa curvatures, which were conditioned by the interim prosthesis (Figure 4).

At six months, from the socket preservation, a periapical radiograph was taken and showed limited bone loss, which was related to the steel wire of the interim prosthesis (Figure 5).

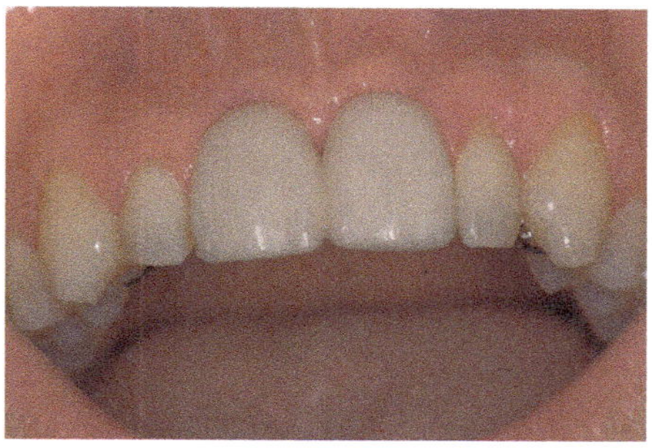

FIGURE 4: Clinical control at three months. The patient showed remarkable healing of the soft tissues, and the gingiva appeared with an excellent color and texture of the tissue too. It also began to outline the proper and harmonious design of the facial mucosa curvatures, which were conditioned by the interim prosthesis.

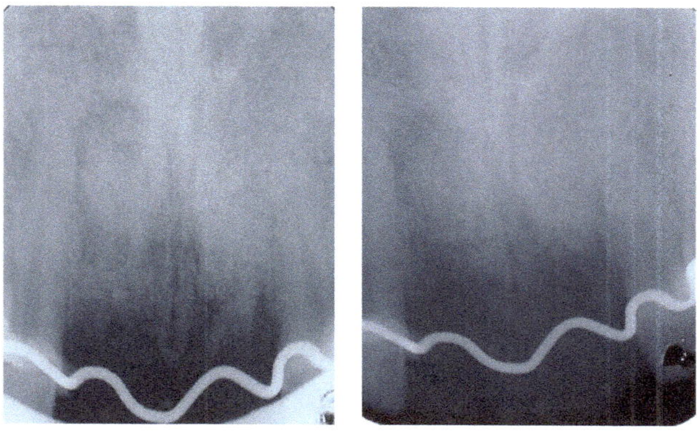

(a) (b)

FIGURE 5: A periapical radiograph was taken at 3 (a) and 6 months (b) from the socket preservation. After 6 months, a limited bone loss was showed related to the steel wire of the interim prosthesis.

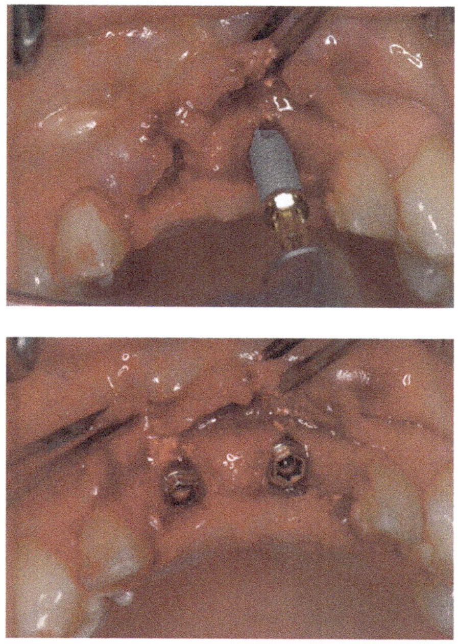

FIGURE 6: Two 13 mm long implants with a 3,75 mm diameter were placed.

Moreover, radiographically, the bone appeared homogenous and with a good radiopacity to show a sufficient remineralization.

An alginate impression with the interim bridge in situ was taken, to construct a surgical template. The patient was satisfied with regard to the esthetic outcome. A thermoplastic vacuum-formed template was then built and two holes corresponding to the cingulum of the maxillary central incisors were performed. The temporary bridge was removed to place two implants. A bone trephine was used to obtain a bone specimen to assess the bone quality and structure. The implant phase, however, was necessary to find the maximum stability in the apical zone [9]. In the presented case, the extracted roots were 11 mm long, and therefore two 13 mm long implants were placed with a 3,75 mm diameter (Nobel Biocare Branemark System) (Figure 6).

After the initial surgical phase, two resin temporary crowns were applied leaving a sufficient space to allow for any swelling. Only after three weeks, the interim crowns were modeled with a slight contact to the soft tissue.

At six months, the implants were uncovered and a resin screw retained prosthesis was constructed with an emergence profile which was suitable for supporting the buccal soft tissue. It also important to remember to avoid any excessive compression, which could lead to a soft tissue shrinkage in the subsequent months of maturation. The occlusal contacts were verified for the presence of a slight contact during maximum intercuspation using shimstock (Almoreshimstock, 8 mm wide, 8 mm thick) in order to protect the implants from any intense forces. Of course, functional loads resulting from lips, tongue, and food bolus will remain [10, 11].

After waiting for another 6 months, we proceeded to the prosthetic finalization. The patient has a good soft tissue maturation induced by the design of temporary crowns. A periapical radiograph was taken to evaluate the proper bone remodeling.

A custom impression of the healed soft tissue, recording and transferring the soft tissue contour with a gingival outline, was taken according to the technique of Hinds, 1997 [12].

Therefore, after trying all the components, the definitive gold-ceramic crowns were delivered with good accuracy as well as a proper emergence profile to support the tissue.

The patient was instructed to maintain good oral hygiene by brushing and flossing.

A year later, the patient was seen to observe overall tissue healing, aesthetics, and radiographic osseointegration of the implants.

This type of rehabilitation used integrates in the morphological and occlusal context of the oral cavity. In this way, this procedure, appropriately managed, is capable of producing the desired implant-prosthetic outcome, ensuring comfort and patient satisfaction (Figure 7) [13].

We recommended the patient a thorough oral hygiene through the use of brush, dental floss, and pipe cleaner.

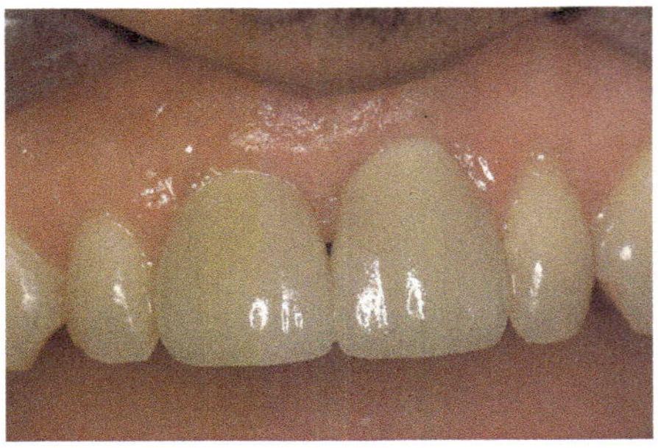

FIGURE 7: Clinical control after 1 year from the surgery.

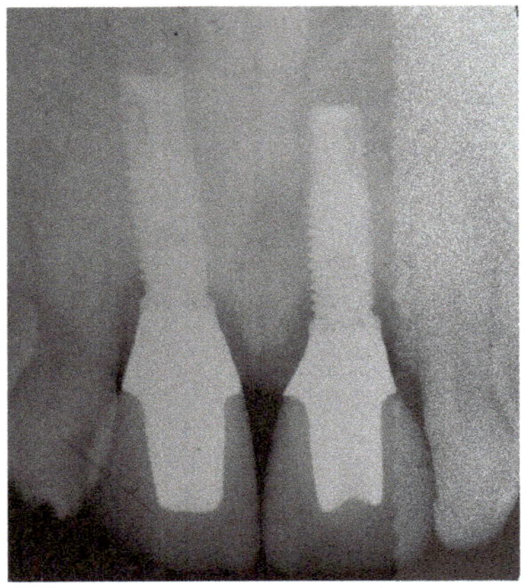

FIGURE 8: Periapical radiograph after 5 years which showed osseointegration of the implants with only a minimal loss of bone height according to the Albrektsson criteria.

The patient was recalled for a clinical control after a three- and five-year period. A new periapical radiograph was taken which showed an excellent osseointegration of the implants with only a minimal loss of bone height according to the Albrektsson criteria and ICOI Consensus Conference, 2007 (Figure 8) [14, 15].

Overall the patient was quite satisfied with the esthetic outcome and had no clinical issues.

## 3. Discussion

With regard to implant-prosthetic rehabilitation after fracture of the upper central incisors, various techniques have been proposed, which include the postextractive immediate loading implant. In this particular case, however, we felt it was necessary to wait for bone healing after the use of a substitute bone graft, without a barrier membrane. In addition to chemical and physical properties of the material, the aesthetic success must not be underestimated.

Moreover, the primary stability of implants was apically searched in the residual native bone and the major axes were placed palatally, in correspondence with the cingulum to maintain the possibility to build a screw-retained crown and to preserve the height and thickness of the facial bone wall. Therefore, the implant shoulder was positioned about 1 mm palatal to the point of emergence at the adjacent teeth. When the implant is placed too facially, a resorption of the facial bone wall could occur with a subsequent recession. With the implant positioned too palatally, an implant crown with a ridge-lap design might be needed.

The position of the implant must be chosen by using a 3D position, which respects the comfort zone, as stated by Belser et al. [16]. Therefore, the key issues were then the distance of the implants from the adjacent teeth, as well as the orofacial and the apicocoronal position. Care must be taken in the mesiodistal remaining space between the implant and the adjacent teeth: a minimum of a 1.5 mm space must be left for the maturation of the papilla. The formation of the papilla does not depend on the implants, but on the underlying bone support; in fact, soft tissue follows the bone in its process of remodeling. It has been shown that the average thickness of soft tissue is 4.3 mm ± 1 mm. The Authors observed that the presence of the papilla depends on the distance between the bone crest and the contact point: when this distance is ≤5 mm there will always be a complete maturation of the papilla. It has been shown that, when this distance increases to 6 mm, in 56% of cases this will cause an opened papilla with the presence of the classic "black hole" (Tarnow et al. 1992) [17]. Therefore, when making a prosthetic restoration on implants in the frontal area, the contact point must be brought as apically as possible, to avoid the loss of soft tissue. At the same time, when the mesiodistal distance between the tooth and the implant is less than 1.5 mm, there will be loss of the papilla in that area. Equally, a minimum distance of 3 mm between the two adjacent implant's emergences was required [18].

Therefore, prosthetic phase is extremely important.

In this case, we could ask if a barrier it is necessary for the alveolar ridge preservation and the answer is indeterminate at this time. The results between the studies regarding the use of any barrier are almost similar; no clear benefit was demonstrated with or without a barrier. Use of a barrier may prove beneficial in cases where extraction socket walls are partially or completely missing [19, 20].

To make sure of obtaining a good bone growth, we have performed a sample of bone from the site analyzing it histologically. Microscopic findings of implanted bone showed fragments of bone embedded in fibrous tissue; the same fragments at higher magnification showed fibroblasts, calcifications, fragments of bone tissue, and traces of grafted material (Figure 9) [21].

However, additional controlled and comparative studies are needed to confirm or refute these findings.

Another important matter is whether the addition of growth factors could provide a benefit for alveolar ridge preservation procedures [19].

However, a small number of studies have evaluated the use of growth factors for alveolar ridge preservation after tooth extractions, and there was significant heterogeneity in the condition of the host extraction socket and bone at time of graft placing [22]. Use of growth factors may give benefits in cases of extreme alveolar defects after tooth extractions, but more studies have to confirm that. Lastly, the cost/benefit ratio of these products must be considered.

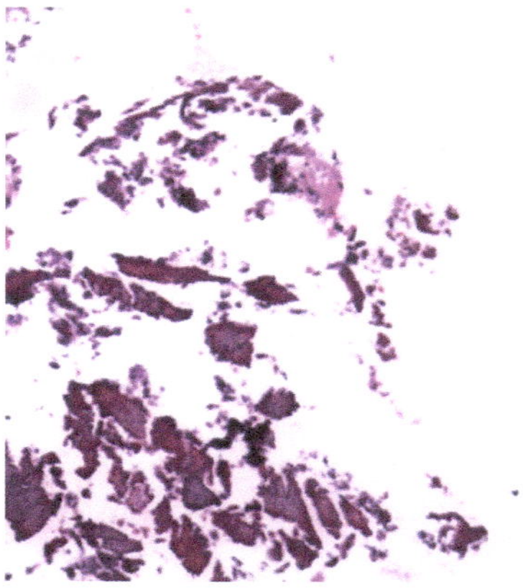

(a)

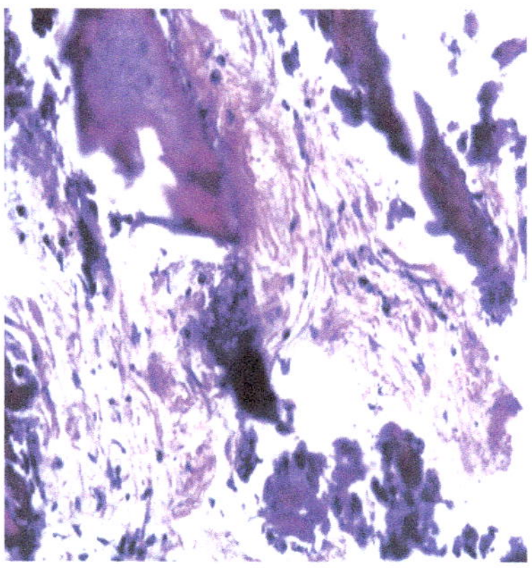

(b)

Figure 9: (a) Microscopic findings of implanted bone showing fragments of bone embedded in fibrous tissue (hematoxylin and eosin 106x). (b) The same fragments at higher magnification showing fibroblasts, calcifications, fragments of bone tissue, and traces of grafted material (hematoxylin and eosin 430x).

## 4. Conclusion

In this report, it has been showed how graft material can be used in extraction sockets without a barrier membrane ensuring nevertheless a good support for the implant prosthetic rehabilitation. Inspite of the nonuse of membranes, the target was obtained, so the question we asked for is that using a grafting material not completely resorbable or with a slow resorption as Bio-Oss, in this technique of resorption prevention, might suggest that the use of membrane does not affects the result with the biological and financial savings of a membrane.

In agreement with literature, our case also shows, that with regards to socket preservation, bone loss was limited without affecting the clinical outcome. Therefore, this specific technique could also be used in an aesthetic area that may be a challenge. Our results show that over a period of time the clinical outcome remained stable.

## Conflict of Interests

The authors declare that they have no conflict of interests.

## References


[1] I. Darby, S. T. Chen, and D. Buser, "Ridge preservation techniques for implant therapy," *The International Journal of Oral & Maxillofacial Implants*, vol. 24, pp. 260–271, 2009.

[2] M. G. Araújo, J. L. Wennström, and J. Lindhe, "Modeling of the buccal and lingual bone walls of fresh extraction sites following implant installation," *Clinical Oral Implants Research*, vol. 17, no. 6, pp. 606–614, 2006.

[3] G. Sammartino, O. Trosino, A. E. Di Lauro, M. Amato, and A. Cioffi, "Use of piezosurgery device in management of surgical dental implant complication: a case report," *Implant Dentistry*, vol. 20, no. 2, pp. e1–e6, 2011.

[4] F. Vignoletti, P. Matesanz, D. Rodrigo, E. Figuero, C. Martin, and M. Sanz, "Surgical protocols for ridge preservation after tooth extraction. A systematic review," *Clinical Oral Implants Research*, vol. 23, no. 5, pp. 22–38, 2012.

[5] R. Horowitz, D. Holtzclaw, and P. S. Rosen, "A review on alveolar ridge preservation following tooth extraction," *Journal of Evidence-Based Dental Practice*, vol. 12, no. 3, pp. 149–160, 2012.

[6] C. Maiorana, M. Beretta, S. Salina, and F. Santoro, "Reduction of autogenous bone graft resorption by means of bio-oss coverage: a prospective study," *International Journal of Periodontics and Restorative Dentistry*, vol. 25, no. 1, pp. 19–25, 2005.

[7] M. G. Araújo and J. Lindhe, "Ridge preservation with the use of Bio-Oss collagen: a 6-month study in the dog," *Clinical Oral Implants Research*, vol. 20, no. 5, pp. 433–440, 2009.

[8] G. Calesini, C. Micarelli, S. Coppè, and A. Scipioni, "Edentulous site enhancement: a regenerative approach for the management of edentulous areas—part 1. Pontic areas," *International Journal of Periodontics and Restorative Dentistry*, vol. 28, no. 5, pp. 517–524, 2008.

[9] V. Bruno, M. Badino, R. Sacco, and S. Catapano, "The use of a prosthetic template to maintain the papilla in the esthetic zone for immediate implant placement by means of a radiographic procedure," *Journal of Prosthetic Dentistry*, vol. 108, no. 6, pp. 394–397, 2012.

[10] D. Buser, W. Martin, and U. C. Belser, "Optimizing esthetics for implant restorations in the anterior maxilla: anatomic and surgical considerations," *International Journal of Oral and Maxillofacial Implants*, vol. 19, pp. 43–61, 2004.

[11] M. G. Araújo, F. Sukekava, J. L. Wennström, and J. Lindhe, "Ridge alterations following implant placement in fresh extraction sockets: an experimental study in the dog," *Journal of Clinical Periodontology*, vol. 32, no. 6, pp. 645–652, 2005.

[12] K. F. Hinds, "Custom impression coping for an exact registration of the healed tissue in the esthetic implant restoration," *International Journal of Periodontics and Restorative Dentistry*, vol. 17, no. 6, pp. 585–591, 1997.

[13] U. Covani, G. Chiappe, M. Bosco, B. Orlando, A. Quaranta, and A. Barone, "A 10-year evaluation of implants placed in fresh extraction sockets: a prospective cohort study," *Journal of Periodontology*, vol. 83, no. 10, pp. 1226–1234, 2012.

[14] T. Albrektsson, D. Buser, and L. Sennerby, "Crestal bone loss and oral implants," *Clinical Implant Dentistry and Related Research*, vol. 14, no. 6, pp. 783–791, 2012.

[15] C. E. Misch, M. L. Perel, H. L. Wang et al., "Implant success, survival, and failure: the International Congress of Oral Implantologists (ICOI) pisa consensus conference," *Implant Dentistry*, vol. 17, no. 1, pp. 5–15, 2008.

[16] U. C. Belser, B. Schmid, F. Higginbottom, and D. Buser, "Outcome analysis of implant restorations located in the anterior

maxilla: a review of the recent literature," *The International Journal of Oral & Maxillofacial Implants*, vol. 19, pp. 30–42, 2004.

[17] D. P. Tarnow, A. W. Magner, and P. Fletcher, "The effect of the distance from the contact point to the crest of bone on the presence or absence of the interproximal dental papilla," *Journal of Periodontology*, vol. 63, no. 12, pp. 995–996, 1992.

[18] G. F. Priest, "The esthetic challenge of adjacent implants," *Journal of Oral and Maxillofacial Surgery*, vol. 65, no. 7, pp. 2–12, 2007.

[19] M. El-Ghareeb, P. K. Moy, and T. L. Aghaloo, "The single-tooth dental implant: practical guidelines for hard tissue augmentation," *Journal of the California Dental Association*, vol. 36, no. 11, pp. 869–884, 2008.

[20] B. M. B. Brkovic, H. S. Prasad, M. D. Rohrer et al., "Beta-tricalcium phosphate/type I collagen cones with or without a barrier membrane in human extraction socket healing: clinical, histologic, histomorphometric, and immunohistochemical evaluation," *Clinical Oral Investigations*, vol. 16, no. 2, pp. 581–590, 2012.

[21] G. E. Romanos, C. G. Toh, C. H. Siar, H. Wicht, H. Yacoob, and G. H. Nentwig, "Bone-implant interface around titanium implants under different loading conditions: a histomorphometrical analysis in the Macaca fascicularis monkey," *Journal of Periodontology*, vol. 74, no. 10, pp. 1483–1490, 2003.

[22] C. Schmitt, R. Lutz, H. Doering, M. Lell, J. Ratky, and K. A. Schlegel, "Bio-Oss blocks combined with BMP-2 and VEGF for the regeneration of bony defects and vertical augmentation," *Clinical Oral Implants Research*, vol. 24, no. 4, pp. 450–460, 2013.

# 3

# Foreign Body Induced Neuralgia: A Diagnostic Challenge

**S. Padmashree, Chaitra H. Ramprakash, and Rema Jayalekshmy**

*Department of Oral Medicine & Radiology, Vydehi Institute of Dental Sciences and Research Centre, No. 82, EPIP Area, Whitefield, Bangalore 560 066, India*

Correspondence should be addressed to Chaitra H. Ramprakash; chaitra_hr@yahoo.com

Academic Editors: T. Lombardi, P. Lopez Jornet, and M. W. Roberts

Neuropathic pain is caused by neural injury or painful states associated with either peripheral or central nerve injury. One of the aetiologies of this type of pain is iatrogenic trauma. This case highlights the features of peripheral neuropathic pain caused by foreign body left in the mental foramen following a previous surgical procedure. The foreign body was detected on routine radiographic evaluation. Once the foreign body was removed by surgical intervention, the pain resolved. This stresses the importance of routine radiographic evaluation in proper diagnosis and treatment planning in the management of neuropathic pain. This paper also sheds light on the role of iatrogenic mechanical cause of peripheral neuropathic pain and warrants a tough degree of caution on the part of oral clinicians.

## 1. Introduction

Neuropathic pain is caused by neural injury or painful states associated with either peripheral or central nerve injury. It is defined as pain initiated or caused by a primary lesion or dysfunction in the nervous system [1]. Neuropathic pain felt in the distribution of a nerve or nerves which is induced by the presence of a foreign body is called the foreign body neuralgia. Traumatic implantations have been published with different objects like the fish bone [2], tooth, or metallic restorations [3]. There are multiple causes of foreign body entrapment. It can occur when the soft tissues are lacerated as in the case of penetrating injuries during accidents, which can give rise to a foreign body granuloma [3]. The other causes may be in the form of an overfilling root canal restoration, fractured root canal filling instrument [4], fragment of the restoration left behind in the area during extraction, which are iatrogenic in origin. These entrapped foreign bodies can impinge the nerve and cause either paroxysmal or continuous type of pain or paresthesia, which can be felt in the area of the distribution of that nerve.

This case highlights the features of foreign body neuralgia which posed a diagnostic challenge at the clinical level and was unraveled later.

## 2. Case Report

A 54-year-old female patient presented with a complaint of pain in the right lower back tooth region since 6–9 months. Pain was continuous, dull aching type localized to the right lower jaw region. It increased on chewing food, talking and decreased slightly on taking medication. She gave a history of pain 4 years ago which was sharp, intermittent, and localized in the same region. It increased on chewing food and reduced on massaging the area on the right side of the lower jaw and gradually with time. Hence, she underwent extraction of all the posterior teeth on the right side of the jaw which gave her no relief from the pain. Visiting another dentist, with the same complaints, she was diagnosed with trigeminal neuralgia and medications were prescribed. Even after one year of medication, she did not find relief from the pain. That is when visiting another dentist was decided around 3 years ago. The mental nerve block resulted in pain reduction; hence, she was advised to undergo mental nerve avulsion, which she underwent under local anesthesia.

After the surgery, there was complete reduction in pain, but after 2 months of the procedure, she developed dull aching, burning type of pain in the same region. Hence, she visited our institution with the complaint of pain in the right mandibular premolar region. The patient had no

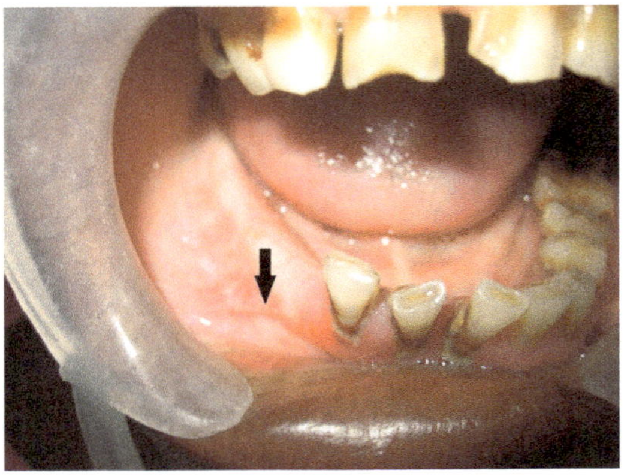

Figure 1: Intraoral photograph showing the previous surgical site which was firm and tender on palpation.

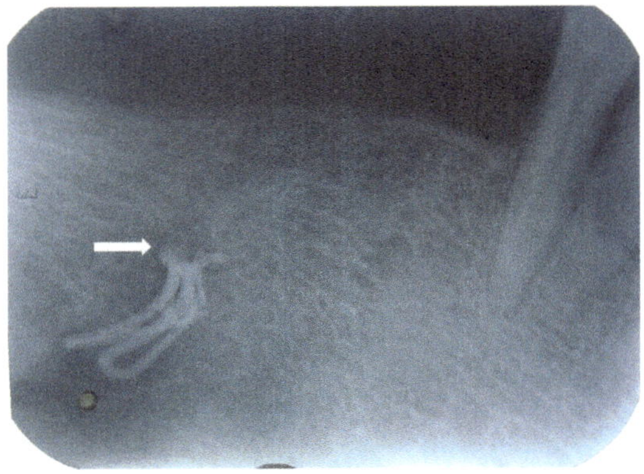

Figure 2: Intraoral radiograph showing the radiopaque foreign body close to the mental foramen.

contributing medical or dental history. On general physical examination, no abnormalities were detected and all the vital signs were within normal limits. The TMJ evaluation revealed no abnormalities. On extraoral palpation, paresthesia was detected in the lower lip on the right side and a part of the chin and the lower part of the cheek on the right side. On intraoral examination, a fibrosed scar was seen in the region of the right mandibular premolar on the alveolar mucosa about 2-3 mm above the buccal vestibule, measuring about 0.5 cm in diameter. The scar was firm and tender on palpation; it could be pinched off from the underlying bone (Figure 1). The general periodontal status of the patient was poor along with generalized enamel hypoplasia secondary to enamel fluorosis.

Taking into consideration the complaint and the presenting symptoms, arriving at a diagnosis was a challenge, as the features were atypical of trigeminal neuralgic pain and no lesion was evident except for the scar which was caused due to the previous surgical intervention. Therefore, provisionally, it was diagnosed as neuropathic pain on the right mental region of the jaw. Traumatic neuroma and infected and retained root stumps in the right premolar region were considered in differential diagnosis, taking into consideration the previous surgical intervention in terms of mental nerve avulsion and extraction of the teeth. As in both cases, the patient may present with continuous type of pain localized to the area of origin. To assess the condition of the mandibular canal and the premolar region of the jaw radiologic examination was essential. Interestingly, on intraoral periapical radiograph, a radiopaque material was detected in the right premolar region well within the substance of the mandible, in the region of the mental foramen on the right side (Figure 2). The same was confirmed on the OPG which revealed the foreign material and the outline of the mental foramen which was not clearly made out on the right side (Figure 3). The importance of radiologic evaluation is quite evident in helping us to arrive at a final diagnosis of foreign body neuralgia in the right mental foramen.

Surgical intervention was planned to explore the right mental foramen under local anesthesia (Figure 4) and the foreign material was retrieved, which consisted of silver points,

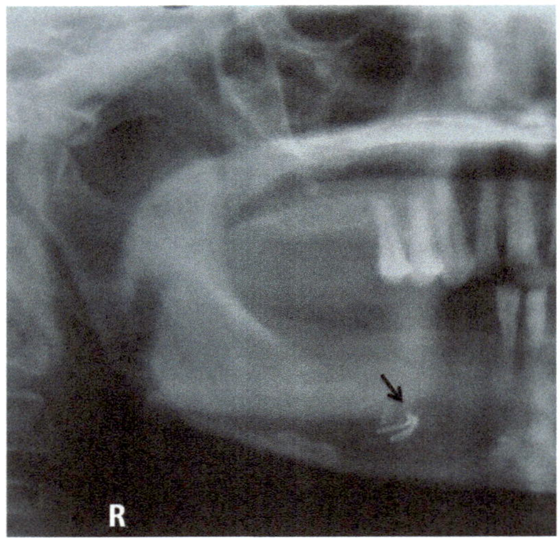


Figure 3: Part of the OPG showing the presence of radiopaque foreign body in the region of right mental foramen.

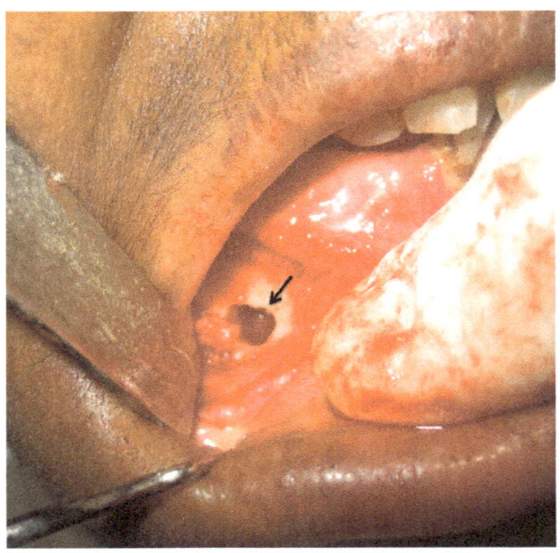

Figure 4: Surgical exploration of the right mental foramen done under local anesthesia.

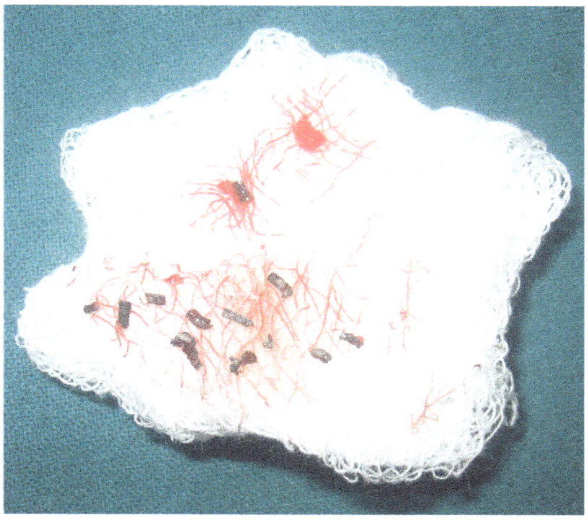

Figure 5: The photograph of the retrieved gutta-percha and silver points.

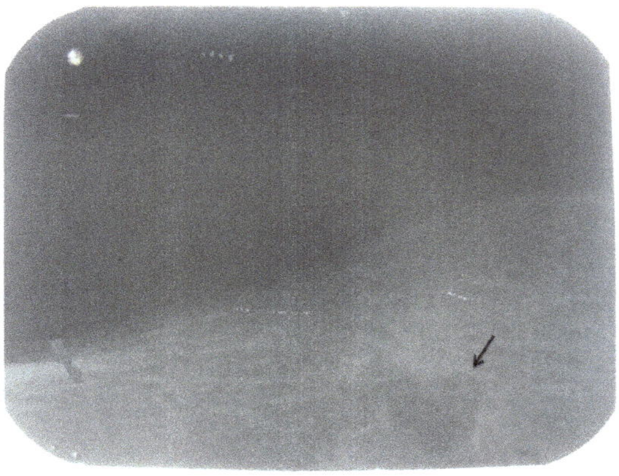

Figure 6: Postsurgical intraoral periapical radiograph showing the enlarged mental foramen with complete absence of the foreign material.

gutta-percha points and restorative material (Figure 5). Postsurgical radiograph reveals enlarged mental foramen and complete absence of the radiopaque material (Figure 6). The surgical site was sutured and the patient was advised to take an analgesic for the day if required and to stop all the other medication. During her first week of the postsurgical recall for suture removal, healing of the surgical site was satisfactory. She was reviewed after three months which revealed completely healed surgical site (Figure 7) and more importantly the patient was free of pain and continues to be on periodic follow up.

## 3. Discussion

Neuropathic pain as defined by International Association for the Study of Pain is a type of pain initiated or caused by a primary lesion or dysfunction in the nervous system [1]. It is caused by neural injury or painful states associated with either peripheral or central nerve injury. Types of neuropathic

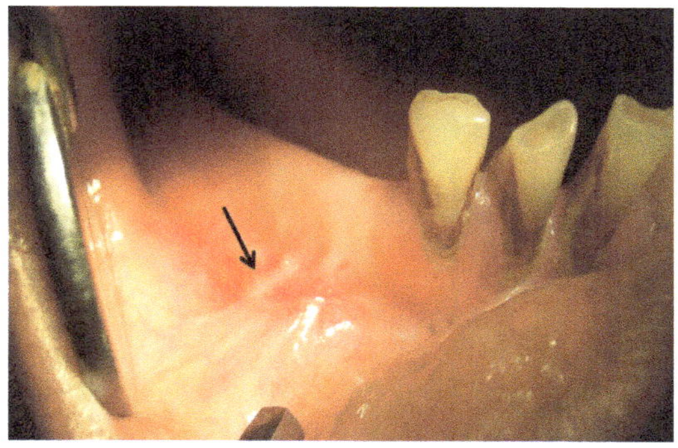

Figure 7: The follow-up intraoral photograph showing complete healing of the surgical site.

Table 1: Classification of the types of neuropathic pain [1].

| Based on anatomic location and etiology | Based on type of pain |
|---|---|
| (i) Peripherally mediated<br>(ii) Centrally mediated<br>(iii) Metabolic polyneuropathies | (i) Paroxysmal/episodic<br>(a) Neurovascular pains<br>(b) Neuralgic pains<br>(ii) Continuous |

pain can be classified based on anatomic location, etiology, and the type of pain experienced by the patients (Table 1).

It has multifactorial etiology, which includes infections, trauma, metabolic abnormalities, chemotherapy, surgery, radiotherapy, neurotoxins, nerve compression, inflammation, and tumor infiltration. The continuous type of neuropathic pain can be caused by foreign bodies' entrapments in the mandibular and submandibular regions which are quite common. These intraosseous entrapments can lead to inflammation and foreign body granuloma formation [3]. This can occur following entrapment of any of the following materials, which could be iatrogenic in origin during the course of any treatment procedures [5]: like amalgam filling, broken injection needle, air turbine bur, endodontic filling material, broken toothbrush bristle, or sometimes tooth displacement.

Foreign body (inflammatory) reaction or injury of inferior alveolar nerve (IAN)/mental nerve may be classified into metallic or nonmetallic, temporary or permanent, and chemicomechanical or thermal in nature [6]. This entrapped foreign body can give rise to paresthesia. Paresthesia is defined as a burning or prickling sensation or partial numbness caused by neural injury [7, 8]. Patients have described it as warm, cold, burning, aching, prickling, tingling, pins and needles, numbness, itching, and formicating. Paresthesia in dentistry can be caused by local or systemic factors. Local factors include traumatic injuries such as mandibular fractures, expanding compressive lesions (benign or malignant neoplasia and cysts [9]), impacted teeth, local infections (osteomyelitis, periapical [10], and peri-implant infections), iatrogenic lesions after teeth extractions, anesthetic injection, endodontic therapy [11] (overfilling and apical surgery), implantology, orthodontic surgery, and preprosthetic surgery. According to Seddon's classification for peripheral nerve injury [12], there are three basic injuries: neurapraxia, axonotmesis, and neurotmesis. Neurapraxia is a temporary conduction block after mild compression of the nerve trunk (i.e. paraesthesia or dysaesthesia of the lip and chin region in case of IAN/mental nerve). Axonotmesis, a more serious condition, results from degeneration of the afferent fibers as a result of internal/external irritation (i.e. anaesthesia), while in neurotmesis the nerve is completely severed which results in permanent paraesthesia. The main mechanism of injury of peripheral nerves is compression. Compression of the arterial blood supply to the nerve results in increased vascular permeability, edema, and ischemia, and the amount of oxygen delivered to the nerve is thereby reduced [13]. The classic response in cases of neuropraxia is paresthesia, but axonotmesis may also occur if the compression lasts long enough; in these cases the recovery can take up to 1 year.

Our case posed a diagnostic challenge as the patient's clinical presentation was atypical of trigeminal neuralgia. If the fibrosed scar was ignored and the high doses of medication were prescribed to manage the neuropathic pain, it would have done more harm to the patient than to help her. The simple routine intraoral radiological examination revealed the actual cause of the pain, thereby aiding us in our diagnosis of a foreign body induced neuralgia. The removal of the cause is the primary management. Hence, we were able to help the patient get rid of her pain with the help of imaging. This case emphasizes the need for routine radiological investigations in the diagnosis of the cases of peripheral neuralgia.

## 4. Conclusion

Patients presenting with sensory symptoms in the distribution of the IAN/mental nerve area should be assessed carefully by proper history recording, taking into consideration any previous surgical intervention. This should be followed by detailed examination and radiological investigation. Diagnosticians should be aware of the presence of a foreign body which can give rise to neuropathic pain. Every effort should be made to avoid any iatrogenic entrapments like the overfilling of root canals, apical surgery, traumatic extraction, fractured fragments of the restoration, and so forth. This case further emphasizes the importance of the radiographic evaluation in diagnosing foreign body induced neuralgia.

## Acknowledgments

The authors are thankful their staff of Department of Oral Medicine & Radiology and Dr. Sham, Professor of oral and maxillofacial surgery, Vydehi Institute of Dental Sciences & Research Centre, for their help and support.

## References

[1] J. P. Okeson, "Bell's orofacial pains," in *The Clinical Management of Orofacial Pain*, Quintessence Publishing, Surrey, Canada, 6th edition, 2005.

[2] C. J. Lin, W. F. Su, and C. H. Wang, "A foreign body embedded in the mobile tongue masquerading as a neoplasm," *European Archives of Oto-Rhino-Laryngology*, vol. 260, no. 5, pp. 277–279, 2003.

[3] V. A. Silveira, E. D. de Carmo, C. E. Colombo, A. S. Cavalcante, and Y. R. Carvalho, "Intraosseous foreign-body granuloma in the mandible subsequent to a 20-year-old work-related accident," *Medicina Oral, Patologia Oral y Cirugia Bucal*, vol. 13, no. 10, pp. E657–E660, 2008.

[4] T. M. S. Marques and J. M. Gomes, "Decompression of inferior alveolar nerve: case report," *Journal of the Canadian Dental Association*, vol. 77, article b34, 2011.

[5] P. Kafas, T. Upile, N. Angouridakis, C. Stavrianos, N. Dabarakis, and W. Jerjes, "Dysaesthesia in the mental nerve distribution triggered by a foreign body: a case report," *Cases Journal*, vol. 2, no. 10, article 169, 2009.

[6] M. M. Gallas-Torreira, M. D. Reboiras-López, A. García-García, and J. Gándara-Rey, "Mandibular nerve paresthesia caused by endodontic treatment," *Medicina Oral*, vol. 8, no. 4, pp. 299–303, 2003.

[7] R. Di Lenarda, M. Cadenaro, and C. Stacchi, "Paresthesia of the mental nerve induced by periapical infection: a case report," *Oral Surgery, Oral Medicine, Oral Pathology, Oral Radiology, and Endodontics*, vol. 90, no. 6, pp. 746–749, 2000.

[8] American Association of Endodontics, *Glossary*, AAE, Chicago, Ill, USA, 1994.

[9] M. Sumer, B. Baş, and L. Yildiz, "Inferior alveolar nerve paresthesia caused by a dentigerous cyst associated with three teeth," *Medicina Oral, Patologia Oral y Cirugia Bucal*, vol. 12, no. 5, pp. E388–E390, 2007.

[10] D. D. Antrim, "Paresthesia of the inferior alveolar nerve caused by periapical pathology," *Journal of Endodontics*, vol. 4, no. 7, pp. 220–221, 1978.

[11] F. K. E. K. Ahlgren, A. C. Johannessen, and S. Hellem, "Displaced calcium hydroxide paste causing inferior alveolar nerve paraesthesia: report of a case," *Oral Surgery, Oral Medicine, Oral Pathology, Oral Radiology, and Endodontics*, vol. 96, no. 6, pp. 734–737, 2003.

[12] H. J. Seddon, "Three types of nerve injury," *Brain*, vol. 66, no. 4, pp. 237–288, 1943.

[13] P. Scolozzi, T. Lombardi, and B. Jaques, "Successful inferior alveolar nerve decompression for dysesthesia following endodontic treatment: report of 4 cases treated by mandibular sagittal osteotomy," *Oral Surgery, Oral Medicine, Oral Pathology, Oral Radiology, and Endodontics*, vol. 97, no. 5, pp. 625–631, 2004.

# 4

# Immediate Provisionalization and Nonfunctional Loading of a Single Implant in the Maxillary Esthetic Zone: A Clinical Presentation and Parameters for Consideration

**Konstantinos X. Michalakis,[1,2,3] Christos D. R. Kalpidis,[4] Yvone Kirmanidou,[5] Hiroshi Hirayama,[1] Pasquale Lino Calvani,[1,6] and Argiris L. Pissiotis[2,3]**

[1] *Division of Graduate and Postgraduate Prosthodontics, Tufts University School of Dental Medicine, Boston, MA 02111, USA*
[2] *Department of Prosthodontics, Division of Removable Prosthodontics, Faculty of Dentistry, Aristotle University School of Health Sciences, 54124 Thessaloniki, Greece*
[3] *Private Practice Limited to Prosthodontics, 54622 Thessaloniki, Greece*
[4] *Private Practice Limited to Periodontics, 54623 Thessaloniki, Greece*
[5] *Private Practice, 54622 Thessaloniki, Greece*
[6] *Private Practice Limited to Prosthodontics, 00198 Rome, Italy*

Correspondence should be addressed to Konstantinos X. Michalakis; konstantinos.michalakis@tufts.edu

Academic Editors: M. N. de Araújo, T. Pereira-Cenci, and G. Schierano

Restoration of single tooth loss with implant supported prosthesis is now considered a highly predictable treatment. However, the maxillary anterior region still presents a challenge for both the prosthodontist and the periodontist because of the inherent difficulties encountered in the provisionalization and harmonic incorporation of the definitive prosthesis into patient's dentogingival complex. This paper presents a clinical case of a single implant placed immediately after the extraction of a maxillary central incisor, followed by immediate provisionalization and nonfunctional loading. The surgical and the restorative techniques are described, and the parameters of consideration for this approach are presented.

## 1. Introduction

Dental implant therapy constitutes a viable treatment modality for both completely [1–4] and partially edentulous patients [5–8]. Furthermore, implants have offered a great service for people, who lost a single tooth due to trauma, carries, internal/external root resorption, or root fracture [9–12]. The biological benefits of not preparing the adjacent teeth for a fixed partial denture fabrication should be emphasized. Conservation of dental tissues, preservation of pulp vitality, respect to periodontium, and maintenance of the residual ridge are the most important factors into consideration.

However, implant treatment had its disadvantages as well. The original protocol, ad modum Brånemark, required an undisturbed healing period of 4 to 6 months, in order for the osseointegration process to take place [3]. Therefore, the provisionalization of a single missing tooth could be a problem, especially in the anterior esthetic area. Originally, removable prostheses were used with negative effects on patient's psychology and an increased risk of force transmissions to the soft tissues overlying the implant. Other alternatives included the fabrication of an etched cast resin-bonded fixed dental prosthesis (Rochette, Maryland or Virginia) [13]. The main advantage of this type of prosthesis is that its fabrication usually requires minimal or no preparation of the abutment teeth. However, high debonding rates [14–16] of these prostheses have been documented, resulting in patient's frustration. Another common disadvantage of both the removable and the etched cast resin-bonded fixed dental prostheses is that their use is very often associated with the loss of the interdental papillae around the definitive implant supported prosthesis [17]. Therefore, the final soft tissue contours of the peri-implant mucosa are far from ideal, jeopardizing the esthetic outcome.

An alternative to the traditional two-stage approach has been presented in the past. This consisted of implant placement and immediate provisionalization. This technique was tested clinically mainly in completely edentulous patients, where cross-arch stabilization was possible, and several studies have reported that the survival rates are similar to those achieved with the unloaded protocol, provided that there was a good bone quality and initial implant stability [18–21]. The "immediate loading" approach was made possible due to changes in the implants' microtopography, achieved with mechanical and/or chemical means [22–26]. This had as a result a faster induction of bone formation onto the alloplastic surface of dental implants, as shown in several animal models and histomorphometric studies in humans [27–29].

This new concept of immediate provisionalization was also applied to single implants, with very good results [30, 31]. It should be emphasized however that, a very careful case selection is essential in order to have a predictable biologic, functional and esthetic outcome.

This paper presents a clinical case involving the extraction of a root fractured maxillary central incisor and immediate placement of an implant, followed by immediate provisionalization and non-functional loading.

## 2. Case Description

A 25-year-old healthy Caucasian woman presented with a metal ceramic restoration on the left maxillary central incisor, that did not satisfy her esthetic demands anymore. In addition, the patient was feeling a dull pain in the area. The patient did not smoke and was healthy. The radiographic examination showed an oversized cast post and core, which occupied three quarters of the root's length (Figure 1). The clinical examination revealed that the metal ceramic restoration was fractured at the buccal marginal area, it had a surface texture that did not match that of the adjacent natural teeth, it was rather opaque, and its margins were placed on the underlying cast post and core instead of on sound tooth structure (Figure 2). Soft tissue inflammation was evident around the crown's marginal area. An 8 mm pocket depth was found at the distal area of the tooth. The examination also demonstrated a discrepancy of the soft tissue contours between the two central incisors, sufficient width of keratinized tissue in the maxillary anterior area and a scalloped thin periodontium [32–34].

Treatment options were presented to the patient after assessment of all clinical and radiographic data. The patient wished to restore the failing tooth with an implant-supported restoration.

Prior to implant surgery, preliminary impressions were obtained by using irreversible hydrocolloid impression material. Diagnostic casts for both the maxillary and mandibular arches were fabricated with type III dental stone and they were mounted in maximal intercuspal position on a semiadjustable articulator. A diagnostic waxing was made and the maxillary cast was duplicated. A surgical stent was

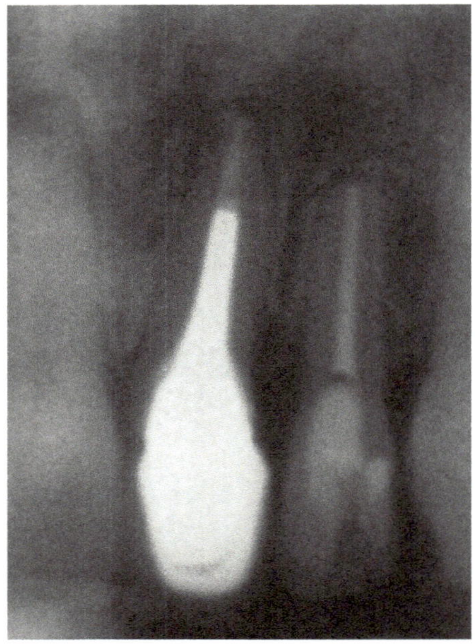

Figure 1: Initial radiograph of maxillary left central incisor.

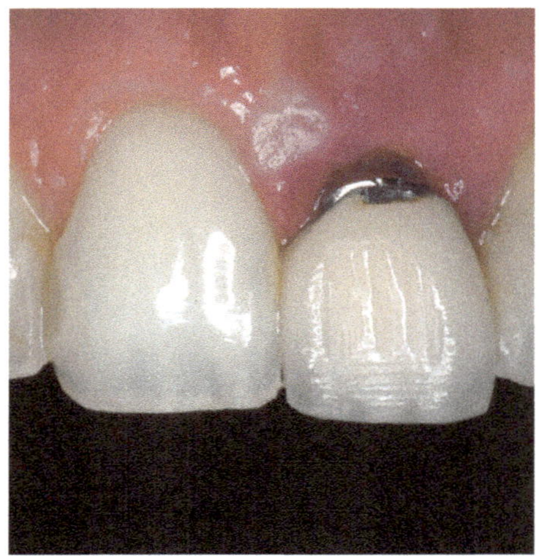

Figure 2: The maxillary left central incisor with a metal ceramic restoration. Its margins were placed on the underlying cast post and core.

then fabricated with clear autopolymerizing polymethylmethacrylate resin. The tooth's cingulum area was marked and an access channel was opened with a 261E-023 laboratory carbide bur (Brasseler, USA). A provisional restoration was also fabricated by using autopolymerizing acrylic resin (GC Unifast III, GC Tokyo, Japan). Two acrylic resin retainers resting on the palatal surfaces of the adjacent teeth were incorporated into the provisional restoration, in order to assist to the orientation of the provisional crown during the surgery. Finally, the provisional restoration was hollowed out and an access hole was opened palatally.

On the day of the surgery, local anesthesia with 4% articaine (1:100,000 epinephrine) (Ubistesin Forte, 3M/ESPE) was delivered and a full thickness flap was raised.

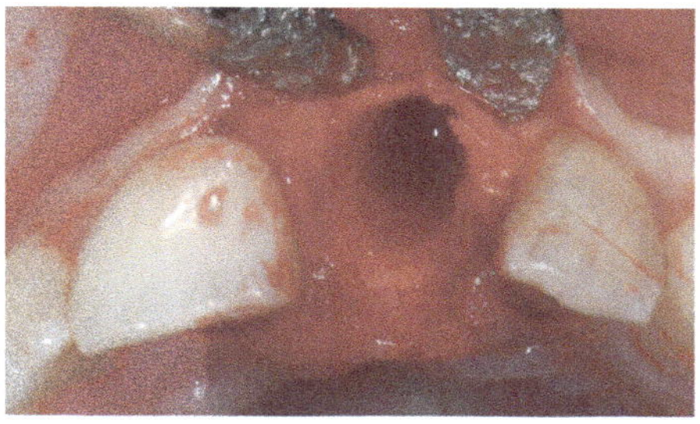

Figure 3: Atraumatic extraction of the maxillary left central incisor.

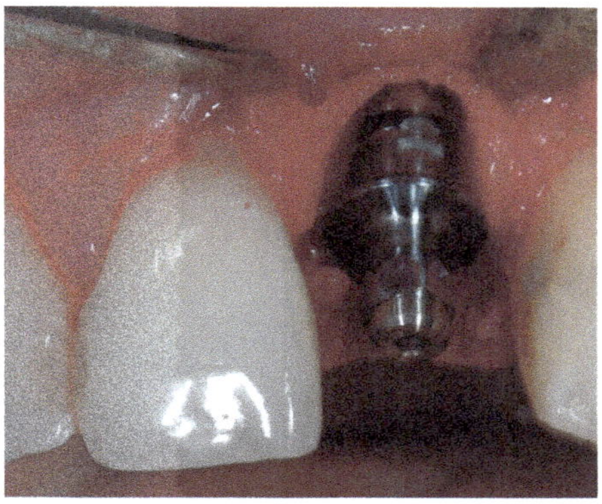

Figure 4: Placement of an Osseotite NT implant in the extraction socket. The platform of the implant was placed 2 mm apically to the cementoenamel junction of the right maxillary central incisor.

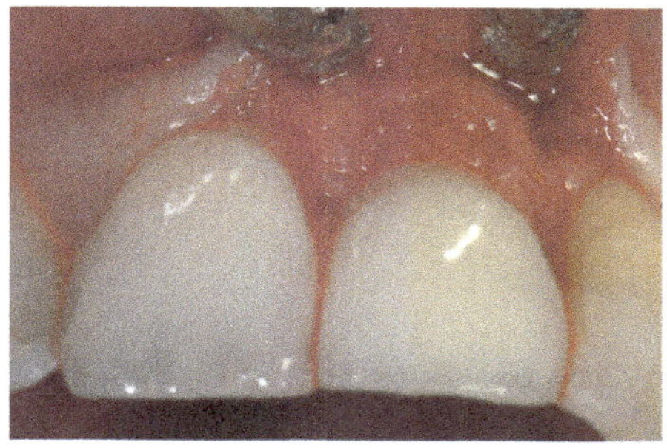

Figure 5: Buccal bone deficiency filled with bovine bone material.

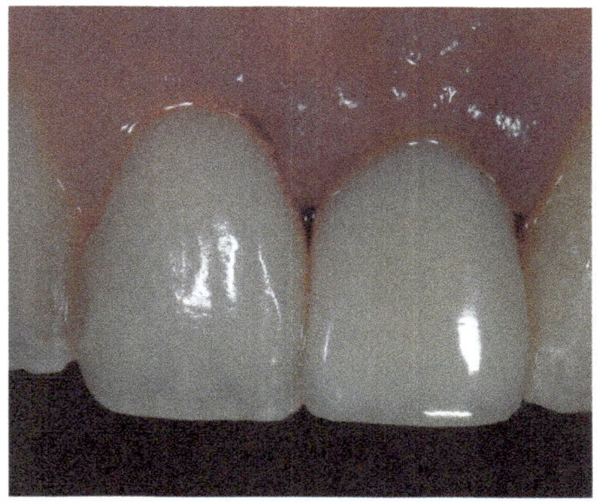

Figure 6: Initial provisional PMMA acrylic resin crown.

An atraumatic tooth extraction was then performed with the use of a periotome, taking extra care to preserve the buccal plate (Figure 3). The osteotomy started with a round bur which was placed into the channel of the surgical stent previously described, and progressed with the 2.3 mm twist drill, the pilot drill, and the 3.25 × 13 mm shaping drill at 500 rpm, with the drill torque test set at 50 Ncm. Attention was given to engage with the drills the palatal wall of the extraction socket. The osteotomy was performed under copious saline irrigation. A 4 × 13 externally hexed Osseotite NT implant (Biomet 3i, Palm Beach Gardens, FL) was placed using 20 rpm at 40 Ncm torque. The platform of the implant was placed 2 mm apically to the cementoenamel junction of the right maxillary central incisor (Figure 4) [35–37].

A temporary metal cylinder was fastened with a titanium screw on the implant and marked in order to be reduced to the proper length. It was then removed, fastened to an implant replica, and cut with a silicon separating disc. It was further reduced and shaped with diamond burs. The final length and shape of the temporary cylinder was checked intraorally, with the provisional restoration in place. Furthermore, the clearance between the temporary cylinder and the provisional restoration was verified. Autopolymerizing polymethyl-methacrylate acrylic resin (Jet, Lang Dental, Wheeling, IL) was added intraorally between the provisional restoration and the temporary cylinder, using the bead-brush technique. After the polymerization was completed, the provisional restoration-temporary cylinder complex was removed and fastened on an implant replica. More autopolymerizing polymethyl-methacrylate acrylic resin was added to support the adjacent soft tissues and the restoration was placed in a pressure pot containing warm water. It was then shaped with laboratory carbide burs and polished with abrasive rubber points (Bredent, Senden, Germany) and pumice. The provisional restoration was fastened on the implant with a torque driver (Anthogyr, Sallanches, France) with a 20 Ncm torque. The palatal access hole was closed with gutta-percha and acrylic resin. Occlusion was checked and any centric and eccentric contacts were eliminated. The acrylic was further polished with abrasive points.

A bone deficiency remained buccally and it was filled with bovine bone mineral (Bio-Oss Collagen, Geistlich) (Figure 5). The flap was sutured in place. Postoperatively, the patient was prescribed 1 g of amoxicillin/clavulanate potassium (Augmentin; GlaxoSmithKline) per day for 6 days and the nonsteroidal analgesic nimesulide (Mesulid; Boehringer Ingelheim) (100 mg, twice a day for 6 days). A 0.2% chlorhexidine (Chlorhexil; Intermed, Greece) rinse was also prescribed and the patient was instructed to use it three times a day for 14 days. The sutures were removed after 10 days (Figure 6). Patient was placed on a soft food diet for 6 weeks.

Two months after implant placement, the provisional restoration was removed and an impression coping was screwed onto the top of the implant. Light-polymerizing resin material (Liquidam; Discus Dental, Culver City, CA) was injected around the impression coping and was immediately polymerized with a UV polymerizing unit, preventing the soft

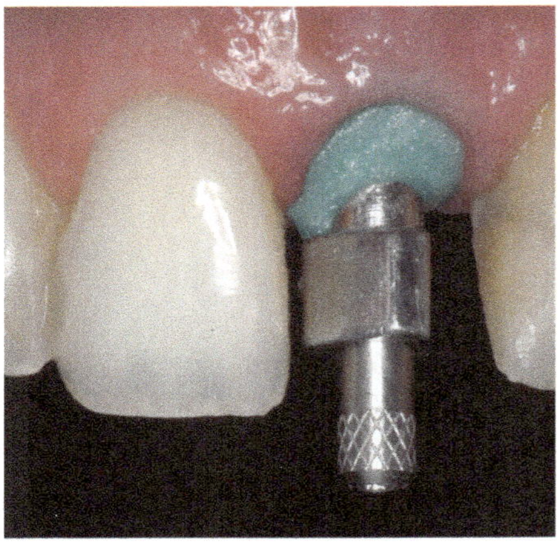

FIGURE 7: The impression coping was modified with light-polymerizing resin material to register the peri-implant soft tissues.

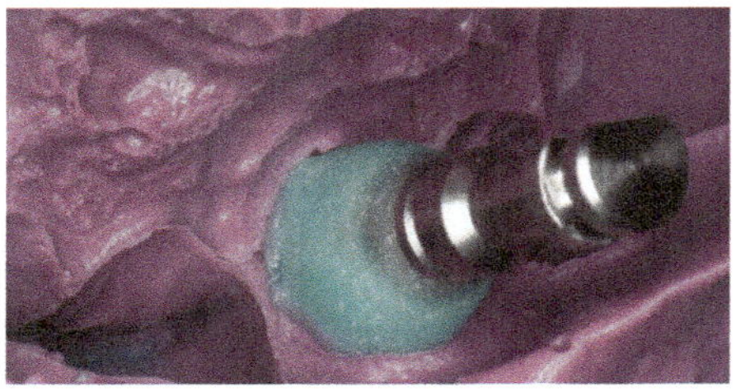

FIGURE 8: The impression coping into the polyether impression material used. Note the amount of light-polymerizing resin material added to support the soft tissues.

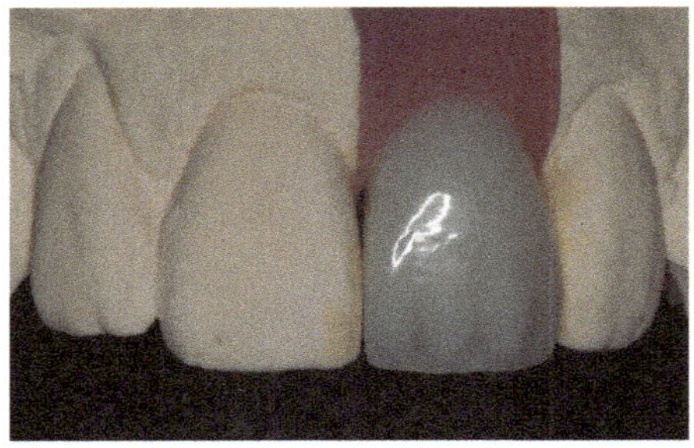

FIGURE 9: A new provisional crown was fabricated with light-polymerizing resin, in order to better support the soft tissue contours mesially and provide a better esthetic result.

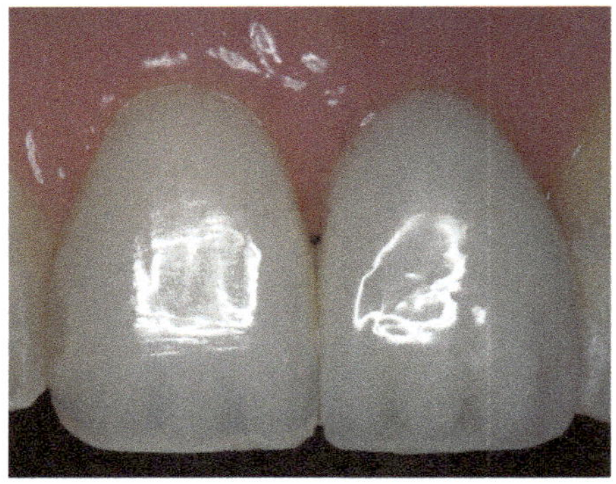

FIGURE 10: Clinical view of the new provisional crown.

tissues from collapsing onto the impression coping (Figure 7). A plastic stock tray and polyether material (Impregum, 3M/ESPE, Seefeld, Germany) were then used for the impression (Figure 8). A new screw-type provisional restoration was fabricated by using a temporary cylinder and light-polymerizing resin (Gradia; GC Tokyo, Japan) (Figure 9). This provisional restoration was fabricated in order to support better the soft tissue contours mesially and provide a better esthetic result (Figure 10). No centric or eccentric contact was given to the crown.

Regular examinations were performed at 3-week intervals for oral hygiene and occlusion evaluation. After 6 months of uneventful healing, a periapical radiograph was taken, showing no areas of radiolucency around the implant. The provisional restoration was removed and a definitive impression was obtained with the method previously described. A definitive cast was fabricated from type IV dental stone and mounted in maximal intercuspal position with the mandibular cast on a semiadjustable articulator. A UCLA abutment with a gold hexed collar was used for the definitive restoration. This was fastened onto the implant replica and waxed to full contour. A silicone key was made and the wax-up was then cut back, invested and cast with high noble alloy. Porcelain was applied and baked in the traditional manner (Figure 11). The restoration was tried-in, and proximal contacts and occlusion were adjusted. After patient's approval, the restoration was returned to the laboratory for the glazing procedure.

After the delivery of the definitive restoration (Figures 12 and 13), the patient was followed every 4 months for the next year. She was then placed on a 6-month recall basis. Soft tissues around the implant supported restoration appeared stable with no signs of inflammation or recession. The interdental papillae looked normal enhancing the optimal esthetic result obtained by the definitive metal ceramic restoration.

## 3. Discussion

The present report demonstrated a successful use of an immediate provisionalization and non-functional loading of a single implant in the maxillary esthetic zone. This approach had a positive psychological impact on this young female patient, as it immediately improved her appearance and confidence. This treatment approach was also based on preliminary data regarding the maintenance of the residual ridge in both height and width and the support of peri-implant tissues with the provisional restoration, including the preservation of the interdental papillae around the definitive restoration [38–40]. It should be mentioned, however, that recent animal histologic research has demonstrated that immediate implant placement cannot prevent bone resorption, which is a physiologic metabolic process after tooth extraction [41, 42]. This has also been confirmed from studies in humans, showing also that the bone resorption of

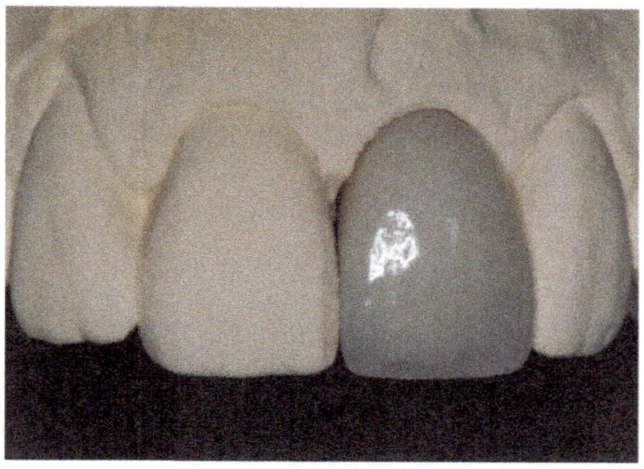

FIGURE 11: A definitive screw retained metal ceramic restoration was fabricated 6 months after implant placement.

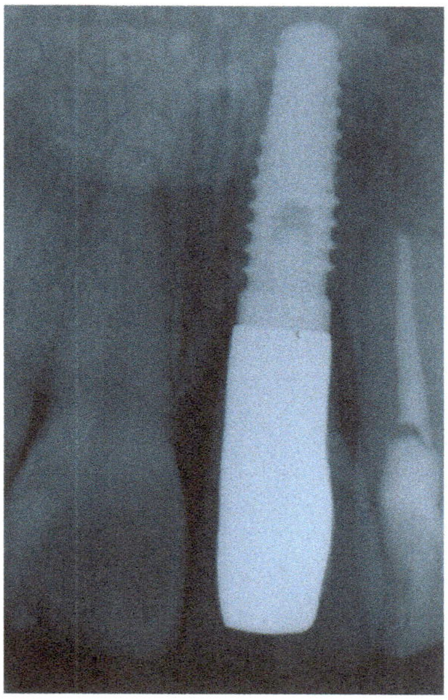

FIGURE 12: Final radiograph obtained at 6 months after implant placement.

the buccal plate is almost double when compared to that of the palatal or lingual plate [43]. Therefore, in the immediate placement approach the engagement of the palatal wall, which is crucial for implant's initial stability, always leaves a space between the implant and the coronal part of the buccal plate. Clinical studies indicate that in spaces with widths up to 2 mm, barrier membranes or regenerative techniques are not needed [44, 45]. This finding justifies the use of bovine bone mineral material without any barrier membrane for the treatment of the buccal bone deficiency after implant placement in the patient presented.

The Osseotite NT implant that was selected for the treatment of the patient presents a greater thread pitch (0.9 mm versus 0.6 mm for cylindric implants) and has the advantage of a taper form which mimics the natural form of the tooth, making it ideal for fresh extraction sites [46–48]. The surface of this type of implants receives a chemical thermal etching with a combination of hydrochloric and sulfuric acids, in order to induce a faster bone formation

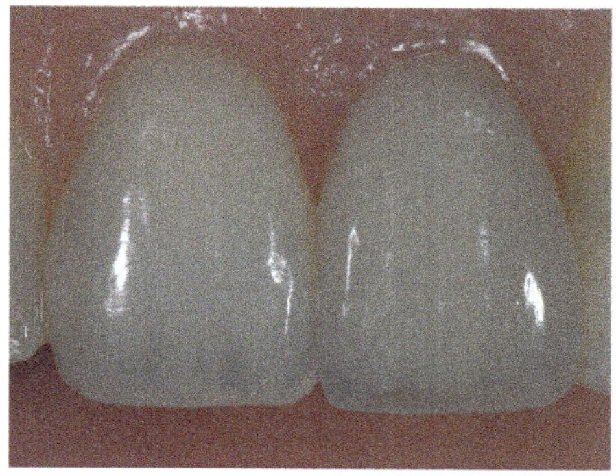

FIGURE 13: Clinical photograph of the definitive metal ceramic crown.

onto it. Histological and 3-year clinical data from multicenter studies confirm that high success rates can be obtained by its use [49–52].

The implant was placed in a more apical position in order to provide adequate space for the harmonic emergence of the prosthetic reconstruction through the soft tissues and its gradual transition from the size of the implant's platform to that of the emergence profile of natural anterior teeth [53]. It should be noted that the greater the difference between the diameter of the implant and the size of the tooth to be restored, the more apical the position of the implant should be in order to provide the appropriate space for the natural emergence of the restoration [36]. A more coronal implant placement may jeopardize the final esthetic result, since the abrupt transition from implant's platform to the restoration's normal contour will have as a result the exertion of big pressure on the surrounding soft tissues [36, 53]. This fact in conjunction with the establishment of the biologic width may ultimately lead to a soft tissue gradual recession and disclosure of the prosthetic components or even of the implant's coronal part. Conversely, if the implant is placed too apically, the respective migration of the microgap signals a bone recession, which is also observed in 1-piece implants [54]. This may cause a soft tissue recession, especially when the bone loss is accompanied by a thin buccal plate [36, 37]. In the patient presented, the cementoenamel junction of the maxillary right central incisor has been used as a reference point for the determination of implant's placement in the apico-coronal direction. In a healthy periodontium, the placement of the implant's platform 2 mm more apically than the cementoenamel junction of the adjacent teeth can be a good starting point [35–37]. It has also been suggested that, for patients with a thin periodontic biotype, the implant's platform should be placed 3-4 mm more apically than the adjacent bone peak [53, 55].

Regarding the labio-palatal dimension, the osteotomy was made after engaging the intact palatal wall of the socket, in order to obtain initial implant stability and to keep a safe distance from the defected and sensitive buccal wall [53, 56]. It should be mentioned, however, that the more palatal the implant is placed, the more space is needed on the vertical axis for a smooth and harmonic emergence of

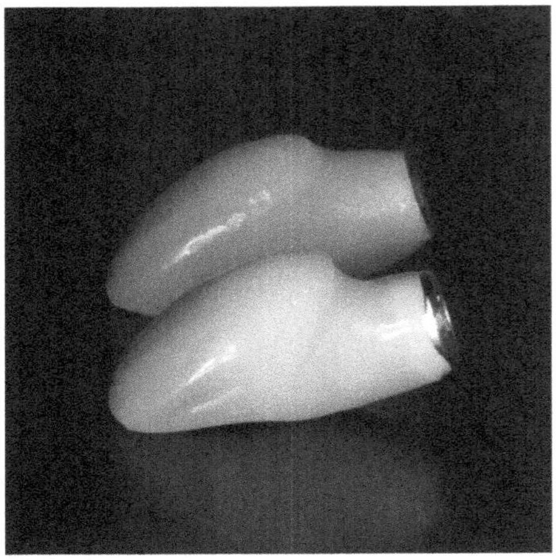

FIGURE 14: The ridge lap observed at the second provisional crown (down) was modified at the definitive crown (up) to facilitate better oral hygiene.

the restoration. Placing this concept in numbers, it can be said that for every 1 mm of palatal displacement, the implant should be placed 1 mm more apically [36, 57]. Nevertheless, a problem to the restoration's natural emergence can be created when the implant is placed too far palatally. In those cases, a restoration with a ridge lap is usually made in order to achieve a natural tooth appearance. However, this approach has negative consequences in dental hygiene [36, 37, 58, 59]. The ridge lap provisional restoration which was fabricated two months after the implant placement was modified at the definitive crown in order to facilitate better access for effective hygiene measures (Figure 14). The decision for a new provisional restoration fabrication was based on clinical data suggesting that a successful functional loading can be obtained two months after implant placement [60, 61].

The clinicians have many restorative options for the implant supported single crown. A screw retained prosthesis was selected for the provisional stage because of the ideal implant placement in relation to the natural contours of the maxillary incisor. Additionally, a cement-retained prosthesis could possibly jeopardize the healing process due to possible cement residues which can cause peri-implant inflammation [62].

A metal-ceramic restoration was the definitive restoration of choice since this was tested during the provisionalization period with no adverse esthetic results. Clinical studies have demonstrated that when the mucosal thickness is greater than 3 mm, no difference between all- and metal-ceramic restorations can be detected by the human eye [63].

The case presented consisted of a maxillary central incisor tooth extraction and immediate non-functional implant loading. This approach preserved both soft and hard tissues, and created a harmonious relationship among the implant, the restoration and the surrounding tissues. What should be emphasized is the necessity of the appropriate case evaluation and selection as well as the careful treatment planning. These parameters along with patient's compliance are of utmost importance for a successful outcome.

## References


[1] P.-I. Brånemark, B. O. Hansson, R. Adell et al., "Osseointegrated implants in the treatment of the edentulous jaw. experience from a 10-year period," *Scandinavian Journal of Plastic and Reconstructive Surgery. Supplementum*, vol. 16, pp. 1–132, 1977.

[2] R. Adell, U. Lekholm, P.-I. Brånemark, and B. Rockler, "A 15-year study of osseointegrated implants in the treatment of the edentulous jaw," *International Journal of Oral Surgery*, vol. 10, no. 6, pp. 387–416, 1981.

[3] P.-I. Brånemark, "Introduction to osseointegration," in *Tissue-Integrated Prostheses: Osseointegration in Clinical Dentistry*, pp. 1–11, Quintessence, Chicago, Ill, USA, 1987.

[4] T. Albrektsson, "A multicenter report on osseointegrated oral implants," *The Journal of Prosthetic Dentistry*, vol. 60, no. 1, pp. 75–84, 1988.

[5] T. Jemt, "Modified single and short-span restorations supported by osseointegrated fixtures in the partially edentulous jaw," *The Journal of Prosthetic Dentistry*, vol. 55, no. 2, pp. 243–247, 1986.

[6] T. Jemt, U. Lekholm, and R. Adell, "Osseointegrated implants in the treatment of partially edentulous patients: a preliminary study on 876 consecutively placed fixtures," *The International Journal of Oral & Maxillofacial Implants*, vol. 4, no. 3, pp. 211–217, 1989.

[7] D. van Steenberghe, "A retrospective multicenter evaluation of the survival rate of osseointegrated fixtures supporting fixed partial prostheses in the treatment of partial edentulism," *The Journal of Prosthetic Dentistry*, vol. 61, no. 2, pp. 217–223, 1989.

[8] J. Gunne, P. Åstrand, K. Ahlén, K. Borg, and M. Olsson, "Implants in partially edentulous patients: a longitudinal study of bridges supported by both implants and natural teeth," *Clinical Oral Implants Research*, vol. 3, no. 2, pp. 49–56, 1992.

[9] T. Jemt, U. Lekholm, and K. Gröndahl, "A 3-year follow-up study of early single implant restorations ad modum Brånemark," *The International Journal of Periodontics & Restorative Dentistry*, vol. 10, no. 5, pp. 340–349, 1990.

[10] A. Schmitt and G. A. Zarb, "The longitudinal clinical effectiveness of osseointegrated dental implants for single-tooth replacement," *The International Journal of Prosthodontics*, vol. 6, no. 2, pp. 197–202, 1993.

[11] A. Ekfeldt, G. E. Carlsson, and G. Börjesson, "Clinical evaluation of single-tooth restorations supported by osseointegrated implants: a retrospective study," *The International journal of oral & maxillofacial implants*, vol. 9, no. 2, pp. 179–183, 1994.

[12] B. Engquist, H. Nilson, and P. Åstrand, "Single-tooth replacement by osseointegrated Brånemark implants-a retrospective study of 82 implants," *Clinical Oral Implants Research*, vol. 6, no. 4, pp. 238–245, 1995.

[13] P. van Thompson, "Resin-bonded fixed dental prostheses," in *Contemporary Fixed Prosthodontics*, pp. 805–829, Mosby-Elsevier, St Louis, Mo, USA, 2006.

[14] D. B. Boyer, V. D. Williams, K. E. Thayer, G. E. Denehy, and A. M. Diaz-Arnold, "Analysis of debond rates of resin-bonded prostheses," *Journal of Dental Research*, vol. 72, no. 8, pp. 1244–1248, 1993.

[15] T. L. Berekally and R. J. Smales, "A retrospective clinical evaluation of resin-bonded bridges inserted at the Adelaide Dental Hospital," *Australian Dental Journal*, vol. 38, no. 2, pp. 85–96, 1993.

[16] N. H. Creugers, R. J. De Kanter, and M. A. Van't Hof, "Long-term survival data from a clinical trial on resin-bonded bridges," *Journal of Dentistry*, vol. 25, no. 3-4, pp. 239–242, 1997.

[17] H. Salama, M. Salama, D. Garber, and P. Adar, "The interproximal height of bone: a guidepost to predictable aesthetic strategies and soft tissue contours in anterior tooth replacement," *Practical Periodontics and Aesthetic Dentistry*, vol. 10, no. 9, pp. 1131–1142, 1998.

[18] P. Schnitman, P. S. Wöhrle, and J. E. Rubenstein, "Immediate fixed interim prostheses supported by two-stage threaded implants: methodology and results," *The Journal of Oral Implantology*, vol. 16, no. 2, pp. 96–105, 1990.

[19] P. A. Schnitman, P. S. Wöhrle, J. E. Rubenstein, J. D. DaSilva, and N.-H. Wang, "Ten years results for Brånemark implants immediately loaded with fixed prostheses at implant placement," *International Journal of Oral and Maxillofacial Implants*, vol. 12, no. 4, pp. 495–503, 1997.

[20] D. P. Tarnow, S. Emtiaz, and A. Classi, "Immediate loading of threaded implants at stage I surgery in edentulous arches: ten consecutive case reports with 1-to 5-year Data," *International Journal of Oral and Maxillofacial Implants*, vol. 12, no. 3, pp. 319–324, 1997.

[21] T. J. Balshi and G. H. Wolfinger, "Immediate loading of Brånemark implants in edentulous mandibles: a preliminary report," *Implant Dentistry*, vol. 6, no. 2, pp. 83–88, 1997.

[22] D. Buser, R. K. Schenk, S. Steinemann, J. P. Fiorellini, C. H. Fox, and H. Stich, "Influence of surface characteristics on bone integration of titanium implants. a histomorphometric study in miniature pigs," *Journal of Biomedical Materials Research*, vol. 25, no. 7, pp. 889–902, 1991.

[23] J. E. Davies, P. Schüpbach, and L. Cooper, "The implant surface and biological response: the changing interface," in *Osseointegration and Dental Implants*, pp. 213–223, Wiley-Blackwell, Ames, Iowa, USA, 2009.

[24] A. Piattelli, M. Paolantonio, M. Corigliano, and A. Scarano, "Immediate loading of titanium plasma-sprayed screw-shaped implants in man: a clinical and histological report of two cases," *Journal of Periodontology*, vol. 68, no. 6, pp. 591–597, 1997.

[25] A. Göransson and A. Wennerberg, "Bone formation at titanium implants prepared with iso- and anisotropic surfaces of similar roughness: an in vivo study," *Clinical Implant Dentistry and Related Research*, vol. 7, no. 1, pp. 17–23, 2005.

[26] G. Mendonça, D. B. S. Mendonça, and F. J. L. Aragão, "Advancing dental implant surface technology: from micron-to nanotopography," *Biomaterials*, vol. 29, no. 28, pp. 3822–3835, 2008.

[27] V. A. Bousdras, S. Sindet-Pedersen, J. L. Cunningham et al., "Immediate functional loading of single-tooth $TiO_2$ grit-blasted implant restorations: a controlled prospective study in a porcine model. part I: clinical outcome," *Clinical Implant Dentistry and Related Research*, vol. 9, no. 4, pp. 197–206, 2007.

[28] V. A. Bousdras, F. Walboomers, J. A. Jansen et al., "Immediate functional loading of single-tooth $TiO_2$ grit-blasted implant restoration. a controlled prospective study in a porcine model. part II: histology and histomorphometry," *Clinical Implant Dentistry and Related Research*, vol. 9, no. 4, pp. 207–216, 2007.

[29] R. J. Goené, T. Testori, and P. Trisi, "Influence of a nanometer-scale surface enhancement on de novo bone formation on titanium implants: a histomorphometric study in human maxillae," *International Journal of Periodontics and Restorative Dentistry*, vol. 27, no. 3, pp. 211–219, 2007.

[30] P. O. Östman, M. Hupalo, R. del Castillo et al., "Immediate provisionalization of nanotite implants in support of single-tooth and unilateral restorations: one-year interim report of a prospective, multicenter study," *Clinical Implant Dentistry and Related Research*, vol. 12, supplement 1, pp. e47–e55, 2010.

[31] P. S. Wöhrle, "Single-tooth replacement in the aesthetic zone with immediate provisionalization: fourteen consecutive case reports," *Practical Periodontics and Aesthetic Dentistry*, vol. 10, no. 9, pp. 1107–1114, 1998.

[32] M. Olsson and J. Lindhe, "Periodontal characteristics in individuals with varying form of the upper central incisors," *Journal of Clinical Periodontology*, vol. 18, no. 1, pp. 78–82, 1991.

[33] M. Olsson, J. Lindhe, and C. P. Marinello, "On the relationship between crown form and clinical features of the gingiva in adolescents," *Journal of Clinical Periodontology*, vol. 20, no. 8, pp. 570–577, 1993.

[34] A. G. Sclar, "Strategies for management of single-tooth extraction sites in aesthetic implant therapy," *Journal of Oral and Maxillofacial Surgery*, vol. 62, supplement 2, pp. 90–105, 2004.

[35] F. A. Chiche and M. A. Leriche, "Multidisciplinary implant dentistry for improved aesthetics and function," *Practical Periodontics and Aesthetic Dentistry*, vol. 10, no. 2, pp. 177–188, 1998.

[36] A. P. Saadoun, M. G. Le Gall, and B. Touati, "Selection and ideal tridimensional implant position for soft tissue aesthetics," *Practical Periodontics and Aesthetic Dentistry*, vol. 11, no. 9, pp. 1063–1074, 1999.

[37] D. Buser, W. Martin, and U. C. Belser, "Optimizing esthetics for implant restorations in the anterior maxilla: anatomic and surgical considerations," *International Journal of Oral and Maxillofacial Implants*, vol. 19, supplement, pp. 43–61, 2004.

[38] R. J. Lazzara, "Immediate implant placement into extraction sites: surgical and restorative advantages," *The International Journal of Periodontics & Restorative Dentistry*, vol. 9, no. 5, pp. 332–343, 1989.

[39] D. A. Garber, M. A. Salama, and H. Salama, "Immediate total tooth replacement," *Compendium of Continuing Education in Dentistry*, vol. 22, no. 3, pp. 210–218, 2001.

[40] S. T. Chen, T. G. Wilson Jr., and C. H. Hämmerle, "Immediate or early placement of implants following tooth extraction: review of biologic basis, clinical procedures, and outcomes," *International Journal of Oral and Maxillofacial Implants*, vol. 19, 1, pp. 12–25, 2004.

[41] M. G. Araújo, F. Sukekava, J. L. Wennström, and J. Lindhe, "Ridge alterations following implant placement in fresh extraction sockets: an experimental study in the dog," *Journal of Clinical Periodontology*, vol. 32, no. 6, pp. 645–652, 2005.

[42] M. G. Araújo, F. Sukekava, J. L. Wennström, and J. Lindhe, "Tissue modeling following implant placement in fresh extraction sockets," *Clinical Oral Implants Research*, vol. 17, no. 6, pp. 615–624, 2006.

[43] D. Botticelli, T. Berglundh, and J. Lindhe, "Hard-tissue alterations following immediate implant placement in extraction sites," *Journal of Clinical Periodontology*, vol. 31, no. 10, pp. 820–828, 2004.

[44] M. Paolantonio, M. Dolci, A. Scarano et al., "Immediate implantation in fresh extraction sockets. a controlled clinical and histological study in man," *Journal of Periodontology*, vol. 72, no. 11, pp. 1560–1571, 2001.

[45] U. Covani, R. Cornelini, and A. Barone, "Bucco-lingual bone remodeling around implants placed into immediate extraction sockets: a case series," *Journal of Periodontology*, vol. 74, no. 2, pp. 268–273, 2003.

[46] F. Daftary, "Dentoalveolar morphology: evaluation of natural root form versus cylindrical implant fixtures," *Practical Periodontics and Aesthetic Dentistry*, vol. 9, no. 4, pp. 469–478, 1997.

[47] A. Meltzer, "Osseotite NT implants for optimal stability and aesthetics," *Implantology*, vol. 1, pp. 5–12, 2003.

[48] C. J. Drago and R. A. Del Castillo, "A retrospective analysis of osseotite NT implants in clinical practice: 1-year follow-up," *International Journal of Periodontics and Restorative Dentistry*, vol. 26, no. 4, pp. 337–345, 2006.

[49] R. J. Lazzara, T. Testori, P. Trisi, R. L. Weinstein, and S. S. Porter, "A human histologic analysis of Osseotite and machined surfaces using implants with 2 opposing surfaces," *International Journal of Periodontics and Restorative Dentistry*, vol. 19, no. 2, pp. 117–187, 1999.

[50] U. Grunder, T. Gaberthuel, N. Boitel et al., "Evaluating the clinical performance of the Osseotite implant: defining prosthetic predictability," *Compendium of Continuing Education in Dentistry*, vol. 20, no. 7, pp. 628–638, 1999.

[51] M. Davarpanah, H. Martinez, R. Celletti, G. Alcoforado, J. F. Tecucianu, and D. Etienne, "Osseotite implant: 3-year prospective multicenter evaluation," *Clinical Implant Dentistry and Related Research*, vol. 3, no. 2, pp. 111–118, 2001.

[52] W. Khang, S. Feldman, C. E. Hawley, and J. Gunsolley, "A multi-center study comparing dual acid-etched and machined-surfaced implants in various bone qualities," *Journal of Periodontology*, vol. 72, no. 10, pp. 1384–1390, 2001.

[53] A. P. Saadoun, M. G. Le Gall, and B. Touati, "Current trends in implantology: part II-treatment planning, aesthetic considerations, and tissue regeneration," *Practical Procedures & Aesthetic Dentistry*, vol. 16, no. 10, pp. 707–714, 2004.

[54] R. P. Kinsel and R. E. Lamb, "Tissue-directed placement of dental implants in the esthetic zone for long-term biologic synergy: a clinical report," *International Journal of Oral and Maxillofacial Implants*, vol. 20, no. 6, pp. 913–922, 2005.

[55] H. Smukler, F. Castellucci, and D. Capri, "The role of the implant housing in obtaining aesthetics: generation of peri-implant gingivae and papillae—part I," *Practical Procedures & Aesthetic Dentistry*, vol. 15, no. 2, pp. 141–150, 2003.

[56] J. C. Kois and J. Y. Kan, "Predictable peri-implant gingival aesthetics: surgical and prosthodontic rationales," *Practical Procedures & Aesthetic Dentistry*, vol. 13, no. 9, pp. 691–698, 2001.

[57] A. S. Weisgold, J. P. Arnoux, and J. Lu, "Single-tooth anterior implant: a word of caution. part I," *Journal of Esthetic Dentistry*, vol. 9, no. 5, pp. 225–233, 1997.

[58] M. Davarpanah, H. Martinez, R. Celletti, and J. F. Tecucianu, "Three-stage approach to aesthetic implant restoration: emergence profile concept," *Practical Procedures & Aesthetic Dentistry*, vol. 13, no. 9, pp. 761–767, 2001.

[59] A. E. El Askary, "Multifaceted aspects of implant esthetics: the anterior maxilla," *Implant Dentistry*, vol. 10, no. 3, pp. 182–191, 2001.

[60] R. J. Lazzara, S. S. Porter, T. Testori, J. Galante, and L. Zetterqvist, "A prospective multicenter study evaluating loading of osseotite implants two months after placement: one year results," *Journal of Esthetic Dentistry*, vol. 10, no. 6, pp. 280–289, 1998.

[61] T. Testori, M. Del Fabbro, F. Bianchi et al., "A multicenter prospective evaluation of 2-months loaded Osseotite implants placed in the posterior jaws: 3-year follow-up results," *Clinical Oral Implants Research*, vol. 13, no. 2, pp. 154–161, 2002.

[62] N. Pauletto, B. J. Lahiffe, and J. N. Walton, "Complications associated with excess cement around crowns on osseointegrated implants: a clinical report," *The International Journal of Oral & Maxillofacial Implants*, vol. 14, no. 6, pp. 865–868, 1999.

[63] R. E. Jung, C. Holderegger, I. Sailer, A. Khraisat, A. Suter, and C. H. F. Hämmerle, "The effect of all-ceramic and porcelain-fused-to-metal restorations on marginal peri-implant soft tissue color: a randomized controlled clinical trial," *International Journal of Periodontics and Restorative Dentistry*, vol. 28, no. 4, pp. 357–365, 2008.

# Management of Horizontal Root Fracture in the Middle Third via Intraradicular Splinting Using a Fiber Post

**Ishani Karhade and Meenal N. Gulve**

*Usha Kiran Bunglow, Anand Nagar, Behind Muktidham, Opp Maharshi Hospital, Nashik Road, Nashik, Maharashtra 422101, India*

Correspondence should be addressed to Ishani Karhade; ishanikarhade@gmail.com

Academic Editor: Hamdi Cem Gungor

Radicular fractures in permanent teeth are uncommon injuries and account for only 0.5–7% of dental traumas. These fractures commonly result from a horizontal impact and are transverse to oblique in direction. Their incidence is more in the middle third of the root than at the apical and cervical thirds. This paper describes a case of complicated crown fracture of maxillary incisors along with horizontal root fracture at the middle third of maxillary right central and lateral incisor. The fractured root fragments of the upper right central and lateral incisor were united with the help of a glass fiber post after receiving an endodontic treatment. The other two incisors were treated endodontically followed by post endodontic restorations. Eventually the four incisors were restored with porcelain fused to metal crowns. A one-year follow-up revealed a well stabilized assembly of the root fragments and the post.

## 1. Introduction

Among all dental traumatic injuries, root fractures account for only 0.5–7% [1–3]. Root fracture is defined as "fracture involving dentin, cement and pulp" [1]. Horizontal root fracture most commonly occurs in the middle third of the root and very rarely in the coronal and apical third [4]. Maxillary central incisors are more prone to traumatic injuries (approximately 68%) probably due to their position in the dental arch. The next in line are the maxillary lateral incisors (27%) followed by mandibular incisors (5%) [5, 6].

Root fracture occurs as a consequence of an impact force on the top of the root and frontal forces affect the compression zone labially and lingually/palatally, thus dividing the root into coronal and apical fragments. This can traumatize the supporting periodontal tissues eventually leading to displacement of the root fragments [7]. Proper clinical and radiographic examination is required for correctly diagnosing root fracture. A clinician must check for mobility of the coronal fragment and the pulp vitality. Radiographically, a radiolucent line is seen separating the apical and coronal fragments [8, 9]. Two or three radiographs taken at different angulations may be sometimes needed to detect the angle of fracture.

The management of horizontal root fracture depends on the location of the fracture and mobility and the vitality of the tooth. Fractures in the apical third usually display no mobility and generally do not require any treatment. Root fracture at the cervical third often requires extraction. When the coronal fragment shows severe mobility, there is no other option but extraction.

Root fractures at the middle third have favourable prognosis. When the coronal fragment is displaced, the initial treatment should be repositioning the fragments, followed by stabilization to allow healing of the surrounding periodontal tissues [1]. With the ever-increasing demand for aesthetics, tooth coloured fiber posts have been introduced, which can be used as a medium to retain the two fractured root fragments in conjunction with bonding agents and composite resins. This report thereby describes a case of horizontal root fracture with displaced fragments, which were united with the help of glass fiber posts followed by core build-up and coronal coverage.

## 2. Case Report

A 19-year-old male patient reported to the department of conservative dentistry and endodontics following trauma to the maxillary anterior region due to a road accident around 20 days back. He complained of fractured maxillary incisors and presented a desire to get them restored in order to have an aesthetic smile. Clinical examination of the patient revealed complicated crown fracture of the upper incisors. An intraoral swelling with a sinus tract was present on the labial gingiva between upper right central and lateral incisor (Figures 1(a) and 1(b)). A radiograph of the maxillary anterior region illustrated horizontal root fracture at the middle third of the upper right central and lateral incisors (Figure 1(c)) but clinically no mobility of the coronal fragment was evident. On the other hand the roots of the upper left central and lateral incisors were intact and endodontic treatment had been done for the upper left central and lateral incisors (Figure 1(c)).

After explaining the treatment plan to the patient and obtaining his consent, endodontic treatment with the upper right central and lateral incisors was initiated. The working length was correctly determined and canals were cleaned, shaped using K files in a step-back manner to an apical file size #60. The remainder of the canals were shaped to obtain a uniform taper from apex towards coronal. An interappointment calcium hydroxide dressing was given and the patient was recalled after 7 days.

On the second visit, when the swelling had resolved, root canals were sectionally obturated with gutta percha cone and AH plus sealer. A gutta percha cone of the same size of the prepared root canal (size #60, with a taper of 2%) was selected and tried into the canal to obtain a snug fit. It was then cut to obtain a section which would be 2-3 mm short of the apical fragment of the root. A suitable plugger which loosely fits 2-3 mm short of the apical root fragment was selected and a stopper was set at this length. The sectioned gutta percha was then coated with AH plus sealer. One end of gutta percha was mounted to a heated plugger and then carried into the canal to the desired length. After this, gutta percha was disengaged from the plugger by slightly rotating the plugger in anticlockwise direction (Figure 1(d)).

After 5 days of recall, the tooth was asymptomatic and the sinus tract healed. Next, glass fiber posts were used to retain the fractured root fragments. Appropriate glass fiber posts were tried into the canals, adjusted to the desired length until they just passively touched the apical gutta percha. Root canals were etched with 37% phosphoric acid gel and dried with paper points. The fiber posts were luted with dual cure resin cement, inserted into the canal without applying any pressure, and then light cured for 40 seconds. The benefit of higher viscosity of the cement in absence of pressure is that it reduces the flow of the resin. Also, the resin was used cautiously only in the amount necessary to achieve a desirable bond between the post and the dentin. Only the post was luted with the cement. Coating the root canal walls with resin cement was precluded to prevent the flow of excess cement laterally between the root fragments.

These fiber posts served as an intraradicular splint, stabilizing the fractured fragments in position. Glass fiber-reinforced posts were used as they exhibit high fatigue strength and high tensile strength and have a modulus of elasticity closer to dentin. Composite cores were built over the posts (Figure 1(e)). The other two incisors (maxillary left central and lateral incisors) received a similar post and core treatment (Figures 1(f)–1(i)). The teeth were then restored with full-coverage porcelain fused to metal crowns (Figures 1(j)–1(m)).

The patient was reevaluated on a regular basis. After 12 months of recall, the patient presented with aesthetically pleasing results and sound periodontium and the fractured root fragments were well retained with the aid of a post (Figures 2(c) and 2(d)).

## 3. Discussion

Root fracture can be a consequence of dental trauma causing a complex injury to the cementum, dentin, pulp, and the periodontal tissues [10]. Such injuries can occur due to road accidents, violence, sport injuries, and so forth. Maintaining "the physiological and functional integrity" is the main goal while treating traumatized teeth.

Four types of conservative endodontic treatment that have been commonly described [11, 12] are (i) cleansing and gutta percha (GP) filling of the root canal of the coronal fragment only; (ii) cleansing and filling of the root canal in both fragments; (iii) cleansing and GP filling of the root canal of the coronal fragment and surgical removal of the apical fragment; and (iv) treatment of the root canal with calcium hydroxide followed by filling with GP. Recently, different types of post materials have been introduced into the dental practice such as carbon fiber, quartz, and glass fiber. The fiber posts offer several advantages such as a suitable elastic modulus, aesthetics, good bonding between post and cement, lower chair side time, and minimal tissue removal.

In the present case report, only the apical fragment was endodontically treated and the two fragments were splinted using a glass fiber post to act as an intraradicular splint. After luting the post with resin cement, it was inserted into the root canal passively, without applying pressure. This is because higher viscosity of the resin in absence of pressure reduces its flow. This may prevent the resin from flowing between the root fragments [13].

The conventional metal posts have a high modulus of elasticity [14], whereas the fiber- reinforced posts have a modulus similar to that of the dentin, minimizing the risk of root fractures [15]. According to Gurtu and Singhal [16], the use of a post ensures support and stability to the tooth. It also helps to retain the root fragments by radicular anchoring thereby strengthening the restoration complex which is subjected to tangential stresses. Further, it creates a monoblock between the post, reconstructive material, cement, and the tooth [17]. Post placement, in addition to bonding, provides retention via a friction bond and assists in preventing dislodgement to nonaxial forces [18]. Thus, light-transmitting fiber posts have been widely used to functionally and aesthetically restore the compromised root filled teeth. Teeth, which earlier

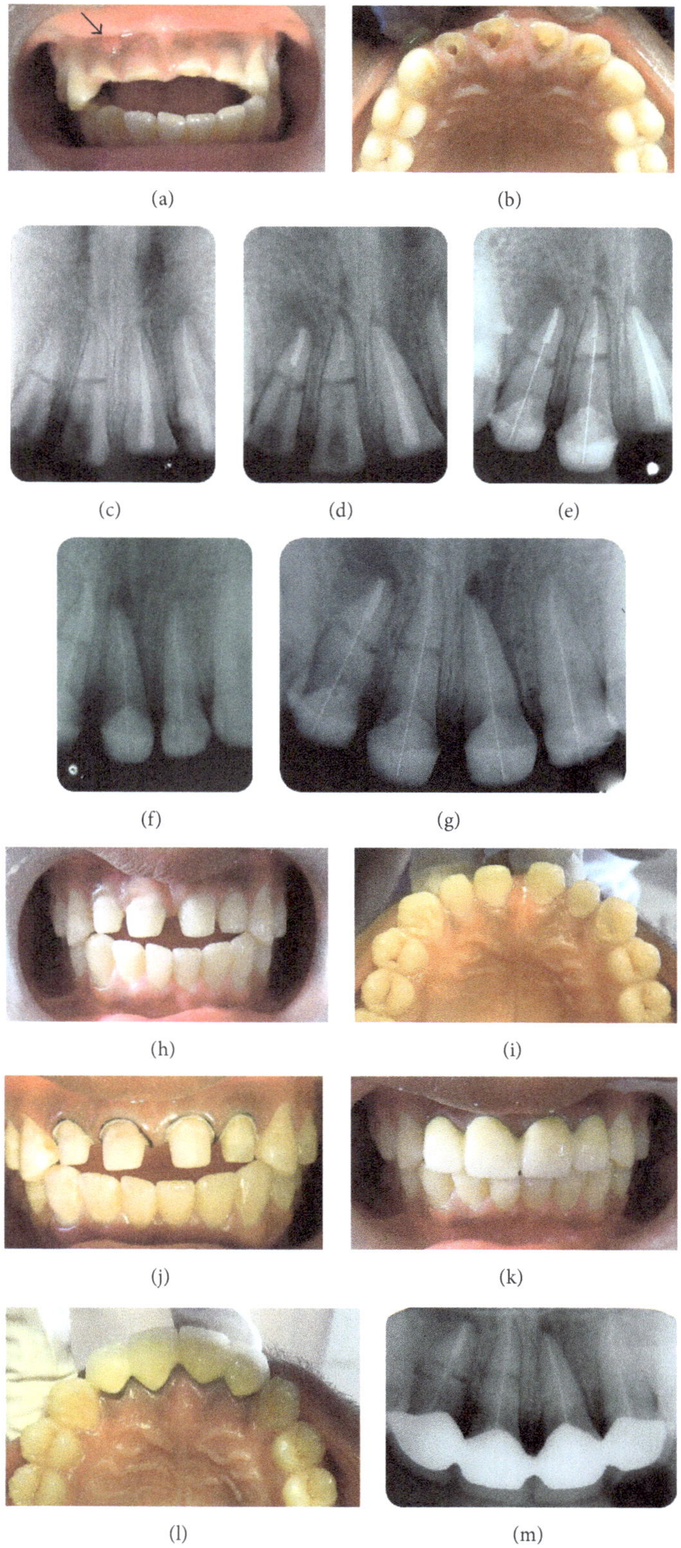


FIGURE 1: Procedural steps. (a) Preoperative clinical photograph (labial view) demonstrating complicated crown fractures of upper central and lateral incisors and the presence of a sinus tract on labial gingiva. (b) Preoperative palatal view. (c) Preoperative radiograph showing horizontal root fracture at the middle third of upper right central and lateral incisors. (d) Sectional obturation using gutta percha cone and AH plus sealer followed by post space preparation. (e) Core build-up following cementation of post. (f) Post and core treatment of maxillary left central and lateral incisors. (g) Radiograph illustrating post and core treatment of the four upper incisors. (h) Clinical photograph after post and core treatment of upper incisors (labial view). (i) Palatal view. (j) Tooth preparation to receive coronal coverage. (k) Cementation of porcelain fused to metal crowns (labial view). (l) Palatal view. (m) Postoperative radiograph after cementation of the crowns.

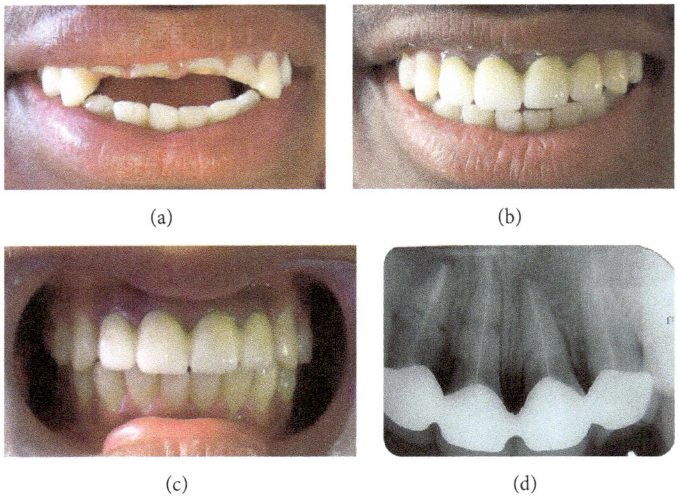


FIGURE 2: (a) Preoperative smile of the patient. (b) Postoperative smile. (c) Clinical photograph after one year of follow-up. (d) Postoperative radiograph after one year of follow-up.

would have been condemned to extraction, could now be strengthened by a sufficiently thick lining of intraradicular reinforcing composite, thereby salvaging them for continued function [19].

Linkow [20] proposed that, by inserting a post through the tooth, deep into the bone and cementing the intradental part to the root canal walls, the fulcrum of movement of a loose tooth is moved deeper into the jaw, the support in the bone is increased, and thus the mobility of the tooth is lessened.

Luting agents including zinc phosphate, zinc polycarboxylate, glass ionomer, and resin modified glass ionomer have been used traditionally. They had disadvantages such as solubility in oral fluids, especially in the presence of acid and lack of true adhesion. Resin modified glass ionomers exhibit hygroscopic expansion and hence their use declined. Nowadays adhesive resin cement has been advocated for cementation of post because it bonds the post to the tooth structure. There is not only chemical adhesion but also micromechanical bonding. However, a disadvantage of this resin cement is its technique sensitivity. Also, the bonding to root canal dentin could be compromised due to the use of various irrigants and eugenol based sealers. Eugenol can prevent or stop the polymerization reaction and can also interfere with bonding [21].

Midroot fractures can heal by different mechanisms. Andreasen and Hjörting-Hansen described four types of healing sequelae [22]: (1) healing with calcified tissue, (2) healing with interproximal connective tissue, (3) healing with interproximal bone and connective tissue, and (4) interproximal inflammatory tissue without healing.

A long-term follow-up is required to check for any possible pathological alterations. Follow-up of this case after one year showed promising results with clinically pleasing aesthetics and radiographic healing with calcified tissue, the fractured line discernible but fragments well stabilized.

## 4. Conclusion

"Preservation of natural dentition and restoration of the oral cavity to a normal functional state" is the primary goal in dentistry. The main aim of treating fractured elements is to keep the tooth steady and maintain its position in the dental arch whenever possible. The improvement in bonding agents and restorative resins and the availability of newer materials like the fiber posts and dual cure resin cement have provided clinicians with different modalities for successfully managing root fractures. Intraradicular splinting using fiber posts can be a good alternative for managing midroot fractures and reestablishing the aesthetics and functional needs of the patients.

## Conflict of Interests

The authors declare that there is no conflict of interests regarding the publication of this paper.

## References

[1] F. M. Andreasen and J. O. Andreasen, "Crown fractures," in *Textbook and Color Atlas of Traumatic Injuries to the Teeth*, pp. 219–256, Munksgaard, Copenhagen, Denmark, 3rd edition, 1994.

[2] E. Davidovich, I. Heling, and A. B. Fuks, "The fate of a mid-root fracture: a case report," *Dental Traumatology*, vol. 21, no. 3, pp. 170–173, 2005.

[3] M. K. Çalişkan, "Prognosis of large cyst-like periapical lesions following nonsurgical root canal treatment: a clinical review," *International Endodontic Journal*, vol. 37, no. 6, pp. 408–416, 2004.

[4] C. M. Bramante, R. Menezes, I. G. Moraes, N. Bernardinelli, R. B. Garcia, and A. Letra, "Use of MTA and intracanal post reinforcement in a horizontally fractured tooth: a case report," *Dental Traumatology*, vol. 22, no. 5, pp. 275–278, 2006.

[5] E. S. Andrade, A. L. P. D. C. Sobrinho, M. G. S. Andrade, and J. L. F. Matos, "Root healing after horizontal fracture: a case report with a 13-year follow up," *Dental Traumatology*, vol. 24, no. 4, pp. e1–e3, 2008.

[6] M. K. Çalişkan and Y. Pehlivan, "Prognosis of root-fractured permanent incisors," *Endodontics and Dental Traumatology*, vol. 12, no. 3, pp. 129–136, 1996.

[7] R. R. Welbury, M. J. Kinirons, P. Day, K. Humphreys, and T. A. Gregg, "Outcomes for root-fractured permanent incisors: a retrospective study," *Pediatric Dentistry*, vol. 24, no. 2, pp. 98–102, 2002.

[8] J. R. Molina, W. F. Vann Jr., J. D. McIntyre, M. Trope, and J. Y. Lee, "Root fractures in children and adolescents: diagnostic considerations," *Dental Traumatology*, vol. 24, no. 5, pp. 503–509, 2008.

[9] M. T. Flores, L. Andersson, J. O. Andreasen et al., "Guidelines for the management of traumatic dental injuries. I. Fractures and luxations of permanent teeth," *Dental Traumatology*, vol. 23, no. 2, pp. 66–71, 2007.

[10] D. N. Mankar, D. N. Jogad, D. A. Chute, D. S. Patil, D. V. Gade, and D. S. Mohkar, "Management of horizontal root fracture: two case reports," *IOSR Journal of Dental and Medical Sciences*, vol. 13, no. 4, pp. 1–4, 2014.

[11] A. E. Michanowicz, "Root fractures. A report of radiographic healing after endodontic treatment," *Oral Surgery, Oral Medicine, Oral Pathology*, vol. 16, no. 10, pp. 1242–1248, 1963.

[12] M. Cvek, "Treatment of non-vital permanent incisors with calcium hydroxide. IV. Periodontal healing and closure of the root canal in the coronal fragment of teeth with intra-alveolar fracture and vital apical fragment. A follow-up," *Odontologisk Revy*, vol. 25, no. 3, pp. 239–246, 1974.

[13] 3M ESPE, RelyX™ Unicem Clicker™, RelyX™ Unicem Aplicap™/Maxicap™ Technical Product Profile, 2007.

[14] D. Assif, E. Oren, B. L. Marshak, and I. Aviv, "Photoelastic analysis of stress transfer by endodontically treated teeth to the supporting structure using different restorative techniques," *The Journal of Prosthetic Dentistry*, vol. 61, no. 5, pp. 535–543, 1989.

[15] G. Á. Galhano, L. F. Valandro, R. M. de Melo, R. Scotti, and M. A. Bottino, "Evaluation of the flexural strength of carbon fiber-, quartz fiber-, and glass fiber-based posts," *Journal of Endodontics*, vol. 31, no. 3, pp. 209–211, 2005.

[16] A. Gurtu and A. Singhal, "Management of horizontal fracture," *Journal of Dental Sciences and Oral Rehabilitation*, pp. 48–50, 2012.

[17] A. Polesel, "Restoration of the endodontically treated posterior tooth," *Giornale Italiano di Endodonzia*, vol. 28, no. 1, pp. 2–16, 2014.

[18] A. Dhingra and D. K. Shrivastav, "Immediate reattachment of fractured crown fragment: a case report," *Endodontology*, pp. 94–96, 2006.

[19] R. Arora, B. Shivakumar, H. M. Rao, and R. Vijay, "Rehabilitation of complicated crown-root fracture by fragment reattachment and intraradicular splinting: case reports," *Journal of International Oral Health*, vol. 5, no. 5, pp. 129–138, 2013.

[20] L. I. Linkow, *Theories and Technique of Oral Implantology-2*, Mosby, St. Louis, Mo, USA, 1970.

[21] N. Garg and A. Garg, "Restoration of endodontically treated teeth," in *Textbook of Endodontics*, pp. 428–453, Boydell & Brewer, 3rd edition, 2010.

[22] J. O. Andreasen and E. Hjörting-Hansen, "Intraalveolar root fractures: radiographic and histologic study of 50 cases," *Journal of Oral Surgery*, vol. 25, no. 5, pp. 414–426, 1967.

# 6

# Multiple Hamartoma Syndrome with Characteristic Oral and Cutaneous Manifestations

**Prashanthi Chippagiri,[1] Spoorthi Banavar Ravi,[2] and Neha Patwa[3]**

[1] *Department of Oral Medicine and Radiology, MS Ramaiah Dental College and Hospital, Bangalore, Karnataka 560010, India*
[2] *Department of Oral Pathology, MS Ramaiah Dental College and Hospital, Bangalore, India*
[3] *Department of Dentistry, Indiragandhi District Hospital, Mandsaur, Madhya Pradesh 458001, India*

Correspondence should be addressed to Prashanthi Chippagiri; drprashanthi.1@gmail.com

Academic Editors: J. Asaumi, D. W. Boston, T. Lombardi, and E. F. Wright

*Aim.* To present a case of Cowden's syndrome and emphasize the importance of continued cancer surveillance in these patients. Cowden syndrome is an inherited autosomal dominant trait with incomplete penetrance and a range of expressivity. It is characterized by multiple hamartomas and neoplasms. Mucocutaneous features include trichilemmomas, oral mucosal papillomatosis, acral keratosis, and palmoplantar keratosis. Here, we report a case of Cowdens syndrome of a 30-year-old female patient who came with a complaint of multiple growths in the oral cavity of a three-month duration. On examination, multiple skin-colored, flat-topped papules over her forehead and right malar bone and multiple papillomatous papules involving all the mucosal surfaces intraorally were observed. This syndrome is associated with the development of several types of malignancies, especially breast carcinoma and thyroid carcinoma, which is why early recognition and regular and vigilant surveillance of individuals with the syndrome are important.

## 1. Background

Cowden syndrome (CS), also termed as multiple hamartoma syndrome, was first described in 1940 by Salem and Steck [1]. Cowden's syndrome was defined and named by Lloyd and Dennis in 1963 referring to their patient Rachael Cowden, who died of breast carcinoma [2, 3]. Weary and coworkers reported 5 more patients in 1972 and suggested the name multiple hamartoma syndrome (MHS) [2, 4].

Cowden's syndrome (CS) is a rare genodermatosis, of autosomal dominant inheritance and variable phenotype, principally characterized clinically by multiple hamartomas of ectodermic, mesodermic, or endodermic origin. It results most commonly from the mutation in the PTEN gene on the arm 10q [5]. Cowden's syndrome is associated with an increased risk of malignancy, particularly cancers of the breast, thyroid, endometrium, and to a lesser extent, renal system [6].

The rare occurrence of this disease and the synchronous association of various malignancies with this disease emphasize the importance of a thorough diagnostic work-up and management of the patients with cowden's syndrome. The present report thus, details the features of a patient who initially presented with oral swellings and was subsequently found to have Cowden's syndrome.

## 2. Case Report

A 30-year-old female patient came with a complaint of multiple growths in the oral cavity of three months duration. Initially, she had noticed only two growths in the right and left retrocomissural areas. Gradually they increased in number, involving the entire oral cavity. The lesions were not associated with any symptoms. Previously, she was prescribed corticosteroid ointment and multivitamins by a local doctor. She found no relief.

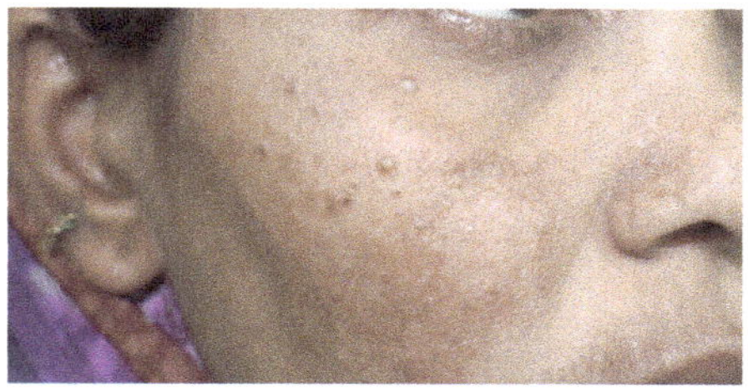

FIGURE 1: Trichilemmomas on the right malar bone.

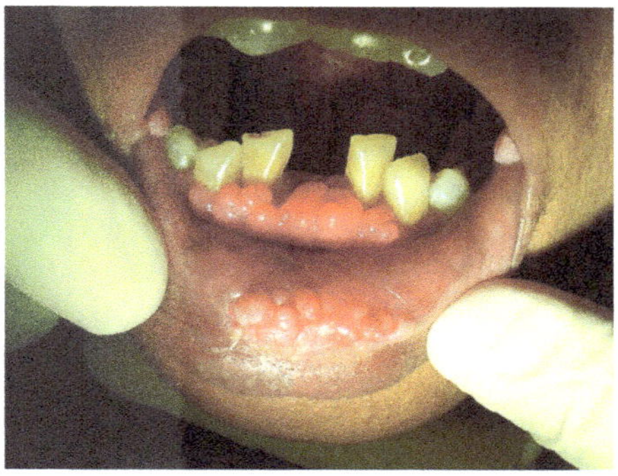

FIGURE 2: Enlarged gingiva having smooth and multiple papillomatous lesions. Multiple papules may also be noticed on the lower labial mucosa.

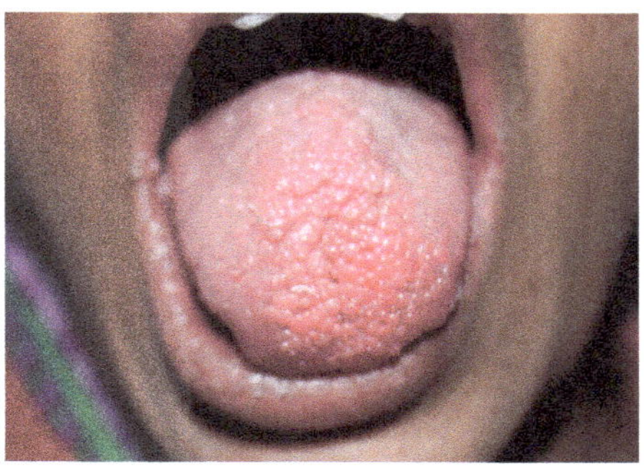

FIGURE 3: Cobblestone appearance of multiple confluent papules on the tongue.

Her medical history reveals a left breast abscess 12 years back which was drained. She also gave a history of a growth in the left lower back region which was excised 10 years back. However, there were no medical records available for proper evidence. Review of the patient's family history was insignificant.

On general physical examination, she was found to be moderately built and nourished with all her vital signs in the normal range. Pallor was noticed on examination of her inferior palpebral conjunctiva. A scar was noticed over the lower back region on the left side.

Extraoral examination revealed the presence of small multiple skin colored, flat topped papules over the skin of her forehead and malar bones, measuring around 1 to 5 mm in diameter (Figure 1). The patient was referred to a dermatologist for evaluation of these lesions and they were diagnosed to be trichilemmomas.

Intraoral examination revealed multiple papillomatous papules involving all the mucosal surfaces. The presence of multiple, confluent lesions produced a cobblestone appearance. The size of the lesions ranged from 1 to 5 mm. The lesions were spherical and they were coral pink in color (Figures 2 and 3). The lesions on the retrocomissural areas were larger in size and paler. On palpation, the lesions were soft to firm in consistency and nontender.

## 3. Discussion of the Diagnosis

A provisional diagnosis of Cowden syndrome was made on the basis of the presence of trichilemmomas and mucosal lesions. There were more than 6 cutaneous papules or trichilemmomas and oral papillomatosis. This case, therefore, fulfilled the diagnostic criteria 1 of the International Cowden Syndrome Consortium.

*The International Cowden Syndrome Consortium proposed a set of diagnostic criteria for diagnosis of Cowden's syndrome, which includes the following:*

*pathognomic criteria:*

(i) facial trichilemmomas

(ii) acral keratosis

(iii) papillomatous papules

(iv) mucosal lesions

*major criteria:*

(i) breast carcinoma

(ii) thyroid carcinoma

(iii) endometrial carcinoma

(iv) macrocephaly

(v) Lhermitte-Duclos disease

*minor criteria:*

(i) thyroid lesions
(ii) mental retardation
(iii) G I Hamartomas
(iv) fibrocystic breast
(v) lipomas
(vi) fibromas
(vii) genitourinary tumors.

*Operational diagnosis in an individual is based on the presence of any one of the following criteria.*

*Criteria 1.* Mucocutaneous lesions alone if

(a) 6+ facial papules with 3+ being trichilemmomas,
(b) cutaneous facial papules and oral mucosal papillomatosis,
(c) oral mucosal papillomatosis and acral keratosis or,
(d) 6+ palmar or plantar keratosis.

*Criteria 2.* Two major criteria with one being Lheimitte-Duclos disease or macrocephaly.

*Criteria 3.* One major and three minor criteria.

*Criteria 4.* Four minor criteria.

Orthopantomogram of the patient only revealed generalized alveolar crestal bone loss. Laboratory investigations performed were complete hematological tests and biopsy of the mucosal lesions. Hematological investigation showed the presence of anemia. Biopsy specimen of papules from lower labial mucosa, buccal mucosa, and gingiva showed hyperplastic stratified squamous epithelium with mild inflammatory evidence in the connective tissue suggestive of nonspecific epithelial hyperplasia.

## 4. Treatment and Management

Surgical excision of the lesions present on the right and left retrocommisural areas, the lower labial lesions, and gingivectomy with surgical contouring of the lower anterior gingiva was performed for esthetic reasons.

Owing to the increased risk of these patients to the benign and malignant thyroid diseases and breast and gastrointestinal cancers, thyroid ultrasonography and thyroid function tests and endoscopy for gastric polyps were performed in this patient. The tests revealed no abnormality. The patient was then referred to a gynaecologist for appropriate screening to rule out malignancies of the endometrium and breast. Mammography was performed. No evidence of malignancy was found from the above tests.

It was decided to follow up the patient closely to monitor the lesions as well as to perform continued cancer surveillance.

## 5. Discussion

Cowden's syndrome is a rare multiple hamartoma disorder [7]. This syndrome is one of a group of heterogeneous disorders known collectively as the *PTEN* hamartoma tumor syndrome (PHTS). Affected individuals usually develop clinical features by their second decade of life [8]; however, there is a considerable heterogeneity in clinical presentation.

Cowden's syndrome is clinically characterised by multiple mucocutaneous hamartomatous lesions and neoplasias of the breast, thyroid gland, and gastrointestinal tract [2, 9]. Mucocutaneous lesions include flesh-colored flat-topped cutaneous facial papules ranging from 1 to 5 mm in diameter, most of which are trichilemmomas. Multiple oral papules are present on gingival, labial, and palatal surfaces of oral cavity. They measure around 1 to 3 mm, and they coalesce to give a cobblestone appearance to the mucosae. Palmoplantar keratosis is another type of mucocutaneous lesions observed in Cowden's syndrome [10]. Because the development of associated malignancy may take several years, these mucocutaneous lesions may serve as important clinical markers in identifying patients at high risk of malignancy of the breast and thyroid [6].

Women with Cowden's syndrome have a 30% to 50% risk for breast cancer. Therefore, women should carry out monthly self-examinations, and professional physical examinations should be performed once every three months. Mammography is suggested to be performed twice a year. Some authors have recommended prophylactic bilateral mastectomy, particularly in women with an extensive fibrocystic breast disease or breast carcinoma [11, 12].

Thyroid should be examined for any abnormalities. Thyroid function tests and ultrasonography of the gland should be performed as baseline diagnostic examinations. Fine needle aspiration or surgical biopsies are indicated if any lesion is identified. In addition, complete blood cell count, liver and renal function tests can be performed at the baseline [2]. Other investigations which could be carried out are gastrointestinal endoscopy, endometrial examination, radionuclide scans to detect any malignancies, molecular genetic analysis for phosphatase and tensin homolog (*PTEN*), and immunohistochemical staining for PTEN.

Treatment for Cowden's syndrome is only cosmetic. The facial papules can be treated physically by $CO_2$-laser ablation, surgical removal, or chemically removed by topical 5-fluorouracil. Systemic therapy with acitretin 0.75 mg/kg/day has been reported to give good cosmetic results for all mucocutaneous lesions [13]. Surgical management of the mucocutaneous lesions includes cryosurgery, electrosurgery, dermabrasion, and laser abrasion.

## 6. Conclusion

Perhaps, the oral lesions could be the only sign of this disease. Hence, the identification of these lesions will help in early recognition of Cowden's syndrome which may in turn facilitate the early diagnosis of cancer. Hence, frequent follow-ups and continued cancer surveillance is vital for long-term survival of these patients.

## Conflict of Interests

The authors declare that there is no conflict of interests.

## Authors' Contributions

Prashanthi Chippagiri contributed by diagnosing the case, advising various investigations, and drafting and critically evaluating the article. Spoorthi Banavar Ravi contributed by conducting a histopathological examination and drafting and critically evaluating the article. Neha Patwa is the first to examine the case and referred the case for diagnosis.

## References

[1] O. S. Salem and W. D. Steck, "Cowden's disease (multiple hamartoma and neoplasia syndrome). A case report and review of the English literature," *Journal of the American Academy of Dermatology*, vol. 8, no. 5, pp. 686–696, 1983.

[2] J. C. Leão, V. Batista, P. B. Guimarães, J. Belo, and S. R. Porter, "Cowden's syndrome affecting the mouth, gastrointestinal, and central nervous system: a case report and review of the literature," *Oral Surgery, Oral Medicine, Oral Pathology, Oral Radiology and Endodontology*, vol. 99, no. 5, pp. 569–572, 2005.

[3] K. M. Lloyd and M. Dennis, "Cowden's disease. A possible new symptom complex with multiple system involvement," *Annals of Internal Medicine*, vol. 58, pp. 136–142, 1963.

[4] P. E. Weary, R. J. Gorlin, W. C. Gentry Jr., J. E. Comer, and K. E. Greer, "Multiple hamartoma syndrome (Cowden's disease)," *Archives of Dermatology*, vol. 106, no. 5, pp. 682–690, 1972.

[5] Y. Takenoshite, S. Kubo, T. Takenchi, and M. Lida, "Oral and facial lesions in Cowden syndrome," *Journal of Oral and Maxillofacial Surgery*, vol. 57, no. 6, pp. 682–687, 1993.

[6] K. Al-Thihli, L. Palma, V. Marcus et al., "A case of Cowden's syndrome presenting with gastric carcinomas and gastrointestinal polyposis," *Nature Clinical Practice Gastroenterology and Hepatology*, vol. 6, no. 3, pp. 184–189, 2009.

[7] C. Eng, "PTEN: one gene, many syndromes," *Human Mutation*, vol. 22, no. 3, pp. 183–198, 2003.

[8] C. Eng, "Will the real Cowden syndrome please stand up: revised diagnostic criteria," *Journal of Medical Genetics*, vol. 37, no. 11, pp. 828–830, 2000.

[9] S. I. Chaudhry, P. J. Shirlaw, P. R. Morgan, and S. J. Challacombe, "Cowden's syndrome (multiple hamartoma and neoplasia syndrome): diagnostic dilemmas three cases," *Oral Diseases*, vol. 6, no. 4, pp. 248–252, 2000.

[10] S. M. Ravi Prakash, G. N. Suma, and S. Goel, "Cowden syndrome," *Indian Journal of Dental Research*, vol. 21, no. 3, pp. 439–442, 2010.

[11] W. Williard, P. Borgen, R. Bol, R. Tiwari, and M. Osborne, "Cowden's disease. A case report with analyses at the molecular level," *Cancer*, vol. 69, no. 12, pp. 2969–2974, 1992.

[12] M. H. Brownstein, M. Wolf, and J. B. Bikowski, "Cowden's disease. A cutaneous marker of breast cancer," *Cancer*, vol. 41, no. 6, pp. 2393–2398, 1978.

[13] F. R. Cnudde, F. Boulard, P. Muller, J. Chevallier, and B. Teron-Abou, "Cowden's disease treated with acitretine," *Annales de Dermatologie et de Venereologie*, vol. 123, no. 11, pp. 739–741, 1996.

# 7

# Laser-Assisted Periodontal Management of Drug-Induced Gingival Overgrowth under General Anesthesia: A Viable Option

**Tupili Muralikrishna,[1] Butchibabu Kalakonda,[1] Sumanth Gunupati,[2] and Pradeep Koppolu[1]**

[1] *Department of Periodontics, Sri Sai College of Dental Surgery, Kothrepally, Vikarabad, Andhra Pradesh 501101, India*
[2] *Department of Periodontics, Narayana Dental College and Hospital, Chinthareddypalem, Nellore, Andhra Pradesh 524003, India*

Correspondence should be addressed to Butchibabu Kalakonda; docbutchi@gmail.com

Academic Editors: A. Epivatianos and T. Hata

Gingival overgrowth/hyperplasia can be attributed to several causes, but drug-induced gingival overgrowth/hyperplasia arises secondarily to prolonged use of antihypertensive drugs, anticonvulsants and immunosuppressants. The management is complex in nature considering the multitude of factors involved such as substitution of drug strict plaque control along with excision of the tissue to be performed under local anesthesia as outpatient. In the recent times, the patient's psychological fear of the treatment with the use of surgical blade and multiple visits has developed the concept of single visit treatment under general anesthesia incorporating a laser as viable option. The present case highlights the new method of management of gingival overgrowth.

## 1. Introduction

Different types of periodontal therapy, both surgical and nonsurgical, have been attempted to either reduce or eliminate pockets associated with drug-induced gingival overgrowth (DIGO). Surgical treatment proved to be the decisive therapy of DIGO. Many of the surgical approaches such as gingivectomy and flap surgery are carried out under local anesthesia but certain cases warrant treatment under general anesthesia. The present case report illustrates management of DIGO under general anesthesia. The management consists of oral hygiene procedures, drug substitution, and a surgical gingivectomy.

## 2. Case Description

A 55-year-old female patient presented to our hospital for evaluation of painless gingival overgrowth in both the upper and lower jaws which is posing her masticatory problems. Patient's medical history revealed that she was hypertensive and was on amlodipine 10 mg once daily for the past 4 years. Intraoral examination revealed generalized diffuse gingival enlargement, fibrotic in nature covering more than 2/3 rd of the crowns with minimal inflammation (Figure 1).

Initial treatment consisting essentially of supragingival scaling was done, and the patient was advised on proper plaque control. The treating physician was consulted for a change in the medication regimen. The physician promptly obliged and put the patient on an alternate regimen of losartan. The review after one week revealed some reduction of the inflammatory component in the lower arch. The clinical diagnosis was suggestive of DIGO. To confirm the diagnosis by histopathological means, a laser-assisted biopsy was suggested. To allay patient's fear about needle and injections, a decision was made to remove the gingival overgrowth for biopsy with a laser.

After appropriate eye protection wear was used, a topical anesthetic gel was applied for 2-3 min. Nd:YAG laser (AT Fidelis, Fotona, Germany) was used with a 300 $\mu$m fiber at 2.75 watts to dissect the overgrowth from its periphery (Figure 2). These laser settings were ideally chosen because peak power was required to penetrate the thick gingiva (Figure 3). The excised tissue was sent for histopathological examination (Figure 4). There was absolutely no bleeding;

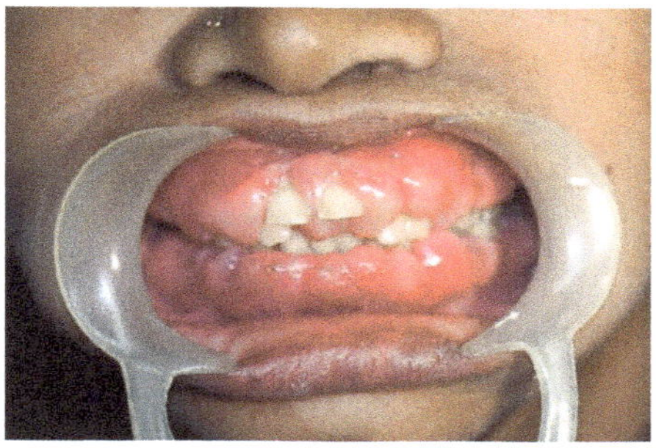

FIGURE 1: Intraoral photograph of amlodipine-induced gingival overgrowth.

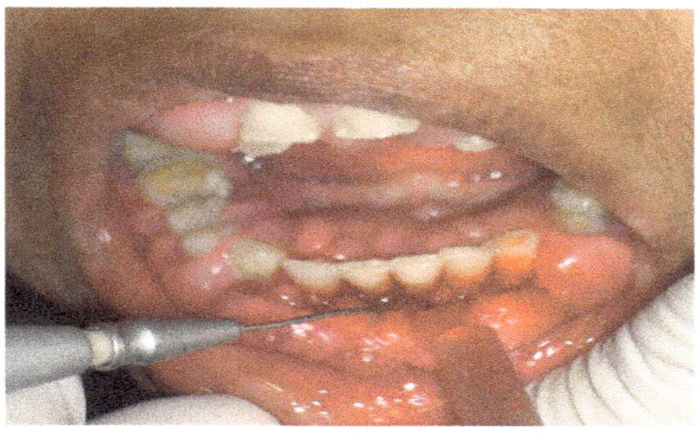

FIGURE 2: Excision of the enlargement for biopsy with a Nd:YAG laser.

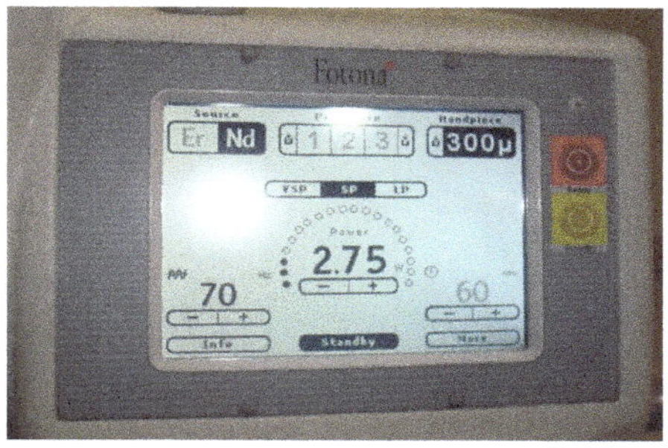


FIGURE 3: Laser settings for excision of the tissue.

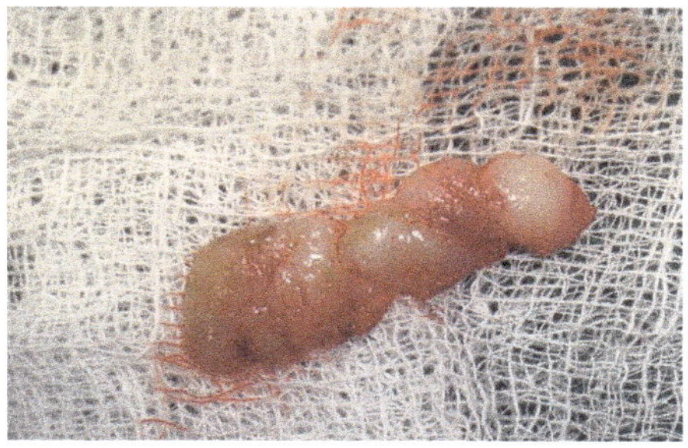

FIGURE 4: Excised specimen sent for histopathological examination.

the patient was comfortable throughout the procedure and was happy that sutures were not necessary.

The histopathological examination on staining the tissue with Hematoxylin and Eosin (H&E) showed hyperkeratotic stratified squamous epithelium with proliferating rete ridges, connective tissue showing abundant plump, and proliferating fibroblasts that are spindle shaped forming a network. Few endothelial lined blood vessels are also observed, suggestive of fibrous gingival hyperplasia (Figure 5).

Considering the cumbersome task of managing a massive gingival enlargement coupled with uncooperative and apprehensive nature of the patient, we decided to perform the surgery under general anesthesia.

Fitness for surgery under general anesthesia was approved by the patient's physician and the anesthetist, and the patient was instructed to report to our hospital a day before the surgery. The patient was thoroughly informed about the surgical procedure, and consent was taken. Preanesthetic medication was given.

Supplemental anesthesia, that is, local infiltration with 2% lidocaine with adrenaline (1 : 100000), was given to minimize bleeding during surgery. External bevel gingivectomy was carried out in both maxillary and mandibular arches using Bard Parker blades nos. 11 and 15. Excised tissue was removed using Gracey curettes and gingivectomy knives (Kirkland and Orban) (Figure 6). Laser was used to recontour the gingiva and aid in hemostasis.

After recovery from general anesthesia, a periodontal dressing Coe-Pack (GC International Inc., Newport Pagnell, UK) was given (Figure 7). The patient was kept under observation aftersurgery and was discharged 3 days after the procedure. There were no postoperative complications, and healing was uneventful (Figure 8). At the most recent followup, after the procedure, no recurrence of the hyperplasia was found.

## 3. Discussion

Fear, inability to cooperate, and trauma associated with injections are the most frequent indications which necessitate the option of general anesthesia. There are hardly few case reports where periodontal surgery was carried out under general anesthesia [1].

In our present case report, the patient underwent excision of her gingival overgrowth under local anesthesia previously and was unwilling to undergo the same procedure once again under local anesthesia as the last surgical procedure left the patient traumatized and made her apprehensive to undergo any further dental treatment. Hence periodontal management under general anesthesia was the viable option considering the massive gingival overgrowth, patient's apprehensive nature, and her medical status.

Many studies emphasize the association between oral hygiene status and the severity of DIGO [2, 3]. Hence this clearly suggests that the degree or severity of gingival enlargement is commensurate with plaque-induced gingival inflammation. In the present case report also the patient's poor plaque control coupled with the massive gingival overgrowth made oral hygiene maintenance a nightmare. There was mild reduction in the inflammatory component of the gingival overgrowth in the upper arch after scaling. Hence the key to manage the DIGO lies in good oral hygiene and patient's compliance.

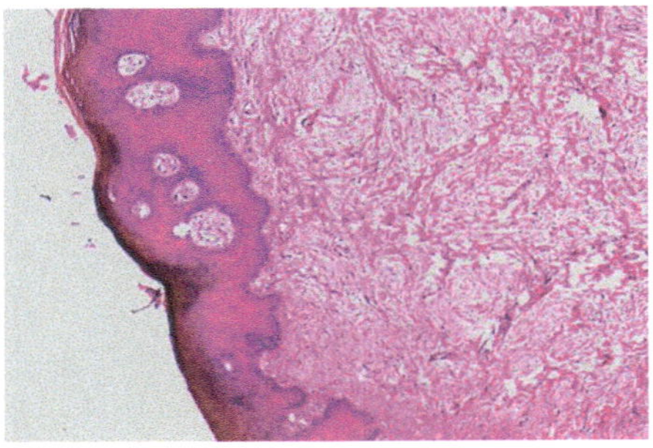

FIGURE 5: Histopathological view of the excised specimen shows stratified squamous epithelium with proliferating rete ridges; connective tissue showing abundant plump and proliferating fibroblasts that are spindle shaped forming a network. Few endothelial lined blood vessels are also observed (H&E, 10x).

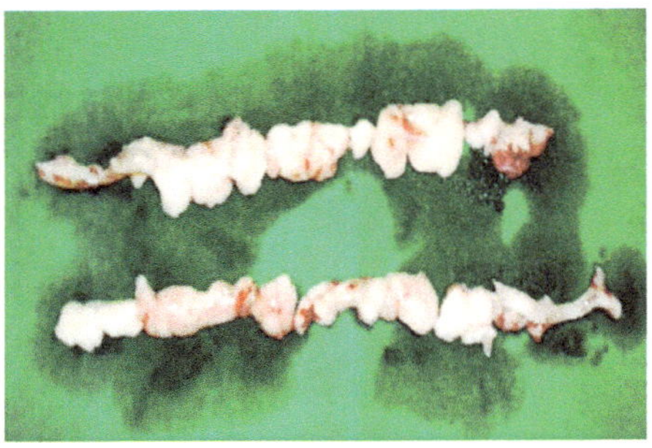

FIGURE 6: Excised tissue after gingivectomy.

Calcium channel blockers are known to cause gingival overgrowth. The prevalence of amlodipine-induced gingival overgrowth was 3.3%, half of nifedipine, that is, 6.3% [3]. As a first line of treatment for reduction of gingival overgrowth and anticipating recurrence after surgery, drug withdrawal or substitution was considered.

Amlodipine was substituted to Losartan 50 mg once daily as per the patient's physician. Patient followup was done for 3 months to notice any advantage of change in medication that might have led to reduction in gingival overgrowth. But unfortunately only mild reduction of gingival overgrowth in the lower anterior teeth had prompted us to opt for a corrective surgery. Literature review and few case reports suggest reduction of gingival overgrowth within weeks to months after drug withdrawal [4, 5]. However, it is unfortunate that not many patients with longstanding gingival overgrowth respond to drug substitution alone [6, 7].

Performing periodontal surgery under general anesthesia involves some amount of risk. Careful selection of patients is mandatory to ensure that the treatment is successful. We have taken into consideration the patient selection criteria given by the American Society of Anesthesiologist (ASA) physical status classification [8]. According to the abovementioned classification, the patient in this present case report was given an ASA class 2 category since she is a wellcontrolled hypertensive patient with blood pressure reading of 140/90 mm Hg.

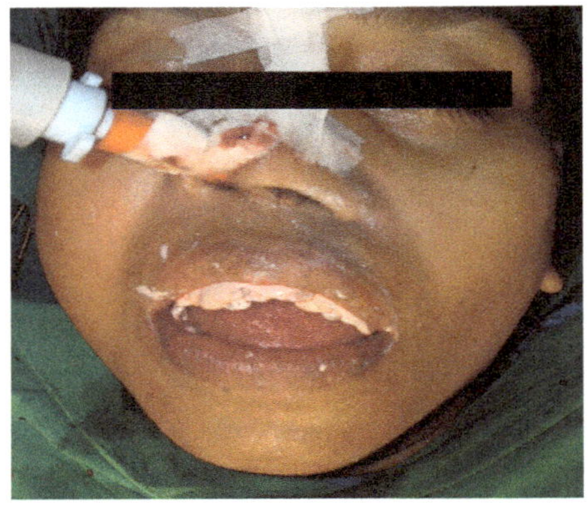

FIGURE 7: Patient at the end of the surgery and after the pack placement.

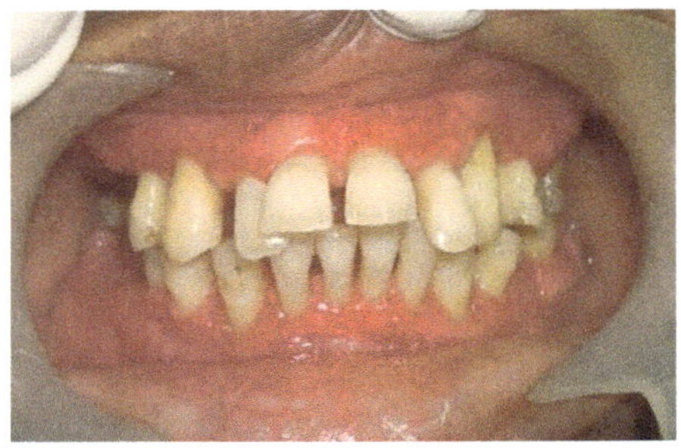

FIGURE 8: Postoperative view depicting uneventful healing.

Preoperative screening was done and a detailed medical history was taken. Thorough evaluation of the patient's respiratory, renal, and cardiovascular systems was done with assessment of blood pressure. The treatment plan for this case is essentially comprised of an external bevel gingivectomy under general anesthesia supplemented by the use of laser to recontour the tissue and aid in hemostasis.

Gingivectomy was considered as the first treatment of choice for DIGO [6]. Various other modalities of treatment for the management of DIGO comprise electrosurgery [9], laser gingivectomy [10], and flap surgery [11]. Considering the massive gingival overgrowth and the operational difficulties such as suturing associated with flap surgery, we considered external bevel gingivectomy as the final option. Also taking into consideration the esthetic outcomes, comparing both flap surgery and scalpel gingivectomy, those treated by the latter method appeared to have a "smoother" gingival surface than when treated with flap procedure [12].

The recovery of the patient after surgery was uneventful. Patient was evaluated for any post surgical bleeding. There are a few studies on recurrence rates after a scalpel gingivectomy but in this present case report, patient followup after 3 months showed no signs of recurrence.

## 4. Conclusion

Periodontal surgery under general anesthesia offers an attractive alternative for patients who are apprehensive or traumatized by earlier dental treatments. General anesthesia could be the preferred option in managing cases with massive gingival enlargements which would otherwise require multiple visits under local anesthesia. But it is imperative for the periodontist to have a sound knowledge before recommending patients to undergo surgical procedures under general anesthesia.

## References

[1] N. Ambalavanan, Vanaja, and U. Arunmozhi, "Hospital periodontal surgery," *Indian Journal of Dental Research*, vol. 16, no. 3, pp. 122–125, 2005.

[2] M. Nakou, J. J. Kamma, A. Andronikaki, and F. Mitsis, "Subgingival microflora associated with nifedipine-induced gingival overgrowth," *Journal of Periodontology*, vol. 69, no. 6, pp. 664–669, 1998.

[3] J. S. Ellis, R. A. Seymour, J. G. Steele, P. Robertson, T. J. Butler, and J. M. Thomason, "Prevalence of gingival overgrowth induced by calcium channel blockers: a community-based study," *Journal of Periodontology*, vol. 70, no. 1, pp. 63–67, 1999.

[4] P. G. Raman, V. N. Mishra, and D. Singh, "Nifedipine induced gingival hyperplasia," *The Journal of the Association of Physicians of India*, vol. 36, no. 3, pp. 231–233, 1988.

[5] A. Khocht and L. C. Schneider, "Periodontal management of gingival overgrowth in the heart transplant patient: a case report," *Journal of Periodontology*, vol. 68, no. 11, pp. 1140–1146, 1997.

[6] R. I. Marshall and P. M. Bartold, "A clinical review of drug-induced gingival overgrowths," *Australian Dental Journal*, vol. 44, no. 4, pp. 219–232, 1999.

[7] J. S. Ellis, R. A. Seymour, J. J. Taylor, and J. M. Thomason, "Prevalence of gingival overgrowth in transplant patients immunosuppressed with tacrolimus," *Journal of Clinical Periodontology*, vol. 31, no. 2, pp. 126–131, 2004.

[8] American Society of Anesthesiologists, "Physical Status Classification," July 2009, http://www.asahq.org/clinical/physicalstatus.htm.

[9] C. R. Walker Jr., C. E. Tomich, and C. E. Hutton, "Treatment of phenytoin-induced gingival hyperplasia by electrosurgery," *Journal of Oral Surgery*, vol. 38, no. 4, pp. 306–311, 1980.

[10] S. Barak and I. Kaplan, "The CO2 laser in the excision of gingival hyperplasia caused by nifedipine," *Journal of Clinical Periodontology*, vol. 15, no. 10, pp. 633–635, 1988.

[11] M. Mavrogiannis, J. S. Ellis, R. A. Seymour, and J. M. Thomason, "The efficacy of three different surgical techniques in the management of drug-induced gingival overgrowth," *Journal of Clinical Periodontology*, vol. 33, no. 9, pp. 677–682, 2006.

[12] A. Pilloni, P. M. Camargo, M. Carere, and F. A. Carranza, "Surgical treatment of cyclosporine A- and nifedipine-induced gingival enlargement: gingivectomy versus periodontal flap," *Journal of Periodontology*, vol. 69, no. 7, pp. 791–797, 1998.

# 8

# An Erupted Dilated Odontoma: A Rare Presentation

**Gaurav Sharma,[1] Amritpreet Nagra,[2] Gurkeerat Singh,[3] Archna Nagpal,[4] Atul Soin,[5] and Vishal Bhardwaj[3]**

[1] *Department of Oral Medicine and Radiology, Sudha Rustagi College of Dental Sciences and Research, Faridabad, Haryana 121002, India*
[2] *Ahead Academy, Rajinder Nagar, New Delhi 11060, India*
[3] *Department of Orthodontics, Sudha Rustagi College of Dental Sciences and Research, Faridabad, Haryana 121002, India*
[4] *Department of Oral Medicine and Radiology, PDM Dental College and Research Institute, Bahadurgarh, Haryana 124507, India*
[5] *Department of Prosthodontics, Kalka Dental College, Meerut 250006, India*

Correspondence should be addressed to Gaurav Sharma; drgaurav7479@rediffmail.com

Academic Editor: Jamil A. Shibli

A dilated odontoma is an extremely rare developmental anomaly represented as a dilatation of the crown and root as a consequence of a deep, enamel-lined invagination and is considered a severe variant of dens invaginatus. An oval shape of the tooth lacking morphological characteristics of a crown or root implies that the invagination happened in the initial stages of morphodifferentiation. Spontaneous eruption of an odontoma is a rare occurrence and the occurrence of a dilated odontoma in a supernumerary tooth is even rarer with only a few case reports documented in the English literature. We present an extremely rare case of erupted dilated odontoma occurring in the supernumerary tooth in anterior maxillary region in an 18-year-old male, which, to the best of our knowledge, is the first ever case reported in English literature.

## 1. Introduction

A dilated odontoma is an extremely rare developmental anomaly that is represented as a dilatation of the crown and root as a consequence of a deep, enamel-lined invagination and is considered a severe variation of dens invaginatus [1]. Proposed theories for origin of dilated odontoma comprise focal growth retardation theory, restricted external pressure, and focal growth stimulation in selected parts of the tooth bud [2]. Dilated odontoma originates during the morphodifferentiation stage of tooth bud formation, but its precise aetiology and genesis are unidentified [2]. Genetic factors have also been implicated as a probable factor for occurrence of dilated odontoma [2]. A dilated odontoma is however not delineated as a separate entity in the existing classification of odontogenic tumors [1]. A tooth with dilated odontoma has a circular or oval shape with a radiolucent interior and presents a single structure, often with a central soft tissue mass [3]. A dilated odontoma in the supernumerary tooth is rare and only a few cases have been reported in the recent literature [1–4]. Spontaneous eruption of an odontoma is a rare occurrence and the occurrence of a dilated odontoma in a supernumerary tooth is even rarer. We present an extremely rare case of erupted dilated odontoma occurring in the supernumerary tooth in anterior maxillary region in an 18-year-old male, which, to the best of our knowledge, is the first ever case reported in English literature.

## 2. Case Report

An 18-year-old male presented to department of oral medicine and radiology with the chief complaint of malformed tooth in his upper front region. The patient was apparently healthy and there was no history of medical or family problem. There was no previous history of trauma to the teeth or jaws. An intraoral clinical examination revealed an anomalous tooth present in area of left maxillary central incisor (Figure 1). There was mild pain which was intermittent but no swelling or mobility was observed. The tooth

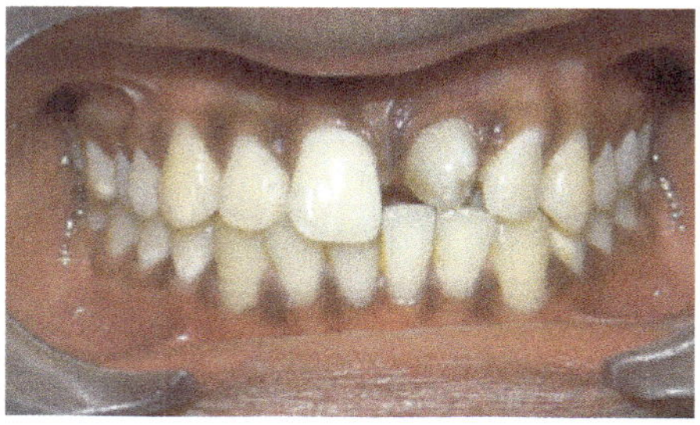

FIGURE 1: Intraoral clinical photograph depicting anomalous maxillary central incisor (frontal view).

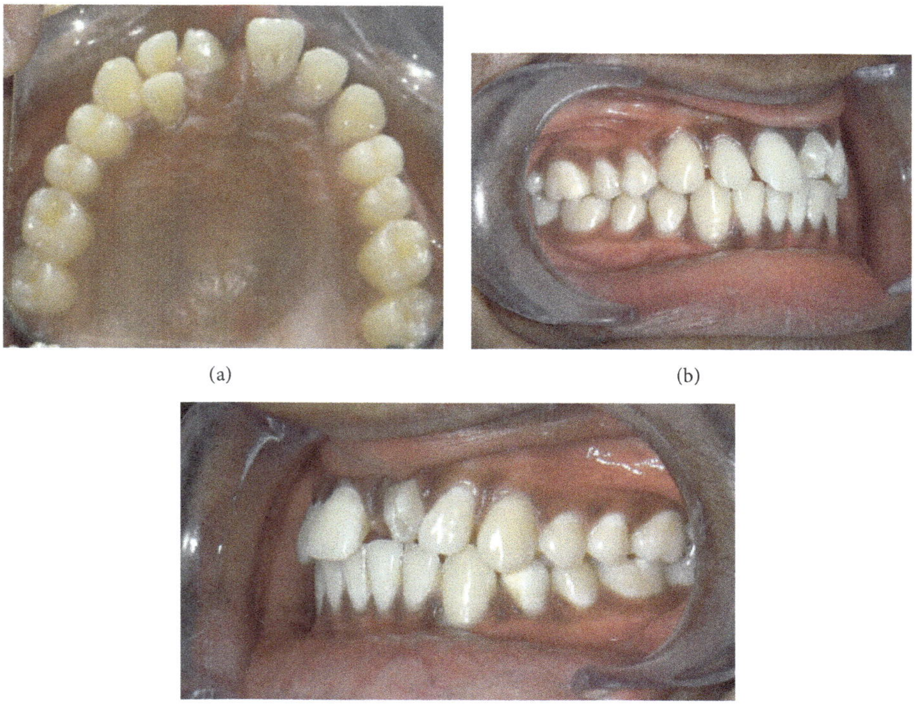

(a) (b) (c)

FIGURE 2: Clinical photographs of erupted dilated odontoma: (a) occlusal view, (b) right lateral view, and (c) left lateral view.

did not respond to an electric pulp test and was tender on percussion. A supernumerary tooth was observed palatally in relation to permanent maxillary lateral incisor region (Figure 2(a)). The patient was advised intraoral periapical radiograph that revealed the presence of impacted permanent maxillary left central incisor (Figure 3(a)). The supernumerary tooth showed an oval radiolucent interior delineated by a well-defined radiopaque border. Patient was advised anterior maxillary occlusal radiograph that showed periapical changes in relation to anomalous supernumerary tooth (Figure 3(b)). The panoramic radiograph further confirmed the presence of impacted maxillary central incisor and supernumerary teeth in anterior maxillary region (Figure 4). Cone beam computerized tomography (CBCT) confirmed the presence of dilated odontoma (Figures 5 and 6). Based on the clinical and radiographic findings, the patient was diagnosed with dilated invaginated odontoma in supernumerary tooth in anterior maxillary region associated with periapical pathology. The diagnosis of supernumerary tooth in palatal region and impacted permanent maxillary central incisor was also done. The supernumerary tooth was subsequently extracted under local anaesthesia with written informed consent from the patient.

Impacted central incisor was surgically exposed using a full thickness mucoperiosteal flap and an attachment was bonded along with looped ligature wire on the labial surface of tooth. Flap was repositioned and a closed eruption was induced by orthodontic traction with a mild force of 60 gm, using elastomeric module. Subsequently, maxillary and mandibular arches were bonded using fixed appliance with $0.022'' \times 0.028''$ slot. Leveling of both arches was continued with sequential arch wires and space was maintained for the central incisor (Figures 7 and 8).

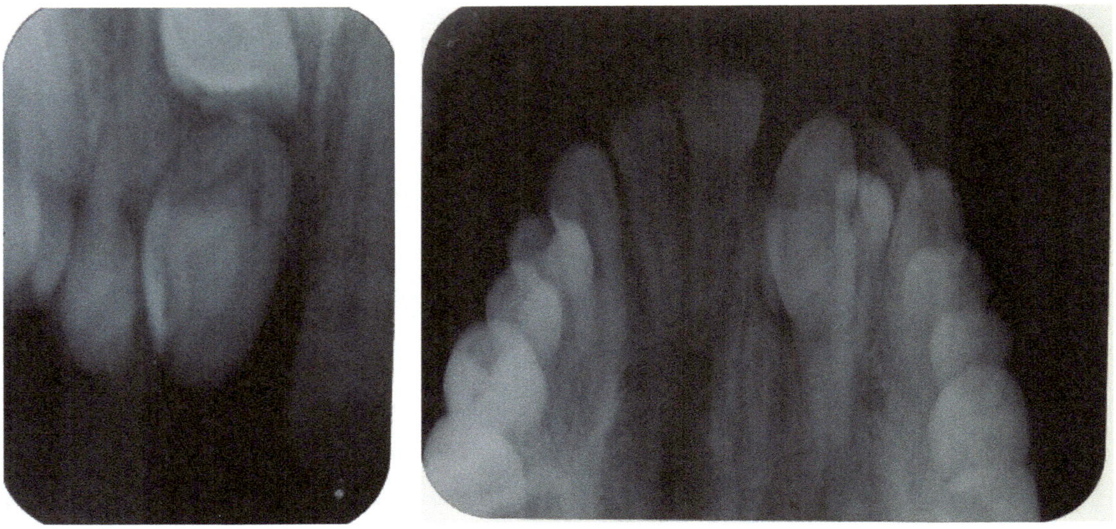

(a) (b)

FIGURE 3: (a) Intraoral periapical radiograph and (b) anterior maxillary occlusal radiograph showing an erupted dilated odontoma with impacted central incisor.

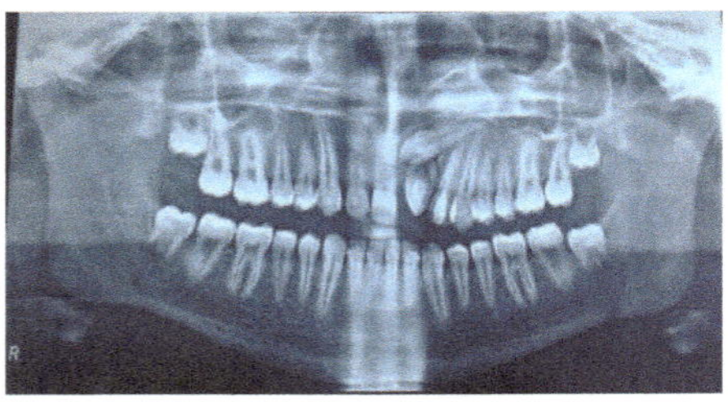

FIGURE 4: Panoramic radiograph showing erupted dilated odontoma and supernumerary incisor with impacted maxillary central incisor.

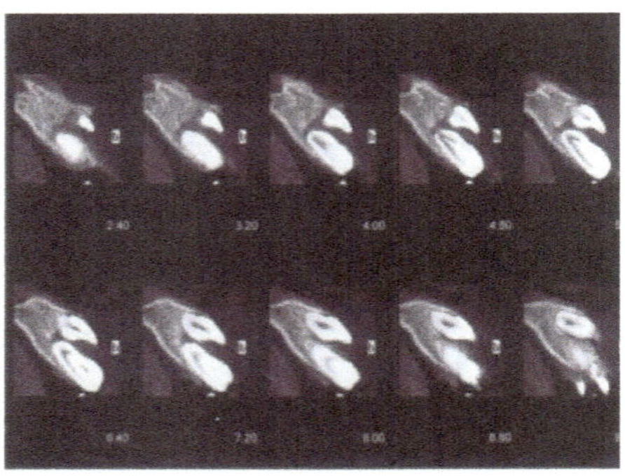

FIGURE 5: Cone beam computer imaging (CBCT) of lateral view depicting dilated odontoma.

After a period of seven months, the impacted central incisor was brought closure to the main arch; then a bracket was bonded on the labial surface of tooth and subsequently the tooth was brought into alignment with 0.012″ NiTi as piggyback on 0.018″ SS base arch wire. The tooth erupted and was guided into occlusion. The patient is still on follow-up (Figure 9).

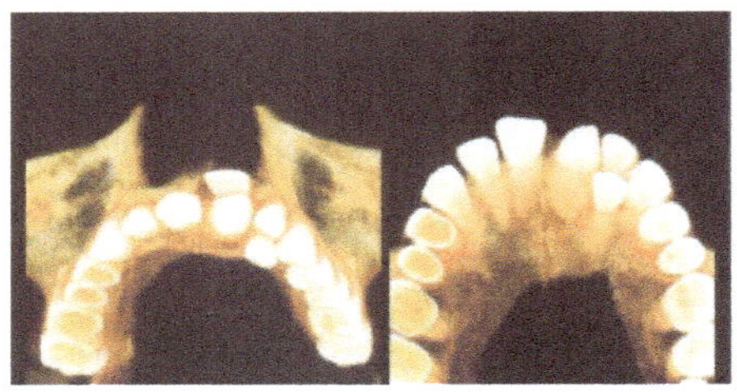

FIGURE 6: CBCT three-dimensional occlusal views depicting dilated odontoma and impacted central incisor.

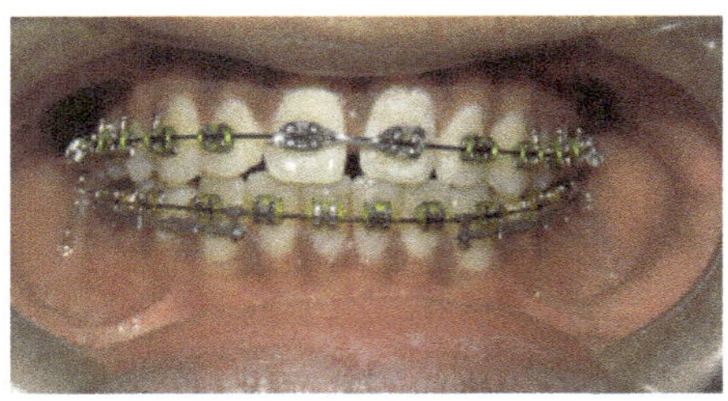

FIGURE 7: Intraoral clinical photograph (orthodontic treatment) depicting maxillary central incisor.

## 3. Discussion

Morphological variations in dental structures involving either the crown or root have often been reported in literature and asymptomatic characteristic nature being identified only on routine radiographs. Dilated odontoma is clinically significant as there is a possibility of the early involvement of pulp [3]. An oval shape of the tooth lacking morphological characteristics of a crown or root implies that the invagination happened in the initial stages of morphodifferentiation [1]. Dens invaginatus represents a rare form of

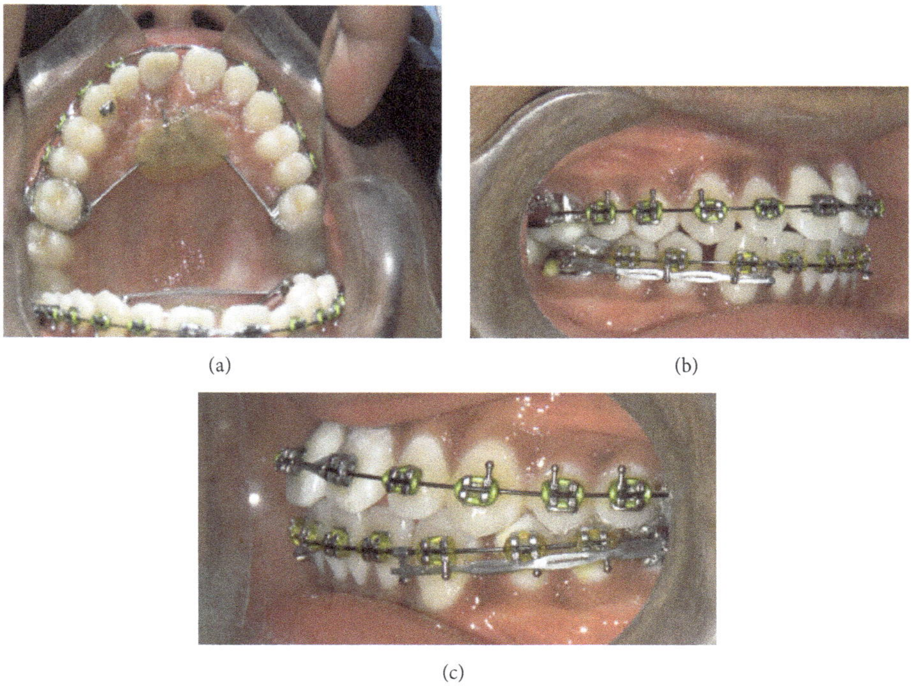

FIGURE 8: Clinical photographs of maxillary central incisor: (a) occlusal view, (b) right lateral view, and (c) left lateral view.

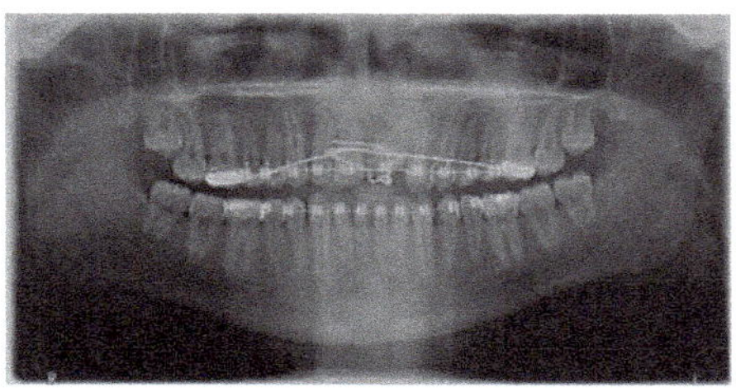

FIGURE 9: Follow-up panoramic radiograph depicting erupted maxillary central incisor.

developmental anomaly with a prevalence of 0.04% with a greater female predilection [3]. The most frequently affected tooth is the maxillary lateral incisors, followed by maxillary central incisors, premolars, canines, and molars [1]. Compound odontomas have radiographic appearances reaching from solitary to multiple small tooth-like denticles in which enamel, dentin, and pulpal tissues are prearranged in a systematized pattern [5]. The most common site of compound odontoma is the anterior maxilla, characteristically over or between the roots of the erupted teeth. Though odontomas are seen frequently and constitute 22% of all odontogenic tumors, erupted odontomas are rare [5]. In the present case, the differential diagnosis of compound odontomas was excluded as they typically present with multiple rudimentary tooth-like structures.

A dilated odontoma has been described as extremely rare type of dens invaginatus [1]. Dilated odontoma is the most advanced condition of density in a tooth due to infolding of the outer tooth surface [5]. This can occur in either the crown or the root during tooth development and may involve the pulp chamber or root canal and lead to the deformity of either the crown or the root [5]. The shape is usually irregular, but the dilated varieties are often well-defined, corticated, round, or oval masses with radiolucent centres. In our case, the patient presented with a deformed crown with an oval shaped radiolucency suggestive of dilated odontoma.

Coronal dens invaginatus has been categorized in 3 groups by Oehlers based on radiographic interpretation according to the degree of invagination. In type I Oehlers classification the enamel lined invagination ends as a blind sac within the crown and is not ranging beyond the cement-enamel junction (CEJ). Type II Oehlers classification represents the enamel-lined invagination extending apically beyond the CEJ but persists within the root. In rare type III Oehlers classification, the enamel-lined invagination extends apically beyond the CEJ and communicates laterally with the periodontal ligament space with no involvement of the pulp [1].

The possibility of the erupted tooth being supernumerary was considered in the current case as the impacted tooth was anatomically similar to the permanent central incisor on a radiographic examination. The above case is unique as the patient also had hyperdontia and there was the presence of a dilated odontoma in an erupted tooth in anterior maxillary region. However, there is no description of an erupted dilated odontoma [6, 7]. Most of dilated odontoma cases have been reported from the posterior mandibular areas and have been impacted frequently. Recently a case report of the occurrence of bilateral odontomas in anterior maxillary teeth with hypodontia and peg laterals was observed [8]. In our case there was a triad of dilated odontoma, supernumerary supplemental incisor, and impacted maxillary central incisor. The authors suggest that the dilated odontomas in concurrence with other dental anomalies should be further investigated for a genetic analysis as it might represent a chromosomal trait.

The association of dens invaginatus with supernumerary tooth is a very rare phenomenon. Extensive PubMed search revealed that only six case reports have been published in English literature till now [9]. However all the cases were of dens invaginatus of milder variety and none of the cases had documented the occurrence of dilated odontoma in a supernumerary tooth. To the best of the authors' knowledge, the present case represents the first case report of an erupted dilated odontoma in a supernumerary tooth. The occurrence of supplemental maxillary incisors is much less common than conical or tuberculate supernumerary teeth. Supplementary maxillary lateral incisor is however more commonly observed as compared to a supplemental maxillary central incisor [8]. In the present case, a supplemental maxillary central incisor was observed palatally. Chronic inflammation at the apical region of the dens invaginatus can lead to a condition called periapical invaginitis [10]. The invagination repeatedly leads to the access of irritants promptly into the pulpal chamber due to a thin permeable membrane [3].

In case of an exceedingly unusual anatomy such as the current case, surgical or endodontic management is not practicable, and extraction is favoured as a last choice of treatment [9]. Amalgamating additional imaging modalities with a comprehensive clinical examination and history is required to achieve an adequate diagnosis and for subsequent management [11]. Extraction was considered in our case in order to facilitate the eruption of the permanent maxillary central incisor in conjunction with orthodontic management. A multidisciplinary approach comprising an oral radiologist, oral maxillofacial surgeon, and orthodontist should be the treatment of choice for these rare morphological variations as an early diagnosis and treatment are very important to prevent physiological, aesthetic, and functional problems.

## Conflict of Interests

The authors declare that they have no conflict of interests regarding the publication of this paper.

## References

[1] Y. Matsusue, K. Yamamoto, K. Inagake, and T. Kirita, "A dilated odontoma in the second molar region of the mandible," *Open Dentistry Journal*, vol. 5, no. 1, pp. 150–153, 2011.

[2] I. Čuković-Bagić, D. Macan, J. Dumančić, S. Manojlović, and J. Hat, "Dilated odontome in the mandibular third molar region," *Oral Surgery, Oral Medicine, Oral Pathology, Oral Radiology and Endodontology*, vol. 109, no. 2, pp. e109–e113, 2010.

[3] R. Jaya, R. S. Mohan Kumar, and R. Srinivasan, "A rare case of dilated invaginated odontome with talon cusp in a permanent maxillary central incisor diagnosed by cone beam computed tomography," *Imaging Science in Dentistry*, vol. 43, no. 3, pp. 209–213, 2013.

[4] K. Yamamoto, Y. Morimoto, T. Kawakami, K. Mishima, H. Shiotani, and M. Sugimura, "A case of dilated odontoma arising in buccal region of 3rd molar tooth of mandible," *Journal of the Japanese Stomatological Society*, vol. 48, pp. 395–399, 1999.

[5] A. Mahmoodi, S. Shahidi, M. Houshyar, and M. Houshyar, "Bilateral cystic lesions associated to maxillary erupted dilated odontomas: a case report," *Journal of Dentistry, Shiraz University of Medical Sciences*, vol. 13, no. 2, pp. 85–89, 2012.

[6] G. Serra-Serra, L. Berini-Aytés, and C. Gay-Escoda, "Erupted odontomas: a report of three cases and review of the literature," *Medicina Oral, Patologia Oral y Cirugia Bucal*, vol. 14, no. 6, pp. E299–E303, 2009.

[7] F. Ide, Y. Ito, T. Muramatsu, I. Saito, and K. Mishima, "Erupted rootless type III dense in dente (dilated odontoma) masquerading as peripheral gingival pathosis," *Oral Surgery*, vol. 6, no. 3, pp. 155–158, 2013.

[8] A. Sebastian, A. Ahsan, A. J. George, and J. Aby, "An unusual triad: bilateral dilated odontoma, hypodontia and peg laterals," *Dental Research Journal*, vol. 10, no. 5, pp. 674–677, 2013.

[9] A. N. Sulabha and C. Sameer, "Association of mesiodentes and dens invaginatus in a child: a rare entity," *Case Reports in Dentistry*, vol. 2012, Article ID 198032, 4 pages, 2012.

[10] S. Kallianpur, U. S. Sudheendra, S. Kasetty, and P. Joshi, "Dens invaginatus (Type III)," *Journal of Oral and Maxillofacial Pathology*, vol. 16, no. 2, pp. 262–265, 2012.

[11] A. Z. Syed, A. Parachuru Venkata, and R. A. Mendes, "'Dilated odontoma': an incidental finding," *BMJ Case Reports*, 2015.

# Removal of a Maxillary Third Molar Displaced into Pterygopalatine Fossa via Intraoral Approach

**Nedim Özer,[1] Fulya Üçem,[2] Alp Saruhanoğlu,[2] Serdar Yilmaz,[1] and Hakkı Tanyeri[2]**

[1] *Department of Oral and Maxillofacial Surgery, Faculty of Dentistry, Istanbul Medipol University, Turkey*
[2] *Department of Oral and Maxillofacial Surgery, Faculty of Dentistry, Istanbul University, Istanbul, Turkey*

Correspondence should be addressed to Alp Saruhanoğlu; saruhanoglualp@yahoo.com

Academic Editors: A. Celebić and A. Markopoulos

The removal of impacted maxillary third molars is one of the most common procedures performed in oral and maxillofacial surgery units with low rates of complications and morbidity. A few cases of accidental displacement of third molars into adjacent anatomical spaces, such as the infratemporal fossa, the pterygomandibular space, the maxillary sinus, buccal space, or the lateral pharyngeal space, during surgical interventions have been reported. In this paper, a case of a maxillary third molar accidentally displaced into the pterygopalatine fossa is presented, and the removal of the tooth via intraoral approach is described.

## 1. Introduction

The removal of impacted maxillary third molars is one of the most common procedures performed in oral and maxillofacial surgery units with low rates of complications and morbidity [1–3]. Most frequently confronted complications are fracture of tuberosity, tooth root fracture, perforation of the maxillary sinus, prolapse of the buccal fat pad, and displacement of the roots or tooth into the maxillary sinus [3–5]. According to the literature, a few cases of accidental displacement of molars into adjacent anatomical spaces, such as the infratemporal fossa, the pterygomandibular space, the maxillary sinus, the buccal space, or the lateral pharyngeal space, during surgical interventions have been reported [3, 5, 6]. However this is the first reported case of maxillary third molar displaced into pterygopalatine fossa. The aim of this case report is to identify potential risk factors and to gather information on the prevention and treatment of this complication.

## 2. Case Report

A 23-year-old girl was referred to our clinic for the assessment of a maxillary left third molar displacement that occurred during surgery performed 1 week earlier. The patient had slight facial swelling and restricted mouth opening. Intraoral examination revealed that the dislodged third molar was not palpable within the soft tissues. Immediately, a panoramic radiograph was taken which revealed that the left maxillary third molar was displaced in a posterior direction possibly in the infratemporal fossa area (Figure 1). For being able to determine the precise position of the tooth, computed tomography (CT) scans were taken. CT revealed that the tooth was located superiorly between the distal margin of maxillary tuberosity and anterior border of lateral pterygoid plate; the root was placed in the antrum of pterygopalatine fossa (Figures 2 and 3). The general anesthesia was the surgeon's choice due to limited working area and patient's psychologic unease that may cause further displacement. The classical maxillary third molar surgery flap design was performed as vertical incision mesial to the first molar and horizontal incision extended to the distal margin of the maxillary tuberosity. Mucoperiosteal flap was reflected. Upon the reflection of the flap the pathway of the displaced third molar has been revealed as the posterior aspect of maxillary sinus area was open to site. Extending through the posterior wall of maxillary sinus and with careful exploring the tooth was reached and exposed with a straight elevator.

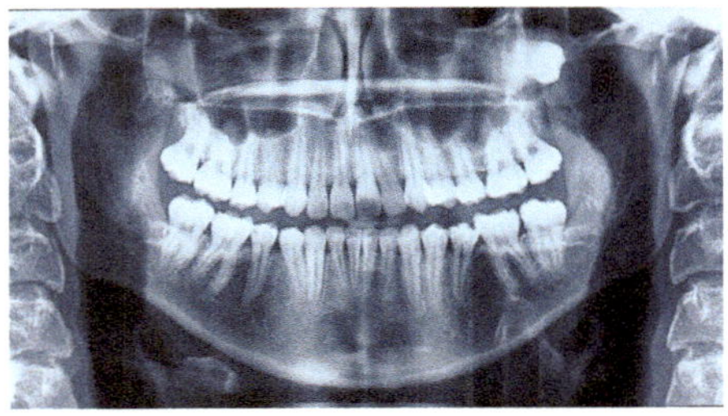

FIGURE 1: A panoramic radiograph revealed that the left maxillary third molar was displaced in a posterosuperior direction.

The granulation tissue around the tooth was removed and the tooth was extracted. Maxillary sinus and deep layers were irrigated with %0.5 saline solution and with Rifocin. The incision was primarily closed. No complication occurred postoperatively after 1 year of followup.

## 3. Discussion

Displacement of maxillary third molars into the neighbouring anatomic spaces is associated with insufficient clinical and radiographic examination, lack of basic principles of surgery such as poor anatomic knowledge, inadequate flap, decreased visibility, and excessive or uncontrolled force applied during extraction [3–6].

Maxillary third molars uncommonly displaced through the periosteum into the infratemporal fossa just adjacent to the lateral pterygoid plate and inferior to the lateral pterygoid muscle [7]. Excessive force application and incorrect use of elevator during the attempt to retrieve the tooth may further displace the tooth upward into the skull base carrying greater risks for morbidity [6, 7].

The access for the surgical removal of the tooth from pterygopalatine fossa is very difficult and has the potential for morbidity because it encloses vital anatomic structures. The pterygopalatine fossa is a complex anatomic structure which has the shape of an inverted cone [8]. It is located lateral to the nasal cavity, anterior/inferior to the middle cranial fossa, inferior to the apex of the orbit, and medial to the infratemporal fossa. The pterygopalatine fossa contains maxillary nerve (second branch of the trigeminal nerve), Vidian nerve, the pterygopalatine ganglion, and the third part of the maxillary artery [8].

Because the exact localization of the displaced tooth is impossible to determine clinically, radiographic examination is indicated [4, 7]. The superimposition of the anatomic structures located at the site of the infratemporal and pterygopalatine fossa may disorient the diagnosis in the case [3–5, 7]. So as to allow to determine the precise and detailed location of the dislodged tooth computed tomography examination is needed [3, 7].

The removal time of the displaced tooth is controversial in the literature [4]. Some authors propose to deliver the displaced tooth immediately because of the risks of infection, foreign body reaction and because of its anatomic location which can have the potential for morbidity [3, 7]. According to some authors, displaced teeth can migrate downwards into the oral cavity, allowing an easy surgical removal [4, 7]. Nonetheless according to others, migration of the tooth is impossible because of fibrosis and anatomical boundaries [3, 4, 7].

In our case, the patient had pain and restricted mouth opening. The cone beam volumetric tomography scan showed clearly that the displaced tooth was just barely stuck inside the pterygopalatine fossa. Because the pterygopalatine fossa encloses vital structures, further displacement could have potential symptoms associated with involvement of the neurovascular structures and pterygopalatine muscles, such as trismus, lateral pharyngeal swelling, hypoesthesia, proptosis, diplopia, pain, and nasal obstruction [9, 10]. Due to being dislodged into the pterygopalatine fossa area, immediate surgery was planned as the patient was referred to our clinic, so as to prevent damage and further complication risks.

Many surgical approaches have been used for the retrieval surgery of displaced maxillary third molar into the infratemporal fossa area such as long incision in the buccal sulcus, Gillies's approach, the Caldwell-Luc approach through the maxillary sinus after removal of the whole posterior wall, and resection of the coronoid process [1–3, 6].

In our case conservative method of surgery via intraoral approach was preferred due to the third molar location, being stuck in the antrum of pterygopalatine fossa. A long incision extending distal to the maxillary tuberosity and a blunt dissection behind the maxillary sinus wall were performed until reaching the tooth. To prevent further dislocation a retractor was placed distal area of the tooth. A soft pressure applied with an elevator, and the tooth was extracted.

As a result if a complication does occur during third molar extraction such in our case, dentists should immediately refer the patient to an oral and maxillofacial surgeon and should not try to remove the displaced root without proper assurance. This is imperative for being able to evaluate the condition of the tooth preoperatively, select adequate instruments and technique, and take good care during extraction and prevent the risk of hemorrhage, neurologic injury, and further displacement of the tooth. Localization with images and proper surgical methods are the keys to retrieving the displaced fragment successfully. There are no certain treatment choices whether immediate or secondary surgery is advantageous for the retrieval of such displaced teeth. The oral and maxillofacial surgeon decides uniquely evaluating the time the patient was referred, location of the

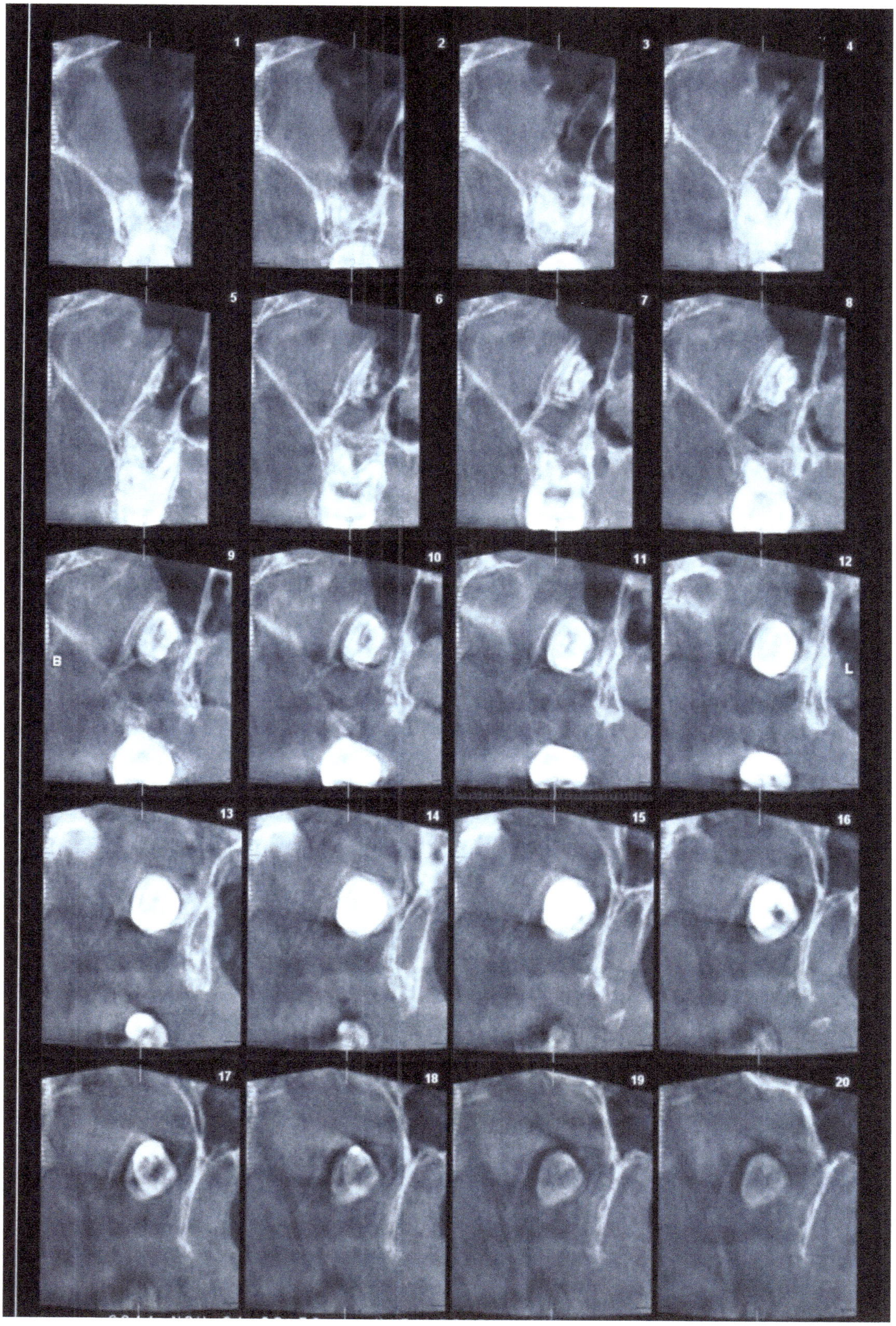


FIGURE 2: CT revealed that the tooth was located superiorly between the distal margin of maxillary tuberosity and the anterior border of lateral pterygoid plate.

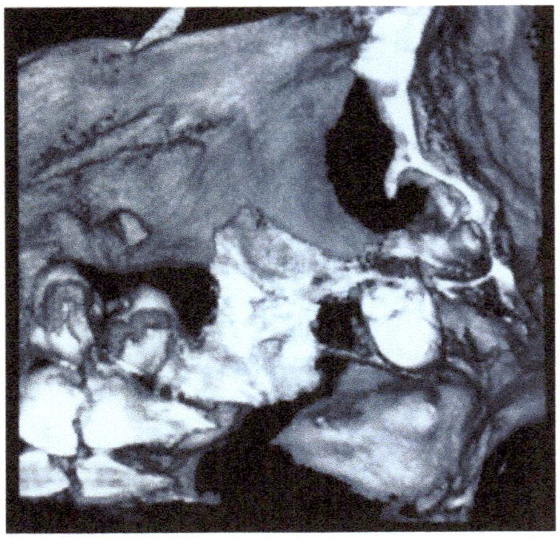

FIGURE 3: CT revealed that the root was stuck in the antrum of pterygopalatine fossa.

tooth, and the patient's psychological conditions all together for the most appropriate surgery approach.

## References

[1] S. R. Gulbrandsen, I. T. Jackson, and E. G. Turlington, "Recovery of a maxillary third molar from the infratemporal space via a hemicoronal approach," *Journal of Oral and Maxillofacial Surgery*, vol. 45, no. 3, pp. 279–282, 1987.

[2] K. Dawson, A. MacMillan, and D. Wiesenfeld, "Removal of a maxillary third molar from the infratemporal fossa by a temporal approach and the aid of image-intensifying cineradiography," *Journal of Oral and Maxillofacial Surgery*, vol. 51, no. 12, pp. 1395–1397, 1993.

[3] C. E. Sverzut, A. E. Trivellato, A. T. Sverzut, F. P. de Matos, and R. B. Kato, "Removal of a maxillary third molar accidentally displaced into the infratemporal fossa via intraoral approach under local anesthesia: report of a case," *Journal of Oral and Maxillofacial Surgery*, vol. 67, no. 6, pp. 1316–1320, 2009.

[4] F. Selvi, S. Cakarer, C. Keskin, and H. Ozyuvaci, "Delayed removal of a maxillary third molar accidentally displaced into the infratemporal fossa," *Journal of Craniofacial Surgery*, vol. 22, no. 4, pp. 1391–1393, 2011.

[5] I. Dimitrakopoulos and M. Papadaki, "Displacement of a maxillary third molar into the infratemporal fossa: case report," *Quintessence International*, vol. 38, no. 7, pp. 607–610, 2007.

[6] M. Patel and K. Down, "Accidental displacement of impacted maxillary third molars," *British Dental Journal*, vol. 177, no. 2, pp. 57–59, 1994.

[7] M. Oberman, I. Horowitz, and Y. Ramon, "Accidental displacement of impacted maxillary third molars," *International Journal of Oral and Maxillofacial Surgery*, vol. 15, no. 6, pp. 756–758, 1986.

[8] P. Janfaza, J. B. Nadol, R. J. Galla, and R. L. Fabian, *Surgical Anatomy of the Head and Neck*, Lippincott Williams & Wilkins, Montgomery, Ala, USA, 2001.

[9] A. N. Akyildiz, M. S. Ozbilen, and N. Goksu, "Hydatid cyst of the pterygopalatine fossa," *Journal of Oral and Maxillofacial Surgery*, vol. 49, no. 1, pp. 87–88, 1991.

[10] K. Gangopadhyay, M. O. Abuzeid, and H. Kfoury, "Hydatid cyst of the pterygopalatine-infratemporal fossa," *Journal of Laryngology and Otology*, vol. 110, no. 10, pp. 978–980, 1996.

# 10

# Oromandibular Limb Hypogenesis Syndrome Type IIB: Case Report of Hypoglossia-Hypodactyly

**Manasa Anand Meundi,[1] Gopakumar R. Nair,[2] Prathima Sreenivasan,[3] and A. C. Raj[4]**

[1] *Department of Oral Medicine, Diagnosis and Radiology, Dayananda Sagar College of Dental Sciences, Shavige Malleshwara Hills, Kumaraswamy Layout, Bangalore 560078, India*
[2] *Department of Oral Medicine, Diagnosis and Radiology, New Horizon Dental College & Research institute, Sakri, Bilaspur 495001, India*
[3] *Department of Oral Medicine, Diagnosis and Radiology, Kannur Dental College, Anjarakkandy post, Kannur 670612, India*
[4] *Department of Oral Medicine, Diagnosis and Radiology, KVG Dental College and Hospital, Vidhyanagar post, Kurunjibagh, Sullia 574327, India*

Correspondence should be addressed to Manasa Anand Meundi; manasaanandmeundi@gmail.com

Academic Editors: N. Brezniak and C. Ledesma-Montes

Hypoglossia-hypodactyly is a rare congenital anomaly affecting the tongue and the limbs. Hall in 1971 classified it under a complex group of disorders called oromandibular limb hypogenesis syndromes. It is an extremely rare condition with around 40 cases reported in the world literature. The cause of the syndrome is unknown. Some type of intrauterine trauma is the most widely accepted etiology. The characteristic features of the syndrome are hypoglossia, limb anomalies of variable degree, and micrognathia of the mandible. This unique case report of hypoglossia-hypodactyly was observed in a patient with normal mandible. In addition, patient also had pulmonary regurgitation. His parents and other siblings were normal. Positive prenatal history of maternal hyperthermia was obtained suspecting it to be the cause of the syndrome.

## 1. Introduction

Hypoglossia is a rare congenital anomaly [1]. It was first described by de Jussieu in 1718 as Aglossia. It may occur in isolation or in conjunction with anomalies of the extremities. Rosenthal in 1932 reported the first case of such an association as "aglossia-adactylia" [2]. Subsequently, similar cases were documented but with variable terminologies like aglossia-congenita, partial adactylia, aglossia-adactylia syndrome, partial anodontia, and microglossia [3]. In 1971, Hall BD coined the term "hypoglossia-hypodactylia syndrome," as he observed that the tongue and limbs were never totally absent. He considered it as a part of classification of oromandibular limb hypogenesis syndromes (OLHS) [4]. The prevalence of hypoglossia-hypodactyly has been documented as less than one per million population [5]. Around 47 cases have been reported so far [1].

The etiology of hypoglossia-hypodactylia (HG-HD) is unknown. Both genetic and environmental factors have been proposed to be responsible for the occurrence [6]. Most cases occur sporadically to unrelated parents with single affectation in the family [3]. Mishima et al. suggest an autosomal dominant or multifactorial inheritance with reduced penetrance and variable expression [1]. Mutation of *Msx 2*, a homeobox gene located in the mesenchyme of branchial arches and limb buds, as well as in the developing teeth and the alveolar ridges, may also be responsible for the clinical manifestations [7].

Environmental factors likely to be the etiology are maternal exposure to radiation and teratogenic drugs, intrauterine trauma/vascular accidents, chorionic villous sampling procedures, and maternal hyperthermia. Membranous strands resulting from amniotic rupture or chorionic villous sampling procedures during early pregnancy may interfere with oral and limb development [3, 8]. Reports of exposure to drugs like Tigan, Benedictine, Imipramine, Diazepam, Chlorpromazine, and Meclizine [2, 3] suggest their involvement, but their effect in the causation of this syndrome has not been proved. Fetal exposure to radiation during first trimester (a crucial period for orofacial development) may result in anomalies at birth [9]. Premature involution or injury to the stapedial artery supplying the first branchial arch may interfere with tongue vasculature [3]. Similarly, intrauterine vascular occlusion from placental fetal vessel thrombosis or emboli, followed by aseptic tissue necrosis, may cause peripheral amputation of the limbs [3]. Hyperthermia is a proven teratogen both in animals and humans. Maternal hyperthermia during first trimester of pregnancy can result even in fetal death [10]. According to Gorlin, intrauterine trauma [6] is the most widely accepted cause of this syndrome.

The three features essential for the diagnosis of this syndrome are [3]

(1) variable reduction in the tongue size (microglossia);

(2) micrognathia of the mandible (or maxilla) in the midline segment;

(3) limb anomalies of varying severity.

Size of the tongue varies from total absence (aglossia) to negligible hypoglossia. It is associated with a small mandible, a receded chin, atrophic mandibular anterior alveolar ridge, and missing incisors. Other oral and extraoral changes observed are enlarged sublingual ridges, defective lower lip, hypertrophic major salivary glands, mandibular cleft in the midline, fibrotic bands connecting the lower lip to the alveolar ridge, and gingival abnormalities [6].

The limb anomalies are extremely variable ranging from syndactyly (incomplete separation of the fingers) to amelia (missing limb) [3, 6]. In general, they tend to be distal to humerus and femur [2]. One or more limbs may be affected with variations seen in the same individual as well as in different patients [2, 3, 6].

Visceral anomalies associated with this syndrome include fused labia majora, imperforate anus, absence of a kidney, and ileal atresias [3].

HG-HD is an extremely rare condition with as few as 47 cases being reported in the world literature [1]. Among them, only three syndromic patients presented with a normal mandible [3, 11]. Yet, they had deficient premaxilla. This paper aims to report an unusual case of hypoglossia-hypodactylia without micrognathia of the mandible or maxilla, who in addition also had pulmonary regurgitation.

## 2. Case Report

A twenty-two-year-old male with extensive limb deformities reported to the department of Oral Medicine, Diagnosis, and Radiology with a chief complaint of unclear speech and difficulty in tongue movements.

The patient's medical history was insignificant. He was the fourth child of normal and unrelated parents. He had four siblings: one brother and three sisters all of whom were normal.

His prenatal history revealed that his mother had four episodes of fever during her first trimester and was medicated for the same. She was unable to remember the names of the medications. She had spontaneous vaginal delivery after

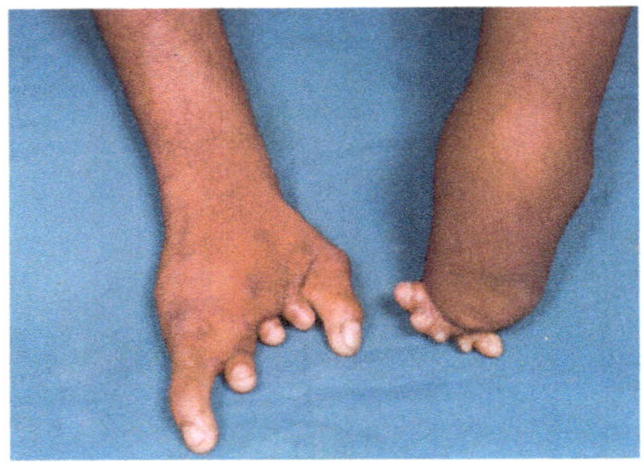

Figure 1: Showing both the upper limbs of the patient. Right limb demonstrates hypoplastic fingers (brachydactyly). The left forearm is absent with five nubbins attached to its distal part.

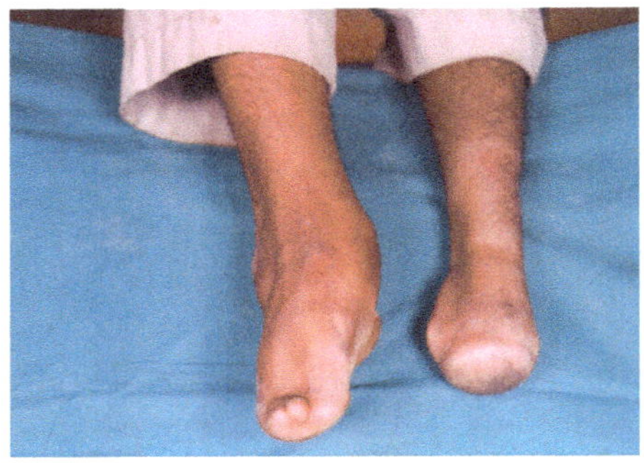

Figure 2: Showing both the lower limbs of the patient; Right foot is hypoplastic, and left foot is absent (apodia) with all the ten toes missing.

thirty-nine weeks of gestation to give birth to a male baby with multiple limb deformities. Patient's family history for congenital abnormalities was negative.

On general examination, a healthy, moderately built male of normal intelligence presented to the clinic with an altered gait. He had anomalies affecting all the four limbs. His right hand showed brachydactyly (short digits) of second to fourth fingers with hypoplastic thumb and little fingers. Finger nails appeared normal (Figure 1). In the left hand, hemimelia (missing half the limb) was observed below the elbow with five nubbins attached to its distal part. Radiograph of the right hand showed hypoplastic second and third metacarpals with deficient second to fourth phalanges. Absence of distal part of the radius and ulna was noted in the left hand radiograph with subluxation of the superior radioulnar joint. Lower limbs were also severely deformed. Right limb showed hypoplastic foot with adactyly (missing digits). Left limb had apodia (missing foot) with adactyly (Figure 2). Radiographically, right limb revealed hypoplasia of the phalanges and first metatarsal bone; left limb revealed absence of tibia, fibula, and both the malleoli. Detailed systemic clinical examinations with appropriate investigations were also performed. Though patient was clinically normal, his chest radiograph showed prominent pulmonary bay. Further, Color Doppler ultrasonography revealed pulmonary artery dilatation with pulmonary regurgitation (Figure 3).

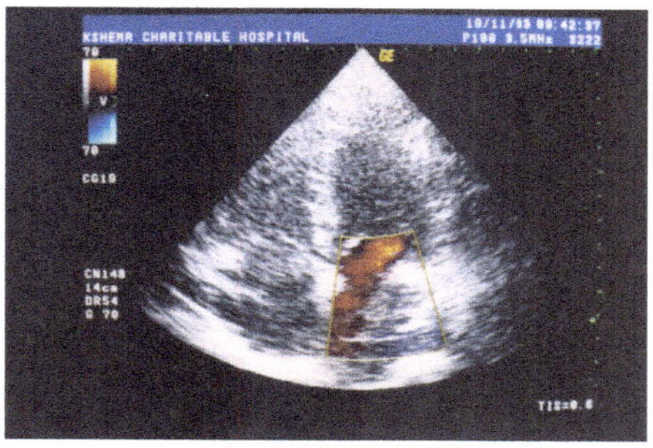


FIGURE 3: Color Doppler ultrasonographic image showing the regurgitation of blood into the left atrium.

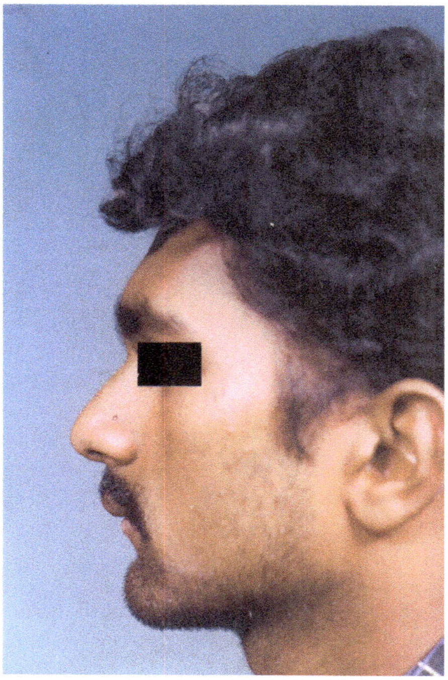

FIGURE 4: Left lateral view of the patient showing convex profile, competent lips, and deep mentolabial sulcus.

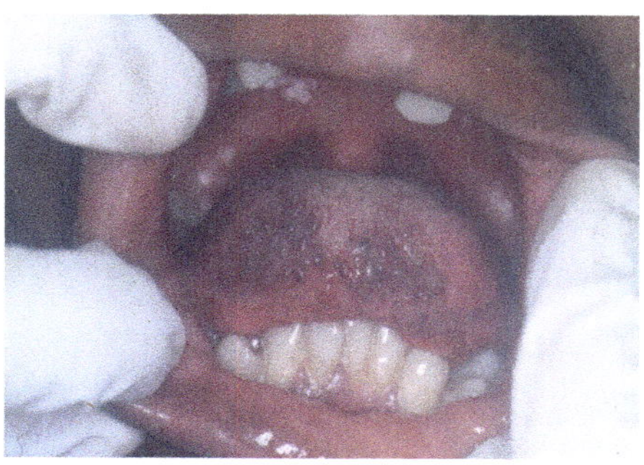

FIGURE 5: Intraoral view of the small tongue showing a poorly defined tip.

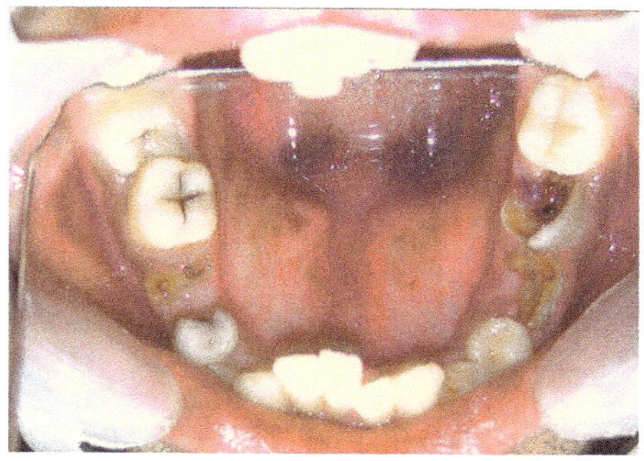

FIGURE 6: Intraoral view of the mandibular arch demonstrates the lingual frenum attaching the blunt tongue tip to the floor of the mouth far behind the incisors. Root stumps of molars are evident. Missing right central incisor may be noted.

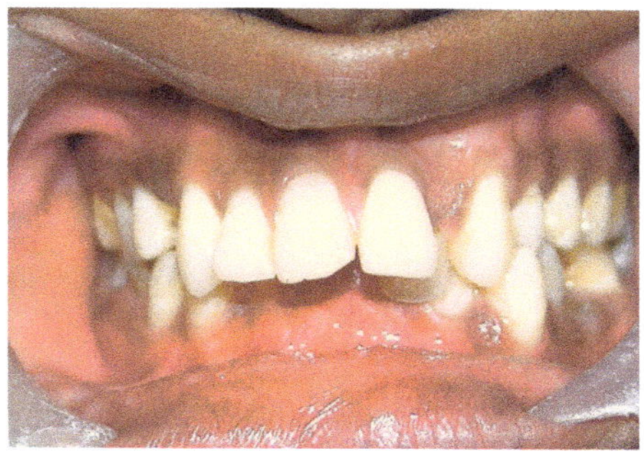

FIGURE 7: Intraoral view of the teeth in occlusion showing anterior deep bite and palatally placed maxillary left lateral incisor.

On extraoral examination, his lips were competent; profile was convex with a deep mentolabial sulcus (Figure 4).

Intraorally, his tongue was hypoplastic; about two thirds the normal size with a rounded tip (Figure 5). The tip was attached to the floor of the mouth by a short lingual frenum and positioned about a centimeter behind the lower incisors (Figure 6). This restricted the protrusive and lateral movements of the tongue. But speech was affected minimally.

Mandibular anteriors were retroclined with congenitally missing right central incisor (Figure 6). There was no radiographic evidence of impaction. Palate was V shaped, high arched, and narrow. Maxillary left lateral incisor was palatally positioned, thus blocking the regular alignment of mandibular anteriors. Anterior deep bite was observed (Figure 7). Root stumps of maxillary left first premolar, mandibular first molars, and mandibular right second molar were present (Figure 6).

Presence of a small tongue in association with extensive limb deformities led to the diagnosis of oromandibular limb hypogenesis syndrome type IIB, hypoglossia-hypodactyly. Although patient complained of altered speech and difficulty in tongue movements, he refused to undergo surgical procedure for the correction of the same. Basic oral rehabilitation procedures like extraction of the root stumps and oral prophylaxis were performed.

## 3. Discussion

OLHS (OMIM 103300) [5] represents a spectrum of disorders affecting the tongue and the limbs. Such patients often present with overlapping clinical features. Hence, in order to simplify the diagnosis, this complex syndrome has been classified twice. Hall's classification [6] is ideal to define the limb anomalies expressed in this patient. Accordingly, this case is OLHS type IIC: hypoglossia-hypodactylomelia, thus expressing the left hemimelia in the diagnosis. Since hypoglossia was the major determinate for the categorization, Chicarilli and Polayes [4] proposed a classification considering both embryologic origin and clinical features. He recognized four major classes, wherein type II represents microglossia as the primary disorder. Accordingly, this case is OLHS type IIB: hypoglossia-hypodactyly.

HG-HD is etiologically heterogeneous. The present case gave a positive prenatal history of maternal fever. Evidence of maternal hyperthermia causing OHLS exists [10, 12]. Maternal fever at/above 102°F between 4–14 weeks of pregnancy results in a range of defects including limb reduction, central nervous system (CNS) defects, facial dysmorphogenesis, and fetal death. Heat induced vascular disruption of the embryo has been implicated in the pathogenesis, The nature of anomalies is related to the extent, duration, and timing of the maternal fever. CNS defects appear to be the most common consequence of gestational hyperthermia. Yet, patients with HG-HD are often born with normal intelligence [10]. Based on this, there is a need to explore maternal hyperthermia as a cause of the syndrome.

Hypoglossia, limb anomalies, and micrognathia are the three characteristic features of the syndrome [3]. Of the three, latter two are often considered diagnostic because assessment of hypoglossia is subjected to observer variability (especially if it is minimal) because tongue is a muscular organ and need to be examined both at rest and during function [3]. The extent of limb deformities varies from syndactyly (incomplete separation of the fingers) to amelia (complete loss of the limb). Severe micrognathia is observed in all the cases of OLHS, due to the osseous defect in the mandibular midline region, and occasionally involves the premaxilla. But this patient of HG-HD presented with a normal mandible. Two similar cases were reported by Lustmann et al. [3], but his patients had a deficient premaxilla instead of mandible. This patient also suffered from pulmonary regurgitation, which probably has never been reported to be associated with this syndrome.

HG-HD syndrome is diagnosed at birth. Though tongue is deficient, in majority of cases, activities like swallowing and speech improve with time. Other muscles substitute for tongue and assist in feeding. Speech therapy improves phonetics. Surgery is desirable only if hypoplasia is severe. Prosthetic limbs would improve the locomotion and enhance the quality of life.

## Conflict of Interest

The authors declared no conflict of interests.

## Acknowledgment

The work was carried out in A. B. Shetty Memorial Institute of Dental Sciences, Nitte University, Deralakatte, Mangalore, India.

## References

[1] K. Mishima, T. Sugahara, Y. Mori, and M. Sakuda, "Case report: hypoglossia-hypodactylia syndrome," *Journal of Cranio-Maxillo-Facial Surgery*, vol. 24, no. 1, pp. 36–39, 1996.

[2] N. C. Nevin, D. Burrows, G. Allen, and D. C. Kernohan, "Aglossia adactylia syndrome," *Journal of Medical Genetics*, vol. 12, no. 1, pp. 89–93, 1975.

[3] J. Lustmann, R. Lurie, P. Struthers, and A. Garwood, "The hypoglossia-hypodactylia syndrome," *Oral Surgery Oral Medicine and Oral Pathology*, vol. 51, no. 4, pp. 403–408, 1981.

[4] Z. N. Chicarilli and I. M. Polayes, "Oromandibular limb hypogenesis syndromes," *Plastic and Reconstructive Surgery*, vol. 76, no. 1, pp. 13–24, 1985.

[5] "Hypoglossia—hypodactyly," 2005, http://www.orpha.net/consor/cgi-bin/OC_Exp.php?Ing=EN&Expert=989.

[6] R. J. Gorlin, M. M. Cohen Jr., and R. C. M. Hennekam, *Syndromes of the Head and Neck*, Oxford University Press, New York, NY, USA, 4 edition, 2001.

[7] F. R. Grippaudo and D. C. Kennedy, "Oromandibular-limb hypogenesis syndromes: a case of aglossia with an intraoral band," *British Journal of Plastic Surgery*, vol. 51, no. 6, pp. 480–483, 1998.

[8] H. V. Firth, P. A. Boyd, P. F. Chamberlain, I. Z. MacKenzie, G. M. Morriss-Kay, and S. M. Huson, "Analysis of limb reduction defects in babies exposed to chorionic villus sampling," *The Lancet*, vol. 343, no. 8905, pp. 1069–1071, 1994.

[9] C. J. Oulis and J. B. Thornton, "Severe congenital hypoglossia and micrognathia with other multiple birth defects," *Journal of Oral Pathology*, vol. 11, no. 4, pp. 276–282, 1982.

[10] J. M. Graham Jr., M. J. Edwards, and M. J. Edwards, "Teratogen update: gestational effects of maternal hyperthermia due to febrile illnesses and resultant patterns of defects in humans," *Teratology*, vol. 58, no. 5, pp. 209–221, 1998.

[11] M. Shear, "Congenital Underdevelopment of the maxilla associated with partial adactylia, partial anodontia and microglossia: report of a case," *The Journal of the Dental Association of South Africa*, vol. 11, pp. 78–83, 1956.

[12] P. Wadhwani, S. Mohammad, and R. Sahu, "Oromandibular limb hypogenesis syndrome, type IIA, hypoglossia-hypodactylia: a case report," *Journal of Oral Pathology and Medicine*, vol. 36, no. 9, pp. 555–557, 2007.

# 11

# Staged Osteotome Sinus Floor Elevation for Progressive Site Development and Immediate Implant Placement in Severely Resorbed Alveolar Bone: A Case Report

**Saad Al-Almaie**

*KFMMC, Dental Department, P.O. Box 946, Dhahran 31932, Saudi Arabia*

Correspondence should be addressed to Saad Al-Almaie; stsralmaie@yahoo.com

Academic Editors: M. A. Polack and J. J. Segura-Egea

This case report discusses osteotome sinus floor elevation (OSFE) and immediate placement in 2 stages in severely resorbed alveolar bone height in which multiple implant placement is not otherwise feasible due to a lack of initial stability. The first implant placed using OSFE without bone grafting prepares the adjacent resorbed sites for further implant placement in the sinus areas, which allows for better initial stability and early functional loading. This process avoids the conventional extensive lateral approach for sinus lifting and bone grafting procedures even in extremely resorbed alveolar bone.

## 1. Introduction

Osteotome sinus floor elevation (OSFE) is a widely practiced technique for elevation of the maxillary sinus prior to implant placement [1, 2]. Summers suggested that OSFE techniques should be performed with immediate insertion of the implant when the remaining bone measures over 6 mm in height [3, 4]. Jensen recommended that the procedure should be performed with simultaneous implant placement when a residual subsinus alveolar bone height (RSBH) of at least 5 mm is present [5]. When less than 5 mm of RSBH is present, primary implant stability may be compromised [6]. The implant is inserted simultaneously with a sinus lift procedure when sufficient primary stabilization can be expected [7, 8].

The osteotome technique is a less invasive method of elevating the sinus floor, reduces the need for more traumatic and expensive procedures, and decreases the risk of damaging the Schneiderian membrane [9]. However, OSFE exhibits a lack of initial stability in severely resorbed alveolar bone [10]. Most cases of prosthetic rehabilitation of the severely posterior maxilla require multiple implants. Attaining initial stability in cases of severely resorbed bone is difficult and is often complicated by fractured residual bone during multiple implant insertion. The reduced initial stability and the delay in further implant placement cause considerable delays in the functional loading of the implant. We report a case of multiple implant insertion on a severely resorbed alveolar bone height in a staged manner in which the first implant is placed by tenting the sinus membrane using OSFE without a bone graft to prepare the adjacent resorbed sites for further implant placement in the sinus areas, which allows for better initial stability and early functional loading.

## 2. Case Report

A 30-year-old male with a noncontributory medical history presented for the replacement of missing upper-left first and second premolars and molars, which were extracted 3 years earlier. The results of blood tests, including a complete blood count, chemistry, and clotting profile, were all within normal limits.

The initial orthopantomogram (Figure 1) revealed an alveolar bone height resorbed edentulous area in the upper-left posterior maxillary region with pneumatization of the maxillary sinus. The residual bone height was 2.5 mm (class D) between the upper first and second molars, 4.5 mm (class C) in the second molar area, and 7 mm (class B) in the second premolar area. The classification of sinus morphology (classes A through E) was initially proposed by Jensen to aid in the selection of the appropriate grafting material or technique at

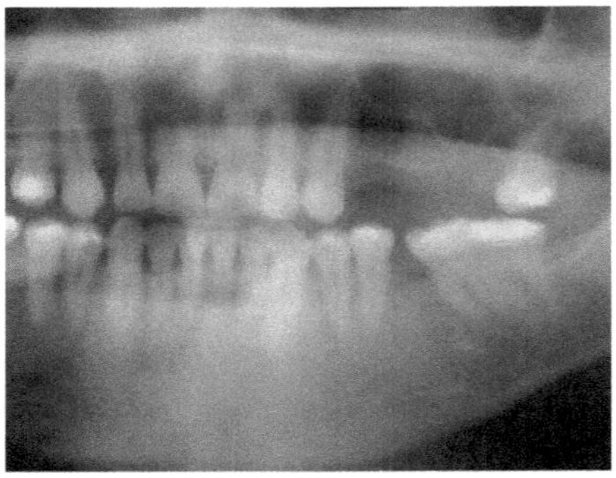

FIGURE 1: Baseline orthopantomogram showing that the subantral bone height was limited at the maxillary posterior left quadrant, with severely resorbed alveolar bone height at the site of the first maxillary molar.

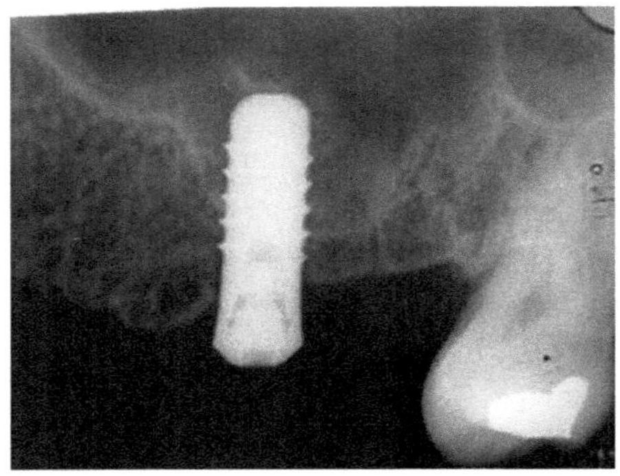

FIGURE 2: Radiograph taken after completion of the OSFE procedure without bone grafting with 8 mm lifting of the sinus membrane and a residual bone height of less than 3.0 mm and the amount of sinus floor elevation.

a specific site [5]. The alveolar ridge was approximately 8 to 10.5 mm in width, and the occlusal clearance was 6 to 7 mm.

In the first stage, the 1st implant was placed at the least alveolar bone height, which was located in the 1st molar area, to obtain maximum lifting of the sinus area and avoid any interference with the Schneiderian membrane in the 2nd stage and prepare the adjacent resorbed sites for further implant placement in the sinus areas. The punch incision was initially preferred (the alveolar ridge was approximately 8 to 10.5 mm in width) but because of the risk of miscalculating the exact alveolar bone height in that critical area, under local anesthesia, a full-thickness flap was elevated using a mid-crestal incision and 2 releasing buccal and palatal incisions of the upper-left first molar. The bone was accessed and marked with a round bur. A 2.2 mm diameter pilot drill was used to the required depth of 0.5 mm below the roof of the sinus. Radiographs were taken with a depth gauge and distance indicator to determine the length of the preparation.

To improve the primary stability in cancellous bone, bone condensation through radial reinforcement was attained by a series of bone condensation devices with a tapered tip and an appropriate diameter of 2.2 mm up to 4.2 mm to widen the implant bed (ITI osteotome instruments for bone condensation, Institut Straumann, Basel, Switzerland). Malleting was performed to fracture the bottom of the sinus cavity using a 4.2 mm angled osteotome with a concave tip (ITI instrument for partial sinus floor elevation, Institut Straumann). A change in the resonance during malleting indicated complete osteotomy. The Valsalva test to assess the patency of the Schneiderian membrane was negative throughout the procedure. A 12 mm long, 4.8 mm diameter, standard neck, and nonsubmerged, SLA, screw-type ITI implant (Institut Straumann) was used. Manual and gentle screwing of the implant facilitated lifting of the sinus membrane to the required implant height, and the initial stability was attained. The surgical site was closed using 4-0 silk sutures. The implant position, osteotomized portions of the sinus floor, and the amount of sinus floor elevation were visible on radiographs (Figure 2). Amoxicillin, 500 mg per 8 h, analgesics, and chlorhexidine mouthwash twice daily for 7 days were prescribed for the patient. The sutures were removed after 10 days, and the patient was followed up once monthly for 3 months.

Three months after the first implant was placed in the upper-left first molar area, a reformatted flythrough image of the maxillary sinus was obtained using computed tomography (CT) and DentaScan; reformatted cross-sectional images were obtained for the radiographic evaluation of the inferior wall of the maxillary sinus and apical border for the first implant at area of the upper-left first molar after the osteotome sinus floor elevation (Figure 3) to reveal the Schneiderian membrane over the apical border projection of the first inserted implant.

Four months after the first implant was placed, punch incisions were used to access the underlying alveolus for further implant placement. These sites required more than 5 mm of faciolingual width and little or no site development. A small envelope incision or tissue punch can be made to expose the bone for the osteotome; however, punch incision can be less traumatic and time consuming, with fewer complications and faster soft tissue healing. By including soft tissue thickness and using a surgical guide in the surgical plan, the procedure was accomplished and resulted in better patient comfort and easier surgical care. Three implants were placed on either side of the first implant. (i) A 12 mm long, 4.1 mm diameter, standard neck, nonsubmerged, SLA, screw-type ITI implant was used in the area of the upper-left second premolar. (ii) A 10 mm long, 4.1 mm diameter, standard neck, nonsubmerged, SLA, screw-type ITI implant was used in the area of the upper-left second molar. Both implants were placed using sinus floor elevation with the osteotome technique. (iii) A 12 mm long, 4.1 mm diameter, standard neck, nonsubmerged, SLA, screw-type ITI implant was placed in the upper-left first premolar area away from the maxillary sinus.

Four months after inserting the implants, radiographs were taken and they showed the implant and surrounding bone under the tented sinus membrane in the upper-left first molar region (Figure 4). The radiographs also showed the transformation of the residual ridge from classes C and D to classes A and B at the medial and distal sides of the implant, respectively. All the implants were loaded and restored with

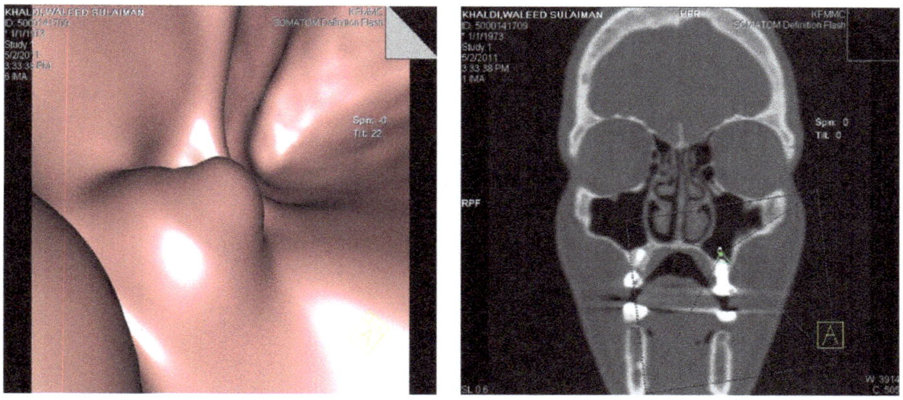


FIGURE 3: The CT and DentaScan reformatted flythrough image of the staged osteotome sinus floor elevation showing the intact Schneiderian membrane over the projection of the apical border of the first implant.

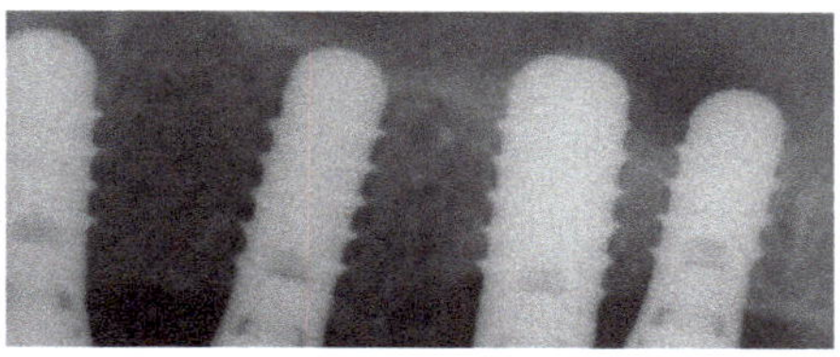

FIGURE 4: Postoperative radiograph of the left maxillary quadrant four months after the placement of three implants with better initial stability medially and distally to the first implant showing the new sinus floor with all the implants appropriately positioned and inclined.

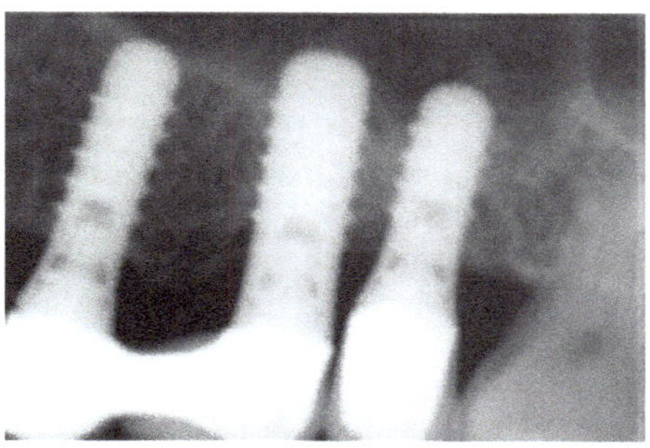

FIGURE 5: Periapical radiograph after 12 months of prosthetic loading showing a stable clinical situation in the area around the apex of the implants.

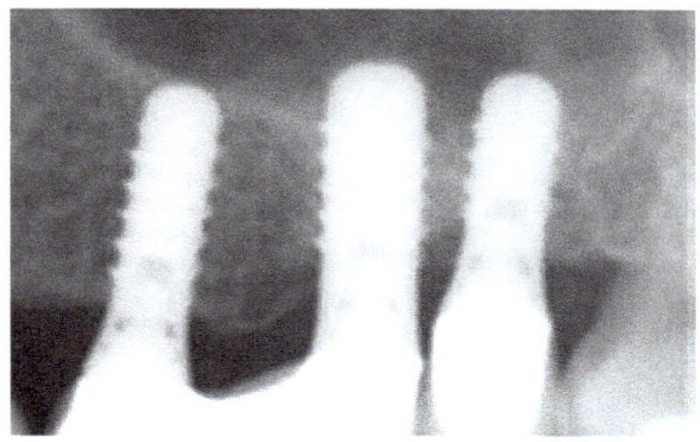

FIGURE 6: Periapical radiograph after two years of prosthetic loading showing a stable clinical situation in the area around the apex of the implants. A dome-shaped structure was apparent at the sites of the first and second molars.

porcelain-metal retainers. Radiographs taken at 12 and 24 months (Figures 5 and 6) showed a stable clinical situation in the area around the apex of the implants. A dome-shaped structure was observed at the sites of the first and second molar areas. Different CT scans, which were obtained after 24 months postoperatively, were used to show the implant, surrounding bone, and new sinus floor using the osteotome sinus floor elevation technique (Figures 7(a) and 7(b)).

## 3. Discussion

In patients with a severely resorbed maxilla, minimally invasive sinus floor elevation with simultaneous implant placement using osteotomes does not appear to be the method of choice. A 2-stage procedure using a lateral window technique [11, 12] or a crestal core approach [13, 14] is preferred. The OSFE procedure involves initial fixation of the implant using the residual alveolar ridge. A residual bone height of less than 4 mm is associated with reduced primary implant stability [15, 16], and a minimum of 5 mm of preoperative bone height has been suggested by many authors [17, 18]. Toffler reported that the primary factor in predicting implant survival using OSFE procedures was the residual height of the alveolar ridge and its ability to stabilize the implant [19].

According to the principles of guided bone regeneration, membrane elevation with space maintenance and blood clot formation may be sufficient to obtain neoformation of bone in the newly created space [20]. Lundgren et al. placed implants protruding into the sinus without introducing a grafting material and showed that all the implants achieved sufficient osseointegration and stability after 1 year of loading [21]. Nedir et al. used an expansion osteotome instead of drills to avoid ovalization of the osteotomy site and to condense the surrounding bone. Implants were often placed deeper with the flared neck resting against the crestal bone, which increased the stability [22].

In the present case report, implant installation was possible with a maxillary bone height of approximately 3 mm using

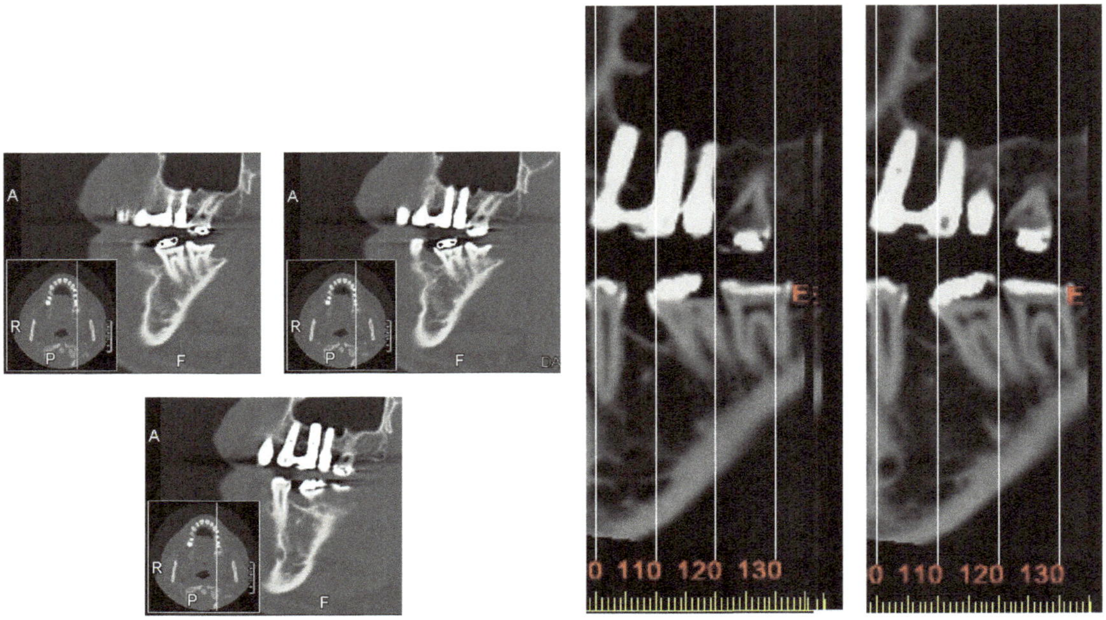


(a) (b)

Figure 7: (a) CT scans showed the implant and surrounding bone and the new sinus floor using the staged osteotome sinus floor elevation technique on the left side 2 years after the operation. (b) Selected magnifying images for CT scans showed the implant, apical borders for these implants, surrounding bone, and the new sinus floor using the staged osteotome sinus floor elevation technique on the left side 2 years after the operation.

relatively long implants (10 and 12 mm sink depth). Initial stability of the first implant was attained by lateral condensation. The lateral condensation technique performed using a series of osteotomes promotes better initial stability [3, 9, 20]. The quality of bone with a dense cortical plate increases the initial stability. In addition to thread engagement, the body design and surface roughness of the implants provided a frictional interface with the receptor site to assist in the mechanical retention by facilitating bone ingrowth during osseointegration [23]. In the presented case, we used the atraumatic, round-shaped end of the ITI implant, which limits the risks of damaging the sinus membrane during the sinus lift osteotome procedure. The convex apex shape of the implant is designed to prevent the tearing of the sinus membrane.

Buser et al. [24] suggested that the omission of tapping in low-density bone would improve primary implant stability. Other authors have proposed using osteotome bone condensation [25] with a smaller than recommended final drill size [26] or placing a submerged implant with its collar in a supracrestal position. Vidyasagar et al. [27] avoided tapping and cervical flaring to improve the primary stability of the implant. Avoiding cervical flaring at the preparation site for a placed dental implant even in low-density bone increases the initial implant stability. In the present case report, tapping and cervical flaring were avoided to increase the initial implant stability. Nedir et al. reported that tapered implants with a reduced thread pitch were placed with good primary stability in the atrophic maxilla of 2 patients using an osteotome sinus floor elevation procedure without grafting material [10].

Biscaro et al. observed signs of osseointegration near the apical third of the implant. A cortical wall was present at the apical end of the implant, which suggests the formation of a new sinus floor [28]. The regenerative properties of the bone beneath the sinus floor resulted in high endo-sinus bone gain. Some researchers have reported successful sinus elevation without bone grafting, and for all the studied implants, the osteotome procedure without grafting material was effective in forming new bone beyond the original limits of the sinus [10, 22, 29, 30]. In the present case report, the least alveolar bone height (less than 3 mm) for the OSFE and immediate placement for just 1 implant was selected because it is a new procedure and any failure would not jeopardize or complicate the entire quadrant if more implants were used. Nevertheless, the lateral window procedure can be used for any Schneiderian membrane perforation or complications that cannot be managed by the 1st stage OSFE procedure. Elevating the Schneiderian membrane with simultaneous implant placement is sufficient for creating bone beyond the natural limit of the sinus, and that was observed in the 3-month radiological study. This procedure created bone beyond the natural limit of the sinus and facilitated further implant placement by conventional OSFE without risking the loss of initial stability or other complications, such as fractures of the antral floor during malleting.

For patients, there are several advantages of staged OSFE for progressive site development and immediate implant placement in severely resorbed alveolar bone compared to the lateral window procedure: less pain and discomfort, a brief recovery, and a shorter time to implant loading. From the doctor's perspective, OSFE is a shorter procedure that can be accomplished in an outpatient setting, requires less surgical skills, time, and equipment, and is free from any meaningful complications. The success of this case in the short term suggests that an atrophic maxilla could be treated with a surgical procedure other than the classic lateral window opening for sinus augmentation. After this procedure is refined, it will likely generate a higher patient and practitioner acceptance rate than the current lateral window procedure. This study does have limitations. It describes just 1 case report and describes an evolving method that will require confirmation regarding its procedural success and failure rates, the quality and quantity of the newly formed bone over time, and implant survival rates.

## 4. Conclusion

Meticulous management of the available residual bone using a staged OSFE in conjunction with immediate implant placement is introduced in this case report. Elevating the Schneiderian membrane with simultaneous implant placement is sufficient to create bone beyond the natural limit of the sinus and allows the antral floor to be amenable to the placement of more implants in the second stage. The attained initial stability favored the early functional loading of the placed implants. The conventional traumatic lateral approach for sinus lifting and grafting procedures can be avoided even in highly resorbed alveolar bone by using this technique. More patients and a longer follow-up period to evaluate the fate of the newly formed bone over time are needed to investigate the reliability of this technique.

## References

[1] M. Chanavaz, "Maxillary sinus: anatomy, physiology, surgery, and bone grafting related to implantology—eleven years of surgical experience (1979–1990)," *The Journal of Oral Implantology*, vol. 16, no. 3, pp. 199–209, 1990.

[2] D. G. Smiler, P. W. Johnson, J. L. Lozada et al., "Sinus lift grafts and endosseous implants. Treatment of the atrophic posterior maxilla," *Dental Clinics of North America*, vol. 36, no. 1, pp. 151–187, 1992.

[3] R. B. Summers, "A new concept in maxillary implant surgery: the osteotome technique," *Compendium*, vol. 15, no. 2, pp. 152–158, 1994.

[4] R. B. Summers, "The osteotome technique: part 2—the ridge expansion osteotomy (REO) procedure," *Compendium*, vol. 15, no. 4, pp. 422–436, 1994.

[5] O. T. Jensen, "Treatment planning for sinus grafts," in *The Sinus Bone Graft*, O. T. Jensen, Ed., pp. 49–68, Quintessence Publishing, Carol Stream, Ill, USA, 1999.

[6] C. M. Ten Bruggenkate and J. P. A. van den Bergh, "Maxillary sinus floor elevation: a valuable pre-prosthetic procedure," *Periodontology 2000*, vol. 17, no. 1, pp. 176–182, 1998.

[7] O. H. Tatum, "Maxillary sinus grafting for endosseous implants," in *Presented at the Annual Meeting of the Alabama Implant Study Group*, Birmingham, Alabama, USA, April 1977.

[8] H. Tatum Jr., "Maxillary and sinus implant reconstructions," *Dental Clinics of North America*, vol. 30, no. 2, pp. 207–229, 1986.

[9] R. B. Summers, "The osteotome technique: part 3—less invasive methods of elevating the sinus floor," *Compendium*, vol. 15, no. 6, pp. 698–710, 1994.

[10] R. Nedir, N. Nurdin, S. Szmukler-Moncler, and M. Bischof, "Osteotome sinus floor elevation technique without grafting material and immediate implant placement in atrophic posterior maxilla: report of 2 cases," *Journal of Oral and Maxillofacial Surgery*, vol. 67, no. 5, pp. 1098–1103, 2009.

[11] P. A. Fugazzotto, "Maxillary sinus grafting with and without simultaneous implant placement: technical considerations and case reports," *The International Journal of Periodontics & Restorative Dentistry*, vol. 14, no. 6, pp. 544–551, 1994.

[12] S. L. Wheeler, R. E. Holmes, and C. J. Calhoun, "Six-Year Clinical and Histologic Study of Sinus-Lift Grafts," *International Journal of Oral and Maxillofacial Implants*, vol. 11, no. 1, pp. 26–34, 1996.

[13] P. A. Fugazzotto, "The modified trephine/osteotome sinus augmentation technique: technical considerations and discussion of indications," *Implant Dentistry*, vol. 10, no. 4, pp. 259–264, 2001.

[14] M. Toffler, "Staged sinus augmentation using a crestal core elevation procedure and modified osteotomes to minimize membrane perforation," *Practical Procedures & Aesthetic Dentistry*, vol. 14, no. 9, pp. 767–776, 2002.

[15] J. M. Hirsch and I. Ericsson, "Maxillary sinus augmentation using mandibular bone grafts and simultaneous installation of implants. A surgical technique," *Clinical oral Implants Research*, vol. 2, no. 2, pp. 91–96, 1991.

[16] F. Bernardello, D. Righi, F. Cosci, P. Bozzoli, M. Soardi Carlo, and S. Spinato, "Crestal sinus lift with sequential drills and simultaneous implant placement in sites with <5 mm of native bone: a multicenter retrospective study," *Implant Dentistry*, vol. 20, no. 6, pp. 439–444, 2011.

[17] T. Kang, "Sinus elevation using a staged osteotome technique for site development prior to implant placement in sites with less than 5 mm of native bone: a case report," *International Journal of Periodontics & Restorative Dentistry*, vol. 28, no. 1, pp. 73–81, 2008.

[18] G. Greenstein and J. Cavallaro, "Transcrestal sinus floor elevation with osteotomes: simplified technique and management of various scenarios," *Compendium of Continuing Education in Dentistry*, vol. 32, no. 4, pp. 12–22, 2011.

[19] M. Toffler, "Osteotome-mediated sinus floor elevation: a clinical report," *International Journal of Oral and Maxillofacial Implants*, vol. 19, no. 2, pp. 266–273, 2004.

[20] A. A. Winter, A. S. Pollack, and R. B. Odrich, "Sinus/alveolar crest tenting (SACT): a new technique for implant placement in atrophic maxillary ridges without bone grafts or membranes," *International Journal of Periodontics & Restorative Dentistry*, vol. 23, no. 6, pp. 557–565, 2003.

[21] S. Lundgren, S. Andersson, F. Gualini, and L. Sennerby, "Bone reformation with sinus membrane elevation: a new surgical technique for maxillary sinus floor augmentation," *Clinical Implant Dentistry and Related Research*, vol. 6, no. 3, pp. 165–173, 2004.

[22] R. Nedir, M. Bischof, L. Vazquez, S. Szmukler-Moncler, and J.-P. Bernard, "Osteotome sinus floor elevation without grafting material: a 1-year prospective pilot study with ITI implants," *Clinical Oral Implants Research*, vol. 17, no. 6, pp. 679–686, 2006.

[23] D. Buser, T. Nydegger, T. Oxland et al., "Interface shear strength of titanium implants with a sandblasted and acid-etched surface: a biomechanical study in the maxilla of miniature pigs,"

*Journal of Biomedical Materials Research*, vol. 45, no. 2, pp. 75–83, 1999.

[24] D. Buser, R. K. Schenk, S. Steinemann, J. P. Fiorellini, C. H. Fox, and H. Stich, "Influence of surface characteristics on bone integration of titanium implants. A histomorphometric study in miniature pigs," *Journal of Biomedical Materials Research*, vol. 25, no. 7, pp. 889–902, 1991.

[25] H. Martinez, M. Davarpanah, P. Missika, R. Celletti, and R. Lazzara, "Optimal implant stabilization in low density bone," *Clinical Oral Implants Research*, vol. 12, no. 5, pp. 423–432, 2001.

[26] D. O'Sullivan, L. Sennerby, and N. Meredith, "Measurements comparing the initial stability of five designs of dental implants: a human cadaver study," *Clinical implant dentistry and related research*, vol. 2, no. 2, pp. 85–92, 2000.

[27] L. Vidyasagar, G. Salms, P. Apse, and U. Teibe, "The influence of site preparation (countersinking) on initial dental implant stability, an in vitro study using resonance frequency analysis," *Stomatologija*, vol. 6, no. 1, pp. 14–16, 2004.

[28] L. Biscaro, A. Beccatelli, and L. Landi, "A human histologic report of an implant placed with simultaneous sinus floor elevation without bone graft," *International Journal of Periodontics & Restorative Dentistry*, vol. 32, no. 4, pp. e122–e130, 2012.

[29] D.-S. Sohn, J.-W. Moon, K.-N. Moon, S.-C. Cho, and P.-S. Kang, "New bone formation in the maxillary sinus using only absorbable gelatin sponge," *Journal of Oral and Maxillofacial Surgery*, vol. 68, no. 6, pp. 1327–1333, 2010.

[30] N. Ferrigno, M. Laureti, and S. Fanali, "Dental implants placement in conjunction with osteotome sinus floor elevation: a 12-year life-table analysis from a prospective study on 588 ITI implants," *Clinical Oral Implants Research*, vol. 17, no. 2, pp. 194–205, 2006.

# 12

# Early Correction of Malocclusion Using Planas Direct Tracks

**Renata Reis dos Santos,[1] Artênio José Isper Garbin,[2] and Cléa Adas Saliba Garbin[3]**

[1] *Universidade Estadual Paulista, UNESP Araçatuba Dental School, Preventive and Social Dentistry, Rua José Bonifácio 1193, Vila Mendonça, Araçatuba16015-050, SP, Brazil*
[2] *Universidade Estadual Paulista, UNESP Araçatuba Dental School, Post-Graduation Program, Rua José Bonifácio 1193, Vila Mendonça, Araçatuba 16018-050, SP, Brazil*
[3] *Universidade Estadual Paulista, UNESP Araçatuba Dental School, Orthodontics and Preventive and Social Dentistry, Rua José Bonifácio, 1193, Vila Mendonça, Araçatuba-16015-050, SP, Brazil*

Correspondence should be addressed to Renata Reis dos Santos; renatar.santos@yahoo.com.br

Academic Editors: C. Landes and J. J. Segura-Egea

The correction of functional posterior crossbite through Planas Direct Tracks has many characteristics that can become advantages. The aim of this study was to present a clinical case showing how to use this procedure for early correction with resources available through public health services. The patient, a 4-year-old girl, arrived to receive treatment due to a functional unilateral crossbite. When the mandible was moved to the centric position, it was observed that the teeth had occlusal trauma. An occlusal adjustment was performed. The adjustment was not sufficient to promote functional equilibrium; thus, Planas Direct Tracks were made, resulting in functional equilibrium and correction of the malocclusion. As shown in the case report, the Planas Direct Tracks were effective for the correction of the posterior crossbite. If malocclusion is considered a public health problem, implementation of low-cost and easy-to-execute techniques is needed.

## 1. Introduction

Neuroocclusal rehabilitation (NOR) can be defined as a subfield of dentistry that studies the etiology of functional and morphological alterations of the stomatognathic system. Its aim is to investigate and eliminate etiological factors and avert the potential for lesions through selective occlusal griding and/or using Planas Direct Tracks. This innovation can be used at any stage of life to correct a crossbite [1].

The crossbite is one of the most common occlusal alterations. It is an abnormal relationship between the buccal or lingual surfaces of the superior teeth and the inferior teeth when the arches are in centric relation and may be unilateral or bilateral. The most common presentation is unilateral with a functional deviation of the mandibula crossed to the side. It can be classified as a dental crossbite, involving only one or more teeth, muscular or functional, in which case there is a possibility of adapting soft tissues through dental interference, or as a skeletal crossbite, in which alterations in the bone development cause asymmetric growth of the maxillaries [2].

Its etiology is a combination of many factors, including skeletal and neuromuscular components; however, the most frequent cause is palatal reduction [3, 4].

Self-correction is rare, and it is believed that early diagnosis and treatment of a posterior crossbite can help to avoid bone base dystrophies with orthopedic or structural alterations [5].

Several treatments have been applied for correction of these problems, and the studies converge on a common point: the therapy is used for deciduous dentition [6, 7].

The Planas Direct Tracks technique is a component of many other neuroocclusal rehabilitation treatments and was developed by Pedro Planas. It constitutes an effective way to correct dental or functional alterations in children during deciduous dentition and the beginning of mixed dentition,

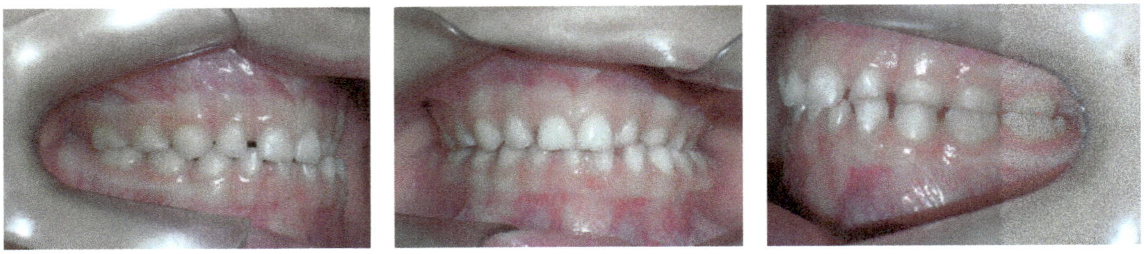

(a) (b) (c)

FIGURE 1: Clinical aspects in centric position. (a) Right side, (b) frontal view, (c) left side.

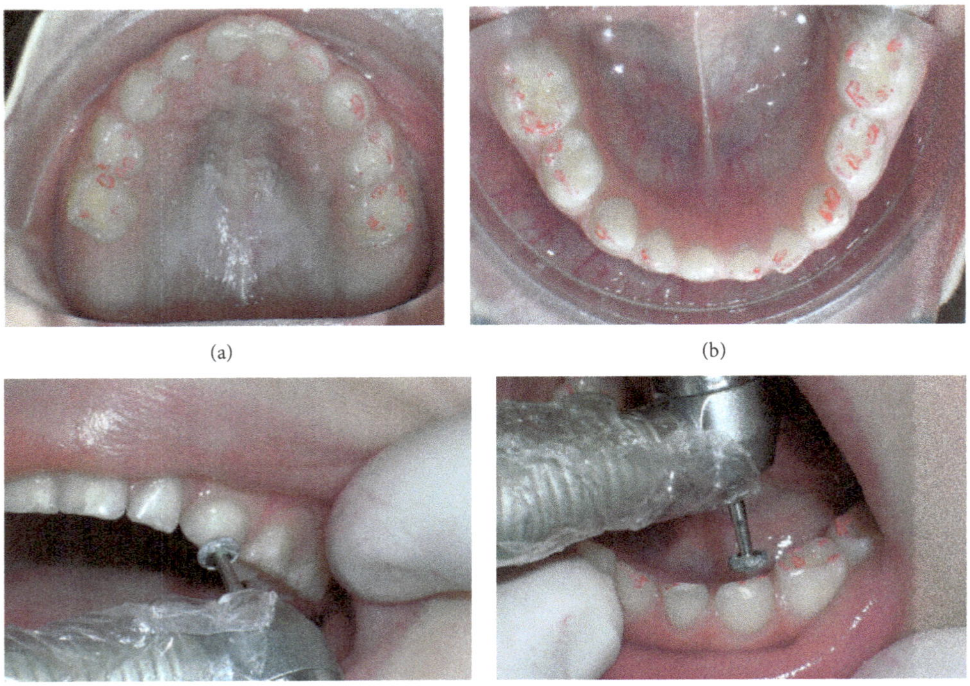

(a) (b) (c) (d)

FIGURE 2: Oclusal view with carbon print and selective wears. (a) Superior oclusal view, (b) inferior oclusal view, (c) selective wears on superior teeth, and (d) selective wears o inferior teeth.

normalizing dental occlusion, mandibular posture, condylar position, and masticatory function [5].

It is recommended as a first measure to facilitate early treatment of posterior crossbite, producing wear on the occlusals to remove the occlusal interference. In cases in which the occlusal wear is not sufficient to eliminate the interferences, the construction of tracks with photopolymerizable resin is suggested [1].

The aim of this study is to present a case report demonstrating how to execute the technique for early correction of crossbite with available resources in a dental public health service facility.

## 2. Description of Case

The patient, JBC, a girl of 4 years and 5 months of age, arrived in search of treatment and showed a functional unilateral posterior crossbite on the left side (Figure 1), no caries lesions, normal soft tissues, and completed deciduous dentition. The crossbite was classified as functional because after mandibular manipulation to the centric position, it was possible to observe premature occlusal contacts.

In this case, it was possible to verify a transversal decrease of the superior arch, which causes a condition of end-to-end biting of the canine teeth and occasional involvement of posterior teeth. In order to avoid discomfort, the patient moved the mandible to one side and then the other side until finding a position that allowed better adaptation, consequently resulting in the functional unilateral posterior crossbite.

Guiding the mandible to the centric position, it was possible to observe that the teeth showed trauma, contributing to mandibular deviation and thus necessitating selective wears. A diamond bur number 3053 with a wheel form was used for high rotation with irrigation (Figure 2).

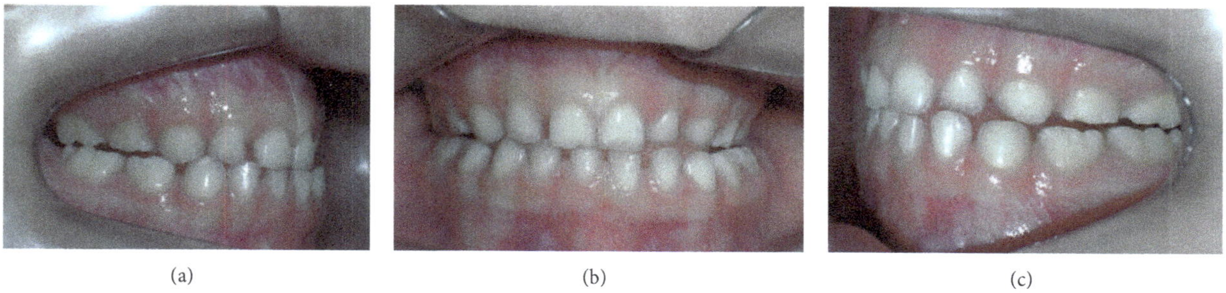


FIGURE 3: Clinical aspects after oclusal adjusts. (a) Right side, (b) front view, and (c) left side.

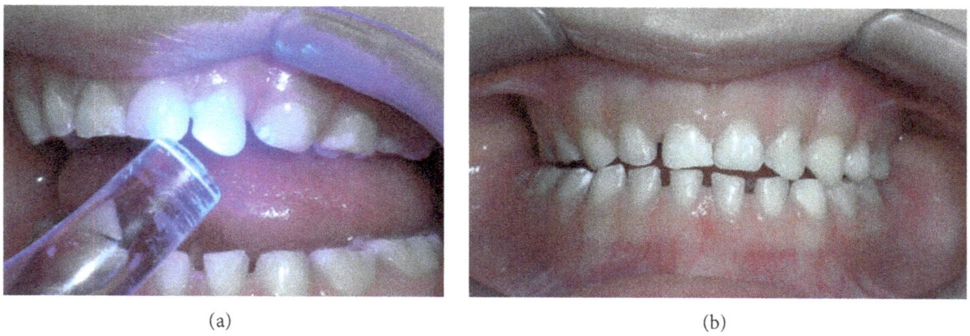


FIGURE 4: Confection of Planas Direct Tracks. (a) Photopolymerization of resin. (b) Front view after confection of Planas Direct Tracks centralizing the median line.

Due the fact that the adjustments were not sufficient to promote the equilibrium to allow the centralization of the median line (Figure 3), Planas Direct Tracks were made on the teeth involved in the crossbite (lateral incisive, canine, and left molars).

The standard procedure was followed using compost resin, conditioning with phosphoric acid at 37% for a duration of 30 seconds, washing and drying, and applying of adhesive and photopolymerized composite resin (Figure 4). The finishing was performed using diamond bur model 1192F and the Enhance bur.

The extension of tracks should be large sufficiently to prevent the mandible from moving back to the comfortable position and should be thick enough to prevent fracture during function. It is suggested that occlusal wears should be made with a 45° angle in the tooth's vertical axis or at an angle greater than 30° to produce inclined planes that allow the mandible to attain an adequate expansion or force during mandibular closing [8].

After application of Planas Direct Tracks, new grinds were made. After treatment, the median line deviation was corrected and there was rehabilitation of functional equilibrium and correction of the malocclusion.

After 6 months, the tracks were evaluated again and reconstruction in one tooth and a new occlusal adjustment were found to be necessary (Figure 5).

## 3. Discussion

Treatments using conventional braces were not effective for correction of the crossbite and did not modify the mandibular movements, probably due to the permanence of occlusal intereferences [9].

Among treatment methods for posterior crossbite, the use of NOR, which includes the use of selective wears and Planas Direct Tracks, is efficient for correction of this anomaly [10]. These procedures are low cost, allowing the treatment of some malocclusions in public health service facilities.

The cases indicated the occlusal adjustments through selective wears show unilateral crossbite, median line deviation, and occlusal interferences in deciduous dentition.

In a longitudinal study conducted by Lindner [11] to evaluate the early unilateral posterior crossbite using selective wears, the 76 children who were evaluated were divided in two groups, treated and untreated. In the untreated group, only 17% showed spontaneous correction of crossbite. Thus, early correction using selective wears is indicated to have a favorable prognosis.

The clinical report showed that the treatment started when the children were 4 years old because early intervention during the deciduous dentition phase may allow avoidance of the formation of several strucutural deformities in permanent dentition. Early diagnosis and correction, together with the physiological positioning of condyles and muscle equilibrium

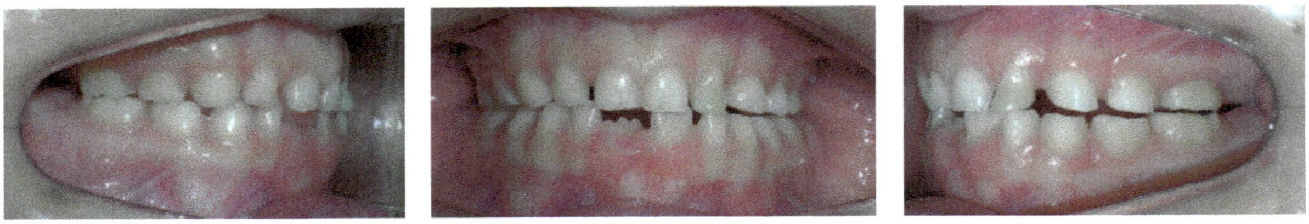

(a) (b) (c)

FIGURE 5: Clinical aspects after six months of treatment. (a) right side, (b) front view and (c) left side.

[1], prevent facial asymmetries in the adult phase [10]. The occlusal adjustment makes rehabilitation of neuromuscular activity possible, preventing masticatory movements during the growing phase. This treatment modifies the standard masticatory cycle, inducing bilateral chewing.

It is important to highlight that during the clinical exam for differential diagnosis between functional or true crossbite, mandibular manipulation should be performed and adjusted to the centric position. Functional crossbites show the meeting of median lines when mandibles stay in the centric position, which demonstrates the presence of occlusal interferences [8, 12].

The inclination of tracks should be made based on the characteristics of each case and should be related to Camper's plane and guide, allowing mandibular movements.

The major advantadge of Planas Direct Tracks is that, in this treatment, patient collaboration is not necessary because its basis is in selective wears and restoration with composite resin that acts continuously after construction. Additionally, it is low cost because sophisticated materials are not necessary for its execution and it is a simple technique that can be performed by general dentists, so it is not necessary to be a specialist in orthodontics [7, 8].

## 4. Conclusion

It can be concluded that Planas Direct Tracks were efficient in the correction of the posterior crossbite in the case report. If malocclusion is considered a public health problem, low-cost techniques that have easy execution are recommended so correction can be performed at an early age.

## References

[1] P. Planas, *Reabilitação Neuroclusal*, Medsi, Rio de Janeiro, Brazil, 2nd edition, 1988.

[2] R. E. Moyers, *Ortodontia*, Guanabara Koogan, Rio de Janeiro, Brazil, 4th edition, 1991.

[3] A. D. S. Andrade, G. H. Gameiro, M. DeRossi, and M. B. D. Gavião, "Posterior crossbite and functional changes: a systematic review," *Angle Orthodontist*, vol. 79, no. 2, pp. 380–386, 2008.

[4] J. J. Warren, R. L. Slayton, T. Yonezu, S. E. Bishara, S. M. Levy, and M. J. Kanellis, "Effects of nonnutritive sucking habits on occlusal characteristics in the mixed dentition," *Pediatric Dentistry*, vol. 27, no. 6, pp. 445–450, 2005.

[5] M. N. Gribel, "Tratamento de mordidas cruzadas unilaterais posteriores com desvio postural mandibular com pistas diretas plana," *Revista Dental Press de Ortodontia e Ortopedia Facial*, vol. 4, pp. 47–54, 1999.

[6] J. E. Harrison and D. Ashby, "Orthodontic treatment for posterior crossbites," *Cochrane Database of Systematic Reviews*, no. 1, Article ID CD000979, 2001.

[7] G. Ramirez-Yañez, "Treatment of anterior crossbite in the primary dentition with esthetic crowns: report of 3 cases," *Pediatric Dentistry*, vol. 33, no. 4, pp. 339–342, 2011.

[8] A. Chibinski, G. Czlusniak, and M. Melo, "Pistas diretas Planas: terapia ortopédica para correção de mordida cruzada funcional," *Revista Clinica de Ortodontia Dental Press*, vol. 4, pp. 64–72, 2005.

[9] Y. Ben-Bassat, A. Yaffe, I. Brin, J. Freeman, and Y. Ehrlich, "Functional and morphological-occlusal aspects in children treated for unilateral posterior cross-bite," *European Journal of Orthodontics*, vol. 15, no. 1, pp. 57–63, 1993.

[10] H. A. Oliveira and G. Ortellado, "Pistas Diretas Planas para a correção de mordida cruzada posterior," *Jornal Brasileiro Ortodontia Ortopedia Facial*, vol. 6, pp. 15–19, 2000.

[11] A. Lindner, "Longitudinal study on the effect of early interceptive treatment in 4-year-old children with unilateral cross-bite," *Scandinavian Journal of Dental Research*, vol. 97, no. 5, pp. 432–438, 1989.

[12] A. C. Chibinski and G. Czlusniak, "Evaluation of treatment for functional posterior crossbite of the deciduous dentition using Planas' direct tracks," *Indian Journal of Dental Research*, vol. 22, no. 5, pp. 654–658, 2011.

# 13

# Rare Giant Granular Cell Ameloblastoma: A Case Report and an Immunohistochemical Study

**Santosh Hunasgi,[1] Anila Koneru,[1] Dinesh Singh Chauhan,[2] and Yadavalli Guruprasad[2]**

[1] *Department of Oral and Maxillofacial Pathology, Navodaya Dental College and Hospital, Raichur, Karnataka 584103, India*
[2] *Department of Oral and Maxillofacial Surgery, AME's Dental College, Raichur, Karnataka 584103, India*

Correspondence should be addressed to Santosh Hunasgi; drsantosh31@gmail.com

Academic Editors: M. H. K. Motamedi and M. J. Wahl

*Aims.* The aim is to present a case of rare giant granular cell ameloblastoma and to review the pertinent literature highlighting the molecular aspects of its pathogenesis by analyzing the expression of CD-68, Bcl-2, and $\beta$-catenin. *Methods.* H and E stained sections showed large odontogenic islands showing peripheral ameloblast-like cells and central stellate reticulum-like cells with extensive granular cell transformation surrounded by fibrous stroma. Polyclonal rabbit anti-CD 68, anti-Bcl2, and anti-$\beta$-catenin were stained immunohistochemically. *Results.* CD-68 showed a moderate to strong staining intensity in granular cells. Moderate staining of Bcl-2 was expressed by the peripheral columnar cells of tumor islands and negative in the granular cells. Expression of $\beta$-catenin was generally weak, except for only the focal areas that showed a moderate staining intensity and weak in peripheral cells. *Conclusion.* The present case of giant granular cell ameloblastoma is a rare entity. Development of monstrous size is indicative of ameloblastomas persistent growth. Granular cell transformation in ameloblastomas probably occurs as a consequence of extensive molecular changes. Immunohistochemical studies help us to know the pathogenesis of this granular cell ameloblastoma. Therefore, an effort has been made here to study the expression of Bcl-2, CD-68, and $\beta$-catenin.

## 1. Introduction

Ameloblastoma is the second most common odontogenic tumor, being clinically and histologically diverse. These tumors have several distinct clinical types, including solid, unicystic, desmoplastic, and peripheral ameloblastomas. Ameloblastomas are further subclassified as follicular, plexiform, granular, basal cell, and acanthomatous [1].

Granular cell ameloblastoma (GCA) is a less common histological subtype of ameloblastoma. The English language literature search has revealed approximately 30 studies regarding this rare subtype of ameloblastoma [2]. It is known to be locally aggressive among all the ameloblastomas and is important to separate GCA from other ameloblastomas because of higher incidence of malignancy and metastases [3].

The granular cells are rich in lysosomal granules, in which there is marked transformation of the cytoplasm, usually of stellate reticulum-like cells, so that it takes a very coarse, granular, and eosinophilic appearance. This "granular change" is thought to be due to a dysfunctional status of neoplastic cells, and the pathogenesis of this tumor seems to be age related. Thus, acquisition of granular cell phenotype has been attributed to an aging or degenerative change in long-standing lesions [4].

Ameloblastomas can show slow and asymptomatic growth, because of this, patient seeks treatment only after the lesion has grown remarkably large size [5]. Therefore neglected ameloblastomas may become enormous and cause gross facial deformities that pose considerable problems in management. In English language literature, 10 cases of giant ameloblastomas (3 cases of Follicular and 7 cases of plexiform) are reported till date [5, 6]. However, there are no cases of giant granular cell ameloblastomas reported.

Thus the purpose of this paper is to present a case of Rare giant granular cell ameloblastoma and to review

TABLE 1: The expression of CD 68, Bcl2, and $\beta$-catenin in the cytoplasm of tumor cells in a granular cell ameloblastoma.

| Examined proteins | Staining intensity | | |
|---|---|---|---|
| | Peripheral cells | Central cells | Granular cells |
| CD 68 | No staining | Weak | Moderate to severe |
| Bcl2 | Moderate to severe | No staining | No staining |
| $\beta$-Catenin | Weak | Moderate to severe | Moderate |

the pertinent literature highlighting the molecular aspects of its pathogenesis by analyzing the expression of CD-68, Bcl-2, and $\beta$-catenin in the present case.

## 2. Case Report

A 39-year-old female patient reported to our hospital with a complaint of a large painless swelling over the left side of the face. She had first noticed the swelling 10 years ago which was painless with minimal extraoral manifestation. The patient neglected the swelling due to its painless nature and slow growth.

On extra oral examination, a large well-defined swelling measuring approximately 12 cm × 10 cm was found in the left cheek, mandible, and submental region (Figure 1). Swelling was soft to firm in consistency with normal overlying stretched skin and no sinus or discharge observed. Intraorally, massive swelling was noticed from 31 to retromolar area, pushing the tongue to the contralateral side. Tongue movements were restricted. Crowding and extrusion of lower left anterior and premolars were observed.

Radiographic examination revealed a multilocular radiolucency, extending from left condyle and coronoid to right central and lateral incisors, with thinning of lower border of mandible (Figure 2). Surgically excised hemimandibulectomy specimen measured 12 × 9 × 10 cm and weighed 1200 grams (Figure 3). A followup of one year showed no recurrence.

## 3. Methods

*3.1. Histopathological Analysis.* H and E stained sections showed large odontogenic islands showing peripheral ameloblast-like cells and central stellate reticulum-like cells with extensive granular cell transformation surrounded by fibrous stroma (Figure 4). The granular cells exhibited coarsely granular eosinophilic cytoplasm and small pyknotic nuclei (Figure 5). Therefore, a final diagnosis of ameloblastoma, granular cell variant, was given. The patient was followed up for 1 year and showed no signs of recurrence.

*3.2. Immunohistochemical Analysis.* Polyclonal rabbit anti-CD-68, anti-Bcl-2, and anti-$\beta$-catenin (Biogenix Life Sciences Limited, CA, USA) were used for immunohistochemistry employing the super sensitive polymer HRP detection system. The sections were later counter-stained with Mayer's hematoxylin. The presence of brown color at the site of target antigen was considered as immunopositive.

The immunoreactivity was assessed based on staining intensity. The staining intensity of positive cells was evaluated visually and classified as follows: weak, moderate, and strong intensity. Finally localization of positively stained cells was also assessed, that is, in peripheral ameloblast-like cells, central stellate reticulum like cells, and granular cells.

## 4. Results

The tumor cells of granular cell ameloblastoma showed positive immunoreactivity to all proteins (Figures 6, 7, and 8). The expression of CD-68, Bcl-2, and $\beta$-Catenin is summarized in Table 1. CD-68 showed a moderate to strong staining intensity in granular cells (Figure 6). Moderate staining of Bcl-2 was expressed by the peripheral columnar cells of tumor islands and negative in the granular cells (Figure 7). Expression of $\beta$-catenin was generally weak, except for only the focal areas that showed a moderate staining intensity and weak in peripheral cells (Figure 8).

## 5. Discussion

This study reports a case of granular cell ameloblastoma that developed at the posterior mandible of a 39-year-old female. Based on a series of 20 cases of granular cell ameloblastoma, this tumor occurs at an average age of 40.7 years with no significant gender predilection and is found predominantly at the posterior region of the mandible particularly around the angle of the mandible. The age and the location of tumor of this case appear to be consistent with the study by Hartman [7].

The term "giant" or "extreme" ameloblastoma is reserved for lesions that are truly large and that cause gross asymmetry and regional dysfunction. Patients with extreme ameloblastomas are usually from rural areas of developing countries who delay the treatment due to fear of surgery [5]. In the present case, the tumor reached an enormous size over 10 years causing gross facial deformity. Till date, there have been ten reported cases of extreme ameloblastoma (Table 2). The maximum size measured was 17 × 15 × 13 cm reported by Acharya et al. [5] where as present case measured 12 × 9 × 10 cm. All reports were of large tumors involving half of the mandible, and histological diagnosis in these ten cases was either follicular or plexiform type of ameloblastoma [5]. To our knowledge, this is the first reported case of giant granular cell ameloblastoma.

Granular cell change in classic ameloblastoma is a well-recognized phenomenon. There has been considerable interest as to the nature of granular cells in ameloblastoma ever

Table 2: A review of clinical features, tumor size, and histopathological type of giant ameloblastomas that were previously reported and the present case.

| SL. no | Year | Age | Sex | Tumor size | Histopathological type |
|---|---|---|---|---|---|
| 1 | 1977 | 57 | M | Mental region to ramus of mandible | Follicular ameloblastoma |
| 2 | 1977 | 62 | F | Right wisdom tooth to left 1st premolar tooth region | Plexiform ameloblastoma |
| 3 | 1985 | 30 | F | $15 \times 14 \times 12$ cm | Plexiform ameloblastoma |
| 4 | 1990 | 33 | M | Right cuspid tooth to left mandibular condyle | Follicular ameloblastoma |
| 5 | 1991 | 39 | F | $11 \times 10 \times 6$ cm | Plexiform ameloblastoma |
| 6 | 1995 | 73 | M | $11 \times 11 \times 14$ cm | Plexiform ameloblastoma |
| 7 | 1997 | 62 | F | $17 \times 15 \times 13$ cm | Plexiform ameloblastoma |
| 8 | 1999 | 53 | F | $15.2 \times 11.4 \times 12$ cm | Plexiform ameloblastoma |
| 9 | 2005 | 53 | M | $14 \times 11 \times 10$ cm | Follicular ameloblastoma |
| 10 | 2011 | 35 | F | $15 \times 12 \times 10$ cm | Plexiform ameloblastoma |
| 11 | Present case | 39 | F | $12 \times 9 \times 10$ cm | Granular cell ameloblastoma |

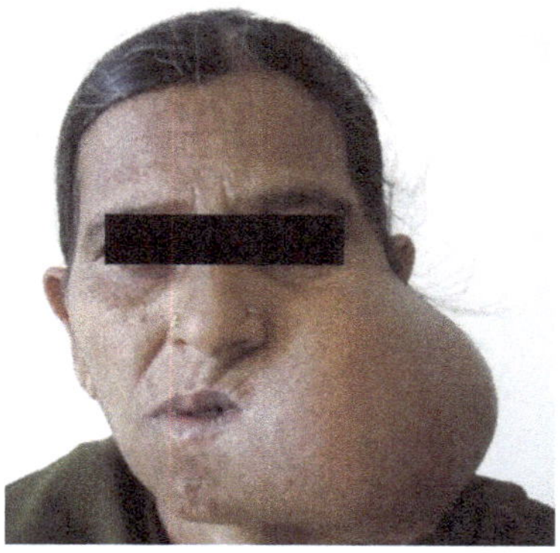

Figure 1: Extra oral examination showed a large well-defined swelling measuring approximately $12 \times 9 \times 10$ cm in the left cheek, mandible and submental region.

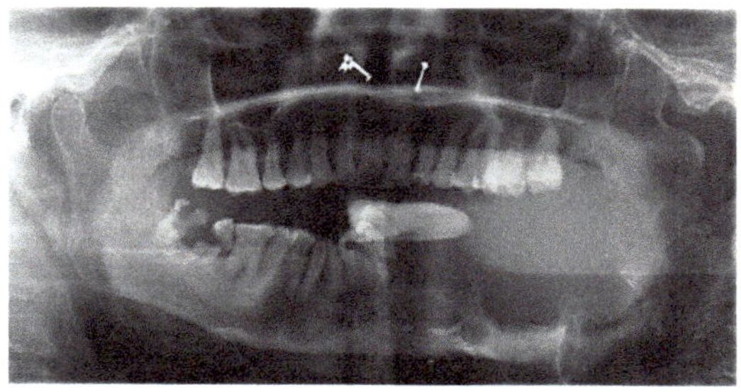

Figure 2: Radiographic examination revealed a multilocular radiolucency, extending from left condyle and coronoid process to right central and lateral incisors with thinning of lower border of mandible.

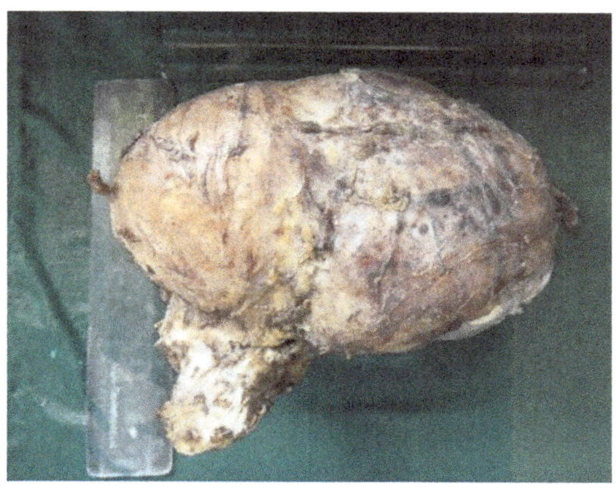

Figure 3: Surgically excised hemimandibulectomy specimen measured $12 \times 9 \times 10$ cm.

since it was recognized. The granular cells acquire small pyknotic nuclei and bulky cytoplasm filled with coarse eosinophilic granules indicating that there is an apoptotic process taking place. Several immunohistochemical studies showed increased apoptotic cells and decreased expression of antiapoptotic factors such as Bcl-2 and p53 proteins in granular cell ameloblastomas [8]. Similarly in the present case, Bcl-2 expression was negative in granular cells.

In granular cell clusters, apoptotic cell fragments with condensed nuclei were phagocytosed by adjacent granular cells and degraded within lysosomes. Therefore, granular cells show positivity for CD-68, lysozyme, and alpha-1-antichymotrypsin indicating cytoplasmic lysosomal aggregates [8]. Similarly in the present case, CD-68 expression was moderate to strong in granular cells.

Cell signaling pathways related to cell proliferation and differentiation are lost or inactive in the granular cells. Hence, the cell signaling molecules such as $\beta$-catenin, BMP-4, and Wnt-2 are altered in granular cells [9]. Similarly in the present case, $\beta$-catenin expression was shown to moderate staining in granular cells. Finally, the immunohistochemical results in the present case highlights that Bcl-2 negativity in granular cells indicating an apoptotic process, CD-68 positivity in granular cells indicating the presence of lysosomal aggregates and $\beta$-catenin cytoplasmic positivity in granular cells indicating an altered cell signaling pathways.

Granular cell ameloblastoma is locally aggressive and has a relatively high chance of recurrence. Recurrence rate for granular cell ameloblastoma was reported to be 33.3%,

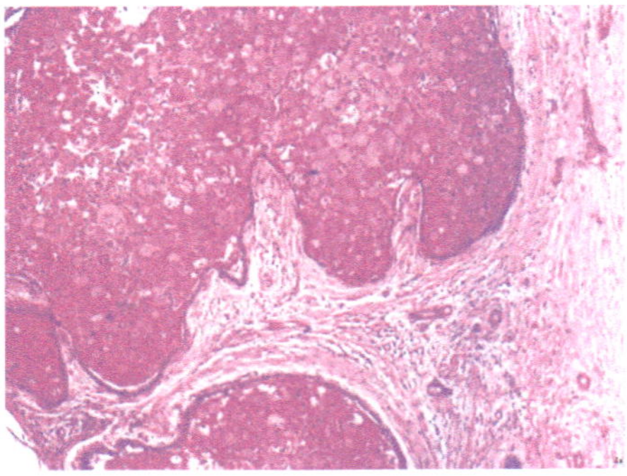

Figure 4: Large odontogenic islands showing peripheral ameloblast-like cells and central stellate reticulum-like cells with extensive granular cell transformation surrounded by fibrous stroma (H and E 20x).

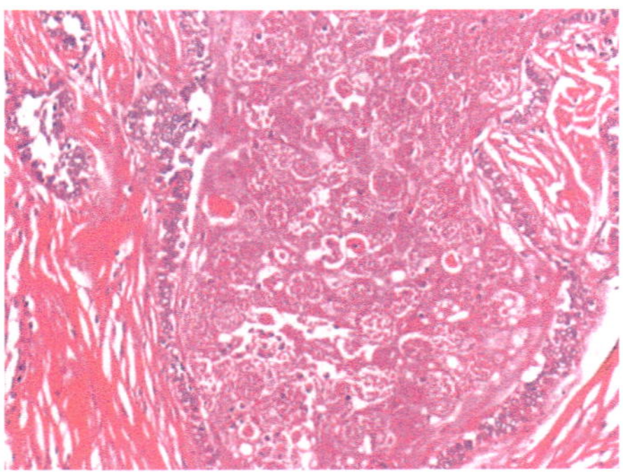

Figure 5: The granular cells exhibited coarsely granular eosinophilic cytoplasm and small pyknotic nuclei (H and E 40x).

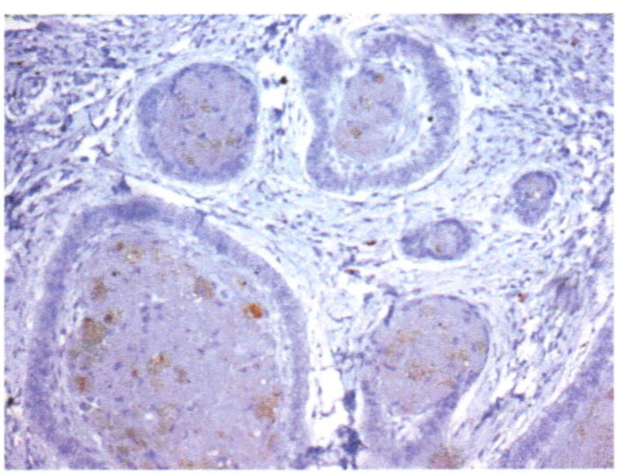

Figure 6: CD-68 showed a moderate to strong staining intensity in granular cells (20x).

which is higher, compared to the more common follicular, plexiform, and acanthomatous subtypes [10]. The present case was followed up for one year and showed no signs of recurrence.

## 6. Conclusion

The present case of giant granular cell ameloblastoma is a rare entity. Development of monstrous size is indicative of

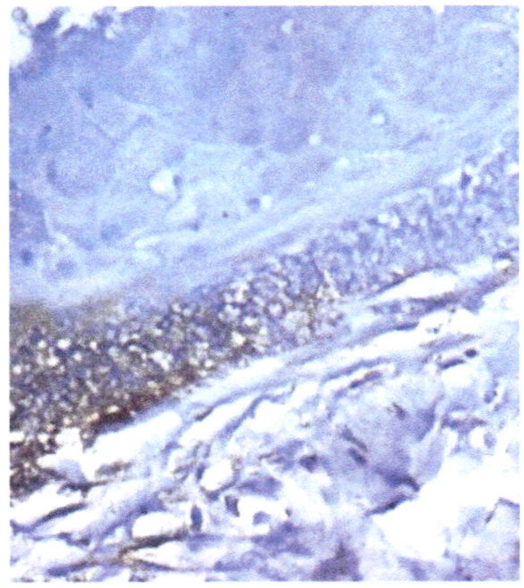

Figure 7: Moderate staining of Bcl-2 was expressed by the peripheral columnar cells of tumor islands and negative in the granular cells (40x).

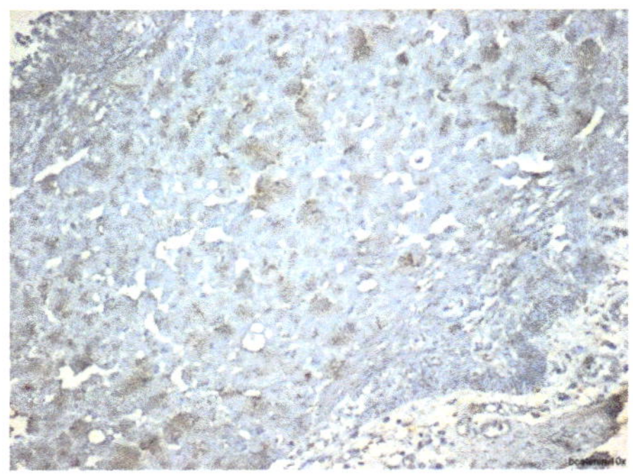

Figure 8: Expression of $\beta$-catenin was generally weak, except for only the focal areas that showed a moderate staining intensity and weak in peripheral cells (20x).

ameloblastomas persistent growth. Granular cell transformation in ameloblastomas probably occurs as a consequence of extensive molecular changes occurring in central stellate reticulum-like cells. Immunohistochemical studies help us to know the pathogenesis of this granular cell ameloblastoma. Therefore, an effort has been made here to study the expression of Bcl-2, CD-68, and $\beta$-catenin. Further studies on a large scale are essential for better understanding of the molecular pathogenesis of ameloblastoma and its subtypes in providing diagnostic and therapeutic benefits.

## References

[1] D. G. Gardner, K. Heikinheimo, M. Shear, H. P. Philipsen, and H. Coleman, "Ameloblastoma," in *World Health Organization Classification of Tumours, Pathology and Genetics of Head and Neck Tumours*, L. Barnes, J. Eveson, P. Reichart, and D. Sidransky, Eds., pp. 296–300, IARC Press, Lyon, France, 2005.

[2] P. Lapthanasupkul, S. Poomsawat, and J. Chindasombatjaroen, "Investigation of basement membrane proteins in a case of granular cell ameloblastoma," *International Journal of Oral Science*, vol. 4, pp. 45–49, 2012.

[3] A. Deshpande, P. Umap, and M. Munshi, "Granular cell ameloblastoma of the jaw: a report of two cases with fine needle aspiration cytology," *Acta Cytologica*, vol. 44, no. 1, pp. 81–85, 2000.

[4] N. Nikitakis, F. Tzerbos, K. Triantafyllou, C. Papadimas, and A. Sklavounou, "Granular cell ameloblastoma: an unusual histological subtype, report and review of literature," *Journal of Oral and Maxillofacial Research*, vol. 4, no. 1, pp. 1–8, 2010.

[5] S. Acharya, A. Joshi, A. Tayaar, and K. Gopalkrishnan, "Extreme ameloblastoma of the mandible with hypoproteinemia. A case report and review of clinicopathological features," *Journal of Clinical and Experimental Dentistry*, vol. 3, no. 4, pp. e343–e347, 2011.

[6] N. Kalavrezos, D. J. Baldwin, and D. M. Walker, "Giant neglected ameloblastoma: single stage treatment and clinicopathological review," *British Journal of Oral and Maxillofacial Surgery*, vol. 46, no. 7, pp. 591–593, 2008.

[7] K. S. Hartman, "Granular cell ameloblastoma. A survey of twenty cases from the Armed Forces Institute of Pathology," *Oral Surgery Oral Medicine and Oral Pathology*, vol. 38, no. 2, pp. 241–253, 1974.

[8] H. Kumamoto and K. Ooya, "Immunohistochemical and ultrastructural investigation of apoptotic cell death in granular cell ameloblastoma," *Journal of Oral Pathology and Medicine*, vol. 30, no. 4, pp. 245–250, 2001.

[9] G. S. A. Sathi, P. P. Han, R. Tamamura et al., "Immunolocalization of cell signaling molecules in the granular cell ameloblastoma," *Journal of Oral Pathology and Medicine*, vol. 36, no. 10, pp. 609–614, 2007.

[10] J. J. V. Pinheiro, V. M. Freitas, A. I. S. Moretti, A. G. Jorge, and R. G. Jaeger, "Local invasiveness of ameloblastoma. Role played by matrix metalloproteinases and proliferative activity," *Histopathology*, vol. 45, no. 1, pp. 65–72, 2004.

# 14

# A Direct Investment Method of Closed Two-Piece Hollow Bulb Obturator

**Suryakant C. Deogade,[1] Sneha S. Mantri,[1] Dinesh Naitam,[2] Gunjan Dube,[3] Pushkar Gupta,[1] and Ashish Dewangan[2]**

[1] *Department of Prosthodontics, Hitkarini Dental College & Hospital, Jabalpur, Madhya Pradesh 482001, India*
[2] *Department of Prosthodontics, Rungta College of Dental Sciences & Research, Bhilai, Chhattisgarh 490024, India*
[3] *Department of Oral Surgery, Hitkarini Dental College & Hospital, Jabalpur, Madhya Pradesh 482001, India*

Correspondence should be addressed to Suryakant C. Deogade; dr_deogade@yahoo.co.in

Academic Editors: R. S. Brown, A. Kasaj, P. Lopez Jornet, and A. Markopoulos

Maxillary defects occur due to surgical treatment of benign and malignant tumors, congenital malformation, and trauma. Prosthetic rehabilitation in such patients is influenced by the size and location of the defect. The most common of all intraoral defects are seen in the maxilla, in the form of an opening into the maxillary sinus and nasopharynx. These defects create disabilities in speech, deglutition, and mastication. The prosthesis which closes such an opening and recreates the functional separation of the oral cavity and sinus and nasal cavities is referred to as an obturator. Numerous techniques of hollow bulb fabrication have been mentioned in the literature from time to time. But there are only a few methods for bulb fabrication in two-piece obturator. This technique describes a direct investment method of waxed-up closed hollow bulb two-piece obturator.

## 1. Introduction

Maxillofacial prosthetics is the branch of prosthodontics concerned with the restoration and/or replacement of the stomatognathic and craniofacial structures with prostheses that may or may not be removed on a regular or elective basis [1]. The most common of all intraoral defects are seen in the maxilla, and it may include hard and soft palate, maxillary sinus, floor of the nasal cavity, and the alveolar ridges [2]. These defects may occur due to surgical resection of benign and malignant tumors, congenital malformation, and trauma [3].

Maxillary intraoral defects due to surgical resection create an open link between the oral and nasal cavities causing difficulty in deglutition, speech, and an unaesthetic appearance. It also results in psychological trauma to the patient [4]. The goals of prosthetic rehabilitation for such patients are to fabricate obturators which separate the nasal and oral cavity and improve deglutition, speech, mastication, and esthetics [2, 3].

An obturator (Latin: obturare, to stop up) is a disc or plate, natural or artificial, which closes an opening or defect of the maxilla as a result of a cleft palate or partial or total removal of the maxilla for a tumor mass [5]. There are numerous techniques described in the literature for the fabrication of open and closed hollow obturators [6–14]. Most of these techniques have their own limitations, such as multiple processing steps while fabrication [15, 16]. All these types of obturators reduce the weight of the prosthesis while properly extending into the defect. Open hollow obturators tend to accumulate nasal secretions leading to odour and added weight [4, 17, 18]. Hence, these require frequent cleaning. Also, it is difficult to polish and clean the internal surface from saliva, mucous crusts, and food accumulation. Where as in closed hollow bulb obturators, pooling of moisture is eliminated. Also, it extends superiorly into the defect, thereby reducing the air space [19].

In this case report, the patient was having severely restricted mouth opening, which required the fabrication of two-piece obturator prosthesis. The fabrication method

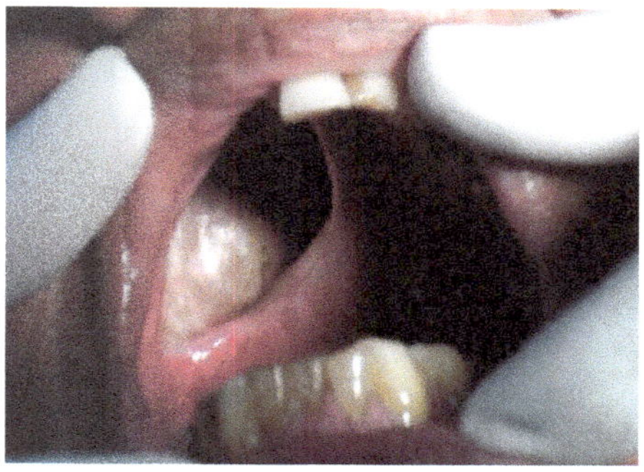

FIGURE 1: Intraoral defect.

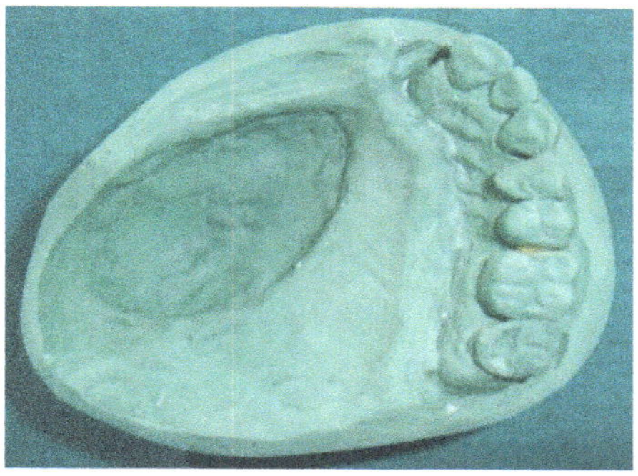

FIGURE 2: Definitive cast.

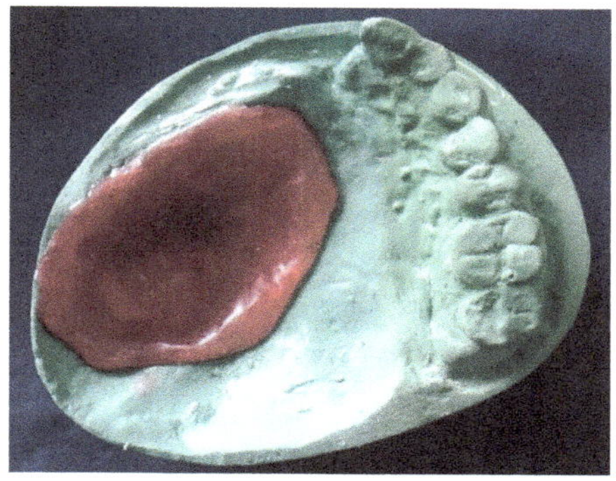

FIGURE 3: Adaptation of a layer of wax.

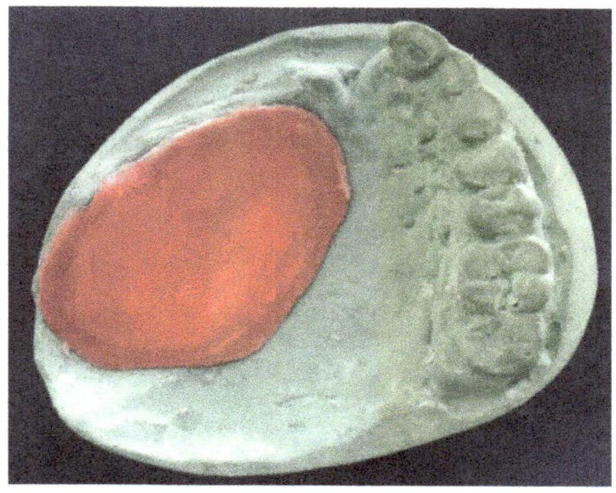

FIGURE 4: Sealed wax lid.

of the two-piece closed hollow bulb obturator with direct investment method is described in this report.

## 2. Case Report

A 70-year old-man was reported to the Department of Prosthodontics, Hitkarini Dental College and Hospital, Jabalpur, India, with a complain of difficulty in speech, deglutition, and mastication. The patient was operated on with maxillectomy to the right side to treat squamous cell carcinoma about four months back. He was wearing on interim obturator prosthesis since four months and demanded a definitive prosthesis. The mouth opening of the patient was severely restricted due to postsurgical scar formation and radiation therapy (Figure 1). Hence, the decision was taken to fabricate a two-piece obturator prosthesis where the obturator was fabricated separately by direct investment technique. Also the magnets were chosen as a method of retention between the obturator and the basic prosthesis. However, only the technique of an obturator fabrication is described.

## 3. Procedure

Preliminary impression of maxillary arch along with defect was made using irreversible hydrocolloid (Dentalgin; Prime Dental Products, Mumbai, India), and the cast was poured with type II gypsum material. After that, the special tray was fabricated with an autopolymerizing acrylic resin (DPI cold cure; Dental Products of India, Mumbai, India), and the definitive impression was made with medium viscosity poly (vinyl siloxane) impression material (Reprosil; DENTSPLY DeTrey GmbH, Konstanz, Germany). All the conventional prosthodontic protocols of boxing and pouring the impression were applied with type III gypsum material (Kalstone; Kalabhai Karson, Mumbai, India) to create a definitive cast (Figure 2). An additional cast was duplicated for the fabrication of closed hollow bulb separately.

The basic prosthesis was fabricated on the master cast by a conventional manner. The procedure of hollow bulb fabrication on the duplicated cast is as follows.

(1) Undercuts in the defect area were blocked out with the plaster of Paris.

(2) A 2 mm thick base plate wax was adapted over the defect area of the duplicated cast (Figure 3).

(3) Then, modeling clay was packed into the defect part, and a tinfoil was kept over it. A 4 mm thick wax lid was adapted on the tinfoil.

(4) After that, already fabricated waxed-up denture was seated over it to maintain the palatal contour. The waxed-up denture was then removed, and the wax lid was sealed on it after removing the clay (Figure 4).

(5) The waxed bulb was then removed carefully, and flasking and dewaxing procedures were completed in a conventional manner (Figures 5, 6, and 7). The mold space was packed with heat-polymerizing acrylic material (DPI, Mumbai, India) (Figure 8).

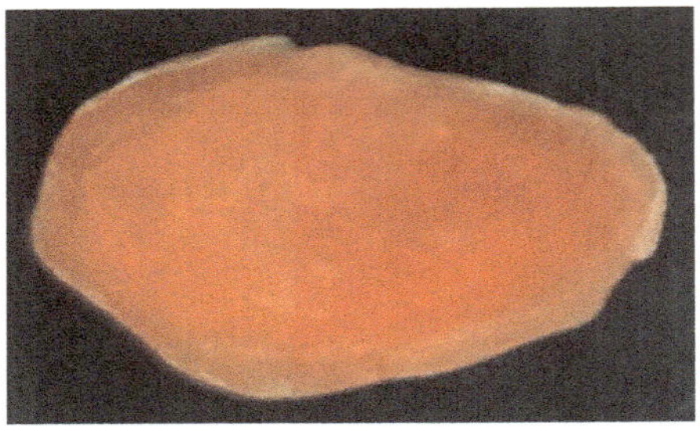

FIGURE 5: Waxed-up bulb.

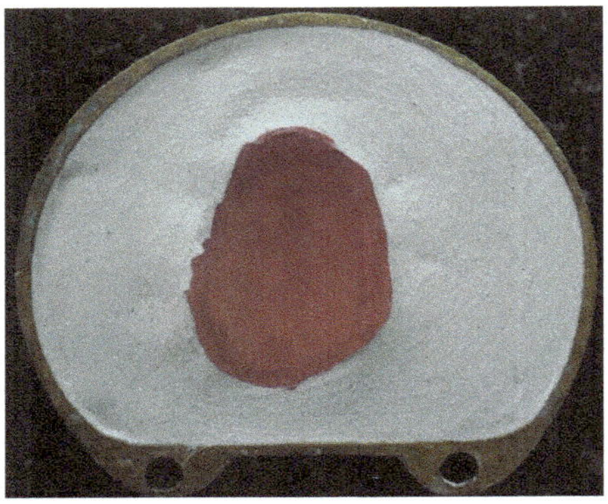

FIGURE 6: Flasking of waxed-up bulb.

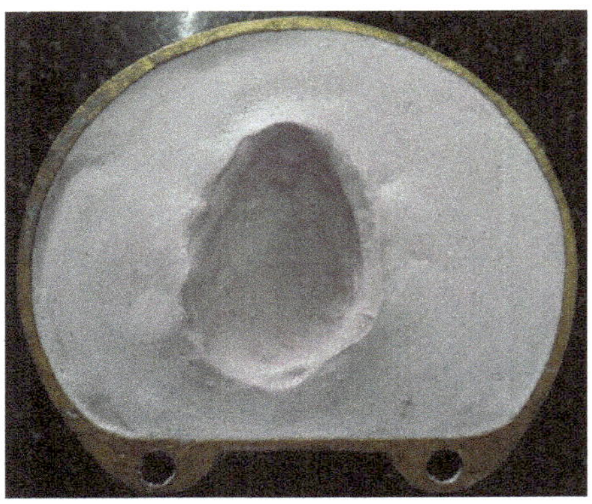

FIGURE 7: Dewaxing of waxed-up bulb.

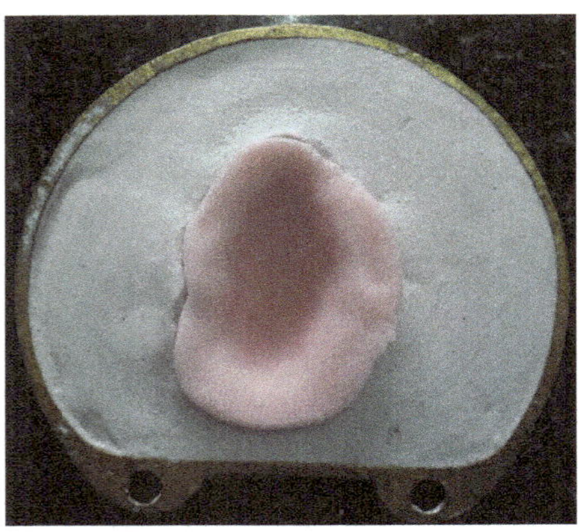

FIGURE 8: Packing with heat-cured PMMA.

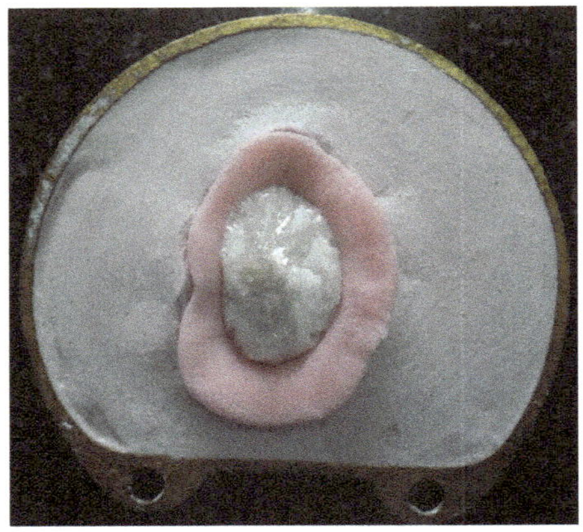

FIGURE 9: A pouch of packed salt.

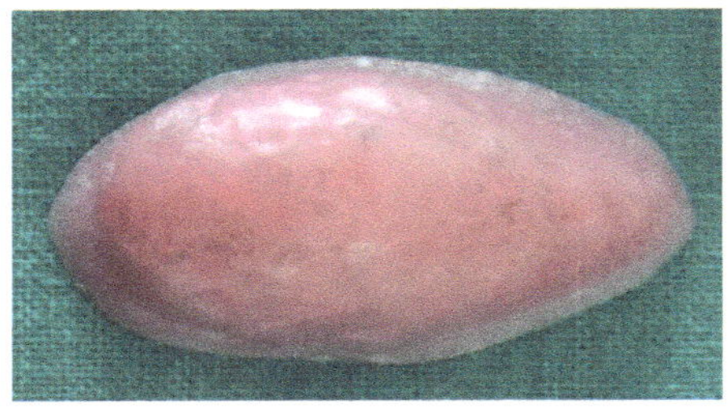

FIGURE 10: Defect side view of bulb.

(6) During packing of material, a pouch of salt was used to hollow the bulb by lost salt technique (Figure 9). Curing procedures were performed according to the manufacturer's instructions.

(7) The cured bulb was then retrieved after deflasking, and the salt was removed after drilling 2 mm holes in the lid portion. The holes were drilled at the future location of magnet attachment.

(8) Then, a pair of commercially available closed-field magnets (Cobalt-Samarium, Ambika Corporation, New Delhi, India), 5 mm in diameter and 2 mm in thickness, was positioned with the help of autopolymerizing acrylic resin, and finishing and polishing were carried out in the conventional manner.

(9) Care was taken not to over thin the bulb, because perforation may occur during the finishing and polishing of the prosthesis.

(10) The finished and polished bulb was then checked on the master cast for its proper fit (Figures 10, 11, and 12). After performing adjustments, the bulb was checked in patient's mouth (Figure 13).

(11) Then the bulb was kept on the cast, and a marking was done on the top portion of magnets with a copying pencil. The finished and polished prosthesis was then tried to seat on the cast. The marks transferred on the tissue surface of the prosthesis determined the position of the countermagnets.

(12) A provision of space was done in the tissue surface of the prosthesis, and the countermagnets were kept

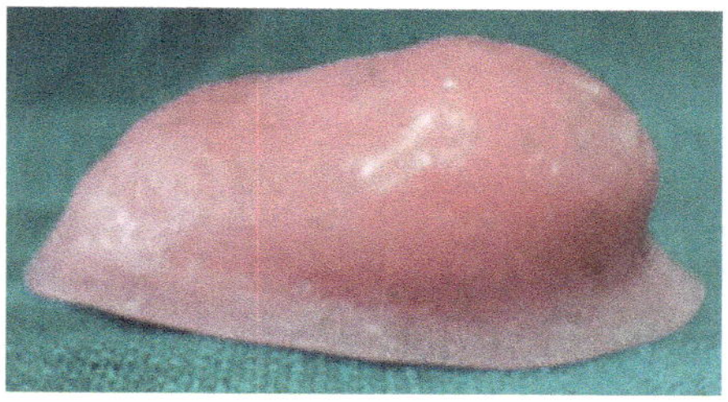

Figure 11: Lateral view of bulb.

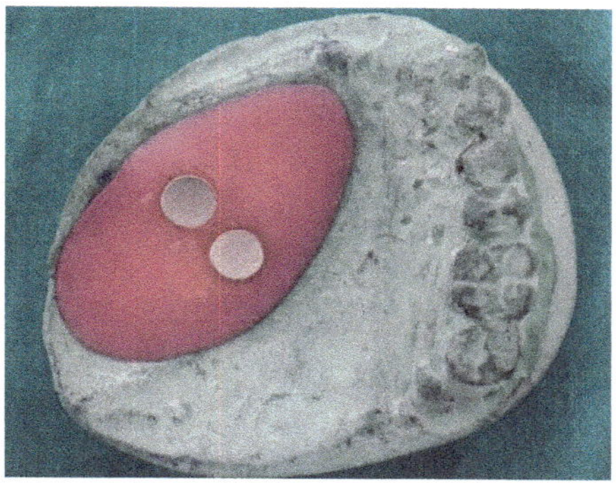

Figure 12: Finished bulb with magnets.

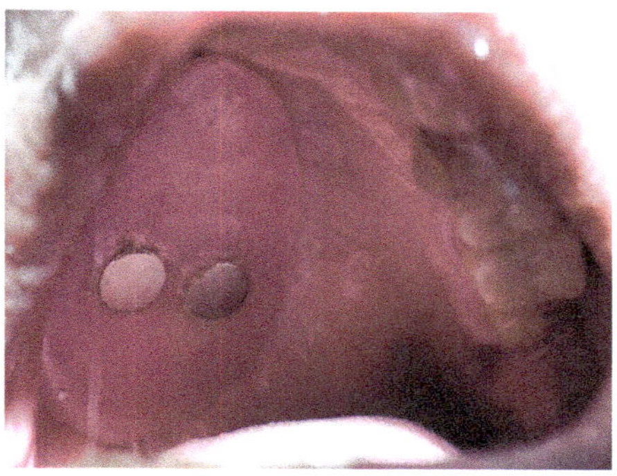

Figure 13: Bulb in patient's mouth.

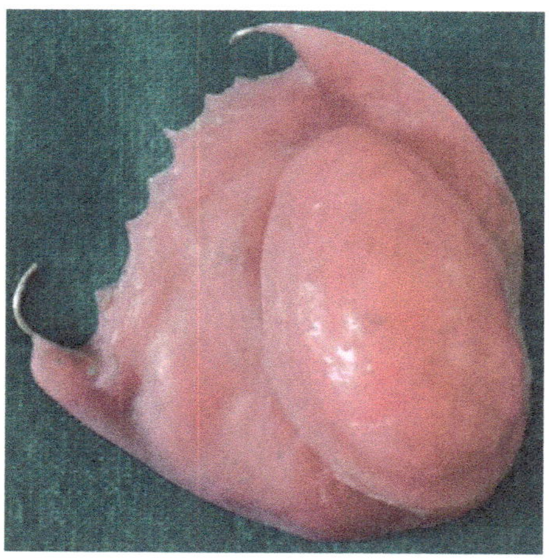

Figure 14: Bulb with prosthesis.

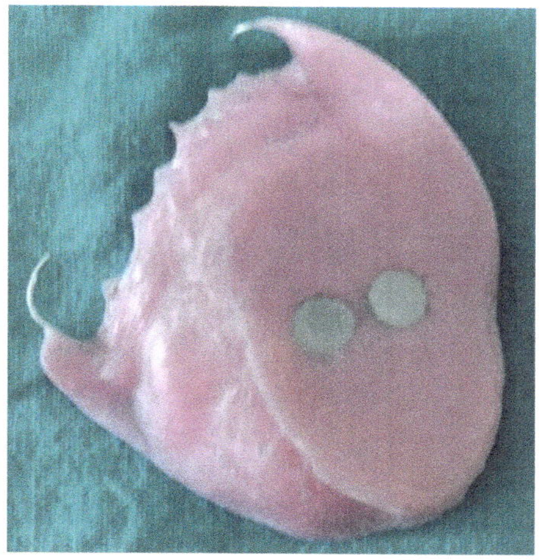

Figure 15: Tissue surface with magnets.

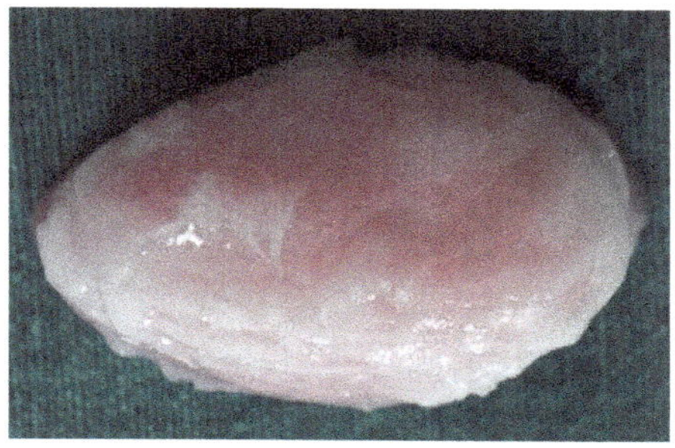

Figure 16: Bulb with soft liner.

over the magnets of the bulb. These were fixed to the prosthesis with the help of self-cure acrylic resin (Figures 14 and 15). After that, a temporary liner (PermaSoft, Soft Denture Liner, DENTSPLY, Austenal) was applied and placed in patient's mouth (Figure 16). After one week, it was replaced with the permanent liner. The patient was educated about positioning, removal, and cleaning of the obturator prosthesis. Patient's demands were fulfilled (Figure 17).

## 4. Discussion

The design and fabrication of the bulb portion is the most important and demanding task for the success of an obturator prosthesis [5, 20]. Numerous articles are mentioned in the literature describing techniques for the fabrication of hollow obturators to lighten the weight of the prostheses. But only few describe the closed hollow bulb in two-pieced obturator prosthesis. A two-piece obturator is given only when the maxillary defect is large with more undercuts, and when the prosthesis is large such that it interferes with its insertion. It is also preferred in those patients who show severely restricted mouth opening due to postsurgical scar formation and radiation therapy [5, 21, 22].

The technique described in this procedure can be applied to complete or partially edentulous patients who have had severely restricted mouth opening. In severe trismus, it

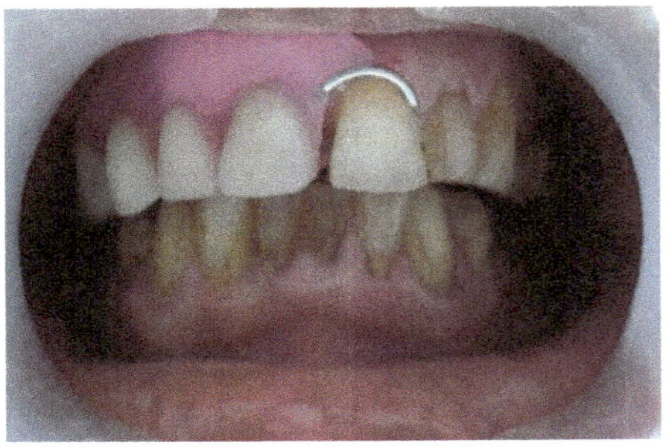

FIGURE 17: Prosthesis in patient's mouth.

becomes very difficult for a patient to insert and remove the prosthesis in a single piece. Hence, it is always better to construct a two-piece obturator for an easy and convenient insertion and removal of prosthesis by the patient. The technique described here utilizes a duplicated cast for the fabrication of bulb separately. The carving and finishing of the waxed-up bulb does not destroy the master cast in this way. Even, the minor adjustment can be done after finishing and polishing the cured bulb. The attachment of retentive means like magnets becomes easy and convenient by this technique. Also, hollowing of the obturator becomes very easy and straightforward. Furthermore, the future relining with permanent soft liner material becomes an easy job.

This technique really works in two-piece obturator due to its ease of fabrication. Even the strength of the bulb is maximized through heat processing of the acrylic resin while minimizing porosity and increasing durability. The thickness of the bulb is easily controlled, which allows for a lightweight prosthesis. The best part of this technique is that the accuracy is assured.

## 5. Conclusion

The hollow bulb obturator given to the patient rehabilitated his function by improving masticatory efficiency and phonetics by adding resonance to the voice. Thus, it improved the clarity of speech and the esthetics of the patient. It improved the comfort of the patient by decreasing the weight of the prosthesis. The two-piece prosthesis was easily tolerated by the patient and made convenient in terms of easy insertion and removal of the prosthesis.

Simplicity of fabrication and assurance of accuracy are the basic advantages of this technique. The technique provides control of the thickness of the hollow bulb, subsequently reducing the overall weight. Patient's functional and esthetic requirements were fulfilled satisfactorily. It improved the morale of the patient greatly.

## References

[1] "Glossary of posthodontic terms," *Journal of Prosthetic Dentistry*, vol. 94, pp. 10–92, 2005.

[2] K. S. McAndrew, S. Rothenberger, and G. E. Minsley, "An innovative investment method for the fabrication of a closed hollow obturator prosthesis," *The Journal of Prosthetic Dentistry*, vol. 80, no. 1, pp. 129–132, 1998.

[3] G. E. Minsley, D. W. Warren, and V. Hinton, "Physiologic responses to maxillary resection and subsequent obturation," *The Journal of Prosthetic Dentistry*, vol. 57, no. 3, pp. 338–344, 1987.

[4] T. D. Taylor, *Clinical Maxillofacial Prosthetics*, Quintessence Publishing, 2000.

[5] V. A. Chalian, J. B. Drane, and S. M. Standish, *Maxillofacial Prosthetics. Multidisciplinary Practice*, The Williams & Wilkins, Baltimore, Md, USA, 1971.

[6] R. P. Desjardins, "Obturator prosthesis design for acquired maxillary defects," *The Journal of Prosthetic Dentistry*, vol. 39, no. 4, pp. 424–435, 1978.

[7] V. Matalon and H. LaFuente, "A simplified method for making a hollow obturator," *The Journal of Prosthetic Dentistry*, vol. 36, no. 5, pp. 580–582, 1976.

[8] A. Schneider, "Method of fabricating a hollow obturator," *The Journal of Prosthetic Dentistry*, vol. 40, no. 3, p. 351, 1978.

[9] Y. Tanaka, H. O. Gold, and S. Pruzansky, "A simplified technique for fabricating a lightweight obturator," *The Journal of Prosthetic Dentistry*, vol. 38, no. 6, pp. 638–642, 1977.

[10] B. H. Habib and C. F. Driscoll, "Fabrication of a closed hollow obturator," *Journal of Prosthetic Dentistry*, vol. 91, no. 4, pp. 383–385, 2004.

[11] P. G. Patil and S. P. Patil, "Fabrication of a hollow obturator as a single unit for management of bilateral subtotal maxillectomy," *Journal of Prosthodontics*, vol. 21, no. 3, pp. 194–199, 2012.

[12] S. Elangovan and E. Loibi, "Two-piece hollow bulb obturator," *Indian Journal of Dental Research*, vol. 22, no. 3, pp. 486–488, 2011.

[13] T. V. Padmanabhan, V. A. Kumar, K. K. Mohamed, and N. Unnikrishnan, "Prosthetic rehabilitation of a maxillectomy with a two-piece hollow bulb obturator. A clinical report," *Journal of Prosthodontics*, vol. 20, no. 5, pp. 397–401, 2011.

[14] V. I. Shambharkar, S. B. Puri, and P. G. Patil, "A simple technique to fabricate a surgical obturator restoring the defect in original anatomical form," *Journal of Advanced Prosthodontics*, vol. 3, pp. 106–109, 2011.

[15] M. Al-Athel, R. Jagger, and D. Jagger, "Effect of ageing on the bond strength of a permanent denture soft lining material," *Journal of Oral Rehabilitation*, vol. 29, no. 10, pp. 992–996, 2002.

[16] S. M. Ortegon, J. W. Martin, and J. S. Lewin, "A hollow delayed surgical obturator for a bilateral subtotal maxillectomy patient: a clinical report," *Journal of Prosthetic Dentistry*, vol. 99, no. 1, pp. 14–18, 2008.

[17] P. Phankosol and J. W. Martin, "Hollow obturator with removable lid," *The Journal of Prosthetic Dentistry*, vol. 54, no. 1, pp. 98–100, 1985.

[18] B. Rilo, J. L. Dasilva, I. Ferros, M. J. Mora, and U. Santana, "A hollow-bulb interim obturator for maxillary resection. A case report," *Journal of Oral Rehabilitation*, vol. 32, no. 3, pp. 234–236, 2005.

[19] B. H. Habib and C. F. Driscoll, "Fabrication of a closed hollow obturator," *Journal of Prosthetic Dentistry*, vol. 91, no. 4, pp. 383–385, 2004.

[20] F. Keyf, "Obturator prostheses for hemimaxillectomy patients," *Journal of Oral Rehabilitation*, vol. 28, no. 9, pp. 821–829, 2001.

[21] R. P. Desjardins, "Obturator prosthesis design for acquired maxillary defects," *The Journal of Prosthetic Dentistry*, vol. 39, no. 4, pp. 424–435, 1978.

[22] V. A. Chalian and M. O. Barnett, "A new technique for constructing a one-piece hollow obturator after partial maxillectomy," *The Journal of Prosthetic Dentistry*, vol. 28, no. 4, pp. 448–453, 1972.

# 15

# Surgical Orthodontic Treatment of Severe Skeletal Class II

**Fahad F. Alsulaimani,[1] Maisa O. Al-Sebaei,[2] and Ahmed R. Afify[1]**

[1] *Orthodontic Division, Department of Preventive Dental Sciences, Faculty of Dentistry, King Abdul-Aziz University, Jeddah, Saudi Arabia*
[2] *Oral and Maxillofacial Surgery Department, Faculty of Dentistry, King Abdul-Aziz University, Jeddah, Saudi Arabia*

Correspondence should be addressed to Fahad F. Alsulaimani; fahad_alsulaimani@yahoo.com

Academic Editors: I. Anic and G. Gómez-Moreno

This paper describes an adult Saudi male patient who presented with a severe skeletal class II deformity. The case was managed with a combination of presurgical orthodontic treatment followed by a double jaw orthognathic surgery and then another phase of orthodontic treatment for final occlusal detailing. Extraction of the four first premolars was done during the presurgical orthodontic phase of treatment to decompensate upper and lower incisors and to give room for surgical setback of the maxillary anterior segment. Double jaw surgery was performed: bilateral sagittal split ramus osteotomy for 8 mm mandibular advancement combined with three-piece Le Fort I maxillary osteotomy, 6 mm setback of the anterior segment, 8 mm impaction of the maxilla, and 5 mm advancement genioplasty. Although the anteroposterior discrepancy and the facial convexity were so severe, highly acceptable results were obtained, both esthetically as well as occlusally.

## 1. Introduction

Orthognathic surgery is considered for the treatment of dentofacial skeletal deformities for more than 100 years ago. Interestingly, the first jaw deformity correction was performed without anesthesia in the United States by Simon Hullihen, an American general surgeon, in the mid of the 19th century.

Dentofacial skeletal deformities always cause severe functional and esthetic problems to the patient. In adult severe cases, the combined approach, orthodontic and orthognathic surgery, is always the treatment of choice, and the results obtained usually ensure a better esthetic, functional, and stable results [1–5].

Class II skeletal deformity is characterized by an exaggerated sagittal distance between the maxilla and the mandible, which could be the result of maxillary prognathism, mandibular retrognathism, or both.

Presurgical orthodontic decompensation is essential to enable the surgeon to make a considerable amount of surgical correction, otherwise the esthetic and functional outcome of the entire procedure will not be that ideal [1–3].

## 2. Case Report

A 21-year-old Saudi male was referred to the orthodontic clinic, Faculty of Dentistry, King Abdul-Aziz University for the treatment of “Bothering anterior teeth.” At the first consultation visit, the patient expressed his great concerns about his anterior teeth in addition to his severely retruded chin. His medical history was nonrelevant except for a scar resulting from closure of an upper-left unilateral cleft lip.

The clinical examination of the patient revealed a severe skeletal class II pattern with a severe mandibular retrognathism. The frontal facial view showed a mesofacial pattern, slightly deviated nose to the right, an excessive lower face height, and an interlabial gap of 21 mm. The interpupillary line was parallel to the occlusal plan, and the lips were incompetent at rest with the lower lip resting behind the upper incisors. At rest, there is a 10 mm incisal show in addition to 4 mm of the gum. The lips are incompetent at rest with a short upper lip, while the lower lip is resting behind the upper incisors. The upper midline is deviated to the right by 3 mm. Upon smiling, there was a severe gingival show around 12 mm. The lateral view of the face revealed an average nose, a normal nasolabial angle, a convex profile,

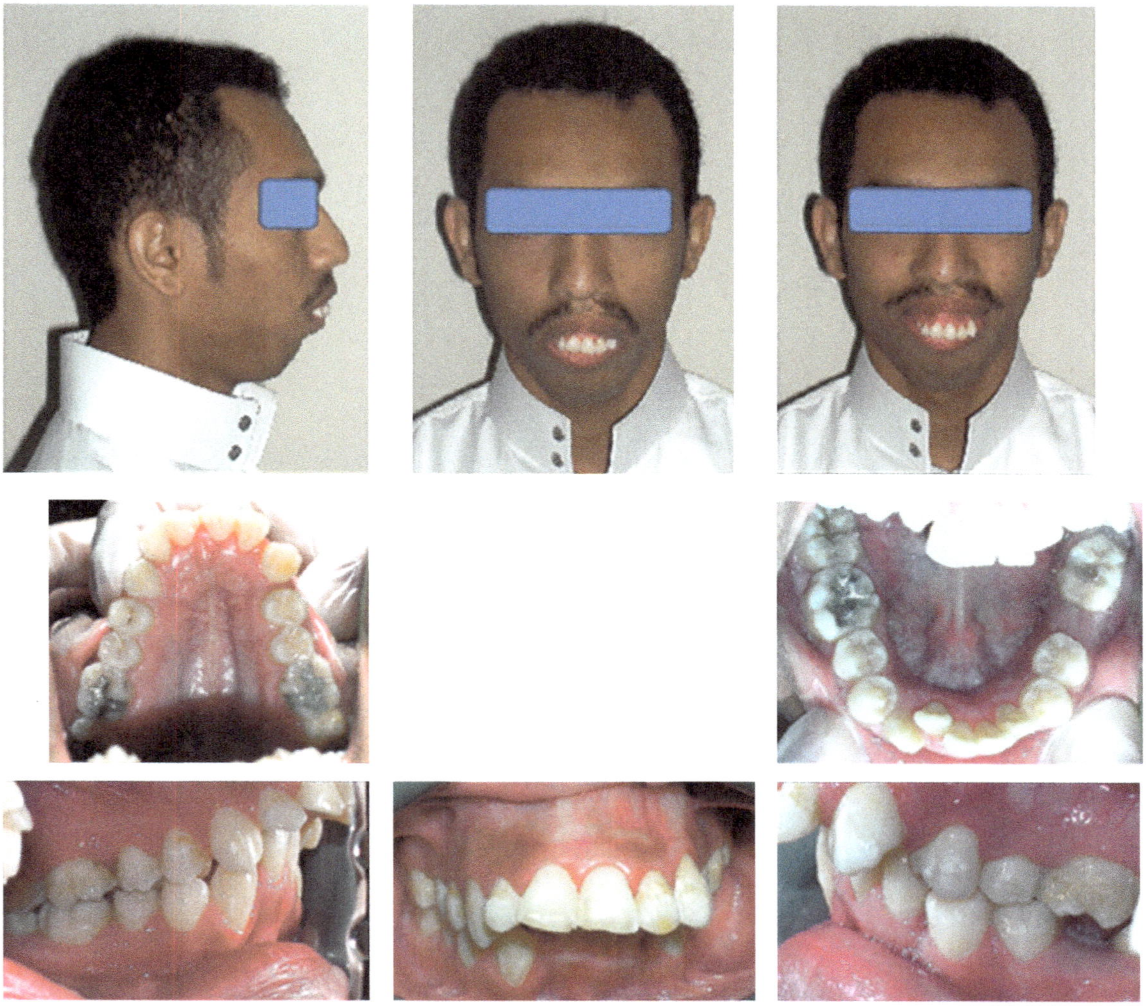

FIGURE 1: Pretreatment extraoral and intraoral photographs.

a severe mandibular retrognathism, a severely deficient chin (Figure 1).

Intraoral photographs reveal a class II molar and canine relation on the right side, while on the left side it is undetermined due to the missing lower left first permanent molar. The upper arch is V shaped, while the lower arch is U shaped. There is around 5 mm lower anterior crowding, meanwhile there is around 6 mm anterior spacing in the upper arch. There is an excessive overjet, almost 15 mm. There is an exaggerated lower curve of Spee causing an impinging overbite with markedly distinct occlusal planes in the anterior and posterior segments (Figure 2).

Radiographically, the panoramic view revealed a normal bony trabeculation, the full number of permanent teeth except for an extracted lower-left first molar, and impacted upper and lower third molars. Cephalometric analysis revealed that the patient had a severe skeletal class II, and the ANB angle was 16° which is more resorted to the lower jaw. Upper incisor position was proclined and protruded, while the lower incisors were more severely proclined and protruded. Vertically, the patient had an increased lower face height. The chin was markedly deficient (Table 1).

After a complete diagnosis of the case, the patient was informed by the detailed treatment plan, and it was explained to the patient that the presurgical orthodontic preparation "decompensation" of the dentition will worsen the deformity and that the malocclusion, facial profile, and speech will be temporarily worsened. The patient was further informed that this presurgical treatment only improves the bony support for the teeth, and all the facial and profile changes will result after the upcoming surgical procedures.

## 3. Diagnosis

*3.1. Treatment Objectives.* The treatment objectives were to improve the patient's facial esthetics: patient's facial profile, mandibular retrognathism, increased lower third of the face, gummy smile, incompetent lips, dental midline shift, and normalizing the overbite and overjet.

*3.2. Treatment Plan.* Presurgical orthodontic phase aimed to decompensate upper and lower incisors via extraction of the four first premolars. Anchorage was maximized in the upper

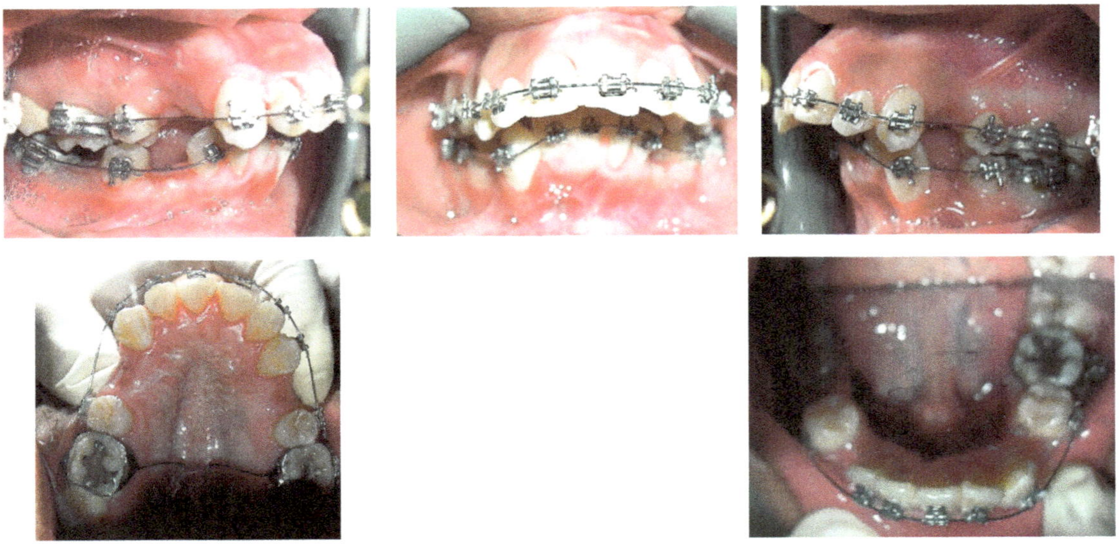

FIGURE 2: Presurgical intraoral photographs.

TABLE 1: Cephalometric analysis.

| Area of study | Measurement | Mean | Pretreatment | Posttreatment |
|---|---|---|---|---|
| Sagittal relationship | SNA | 82° | 87° | 84° |
| | SNB | 80° | 71° | 75° |
| | ANB | 2° | 16° | 9° |
| | N Pg/FH | 87° | 73° | 86° |
| | Wits appraisal | −1–0 mm | 26 mm | 5 mm |
| | Pg to NB dist. | 2-3 mm | 0 mm | 3 mm |
| Vertical relationship (divergency) | Mand. Pl. to FH | 25° | 39° | 33° |
| | Mand. Pl. to SN | 32° | 48° | 45° |
| | *Y* axis S Gn/SN | 60°–66° | 77° | 63° |
| | Lower face height | 64 mm | 85 mm | 74 mm |
| Dental relationship (incisor position) | U Inc. to SN | 103° | 119° | 109° |
| | U Inc. to NA | 22° | 32° | 25° |
| | U Inc. to NA dist. | 4 mm | 6 mm | 3 mm |
| | U Inc. to L Inc. | 130°–132° | 86° | 109° |
| | L Inc. to Mand. | 90° | 105° | 95° |
| | L Inc. to NB | 25° | 44° | 36° |
| | L Inc. to NB dist. | 4 mm | 10 mm | 10 mm |
| Soft tissue relationship | Upper lip to E-line | −4 mm | 9.3 mm | 3.8 mm |
| | Lower lip to E-line | −2 mm | 7 mm | 0 mm |
| | Nasolabial angle | 90°–110° | 77° | 93° |

arch through the use of transpalatal arch (TPA) in addition to including the upper second molars.

### *3.3. Treatment Progress*

*3.3.1. Presurgical Orthodontic Treatment.* In general, the goal of presurgical orthodontics is to position the teeth, allowing an optimal surgical correction of the jaw bones. This will make the malocclusion look worse presurgically, but it will show the true entity of the skeletal problem, thus facilitating an optimal surgery [4]. Our aims from the presurgical treatment were to decompensate the upper and lower incisors and to level and align both arches and relief of crowding in the lower arch. Upper and lower first premolars were extracted to get space for retracting the lower incisors, alleviation of lower arch crowding, uprighting the upper incisors, and severing dental class II relation. The patient received 0.018-inch Roth edgewise appliance. Initial leveling was accomplished with 0.016-inch nickel-titanium (Ni-Ti) arch wires. Anchorage was maximized in the maxillary arch by inserting a TPA in addition to bonding the 2nd molars. After initial leveling and alignment, the upper and lower cuspids were retracted; lower

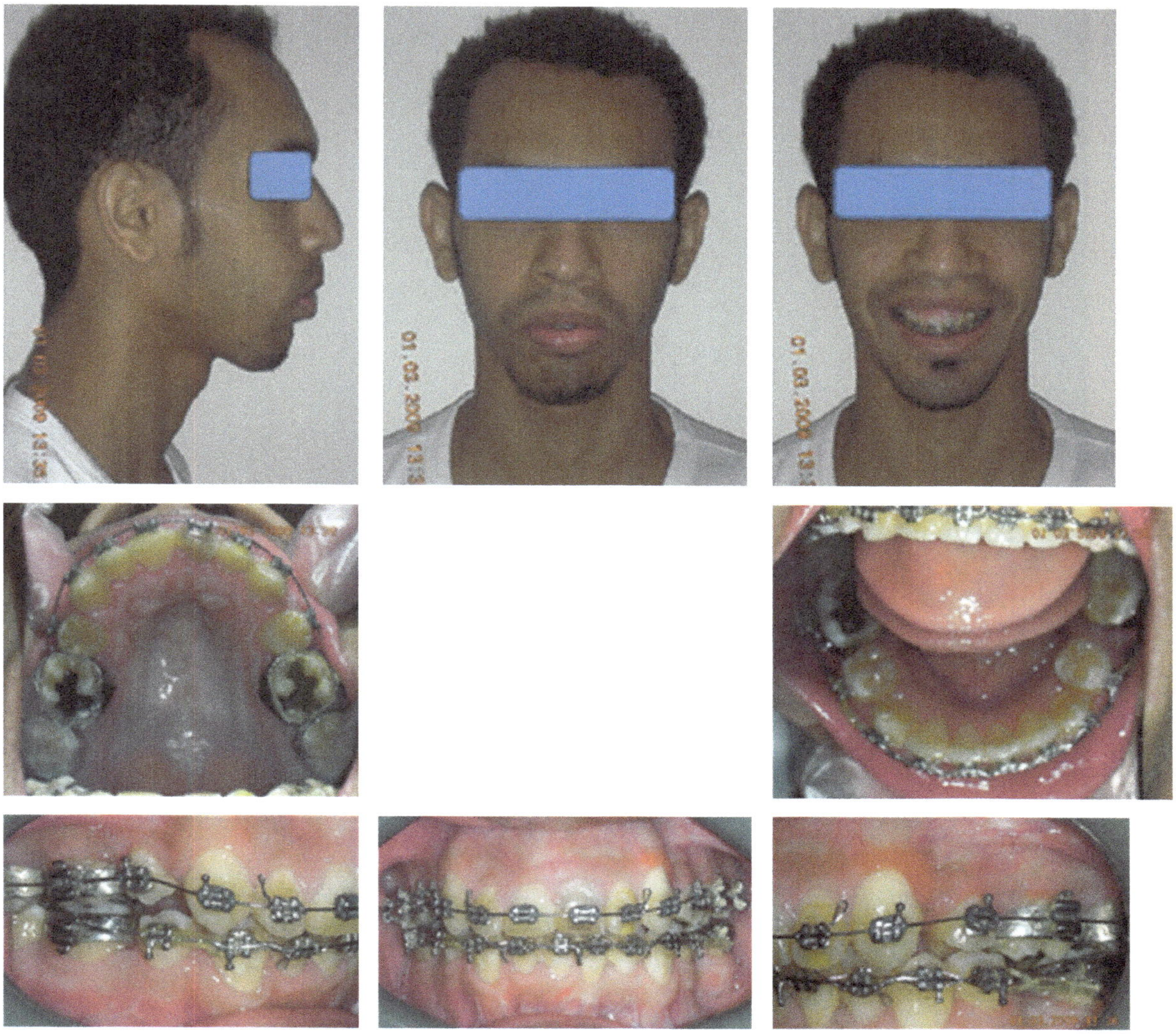

FIGURE 3: Postsurgical extraoral and intraoral photographs.

incisors were decompensated, and a space left in the upper premolars area for anterior maxillary was set back.

### 3.3.2. Orthognathic Surgery

*Preoperative Surgical Planning.* Upper and lower impressions were taken, and study casts were prepared. The models were mounted on a semi-adjustable articulator using a face-bow transfer. A full orthognathic model surgery was performed. Final and intermediate splints were fabricated using orthodontic cold-cure resin.

*Surgery.* A standard bilateral sagittal split incision was performed, and the medial aspect of the mandible was exposed. After identifying and protecting the inferior alveolar neurovascular bundle, a bilateral sagittal split osteotomy was performed with a surgical saw.

A standard Le Fort I incision was performed in the mucosa. This was followed by a Le Fort I osteotomy using a surgical saw. The maxilla was downfractured and mobilized. A 3-piece maxillary osteotomy was performed using the surgical saw followed by a thin osteotome by cutting bilaterally in the mesial and distal of the extraction socket of the upper first bicuspid. A strip of bone measuring 6 mm was removed from each side. This was done to facilitate the posterior repositioning of the anterior segment of the maxilla.

The maxillary segments were aligned and positioned in the intermediate splint. The patient's occlusion was placed into the intermediate splint, and the patient was placed in an intermaxillary fixation with wires and elastics. The maxilla was fixated in the new position using mini titanium alloy plates and 2.0 screws in the areas of the pyriform rim and maxillary buttress. The intermaxillary fixation and intermediate splint were removed.

Attention was then drawn back to the mandible where the bilateral sagittal split osteotomy was completed, the mandible was advanced to 8 mm, and the patient was placed in proper occlusion using the final splint. The mandible was fixated

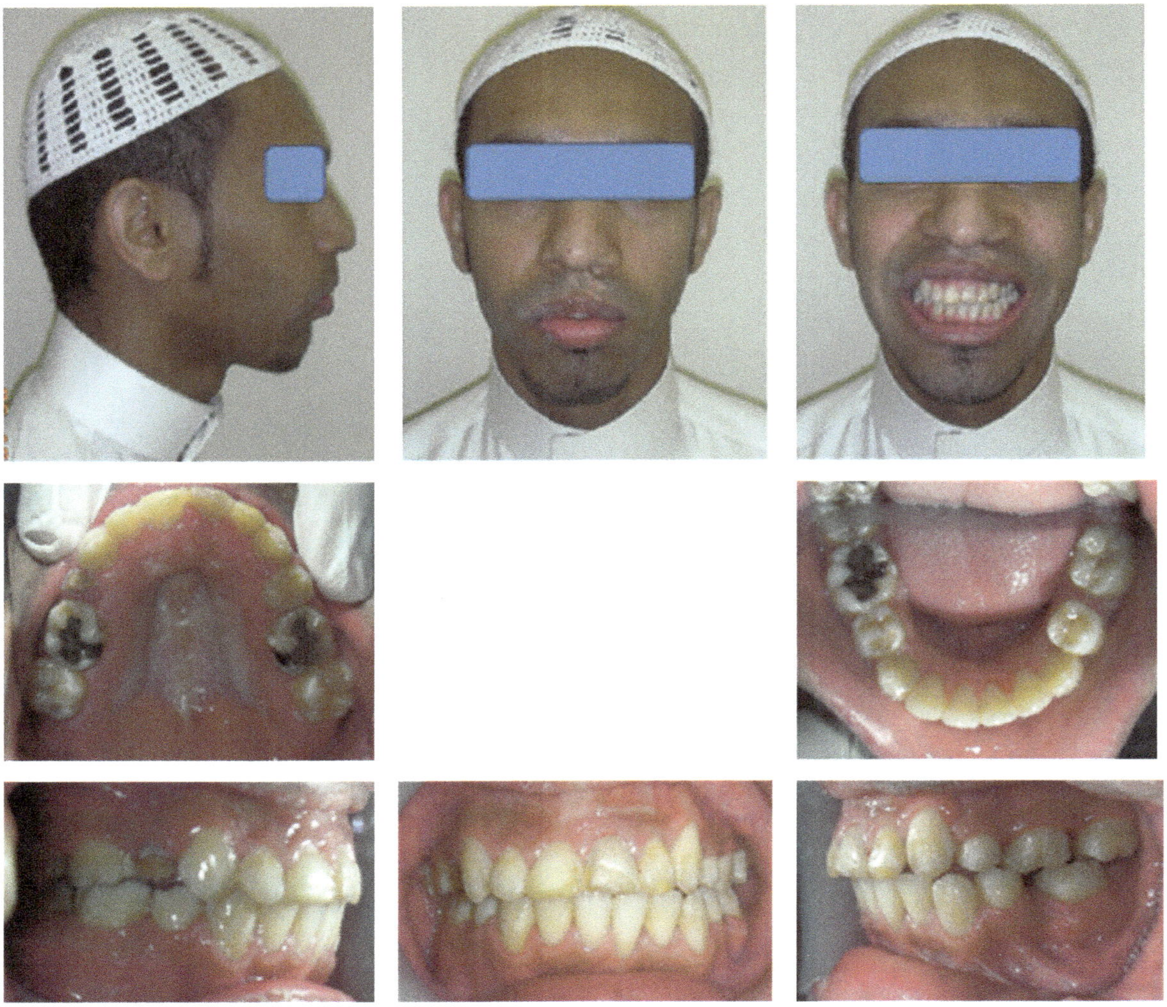

FIGURE 4: Posttreatment extraoral and intraoral photographs.

using mini titanium plates and 2.0 screws. The intermaxillary fixation was removed, and the occlusion was checked to be as predetermined in the model surgery preoperatively. The occlusion was passive and reproducible. An anterior 5 mm advancement genioplasty was performed. The intermaxillary fixation was placed again using elastics.

*Postoperative Care*. The wound was checked daily for one week for signs of ischemia. The splint was kept in place for 4 weeks, and the patient was placed on a liquid and pureed diet and sinus precautions. The splint was removed in the clinic, and the occlusion was checked. It was stable and reproducible.

*3.3.3. Postsurgical Orthodontic Treatment*. Postsurgical orthodontics was continued after surgery to close minor spaces distal to the cuspids in the upper and lower arches. The goals of this phase of treatment were to rehabilitate and restore the neuromuscular function and get final occlusal settling. Occlusal function and settling was greatly improved through the use of intermaxillary elastics. Occlusal selective grinding was also done to finalize the occlusion. The postsurgical phase of orthodontic treatment continued for 8 months (see Figure 3).

## 4. Results

Both the gummy smile and lips incompetence were greatly improved. The patient profile showed a marked improvement.

Although the occlusion and facial esthetics were greatly improved, the results were not that perfect. The patient started to develop some carious lesions. In addition to this, the patient started to feel distressed due to the lengthy treatment time. That is why we decided to debond, although the results were less than ideal, to enhance both the dental brushing as well as the fast psychological adaptation (see Figure 4).

## 5. Discussion

The surgical correction of such severe dentofacial deformities is a functional and esthetic surgery that affects patients'

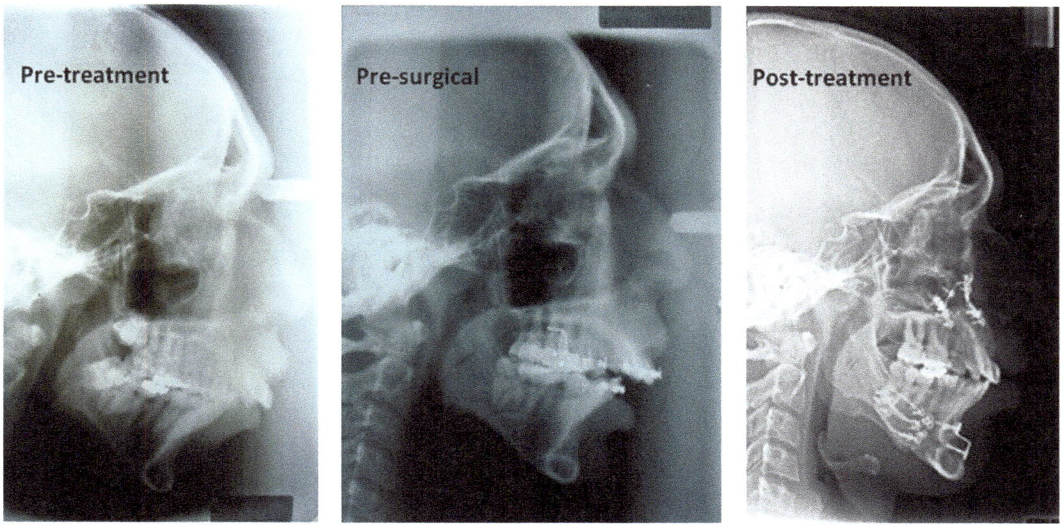


(a) (b) (c)

FIGURE 5: Pretreatment, presurgical and posttreatment lateral cephalograms.

self-perception. The patient appreciated the improvement in his facial appearance after orthognathic surgery that was associated with a noted improvement in his psychosocial adjustments.

Although there is new trends in the management of skeletal dentofacial deformities to start surgery then proceed the postsurgical phase of orthodontic treatment, we still believe in the presurgical orthodontic preparation as it adapts the occlusion greatly to the new postsurgical position and consequently a better opportunity for a more stable occlusion. Those who believe in starting with surgery are concerned about the severity of deterioration of both the facial profile and function during the period of presurgical orthodontics (see Figure 5).

Orthognathic surgery is only one part of the process to correct a dentofacial deformity. The process starts with the initial diagnosis, followed by a treatment plan, and then patient consent. Treatment generally begins with a dental assessment to correct decay, followed by orthodontic decompensation in preparation for surgical intervention. Orthognathic surgery is followed by postoperative orthodontia to maximize the occlusal relationship.

## References

[1] P. M. Sinclair, "Orthodontic considerations in adult surgical orthodontic cases," *Dental Clinics of North America*, vol. 32, no. 3, pp. 509–528, 1988.

[2] K. Dryland Vig and E. Ellis, "Diagnosis and treatment planning for the surgical-orthodontic patient," *Clinics in Plastic Surgery*, vol. 16, no. 4, pp. 645–658, 1989.

[3] W. W. Neeley, C. Dolce, J. P. Hatch, J. E. Van Sickels, and J. D. Rugh, "Relationship of body mass index to stability of mandibular advancement surgery with rigid fixation," *American Journal of Orthodontics and Dentofacial Orthopedics*, vol. 136, no. 2, pp. 175–184, 2009.

[4] R. Sabri, "Orthodontic objectives in orthognathic surgery: state of the art today," *World Journal of Orthodontics*, vol. 7, no. 2, pp. 177–191, 2006.

[5] T. Kitahara, A. Nakasima, S. Kurahara, and Y. Shiratsuchi, "Hard and soft tissue stability of orthognathic surgery," *Angle Orthodontist*, vol. 79, no. 1, pp. 158–165, 2009.

# Odontogenic Fibromyxoma of Maxilla: A Rare Case Report

**G. Siva Prasad Reddy,[1] B. Surya Kumar,[2] Radhika Muppa,[3] Shravan Kumar Regonda,[1] and Harish Kumar TVS[1]**

[1] *Department of Oral and Maxillofacial Surgery, Panineeya Institute of Dental Sciences, Road No. 5, Kamala Nagar, Dilsukhnagar, Hyderabad, Andhra Pradesh 500060, India*
[2] *Department of Dental Surgery, Mediciti Hospital, Near Secretariate, Hyderabad, India*
[3] *Department of Pedodontics, Panineeya Institute of Dental Sciences, Hyderabad, India*

Correspondence should be addressed to G. Siva Prasad Reddy; gspreddy@yahoo.com

Academic Editors: A. Epivatianos, C. S. Farah, and L. J. Oesterle

Fibromyxoma is a rare odontogenic tumour which is benign, but locally aggressive. The etiology of these tumours is unknown, but because of its limitation to the teeth bearing areas and occasional presence of odontogenic epithelial fragments within the tumour which suggest that it is of odontogenic origin. It is a slow growing painless tumour that frequently occurs in second and third decades of life. Females are more commonly affected than males. The tumour can cause gradual expansion of the cortical plates and cause loosening and displacement of teeth, although root resorption may be rare. The surgical treatment of these tumours consists of complete enucleation or radical excision. The aim of this paper is to present the rarity of a fibromyxoma of the maxilla.

## 1. Introduction

Fibromyxoma is a benign tumour of ectomesenchymal origin with or without odontogenic epithelium [1]. The term myxoma was first used by Virchow in 1863, but the term fibromyxoma was described by Dietrich et al. [2]. The tumour occurs in soft and bony tissues. Earlier, the bone myxomas were subclassified into osteogenic and odontogenic entities [3]. Myxomas can be found in heart, skin, and subcutaneous tissue and centrally in the bone, but myxomas of the jaws are encountered rarely. It accounts for only 1% to 3% of all cysts and tumors of the jaws [4]. Mandible is more frequently affected than the maxilla. They frequently occur in 2nd and 3rd decades of life. Females are more commonly affected than males. Some studies reveal a lack of sex predilection and equal frequency of the maxillary and mandibular involvements [5]. The myxomas usually appear as solitary growths, and they are extremely rare in children under the age of 12 years [6]. The size of the tumour varies, and it may reach up to 4 cm in diameter. Small myxomas are treated conservatively with curettage followed by cauterization. Larger tumours may require extensive resection, as recurrence rates as high as 25% have been reported. Fibromyxoma of the jaw appears to have a better prognosis than does fibromyxoma occurring in the long bones of the skeleton.

## 2. Case Report

A 12-year-old female patient visited our unit with a chief complaint of swelling on left side of the face since 6 months. Extraoral examination revealed diffuse swelling over the left cheek involving lateral part of the nose and infraorbital region (Figure 1). Skin over the swelling was normal without any tenderness or surface discolouration. Intraoral examination revealed a firm to hard swelling with buccal cortical plate expansion in relation to left upper canine-premolar region. Mucosa over the swelling was normal without any draining sinuses. The palatal aspect was devoid of any such swelling, and the mucosa appeared normal. Upper left central incisor and canine teeth were tilted, and the lateral incisor was missed. Orthopantomograph revealed an ill-defined mixed radiolucency in the left maxilla with displacement of adjacent teeth (Figure 2). Computed tomography sections showed

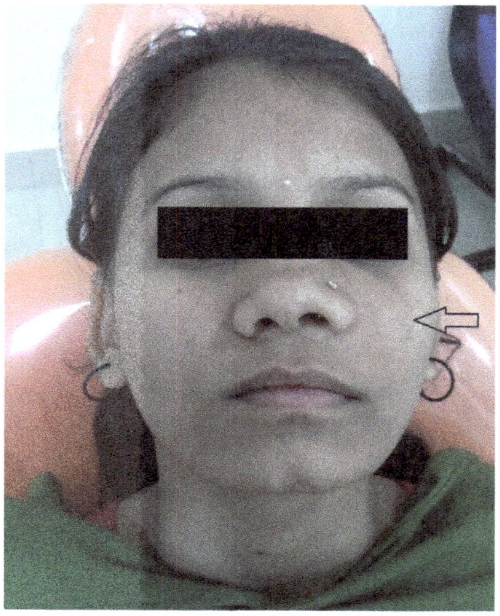

FIGURE 1: Preoperative frontal view showing swelling on left side of the face.

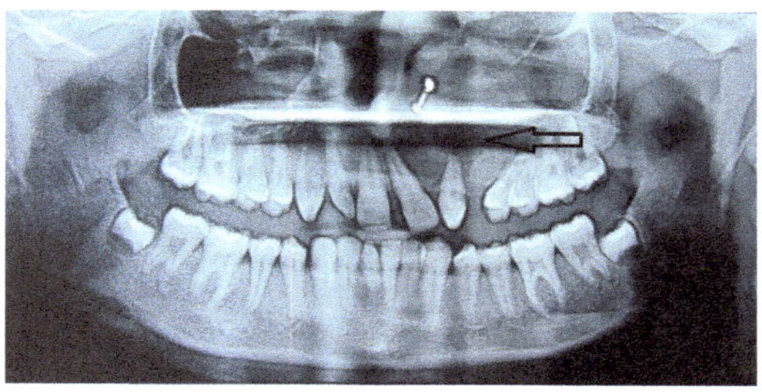

FIGURE 2: Orthopantomograph showing ill-defined mixed radiolucency in the left maxilla with displacement of the adjacent teeth.

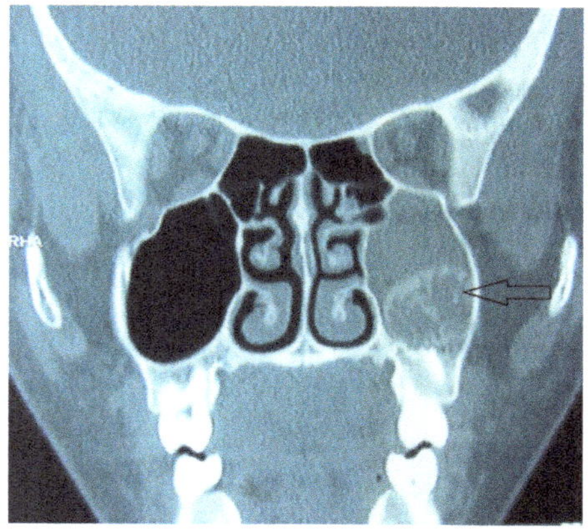

FIGURE 3: Coronal CT scan section showing the lesion completely obliterating the left maxillary sinus.

the lesion completely obliterating the left maxillary sinus with intact palatal bone and posterior wall of the sinus (Figures 3, 4(a), and 4(b)). An incisional biopsy was performed under local anesthesia, and the histopathological examination revealed the lesion as fibromyxoma. Complete curettage and enucleation of the lesion was then performed by an intraoral approach under general anesthesia (Figures 5 and 6). The enucleated tumour mass was submitted to oral and Maxillofacial Pathology Department (Figure 7). The histopathology showed spindle-shaped fibroblasts in loose myxoid tissue and confirmed the diagnosis (Figure 8). Patient came for regular followups, and there was no recurrence of the lesion with good intraoral healing (Figure 9).

## 3. Discussion

Fibromyxoma is a rare aggressive intraosseous lesion derived from embryonic mesenchymal tissue associated with odontogenesis. The maxilla and anterior region of the mandible are rarely affected. When found in the maxilla it usually behaves more aggressively than that of the mandible. It involves the zygoma, maxillary sinus, and even the orbits.

Evidence that may support the odontogenic origin of fibromyxoma of the jaws was contributed by Thoma in 1934. He stated that the greater portion of myxomas that occur in the jaws are derived from embryonic tissues of the dental papilla, the dental follicle, or the periodontal membrane [7, 8]. Most myxomas are asymptomatic, although some patients present with progressive pain in lesions involving the maxilla and maxillary sinus, with eventual neurologic disturbances.

Radiographically, the fibromyxomas present themselves as multilocular or unilocular radiolucency with well-defined borders. Most of them are multilocular. Radiological investigations reveal homogenous radiolucencies with different appearances like honey comb, soap bubble, or tennis racket [1, 9]. Differential diagnosis for a unilocular radiolucency can be any cyst, and for a multilocular radiolucency it can be ameloblastoma, central hemangioma, and odontogenic keratocyst. An aspiration biopsy would be nonproductive.

Grossly the tumour is greyish-yellow multinodular tissue. Its consistency varies. Some portions of the tumour may be sticky, gelatinous, or semisolid, and others may be firm. The surface of the tumour is shiny and glistening.

Histologically the fusiform or stellate cells are elongated, having cytoplasmic processes stretching in various directions. It contains few cells that lie in a myxoid ground substance being elongated with spindle-shaped nuclei and having the appearance of fibrocytes. It is of diagnostic challenge to the examiners because it is difficult to differentiate from the other odontogenic tumours. Mitotic figures are rarely seen. The ultrastructural studies of an odontogenic myxoma demonstrate the presence of two basic functional types of cells: secretory and nonsecretory. The secretory cell type is the principal tumour cell and resembles the fibroblast [10].

The tumour is not radiosensitive, and hence surgery is the only treatment of choice. The surgical treatment of the fibromyxoma involves enucleation and curettage, radical excision, en bloc resection. The avoidance of recurrence is strongly related to the complete resection of the lesion. Thomas has stated that recurrence of fibromyxoma is uncommon if enucleation is complete. Myxomas or fibromyxomas show a recurrence rate between 25% and 43%. Harder et al.

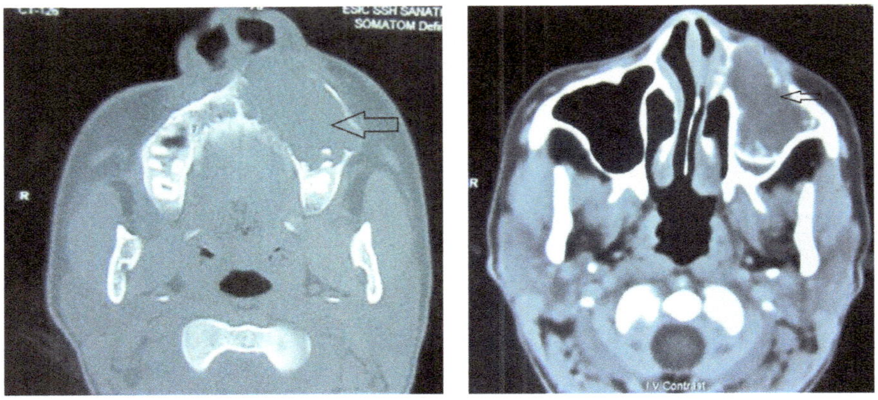

(a) (b)

FIGURE 4: Axial CT Scan sections showing the lesion perforating the anterior wall of the antrum and its extension in to the nasal cavity.

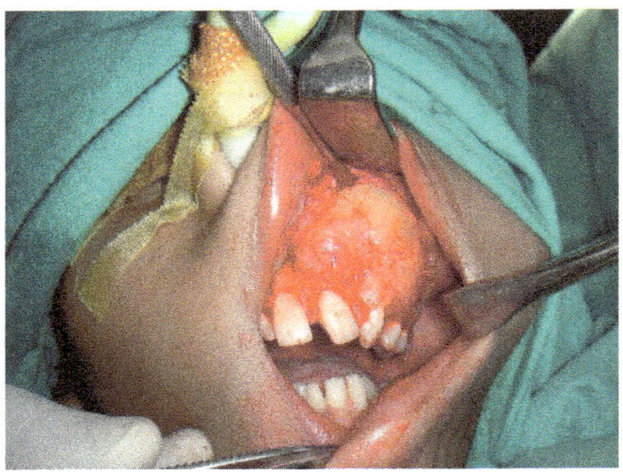

FIGURE 5: Exposure of the tumour by an intraoral approach.

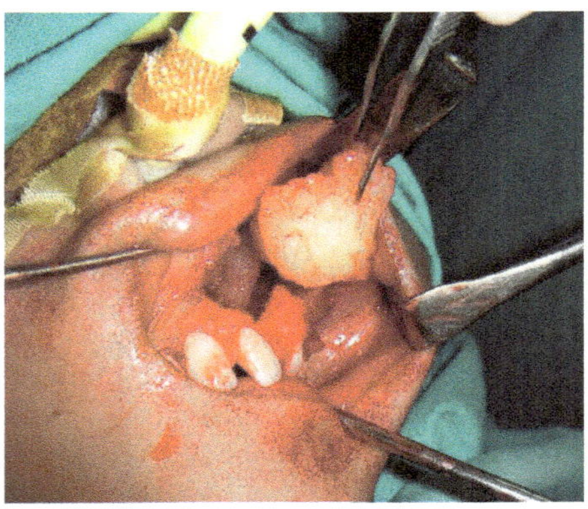

FIGURE 6: Curettage and complete removal of the lesion.

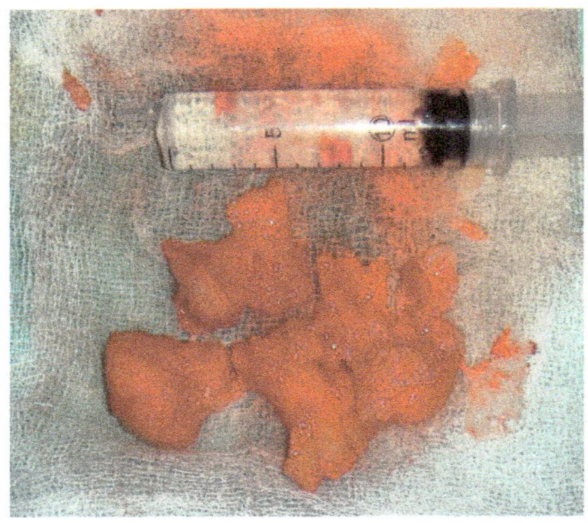

FIGURE 7: Gross appearance of the tumour mass.

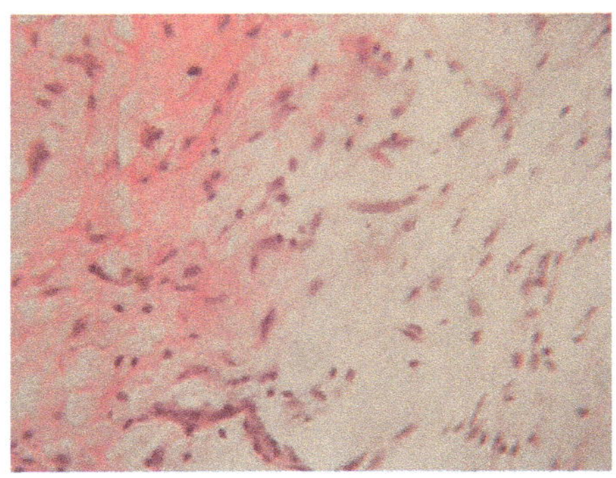

FIGURE 8: Histopathological examination showing spindle-shaped fibroblasts in loose myxoid tissue.

stated that rate of recurrence varies widely as does the choice of treatment. Their study supports conservative surgery as the appropriate treatment for odontogenic myxomas, as they have found no evidence of malignant change or increasingly aggressive behaviour in any of the recurrences [8].

Chen et al. proposed conservative treatment as the preferred method for excision with extensive resection reserved for large tumors. In the long bones the tumour is frequently malignant and tends to recur with great frequency after removal, but fibromyxomas of the jaws appear to have a better prognosis.

## 4. Conclusion

In conclusion, fibromyxomas of the jaws are rare but not uncommon. The prime treatment considerations include the

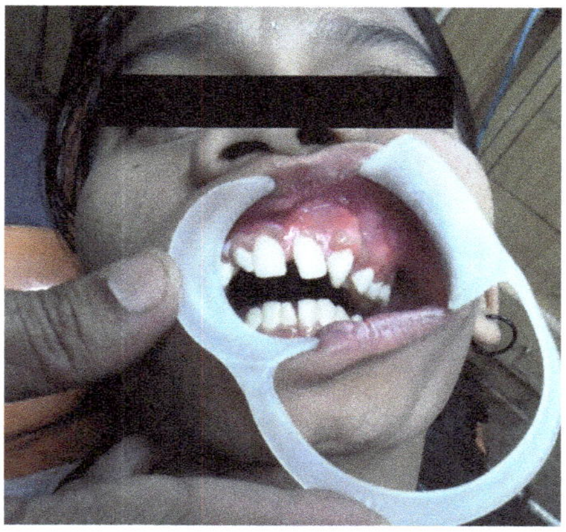

FIGURE 9: Postoperative image showing intraoral healing.

age of the patient and recurrence of the lesion. The tumour is not radiosensitive, and surgery is the only choice of treatment. In this young unmarried girl as the extent of lesion is confined to the maxillary sinus, we have opted for an intraoral conservative surgical approach.

## Acknowledgment

We sincerely thank Dr. Vittal Kavuri MD Chief anaesthesiologist, Mediciti Hospital, Hyderabad for his support and contribution in the surgical intervention of this patient.

## References

[1] A. Shah, P. Lone, S. Latoo et al., "Odontogenic myxoma of the maxilla: a report of a rare case and review on histogenetic and diagnostic concepts," *National Journal of Maxillofacial Surgery*, vol. 2, no. 2, pp. 189–195, 2011.

[2] E.-M. Dietrich, S. Papaemmanouil, G. Koloutsos, H. Antoniades, and K. Antoniades, "Odontogenic fibromyxoma of the maxilla: a case report and review of the literature," *Case Reports in Medicine*, vol. 2011, Article ID 238712, 5 pages, 2011.

[3] B. H. Hendler, N. A. Abaza, and P. Quinn, "Odontogenic myxoma. Surgical management and an ultrastructural study," *Oral Surgery Oral Medicine and Oral Pathology*, vol. 47, no. 3, pp. 203–217, 1979.

[4] G. C. Shivakumar and S. Sahana, "Fibromyxoma of the maxilla: a case report," *International Journal of Medical Sciences*, vol. 9, no. 1, pp. 36–41, 2010.

[5] S. Berry and R. Puri, "Fibromyxoma of the maxilla," *Otolaryngology*, vol. 135, no. 2, pp. 330–331, 2006.

[6] D. R. James and V. S. Lucas, "Maxillary myxoma in a child of 11 months. A case report," *Journal of Cranio-Maxillofacial Surgery*, vol. 15, no. 1, pp. 42–44, 1987.

[7] E. Bucci, L. L. Muzio, M. D. Mignogna, and G. De Rosa, "Odontogenic myxoma: report of a case with peculiar features," *Journal of Oral and Maxillofacial Surgery*, vol. 49, no. 1, pp. 91–94, 1991.

[8] F. Harder, "Myxomas of the jaws," *International Journal of Oral Surgery*, vol. 7, no. 3, pp. 148–155, 1978.

[9] B. O. Abiose, H. A. Ajagbe, and O. Thomas, "Fibromyxomas of the jawbones—a study of ten cases," *British Journal of Oral and Maxillofacial Surgery*, vol. 25, no. 5, pp. 415–421, 1987.

[10] L. I. Goldblatt, "Ultrastructural study of an odontogenic myxoma," *Oral Surgery Oral Medicine and Oral Pathology*, vol. 42, no. 2, pp. 206–220, 1976.

# 17

# Genetic Mapping in Papillon-Lefèvre Syndrome: A Report of Two Cases

**Kaustubh Suresh Thakare,[1] M. L. Bhongade,[1] Pretti Charde,[1] Shweta Kale,[2] Priyanka Jaiswal,[1] B. K. Somnath,[1] and Sunil Pendor[1]**

[1] *Department of Periodontology & Implantology, Sharad Pawar Dental College and Hospital, Wardha, Maharashtra 442001, India*
[2] *Department of Prosthodontics, Sharad Pawar Dental College and Hospital, Wardha, Maharastra 442001, India*

Correspondence should be addressed to Kaustubh Suresh Thakare; kaustubhthakaremds@gmail.com

Academic Editors: P. Lopez Jornet and E. F. Wright

Papillon-Lefevre syndrome (PLS) is a rare autosomal recessive heterogeneous trait which is characterized by erythematous palmoplantar hyperkeratosis, early-onset periodontitis, and associated calcification of dura mater. The etiology of PLS is multifactorial with genetic, immunological, and microbial factors playing a role in etiopathogenesis. Recently identified genetic defect in PLS has been mapped to chromosome 11q14–q21, which involves mutations of cathepsin C. This paper presents a report of 2 cases of Papillon-lefevre syndrome in which diagnosis is based on clinical presentation and genetic mapping.

## 1. Introduction

Papillon-Lefèvre syndrome (PLS) is a rare autosomal recessive heterogeneous trait which was first described in 1924 by two French physicians, Papillon and Lefèvre [1]. It is characterized by erythamatous palmoplantar hyperkeratosis, early-onset periodontitis, and associated calcification of dura mater [2]. This disease usually has its onset between the ages of 1 and 4 affecting males and females equally. Its prevalence is estimated to be 1 to 4 per million in the general population with carrier rate of 2 to 4 per 1000. Consanguineous marriage is determined in 20 to 40% of patients with PLS [3].

Cutaneous changes include well-demarcated erythematous hyperkeratotic lesions on the palms, soles, dorsum of the hands, and the interphalangeal joints. Other regions, including the eyelids, cheeks, knees, elbows, thighs, labial commissures, external malleolus, toes, and dorsal fingers may also be involved [1].

The second major feature of PLS is severe periodontitis, which starts at the age of 3 or 4 [4]. Periodontal effects appear almost immediately after tooth eruption when gingiva becomes erythematous and oedematous. The primary incisors are usually affected first and can display marked mobility by the age of 3. By the age of 4 or 5 years, all the primary teeth may have exfoliated [5]. After exfoliation, the inflammation subsides and the gingiva appears healthy. However, with the eruption of the permanent dentition, the process of gingivitis and periodontitis is usually repeated, and there is subsequent premature exfoliation of the permanent teeth at the age of 12 to 15 [6, 7]. There is a dramatic alveolar bone resorption, which leads to a "floating-in-air appearance" in the dental imaging [8].

The etiology of PLS is multifactorial with genetic, immunological, and microbial factors playing a role in etiopathogenesis. Recently identified genetic defect in PLS has been mapped to chromosome 11q14–q21, which involves mutations of cathepsin C [6, 9]. Studies in PLS patients have shown more than 90% reduction in cathepsin C activity [9]. Another important etiologic factor is an alteration of host defense owing to the decreased function of lymphocytes, polymorphonuclear leukocytes (PMNs), or monocytes [10]. Gram-negative microbial polysaccharides are generally recognized to be a primary factor in the etiology of periodontitis including periodontitis in LPS [11, 12]. The present case series report two cases of PLS in pediatric patients which are treated with multidisciplinary approach.

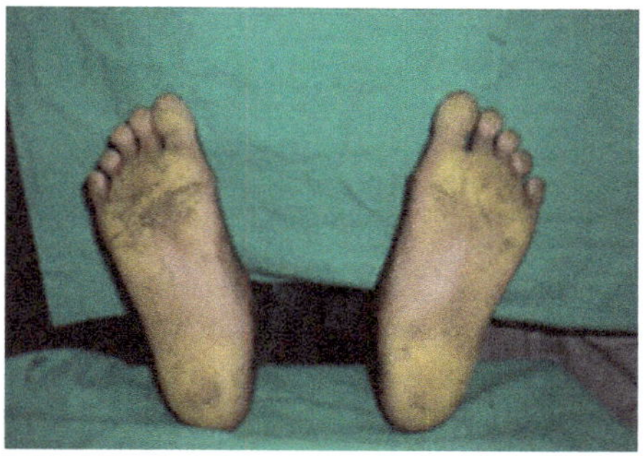

Figure 1: Plantar keratosis.

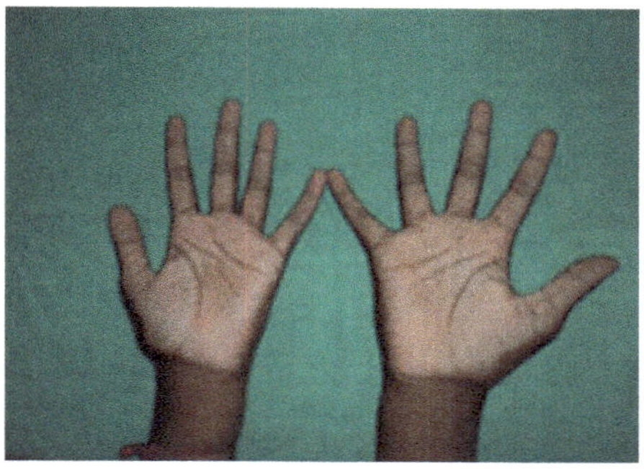

Figure 2: Palmar keratosis.

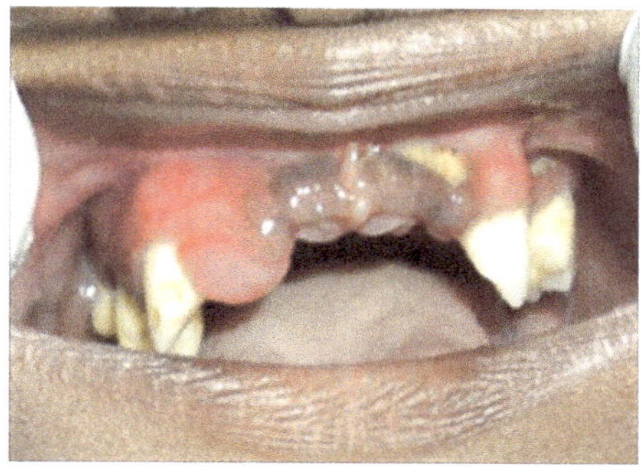

Figure 3: Initial clinical appearance with severe gingival inflammation and loss of several teeth.

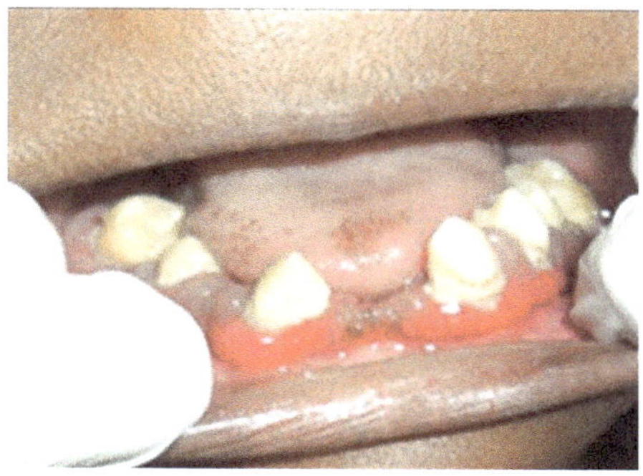

Figure 4: Initial clinical appearance with severe gingival inflammation and loss of several teeth.

## 2. Presentation of Cases

*2.1. Case 1.* A 14-year-old female patient reported to the department of periodontics and implantology, in 2011, with chief complaint of teeth mobility and difficulty in mastication of 2 years due to loss of permanent teeth.

Past dental history revealed early shedding of deciduous dentition and loss of many of the permanent teeth 1 year ago due to excessive mobility. She also gave a history of thickening of the skin of the palms and soles since childhood. The rest of the family members including parents and one sibling were apparently normal.

Intraoral examination revealed that teeth numbers 13, 14, 17, 24, 27, 33, 34, 35, 37, 43, 45, and 47 were present. All the teeth were pathologically migrated. Twenty seven, 34, and 43 were grade-II mobile while the rest of the present teeth were grade III mobile. The gingiva around the teeth was inflamed, swollen, and tender while the oral mucosa covering the edentulous area appeared normal (Figures 3 and 4). Generalized plaque accumulation with halitosis was present. In addition, deep periodontal pockets and exudation were also observed. A panoramic radiograph was obtained which showed severe alveolar bone loss with about 10 to 15% bone remaining around the teeth present and impacted 28, 38, and 48 (Figure 5).

Extraoral examination revealed increased keratinization of the skin of the palmar and plantar surfaces as well as the skin over the dorsal surfaces of the joints of the hands; the keratinized skin was clearly demarcated from adjacent normal skin. Deep fissures were present on the soles of her feet (Figures 1 and 2). There was associated hyperhidrosis of palms and soles resulting in a foul-smelling odor. Her nails and hair were normal.

*2.2. Case 2.* A 13-year-old male patient reported to the department of periodontics and implantology, in 2012, with chief complaint of teeth mobility, aesthetic problems, and difficulty in mastication.

The past dental history revealed that his deciduous teeth had erupted normally but exfoliated gradually by the age of 4–6. Similarly, his permanent teeth too were lost prematurely after having erupted normally.

On intraoral examination, it was found that the patient's central incisors, mandibular lateral incisors, and all permanent first molars and maxillary second molars were missing. The teeth numbers 12, 13, 14, 15, 22, 23, 24, 25, 32, 33, 34, 35, 37, 42, 43, 45, 44, 45, and 47 were present. Mobility was present in all the permanent teeth that were present. The gingiva in relation to the existing permanent teeth was red, soft, and edematous, with deep periodontal pockets and bleeding on probing. OPG of the patient showed severe alveolar bone loss in relation to the existing permanent teeth up to the level of the apical third of roots, giving the teeth a "floating in air" appearance.

On extraoral examination, there were symmetrical, well-demarcated, keratotic, and confluent plaques affecting the skin of the palms and soles, which extended to the dorsal surface of the finger joints. The skin was dry and rough on palpation. The hair and nails appeared normal.

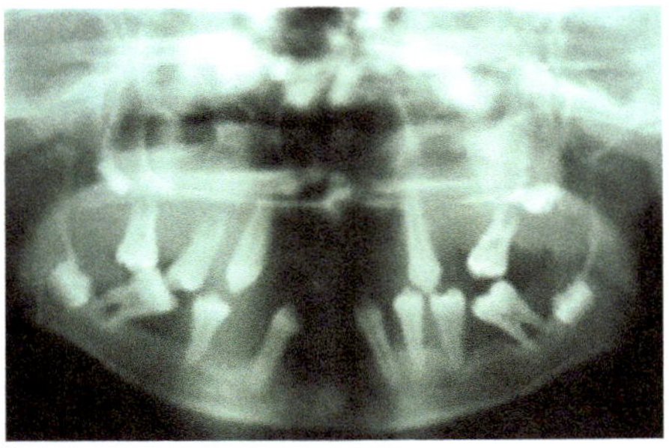

FIGURE 5: Panoramic radiograph showing "floating teeth appearance."

In both cases based on the history, clinical examination, and radiographic examination, a provisional diagnosis of Papillon-Lefèvre syndrome was made. For the conformation of the diagnosis, dermatological consultation was advised and blood samples were sent for genetic mapping (Super Religare Laboratories Ltd., Nagpur, Maharashtra, India). Result of the genetic mapping revealed abnormal gene at 11q14.1–q14.3 in both cases. This gene is commonly defective in patients with Papillon-Lefèvre syndrome, which confirmed the diagnosis of the cases.

## 3. Treatment

A multidisciplinary approach is important in the management of patients with LPS. For cutaneous lesions, patients were referred to the dermatologist for dermal treatment and were treated with topical keratolytic 5% salicylic acid in combination with 10% urea and in combination with topical 8-methoxypsoralen-ultraviolet, A photochemotherapy acitretin 4 (10 mg/day) (PUVA) was initiated.

Periodontal therapy consisting of antibiotic amoxicillin (500 mg, thrice daily) and metronidazole (400 mg, thrice daily) for one week along with a mouth rinse (0.2% chlorhexidine gluconate, 10 mL twice daily) was prescribed to the patients, and the patients were educated for oral hygiene. Teeth involved with severe periodontitis were extracted and some teeth were retained for prosthetic treatment (overdenture). The patients were referred to the prosthetic department and prosthesis was planned. The patients follow-up trials were carried out and prosthetic appliances were delivered to the patient.

## 4. Discussion

Papillon-Lefèvre syndrome is a rare disorder that is inherited in an autosomal recessive manner; that is, both parents are phenotypically healthy and there is no family history of the disease, other than the affected person and possibly some siblings. Both parents must carry the autosomal gene for the syndrome to appear in their offspring. When 2 such carriers mate, there is a 25% chance of producing affected offspring [13, 14].

The exact etiology of Papillon-Lefèvre syndrome is still obscure; however, genetic, immunologic, and microbiologic factors have all been linked to the development of the syndrome. A defect of immune-mediated mechanisms including an impairment of neutrophil chemotaxis, phagocytosis, and bactericidal activities accompanied by a decrease in cell migration, reduced lymphocyte response to pathogens, depression of helper/suppressor T-cell ratio, deficient monocytic function, elevation of serum IgG, and degenerative changes of plasma cells is observed [15].

*Aggregatibacter actinomycetemcomitans* was reported to have a significant role in the progression of periodontal involvements [16]. Other microbiological agents including *Porphyromonas gingivalis, Fusobacterium nucleatum, and Treponema denticola* have also been suggested to have causal effects [17].

Recently, genetic examinations point to the Papillon-Lefèvre syndrome gene locus in these patients. The gene responsible for it has been localized to chromosome 11q14–q21 where the cathepsin C gene is, encoding a lysosomal protease, in the interval between D11S4082 and D11S931. Subsequently, inactivating mutations were identified in this gene and an almost total loss of cathepsin C activity was shown in patients with Papillon-Lefèvre syndrome. Mechanistically, deficient activation of leukocyte serine proteinases due to lack of cathepsin C gene activity could possibly explain the severe periodontitis in PLS.

PLS should be differentiated from other conditions showing similar oral or cutaneous clinical features. Diseases with oral manifestations such as acrodynia, hypophosphatasia, histiocytosis X, cyclic neutropenia, and Takahara syndrome are also associated with periodontitis and premature loss of teeth. PLS is differentiated from these other conditions by the presence of palmoplantar hyperkeratosis. PLS can also be distinguished from palmoplantar keratoderma of Unna thost, Malde Meleda, Howel-Evans syndrome, keratosis punctata, keratoderma hereditarium mutilans (Vohwinkel syndrome), and Greither syndrome as these entities are not associated with periodontal disease.

## 5. Conclusion

Even though PLS is an extremely rare condition it is associated with lifelong psychological and social impacts on the growing children such as depression including hopelessness, aimlessness, social phobia, and a fear of communicating with people outside their family. Combined cooperation from dermatologists, pediatrician, periodontists, and prosthodontists is critical for the overall care of patients suffering from PLS.

## References

[1] M. M. Papillon and P. Lefèvre, "Two cases of symmetrically familiar palmer and plantar hyperkeratosis (Meleda disease) within brother and sister combined with severe dental alterations in both cases," *Bulletin de la Société Française de Dermatologie et de Syphiligraphie*, vol. 31, pp. 82–84, 1924.

[2] A. K. Valeshabad, A. Mazidi, R. K. Valeshabad et al., "Papillon-Lefèvre syndrome: a series of six cases in the same family," *ISRN Dermatology*, vol. 2012, Article ID 139104, 4 pages, 2012.

[3] T. C. Hart and L. S. Shapira, "Papillon-Lefèvre syndrome," *Periodontology*, vol. 6, no. 1, pp. 88–100, 2000.

[4] S. Kressin, A. Herforth, S. Preis, V. Wahn, and H. G. Lenard, "Papillon-Lefèvre syndrome—successful treatment with a combination of retinoid and concurrent systematic periodontal therapy: case reports," *Quintessence International*, vol. 26, no. 11, pp. 795–803, 1995.

[5] T. C. Hart, P. S. Hart, D. W. Bowden et al., "Mutations of the cathepsin C gene are responsible for Papillon-Lefevre syndrome," *Journal of Medical Genetics*, vol. 36, no. 12, pp. 881–887, 1999.

[6] E. Haneke, "The Papillon-Lefevre syndrome: keratosis palmoplantaris with periodontopathy. Report of a case and review of the cases in the literature," *Human Genetics*, vol. 51, no. 1, pp. 1–34, 1979.

[7] C. Toomes, J. James, A. J. Wood et al., "Loss-of-function mutations in the cathepsin C gene result in periodontal disease and palmoplantar keratosis," *Nature Genetics*, vol. 23, no. 4, pp. 421–424, 1999.

[8] V. K. Mahajan, N. S. Thakur, and N. L. Sharma, "Papillon-Lefèvre Syndrome," *Indian Pediatrics*, vol. 40, no. 12, pp. 1197–1200, 2003.

[9] M. D'Angelo, V. Margiotta, P. Ammatuna, and F. Sammartano, "Treatment of prepubertal periodontitis. A case report and discussion," *Journal of Clinical Periodontology*, vol. 19, no. 3, pp. 214–219, 1992.

[10] H. E. Schroeder, R. A. Seger, H. U. Keller, and E. M. Rateitschak-Pluss, "Behavior of neutrophilic granulocytes in a case of Papillon-Lefevre syndrome," *Journal of Clinical Periodontology*, vol. 10, no. 6, pp. 618–635, 1983.

[11] T. E. van Dyke, M. A. Taubman, J. L. Ebersole et al., "The Papillon-Lefèvre syndrome: neutrophil dysfunction with severe periodontal disease," *Clinical Immunology and Immunopathology*, vol. 31, no. 3, pp. 419–429, 1984.

[12] M. Umeda, Y. J. Zhang, T. Koseki, and I. Ishikawa, "Clinical, bacteriological, and immunological examination and treatment of two Papillon-Lefevre syndrome patients," *The Journal of the Stomatological Society*, vol. 57, no. 3, pp. 430–440, 1990.

[13] N. Y. Ashri, "Early diagnosis and treatment options for the periodontal problems in Papillon-Lefèvre syndrome: a literature review," *Journal of the International Academy of Periodontology*, vol. 10, no. 3, pp. 81–86, 2008.

[14] F. N. Hattab and W. M. Amin, "Papillon-Lefèvre syndrome with albinism: a review of the literature and report of 2 brothers," *Oral Surgery, Oral Medicine, Oral Pathology, Oral Radiology and Endodontology*, vol. 100, no. 6, pp. 709–716, 2005.

[15] S. A. Janjua and A. Khachemoune, "Papillon-Lefèvre syndrome: case report and review of the literature," *Dermatology Online Journal*, vol. 10, no. 1, 2004.

[16] A. Stabholz, N. S. Taichman, and W. A. Soskolne, "Occurrence of Actinobacillus actinomycetemcomitans and anti-leukotoxin antibodies in some members of an extended family affected by Papillon-Lefèvre syndrome," *Journal of Periodontology*, vol. 66, no. 7, pp. 653–657, 1995.

[17] R. K. Hall, Ed., *Paediatric Orofacial Medicine and Pathology*, Chapman & Hall Medical, London, UK, 1st edition, 1994.

# 18

# Idiopathic Gingival Fibromatosis Rehabilitation: A Case Report with Two-Year Followup

**Mahesh Jayachandran,[1] Shalini Kapoor,[2] and Rethi Mahesh[1]**

[1] *Noorul Islam College of Dental Sciences, Aralammoodu PO, Thiruvananthapuram, Kerala 695123, India*
[2] *SGT Dental College, Hospital & Research Institute, Gurgaon, Delhi, India*

Correspondence should be addressed to Mahesh Jayachandran; dr.maheshj@yahoo.co.in

Academic Editors: G. Schierano and L. C. Spolidorio

Gingival enlargements are quite common and may be either inflammatory, noninflammatory, or a combination of both. Gingival hyperplasia is a bizarre condition causing esthetic, functional, psychological, and masticatory disturbances of the oral cavity. Causes of gingival enlargement can be due to plaque accumulation, due to poor oral hygiene, inadequate nutrition, or systemic hormonal stimulation (Bakaeen and Scully, 1998). It can occur as an isolated disease or as part of a syndrome or chromosomal abnormality. A progressive fibrous enlargement of the gingiva is a facet of idiopathic fibrous hyperplasia of the gingiva (Carranza and Hogan, 2002; Gorlin et al., 1976). It is described variously as *fibromatosis gingivae, gingivostomatitis, hereditary gingival fibromatosis, idiopathic fibromatosis, familial elephantiasis,* and *diffuse fibroma*. We present a case of idiopathic gingival fibromatosis with its multidisciplinary approach of management.

## 1. Introduction

Idiopathic gingival fibromatosis is characterized by a slowly progressive, benign enlargement, which affects the marginal gingiva, attached gingiva, and interdental papilla. The fibromatosis may potentially cover the exposed tooth surfaces, causing esthetic and functional problems, and in extreme cases may distort the jaws. Gingival tissues surrounding both the maxillary detention and the mandibular dentition may be affected. The hyperplasic gingiva usually presents a normal color and has a firm consistent with abundant stippling [1]. Buccal and lingual tissues may be involved in both the mandible and the maxilla. This anomaly is classified into two types according to its form—the nodular form and the symmetric form. The localized nodular form is characterized by the presence of multiple enlargements in the gingiva. The symmetric form which is the most common type of this disorder results in uniform enlargement of the gingiva. The degree of enlargement may vary from mild to severe. As a result, the teeth become buried, to varying degrees, beneath the redundant hyperplastic tissues. The gingival tissues are usually pink and nonhemorrhagic and have a firm, fibrotic consistency [1, 2]. Most cases of hereditary gingival fibromatosis appear to be inherited in an autosomal-dominant manner, although autosomal recessive inheritance has also been reported. Autosomal-dominant forms of gingival fibromatosis, which are usually nonsyndromic, have been genetically linked to the chromosomes 2p21-p22 and 5q13-q22 [3–5]. In modern times, a mutation in the Son of sevenless-1 (*SOS-1*) gene has been suggested as a possible cause of isolated (nonsyndromic) gingival fibromatosis [3]. However, no definite linkage has been established. Diffuse gingival enlargement is also found to be associated with syndromes like Cross syndrome, Rutherford syndrome, Ramen syndrome, Zimmerman Laband syndrome, and Juvenile hyaline syndrome [1, 2, 6] (Table 1).

## 2. Case Report

A 30-year-old woman reported complaining of disfigurement of face due to swelling in gums since seven years, which was causing functional and masticatory difficulty. She presented with a generalized severe gingival overgrowth, involving the maxillary and mandibular arches and covering almost the

Table 1: Syndromes associated with gingival fibromatosis [6].

| Syndrome | Clinical features | Mode of inheritance |
|---|---|---|
| Laband syndrome | Syndactily, nose, and ear abnormalities, hyperplasia of the nails, and terminal phalanges | Dominant |
| Rutherfurd syndrome | Corneal dystrophy | Dominant |
| Cross syndrome | Microphthalmia, mental retardation, and pigmentary defects | Recessive |
| Ramon syndrome | Hypertrichosis, mental retardation, delayed development epilepsy, and cherubism | Recessive |

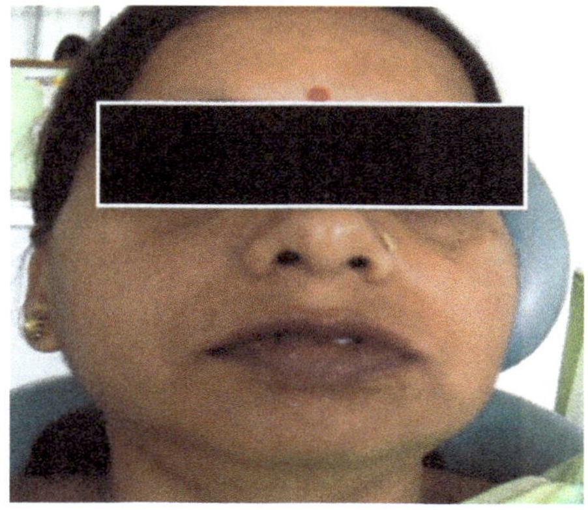

Figure 1: Preoperative photograph with fullness of face.

whole dentition. The patient was also concerned about the progressively increasing space between her upper front teeth and their movement away from their original positions. Extra oral examination (Figure 1) revealed a convex profile with bimaxillary protrusion, incompetent lips, and malocclusion.

Patient's medical and family history was noncontributory. The patient was not receiving any antiepileptic, antihypertensive, or immunosuppressive medications that could contribute to the gingival enlargement. Past dental history reveals that patient got surgical treatment (gingivectomy) done for the same twice, but the condition had reoccurred.

Intraoral examination revealed enlargement of the gingiva on both buccal and lingual/palatal sides with pinkish red, fibrous inconsistency and absence of stippling. Gingival enlargement enclosed the major surface of the teeth present except the incisal/occlusal surfaces. Severe diffuse enlargement involving the marginal, interdental, and attached gingiva of both arches, covering almost all the surfaces of the teeth, was found. There was generalized spacing in the dentition with proclined maxillary anteriors (Figure 2).

Clinical examination revealed mobility in all the teeth present and severe pathologic migration, especially of the upper anterior teeth. There were deep pockets present and there was an increase in the intermaxillary rest position. Physical examination of the whole body and blood investigations were advised to eliminate any medical abnormalities.

The radiographic findings corroborated those of the clinical examination and revealed severe generalized alveolar bone loss, which could be attributed to the local factors which must have exaggerated the hyperplastic condition. The peripheral blood results were normal and correlated with an absence of any history of systemic disease. Based on all these findings, a provisional diagnosis of idiopathic gingival enlargement was made.

*2.1. Treatment.* Treatment decided was full mouth undisplaced flap surgery.

*2.1.1. Surgical Stage.* After routine phase one periodontal therapy a treatment plan was formulated which comprised of quadrant-wise undisplaced flap surgery (the only treatment of choice in this condition as we had to treat the patient's underlying periodontal disease). The treatment procedure was explained to the patient and written consent was obtained. The surgery was planned under local anesthesia containing 2% lignocaine with 1 : 200000 epinephrine. Undisplaced flap surgery was performed to excise desired quantity of soft tissue. The wound was irrigated with betadine and a Coe-Pak (noneugenol, hard, and fast set) was given for seven days. Patient was advised to take analgesics and rinse twice daily with 0.2% chlorhexidine mouthwash. The excised tissue was sent for histopathological evaluation.

*2.1.2. Histopathological Report.* The sections revealed moderately dense collagenous connective tissue with collagen bundles arranged in a haphazard manner. Connective tissue was relatively avascular along with scanty inflammatory cell infiltrate showing dense wavy bundles of collagen fibers containing numerous fibrocytes and fibroblasts. The overlying epithelium was hyperplastic with elongated rete ridges. The histopathologic features led to the final diagnosis of idiopathic gingival fibromatosis.

*2.1.3. Maintenance Phase.* The case was followed up for 6 weeks postoperatively and then every 3 months for 2 years. The mobility of the teeth was reduced to physiologic at the end of 3 months. No recurrence was observed within 2 years. Patient is still following the follow-up regime. Mild recurrence in the right maxillary posterior palatal segment was seen after 1 year (Figure 3).

## 3. Discussion

This paper reports a case of idiopathic gingival fibromatosis. It may be congenital or hereditary. Gingival overgrowth varies from mild enlargement of isolated interdental papillae to segmental or uniform and marked enlargement affecting one or both jaws [7]. In the present case, patient had no history of any systemic disease, hypertrichosis, mental retardation, epilepsy, or medication which could contribute to gingival overgrowth. She also did not give history of pregnancy. General physical examination of the patient

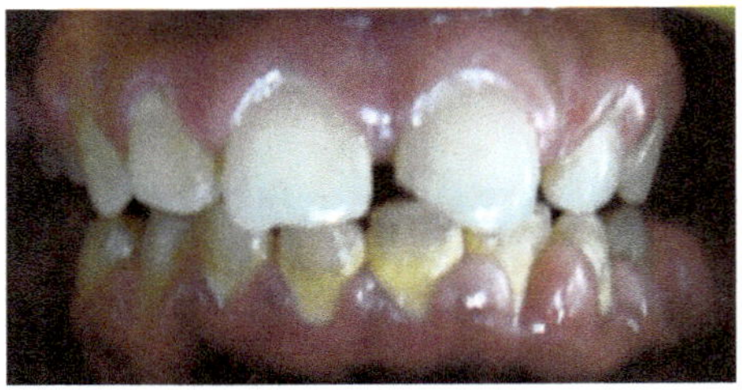

(a) Frontal view

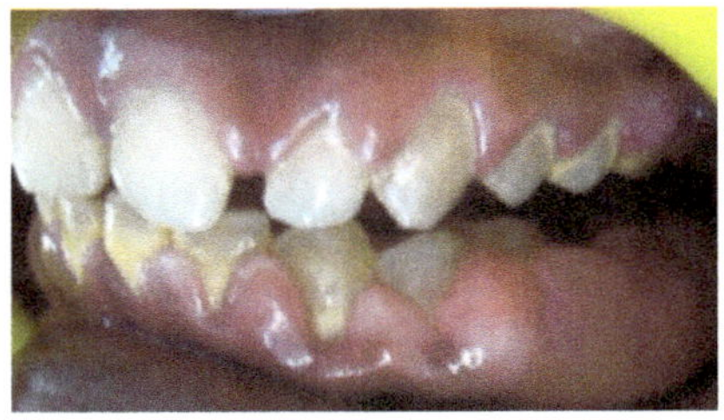

(b) Facial view

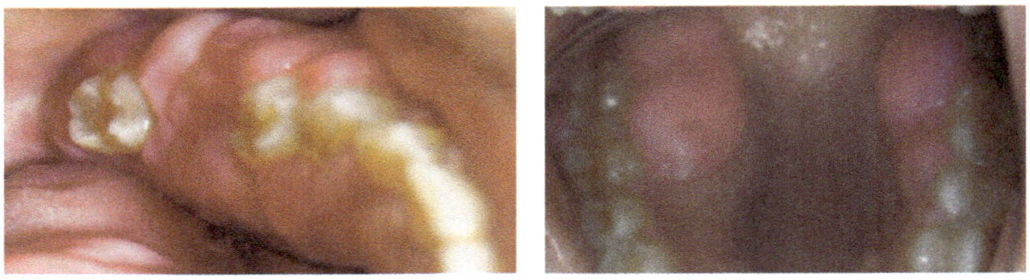

(c) Mandibular arch fibromatosis

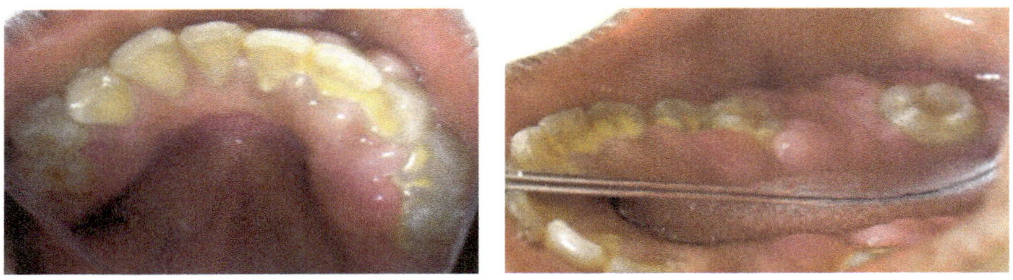

(d) Maxillary arch fibromatosis

FIGURE 2: Preoperative intraoral picture of generalized gingival fibromatosis.

revealed no syndromic association which could contribute to gingival overgrowth. The clinical, histopathological features and systemic examination excluded the diagnosis of neoplastic enlargement, hereditary gingival fibromatosis, Wegener's granulomatosis, acanthosis nigricans, and idiopathic variety [5, 8].

The precise mechanism of idiopathic gingival fibromatosis is unknown, but it is seen often to confine to the fibroblasts which harbor in the gingivae. The hyperplastic response does not involve the periodontal ligament and occurs peripheral to the alveolar bone within attached gingivae [7]. The continuing recurrence of the enlargement after repeated surgery and a permanent remolding of tissues after extraction of teeth suggest the importance of the presence of teeth and the gingival crevice environment in the pathogenesis of gingival fibromatosis [7]. In our case classically in those sites where extraction has been done there was no gingival overgrowth present.

There is inconsistency in the literature as to the cellular and molecular mechanisms that lead to gingival fibromatosis. Some authors report an increase in the proliferation of gingival fibroblasts [9], whereas others report slower-than normal growth [10]. Increased collagen synthesis rather than decreased levels of collagenase activity may be involved [9]. The constant increase in the tissue mass can result in delayed eruption and displacement of teeth, arch deformity, spacing, and migration of teeth. The condition is not painful until the tissue enlarges to partially cover the occlusal surface of the molars, thereby getting traumatized during mastication. In the present case, enlargement was not found to cover the occlusal surface, although due to massive gingival enlargement, the patient experienced difficulty in speech and maintaining oral hygiene measures. This could have resulted in the accumulation of materia alba and plaque, which could have further complicated the existing situation.

The surgical treatment of choice is the gingivectomy, which was first advocated for drug-induced gingival enlargement in 1941. As there is, in nearly all circumstances, adequate attached gingiva, there is little fear of creating mucogingival problem with this technique. However, in this case we opted for undisplaced flap procedure to treat the patient's periodontal disease as well as to improve esthetics. Since the literature reports high recurrence rate after surgery present case has been monitored closely for improvement in her periodontal condition for two years with a mild recurrence in the right maxillary posterior palatal segment. Patient was advised to maintain good oral hygiene to minimize the effect of inflammation on fibroblasts.

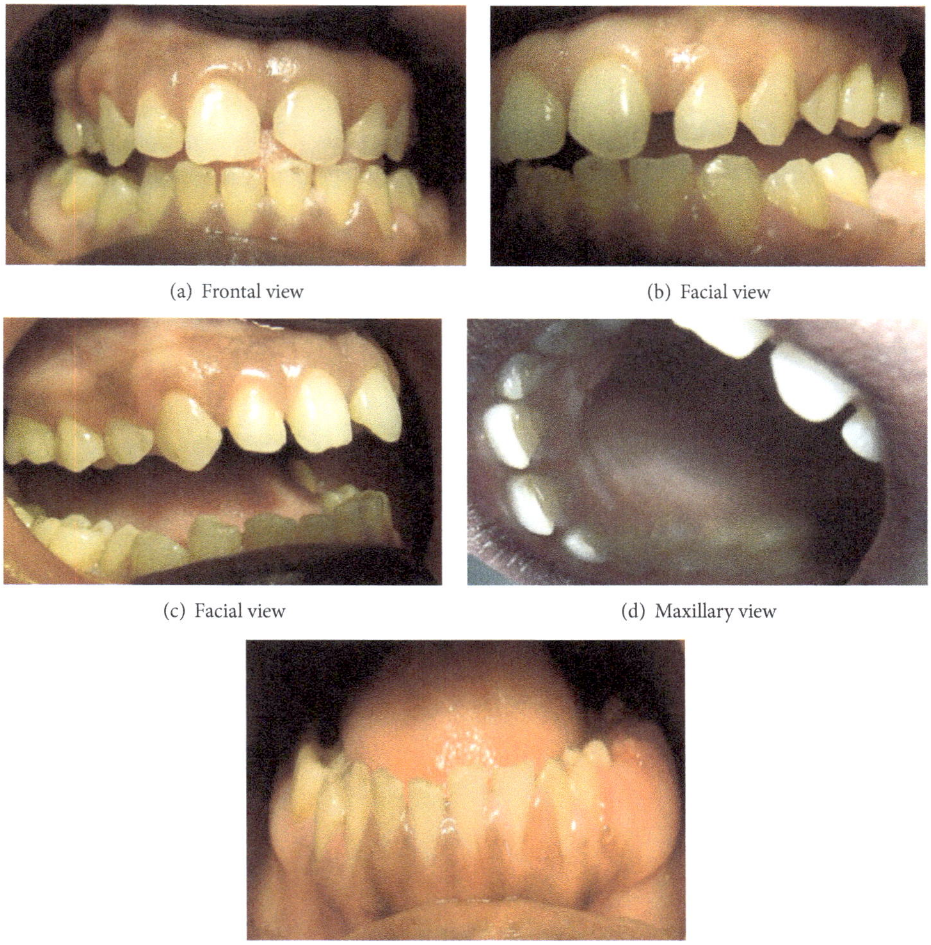

(a) Frontal view

(b) Facial view

(c) Facial view

(d) Maxillary view

(e) Mandibular view

FIGURE 3: Postoperative intraoral picture of generalized gingival fibromatosis.

## 4. Conclusion

Our present case was of nonsyndromic idiopathic gingival enlargement, with its surgical management and followup for a period of two years. Treatment was undisplaced flap surgery, which appreciably improved the patient's aesthetic and masticatory competence as well as her periodontal condition.


## Acknowledgment

This study was self-funded by the authors and our institution and there is no conflict of interests.


## References


[1] F. A. Carranza and E. L. Hogan, "Gingival enlargement," in *Clinical Periodontology*, M. G. Newman, H. H. Takei, and F. A. Carranza, Eds., pp. 279–296, Saunders, Philadelphia, Pa, USA, 9th edition, 2002.

[2] G. Bakaeen and C. Scully, "Hereditary gingival fibromatosis in a family with the Zimmermann-Laband syndrome," *Journal of Oral Pathology and Medicine*, vol. 20, no. 9, pp. 457–459, 1998.

[3] T. C. Hart, D. Pallos, L. Bozzo et al., "Evidence of genetic heterogeneity for hereditary gingival fibromatosis," *Journal of Dental Research*, vol. 79, no. 10, pp. 1758–1764, 2000.

[4] T. C. Hart, D. Pallos, D. W. Bowden, J. Bolyard, M. J. Pettenati, and J. R. Cortelli, "Genetic linkage of hereditary gingival fibromatosis to chromosome 2p21," *American Journal of Human Genetics*, vol. 62, no. 4, pp. 876–883, 1998.

[5] T. C. Hart, D. Pallos, L. Bozzo et al., "Evidence of genetic heterogeneity for hereditary gingival fibromatosis," *Journal of Dental Research*, vol. 79, no. 10, pp. 1758–1764, 2000.

[6] R. J. Gorlin, J. J. Pinborg, and M. M. Cohen Jr., *Syndromes of the Head and Neck*, McGraw Hill, New York, NY, USA, 2nd edition, 1976.

[7] P. S. Tiwana, I. J. De Kok, D. S. Stoker, and L. F. Cooper, "Facial distortion secondary to idiopathic gingival hyperplasia: surgical management and oral reconstruction with endosseous implants," *Oral Surgery, Oral Medicine, Oral Pathology, Oral Radiology and Endodontology*, vol. 100, no. 2, pp. 153–157, 2005.

[8] R. Chaturvedi, "Idiopathic gingival fibromatosis associated with generalized aggressive periodontitis: a case report," *Journal of the Canadian Dental Association*, vol. 75, no. 4, pp. 291–295, 2009.

[9] K. Shirasuna, M. Okura, K. Watatani, Y. Hayashido, M. Saka, and T. Matsuya, "Abnormal cellular property of fibroblasts from congenital gingival fibromatosis," *Journal of Oral Pathology*, vol. 17, no. 8, pp. 381–385, 1988.

[10] D. A. Tipton, K. J. Howell, and M. K. Dabbous, "Increased proliferation, collagen, and fibronectin production by hereditary gingival fibromatosis fibroblasts," *Journal of Periodontology*, vol. 68, no. 6, pp. 524–530, 1997.

# 19

# Orthodontic Wire Ingestion during Treatment: Reporting a Case and Review the Management of Foreign Body Ingestion or Aspiration (Emergencies)

**Mohammad Hoseini,[1] Seyed Morteza Saadat Mostafavi,[1] Navid Rezaei,[1] and Ehsan Javadzadeh Boluri[2]**

[1] *Department of Orthodontics and Dentofacial Orthopedics, School of Dentistry, Shahid Sadoughi University of Medical Sciences, Daheye Fajr BLV, Imam Avenue, Yazd 89195/165, Iran*
[2] *School of Dentistry, Shahid Sadoughi University of Medical Sciences, Daheye Fajr BLV, Imam Avenue, Yazd 89195/165, Iran*

Correspondence should be addressed to Seyed Morteza Saadat Mostafavi; saadat175@hotmail.com

Academic Editors: T. Hata and S. R. Watt-Smith

Today orthodontic treatment is in growing demand and is not limited to a specific age or social group. The nature of orthodontic treatment is such that the orthodontic wires and appliances, which are used to apply force and move the teeth, are exposed to the oral cavity. Shaping and replacing these wires in oral cavity are the major assignments of orthodontist on appointments. Therefore, we can say that orthodontic treatment requires working with dangerous tools in a sensitive place like oral cavity which is the entrance of respiratory and digestive systems. In this paper, a case of ingesting a broken orthodontic wire during eating is reported, and also necessary remedial measures at the time of encountering foreign body ingestion or aspiration are provided.

## 1. Introduction

Optional or accidental foreign body ingestion is common. Although in most cases these objects are excreted, in 1% of the cases, complex problems such as gastrointestinal perforation are seen [1, 2] which can sometimes lead to serious risks, including death. In the United States, 1500 people die each year due to foreign body ingestion [3, 4]. Incidence of ingesting dental materials and appliances varies in different studies. It was 3.6% to 27.7% in Tamura's review paper, and the majority belonged to adults. Aspiration or ingestion of orthodontic appliances is less common and depends on the kind of appliance [5]. Orthodontic appliances are usually small and are difficult to use especially when covered with saliva. The risk of objects to fall back into oropharynx and ingested or aspirated is more when the patient is in supine position, and it gets worse if you break the appliance. Depending on the shape, size, and flexibility of the object, some events may have minimal risk, while some may even be fatal. Prevention is the best method, but when happened, an efficient management of the event would be critical to save the patient's life [6]. The aim of this paper is to present a case of orthodontic wire ingestion and consequences and suggests approaches in the face of these events.

## 2. Case Report

The patient is a 29-year-old man who had been treated at a private clinic in the city (Yazd, Iran). Nonextraction treatment plan with 0.18 Roth system (Dentaurum Germany) was accomplished for the patient, and 0.16 Ni Ti arch wire (3M Unitek) was placed, at the finishing phase, on the maxillary teeth. At this time, due to lack of patient compliance, the brackets on left first and second premolars on maxillary arch were debonded. When eating, patient noticed that a piece of wire was ingested and at the same time a gastric irritation was felt. This filling was repeated the following day. The patient referred to a GI specialist. Radiographic images were taken

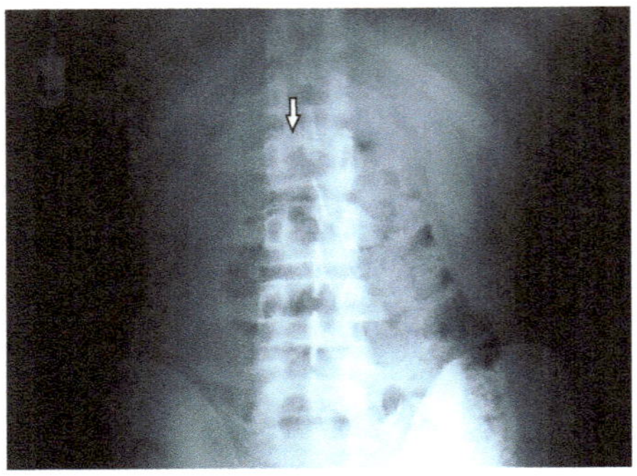

Figure 1: Abdominal radiographic image: presence of orthodontic wire in stomach location.

to track and locate the ingested wire (Figure 1). The wire was found at the lower stomach.

The wire was removed from the stomach under sedation with Midazolam in Shahid Sadooghi Hospital, Yazd, Iran (Figure 2).

Treatment was performed by endoscope including an overtube to prevent esophagus being ruptured by the wire. However, due to relatively large size of the wire, there was some degree of esophageal scratches that required IV chemotherapy (Metronidazole, ceftriaxone, Pantoprazol) with a 24 hr NPO. Burning sensation continued for a while. Treatment was terminated in 3 months.

## 3. Discussion

Foreign body ingestion and aspiration are potentially life threatening emergencies that may happen in any field of dentistry [1, 2]. Preventing from ingestion and aspiration is the best method and is achievable through following the principals of prevention [3].

Orthodontic wires may break in two situations. First, when the patient is sitting on the dental chair and orthodontist is cutting the end of a newly placed arch wire. Although there are customized end cutting players that hold the cut end, but it may happen for any reason such as using inefficient or inappropriate instrument. Second, as in this case, the patient is discharged, and in everyday life and activities the wire breaks. This may happen where a part of arch wire, due to treatment plan, is unsupported and is exposed to masticatory forces, or negligence in mastication and applying too much force lead to debonding some of brackets.

If a foreign body remains in oropharynx, the patient should be placed in reclined position and encouraged to cough deeply. Immediate priority is to ensure that the airways are clear, if they are not, immediate recognizable signs will appear soon. Orthodontists and general dentists should be able to recognize the signs and symptoms of airway obstruction including choking, inspiratory stridor, and using accessory respiratory muscles to breath. According to Mayo clinic website, the common sign is gripping throat with hands. If the patient did not show this sign, it would be necessary to look for inability to speak; difficulty in breathing; respiratory stridor; inability to cough; blue discoloration on skin, lips, and nails; and loss of consciousness [7]. If deep cough had no benefit, Heimlich maneuver should be performed to open the airways [8]. It is necessary to be successful very quickly. Otherwise, you must notify and summon urgent medical care team. Meanwhile, life support measures such as cricothyroidotomy, if indicated, should be taken to open the airway [9]. We can also make use of bronchoscopy to retrieve foreign bodies within the trachea and bronchial tree.

If there was no issue with the airways, the oral cavity should be inspected to find the foreign body. If you could not find the object, the patient would be informed in relation to the problem. You refer the patient to hospital for taking X-ray and clinical exam [10]. In case of foreign body ingestion, the patient may experience some problems in digestive tract including obstruction consequent perforation, and abscess formation; bleeding and fistulation; and also the object may remain motionless [11]. Obstruction is more likely in the upper esophagus [12]. This may lead to esophageal perforation with secondary mediastinitis. Esophageal obstruction may be in association with aspiration. So, the foreign body must be removed quickly using a fibro-optic endoscope.

If the foreign body reaches the stomach, it will pass through the digestive tract, with a probability of greater than 90%. It may take 10 days [13].

The risk of perforation or obstruction depends on the size and shape of the object. It is higher for a sharp object. In addition, an object longer than 5 cm is unlikely to pass through the duodenum [14, 15]. When an object leaves the stomach into small intestine, it is likely to pass it. The most common location for perforation or obstruction is ileocaecal valve [11, 16]. The risk of obstruction increases with anatomical anomalies such as constrictions and roughness. Removing the object by means of colonoscopy is possible.

Managing a patient who has ingested an object is accomplished with serial radiographic assessment. Patient must be examined and assessed regarding the clinical symptoms of perforation and obstruction such as pain and nausea and also the signs such as tenderness and guarding. There is no evidence that laxatives are useful and may even increase the risk of perforation [12].

Radiographs are useful to confirm the presence of foreign body, assess the size and shape, determine the location, and also to define the moving in or exiting out of the digestive system. If the patient showed the signs of perforation or the object remained for 2 weeks or more, surgical intervention is required.

Orthodontists and general dentists must be able to recognize the signs of airway obstruction due to remaining foreign body in esophagus.

## 4. Conclusion

In addition to this fact that general dentists and orthodontists must provide precautionary measures to prevent from foreign body aspiration and ingestion, they may be informed how to manage these cases.

One of the necessary measures is preparing chair side emergency equipments. If the airway is open, the patient

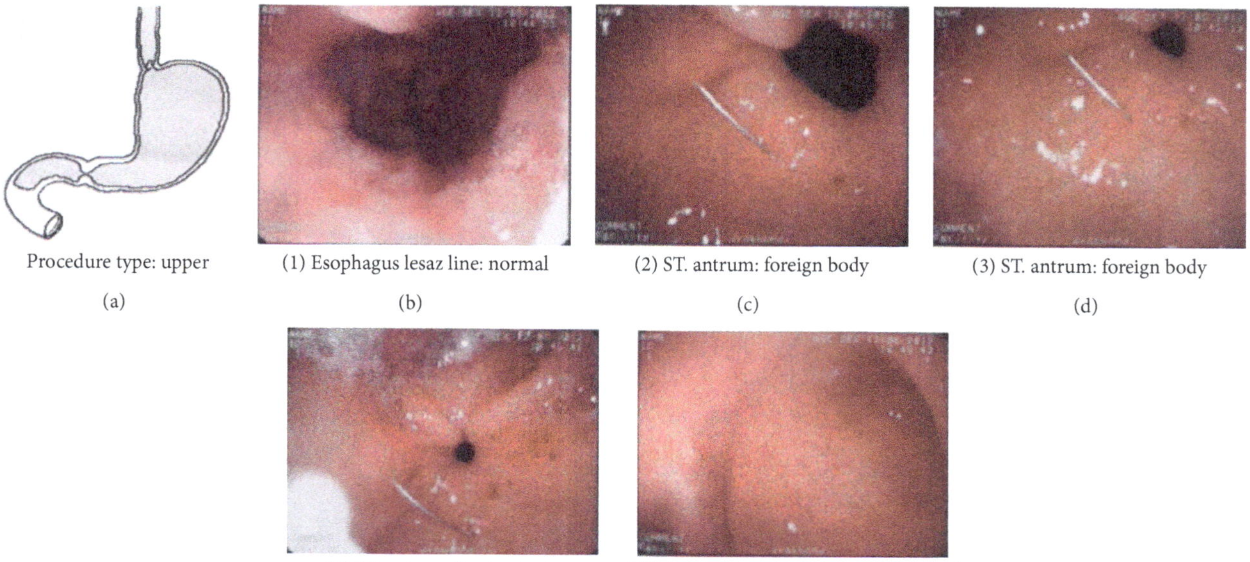

Procedure type: upper (a)

(1) Esophagus lesaz line: normal (b)

(2) ST. antrum: foreign body (c)

(3) ST. antrum: foreign body (d)

(4) ST. antrum: foreign body (e)

(5) ST. antrum greater curvature: normal (f)

FIGURE 2: Endoscopic images of orthodontic wire in antrum of stomach before and after endoscopy.

should be taken to hospital, clinical and radiographic examinations should be performed by qualified persons, and then appropriate treatment should be performed according to diagnosis and location of the foreign body.

## References


[1] A. P. Madrona, J. A. F. Hernández, M. C. Prats, J. R. Riquelme, and P. P. Paricio, "Intestinal perforation by foreign bodies," *European Journal of Surgery*, vol. 166, no. 4, pp. 307–309, 2000.

[2] N. G. Velitchkov, G. I. Grigorov, J. E. Losanoff, and K. T. Kjossev, "Ingested foreign bodies of the gastrointestinal tract: retrospective analysis of 542 cases," *World Journal of Surgery*, vol. 20, no. 8, pp. 1001–1005, 1996.

[3] A. T. Y. Lai, T. L. Chow, D. T. Y. Lee, and S. P. Y. Kwok, "Risk factors predicting the development of complications after foreign body ingestion," *British Journal of Surgery*, vol. 90, no. 12, pp. 1531–1535, 2003.

[4] J. I. Rodríguez Hermosa, J. Roig García, B. Ruiz Feliú et al., "Recurrent ingestion of foreign bodies and abdominal self-injury as a form of attempted suicide," *Gastroenterología y Hepatología*, vol. 9, pp. 529–534, 2004.

[5] N. Tamura, T. Nakajima, and S. Matsumoto, "Foreign bodies of dental origin in the air and food passages," *International Journal of Oral and Maxillofacial Surgery*, vol. 15, no. 6, pp. 739–751, 1986.

[6] N. S. Rohida and W. A. Bhad, "Accidental ingestion of a fractured Twin-block appliance," *American Journal of Orthodontics and Dentofacial Orthopedics*, vol. 139, no. 1, pp. 123–125, 2011.

[7] "Choking: first aid," http://www.mayoclinic.com/health/first-aidchoking/.

[8] H. J. Heimlich, "The Heimlich maneuver: prevention of death from choking on foreign bodies," *Journal of Occupational Medicine*, vol. 19, no. 3, pp. 208–210, 1977.

[9] M. C. Colquhoun, A. J. Handley, and T. R. Evans, *ABC of Resuscitation*, BMJ Publishing, London, UK, 3rd edition, 1995.

[10] A. D. C. Monini, L. G. M. Maia, H. B. Jacob, and L. G. Gandini Jr., "Accidental swallowing of orthodontic expansion appliance key," *American Journal of Orthodontics and Dentofacial Orthopedics*, vol. 140, no. 2, pp. 266–268, 2011.

[11] M. Maleki and W. E. Evans, "Foreign-body perforation of the intestinal tract. Report of 12 cases and review of the literature," *Archives of Surgery*, vol. 101, no. 4, pp. 475–477, 1970.

[12] C. T. Henderson, J. Engel, and P. Schlesinger, "Foreign body ingestion: review and suggested guidelines for management," *Endoscopy*, vol. 19, no. 2, pp. 68–71, 1987.

[13] W. A. Webb, "Management of foreign bodies of the upper gastrointestinal tract," *Gastroenterology*, vol. 94, no. 1, pp. 204–216, 1988.

[14] G. M. Eisen, T. H. Baron, J. A. Dominitz et al., "Guideline for the management of ingested foreign bodies," *Gastrointestinal Endoscopy*, vol. 55, no. 7, pp. 802–806, 2002.

[15] W. A. Webb, "Management of foreign bodies of the upper gastrointestinal tract: update," *Gastrointestinal Endoscopy*, vol. 41, no. 1, pp. 39–51, 1995.

[16] F. M. H. Ziter Jr., "Intestinal perforation in adults due to ingested opaque foreign bodies," *American Journal of Gastroenterology*, vol. 66, no. 4, pp. 382–385, 1976.

# 20

# Surgical Treatment of Congenital True Macroglossia

**Sabrina Araújo Pinho Costa, Mário César Pereira Brinhole, Rogério Almeida da Silva, Daniel Hacomar dos Santos, and Mayko Naruhito Tanabe**

*Department of Oral and Maxillofacial Surgery, Vila Penteado General Hospital, Avenue Ministro Petrônio Portela, 1642, Freguesia do Ó, 02802-120 São Paulo, SP, Brazil*

Correspondence should be addressed to Sabrina Araújo Pinho Costa; binapinho@hotmail.com

Academic Editors: P. Lopez Jornet, A. Mansourian, Y. Nakagawa, and P. I. Varela-Centelles

Macroglossia is a morphological and volumetric alteration of the tongue, caused by muscular hypertrophy, vascular malformation, metabolic diseases, and idiopathic causes and also associated with Down and Beckwith-Wiedemann syndromes. This alteration can cause dental-muscle-skeletal deformities, orthodontic instability, masticatory problems, and alterations in the taste and speech. In this paper we present a case of true macroglossia diagnosed in a female patient, 26 years, melanoderma, no family history of disease, with a history of relapse of orthodontic treatment for correction of open bite, loss of the lower central incisors, and complaint of difficulty in phonation. The patient was submitted to glossectomy under general anesthesia using the "keyhole" technique, with objective to provide reduction of the lingual length and width. The patient developed with good repair, without taste and motor alterations and discrete paresthesia at the apex of the tongue.

## 1. Introduction

Macroglossia is an uncommon condition that can lead to several alterations like dental-muscle-skeletal deformities, orthodontic treatment instability, masticatory, and breathing and phonation problems, characterized by increased size of the tongue, can be caused by congenital malformations or acquired diseases. The most common causes are muscle hypertrophy and congenital vascular malformations, such as lymphangioma and hemangioma, they are also characteristics found in the Beckwith-Wiedemann syndrome, and can be present in the Down syndrome [1–14]. It can be acquired as a result of amyloidosis, myxedema, angioedema, and macromegalia [1, 5, 14–19]. The tongue can also be normal in size but can seem increased when compared with adjacent structures because of anteroposterior mandible or maxillary transverse deficiency or also due to cysts, tumors, and tonsillar hyperplasia that can move up and out the tongue. This last condition is called pseudomacroglossia and must be differentiated from true macroglossia, because its correction is achieved by treating the primary disease [20].

Accurate diagnosis of true macroglossia is obtained through the signs and symptoms of this alteration, which is of fundamental importance for the correct indication for surgical treatment, in order to restore proper function and provide stability for orthodontic treatment [21].

The surgical treatment indicated for the true macroglossia is the reductive glossectomy. Several techniques have been proposed in the literature to enable the reduction of the tongue. Peripheral incisions with marginal resection of tissue have as complications hipomobility and change in the form of the tongue that becomes globular [2, 5, 16, 20, 22]. Incisions V-shaped positioned in the midline of the tongue are effective in reducing the length but are ineffective in reducing the width of the tongue [3, 23, 24]. Elliptical incision positioned in the midline without reaching the apex of the tongue contributes to reducing the width with little influence on its length [25]. Incisions in the form of keyhole combine characteristics of elliptical and V-shaped incisions and are indicated when the reduction of the width and length of the tongue are desirable and its design can be changed according to the specific needs of each case [9, 26, 27].

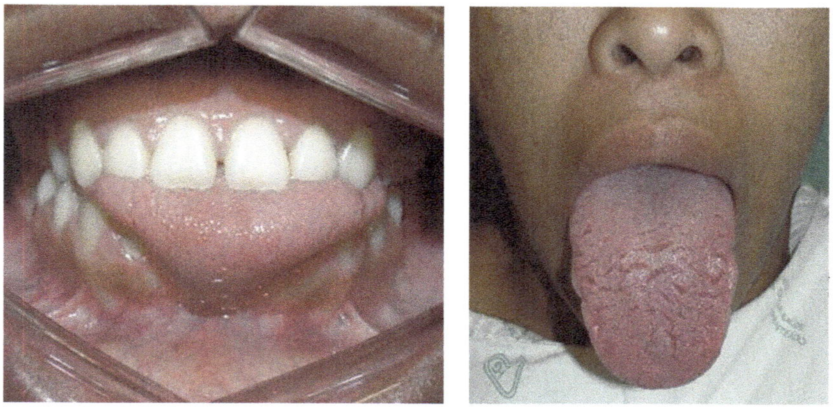

(a) (b)

FIGURE 1: The tongue was increased both in length and in width, with anterior open bite with interposition of the tongue and loss of 31 and 41 teeth.

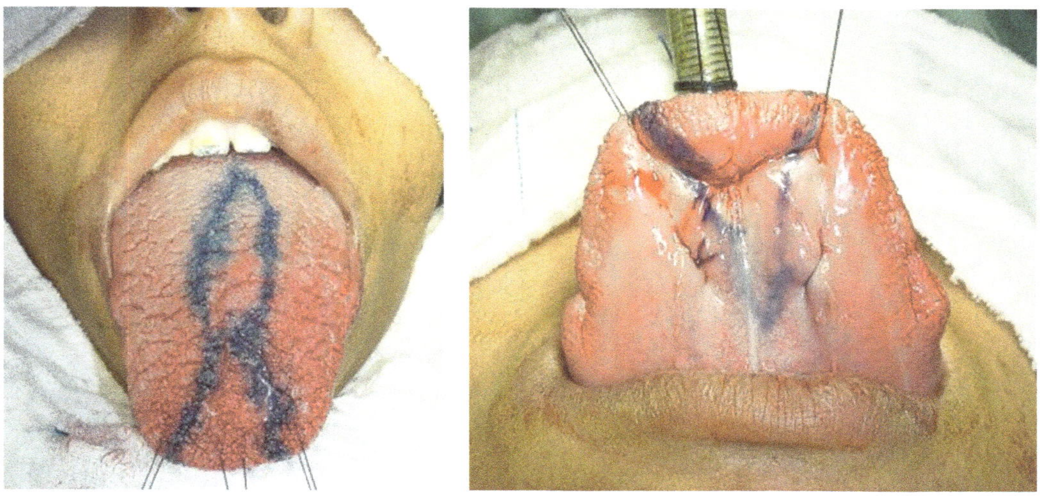

(a) (b)

FIGURE 2: The tongue was pulled out of the oral cavity through three repairs with nylon suture 3-0 fixed to the surgical field to maintain the symmetry between the sides and facilitate the demarcation of the incisions, which was performed which methylene blue.

This paper aims to present a case of true macroglossia treated surgically using the keyhole technique.

## 2. Case Report

Female patient, 26 years, melanoderma, was referred by the Department of phonoaudiology with complain of difficulty in speech and history of orthodontic treatment for correction of anterior open bite that resulted in complete recurrence. No history of systemic diseases or drug allergies or family history of her disease. On physical examination, the tongue was increased both in length and in width, with anterior open bite and interposition of the tongue, impression of the lingual surface of mandible molars on the edges of the tongue, loss of the tooth 31 and 41, occlusion in Class I of Angle, reversion Spee curve in the mandible and marked in the maxilla (Figures 1(a) and 1(b)), with diagnosis of true macroglossia requiring multidisciplinary treatment involving surgery, 1 orthodontics, and fonoaudiology.

The technique chosen for reduction glossectomy was the "keyhole" technique with the goal of reducing the tongue in width and length. The patient underwent general anesthesia nasotracheal intubation, and the tongue was pulled out of the oral cavity through three repairs with nylon suture 3-0 fixed to the surgical field to maintain the symmetry between the sides and facilitate the demarcation of the incisions, which was performed with methylene blue (Figures 2(a) and 2(b)). After infiltration of lidocaine 2% with epinephrine 1 : 200.000, a partial thickness elliptical wedge incision was made in the tongue dorsum, starting at the midline and at 4 mm away from tongue taste buds, as well as, incisions on dorsum and belly anterior tongue using electrocautery, which were united resulting in a full-thickness flap, proceeding the excision of excess tissue (Figures 3(a), 3(b), and 3(c)). The suture

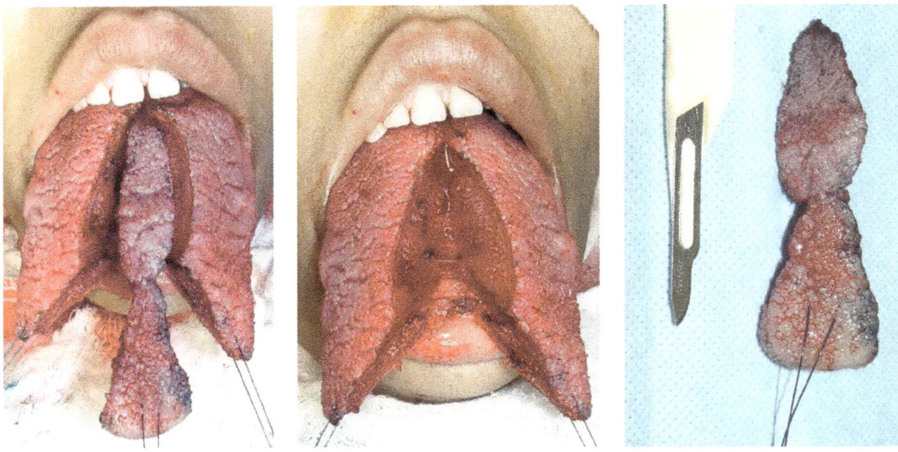

(a) (b) (c)

FIGURE 3: A partial thickness elliptical wedge incision starting at the midline and 4 mm distance from tongue taste buds using electrocautery, the dorsum, and incisions on belly anterior tongue were united resulting in a full-thickness flap, proceeding the excision of excess tissue.

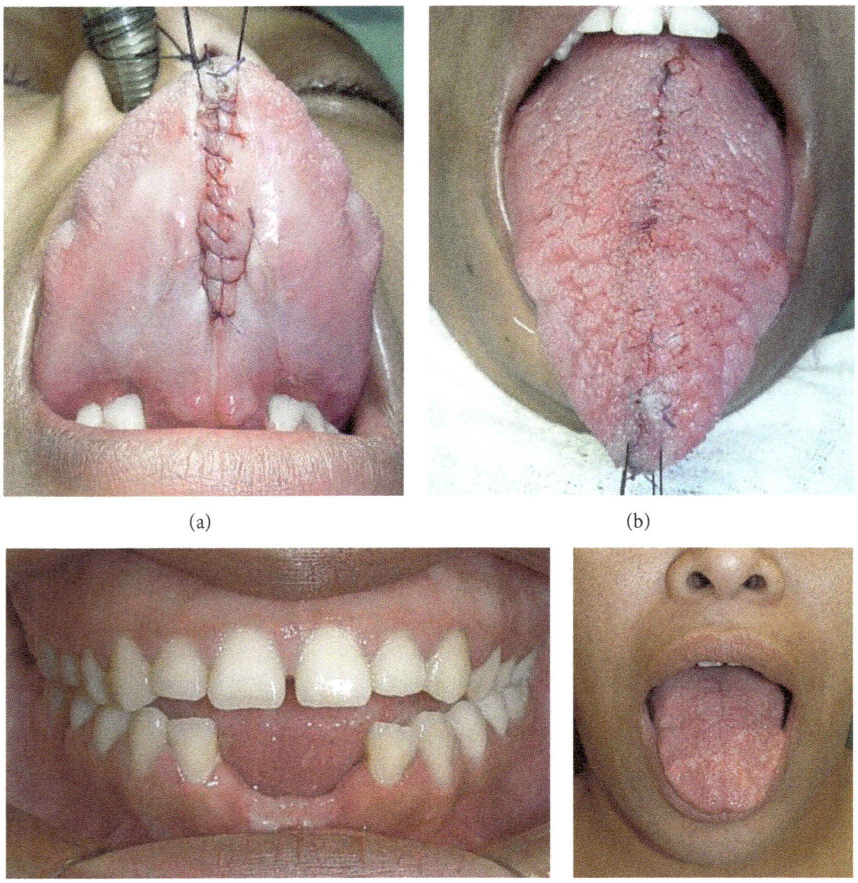

(a) (b)

(c) (d)

FIGURE 4: The suture was made by planes with polyglactin 910 suture 3-0, good tissue repair, perfect symmetry, and no tongue interposition.

was made by planes with polyglactin 910 suture 3-0. In the immediate postoperative period there was slight swelling in the floor of the mouth and on belly anterior tongue, and discrete lingual hypoesthesia, and it evolved after a week without taste or motor alteration and with good tissue repair, perfect symmetry, and no tongue interposition. The patient was referred to orthodontic and fonoaudiology treatment (Figures 4(a), 4(b), 4(c), and 4(d)).

## 3. Discussion

To determine the real need of surgical treatment is of fundamental importance to define the signs and symptoms of true macroglossia. The diagnosis must be based on clinical findings [20].

In cases of true macroglossia, as presented, in the literature several reductive glossectomy techniques are suggested. Each technique has a purpose in accordance with the clinical aspect.

In the presented case the keyhole technique was used which is indicated for reduction of length and width of the tongue, preserving the vasculonervous bundle and with few reports of sensory and functional deficits [9, 25, 28]. Sensitivity, movement, and taste when modified are resolved spontaneously within a few weeks [10, 29] and these observations from the literature were confirmed in our experience.

## 4. Conclusion

Surgical reduction of the tongue is an uncommon procedure, being indicated in specific cases; the keyhole technique allows anterior and median partial resection, technically simple, minimal morbidity, and good functional result.

## Conflict of Interests

There is no conflict of interests regarding this paper.

## References

[1] J. E. Vogel, J. B. Mulliken, and L. B. Kaban, "Macroglossia: a review of the condition and a new classification," *Plastic and Reconstructive Surgery*, vol. 78, no. 6, pp. 715–723, 1986.

[2] R. O. Dingman and W. C. Grabb, "Lymphangioma of the tongue," *Plastic and Reconstructive Surgery and the Transplantation Bulletin*, vol. 27, pp. 214–223, 1961.

[3] J. W. Hendrick, "Macroglossia or giant tongue. Case report," *Surgery*, vol. 39, no. 4, pp. 674–677, 1956.

[4] R. Virchow, "Ueber Makroglossie und pathologische neubildung quergestreifter muskelfasern," *Archiv für Pathologische Anatomie und Physiologie und für Klinische Medicin*, vol. 7, no. 1, pp. 126–138, 1854.

[5] H. T. Butlin, *Diseases of the Tongue*, Lea Brothersand, Philadelphia, Pa, USA, 1885.

[6] J. N. Pannullo, "Congenital macroglossia; report of a case," *Obstetrics and Gynecology*, vol. 7, no. 1, pp. 97–98, 1956.

[7] M. C. Reynoso, A. Hernandez, L. A. Lizcano-Gil et al., "Autosomal dominant congenital macroglossia: further delineation of the syndrome," *Genetic Counseling*, vol. 5, no. 2, pp. 151–154, 1994.

[8] O. P. Gupta, "Congenital macroglossia," *Archives of Otolaryngology*, vol. 93, no. 4, pp. 378–383, 1971.

[9] A. Kacker, C. Honrado, D. Martin, and R. Ward, "Tongue reduction in Beckwith-Weidemann Syndrome," *International Journal of Pediatric Otorhinolaryngology*, vol. 53, no. 1, pp. 1–7, 2000.

[10] A. Davalbhakta and B. G. H. Lamberty, "Technique for uniform reduction of macroglossia," *British Journal of Plastic Surgery*, vol. 53, no. 4, pp. 294–297, 2000.

[11] F. L. Rimell, A. M. Shapiro, D. L. Shoemaker, and M. A. Kenna, "Head and neck manifestations of Beckwith-Wiedemann syndrome," *Otolaryngology*, vol. 113, pp. 262–265, 1995.

[12] M. Elliott, R. Bayly, T. Cole, I. K. Temple, and E. R. Maher, "Clinical features and natural history of Beckwith-Wiedemann syndrome: presentation of 74 new cases," *Clinical Genetics*, vol. 46, no. 2, pp. 168–174, 1994.

[13] P. M. Sokoloski, R. G. Ogle, and D. E. Waite, "Surgical correction of macroglossia in Beckwith-Wiedemann syndrome," *Journal of Oral Surgery*, vol. 36, no. 3, pp. 212–215, 1978.

[14] F. J. N. Dias, J. H. F. Junior, P. A. Faber, and R. G. Toloi, "True macroglossy—a case report," *Revista De Cirurgia e Traumatologia Buco-Maxilo-Facial*, vol. 6, pp. 33–38, 2006.

[15] A. Smith and B. Speculand, "Amyloidosis with oral involvement," *British Journal of Oral and Maxillofacial Surgery*, vol. 23, no. 6, pp. 435–444, 1985.

[16] W. G. Ensign, "Macroglossia as a manifestation of primary systemic amyloidosis; report," *Journal of the American Medical Association*, vol. 149, no. 2, pp. 136–138, 1952.

[17] W. S. Caudell and Y. K. Yoshida, "Macroglossia in primary amyloidosis," *Surgery*, vol. 37, no. 4, pp. 643–649, 1955.

[18] J. J. Kempton and C. Latto, "Neurofibromatosis presenting as macroglossia," *Archives of disease in childhood*, vol. 26, no. 125, pp. 76–77, 1951.

[19] T. Bird and G. O. Clark, "Neurofibromatous macroglossia," *The Journal of Laryngology and Otology*, vol. 69, no. 1, pp. 51–58, 1955.

[20] R. F. García de Guilarte, B. B. Frönher, P. R. Urcelay, R. C. Nájera, B. G. Meli, and J. Enríquez de Salamanca Celada, "An idiopathic case of macroglossia," *Journal of Plastic, Reconstructive and Aesthetic Surgery*, vol. 62, no. 2, pp. e41–e43, 2009.

[21] L. M. Wolford and D. A. Cotrelli, "Diagnosis of macroglossia and indications for reduction glossectomy," *American Journal of Orthodontics & Dentofacial Orthopedics*, vol. 110, pp. 170–177, 1996.

[22] T. Harris, "Chronic intumescence of the tongue," *American Journal of the Medical Sciences*, vol. 7, pp. 17–22, 1830.

[23] T. Harris, "A case of congenital enlargement of the tongue," *American Journal of the Medical Sciences*, vol. 20, pp. 15–18, 1837.

[24] V. P. Blair, *Surgery and Diseases of the Mouth and Jaws*, CV Mosby, St Louis, Miss, USA, 1912.

[25] H. Pichler and R. Trauner, *Mund Und Kieferchirurgie Fur Den Zahndarzt und Studenten*, Urban and Schwarzenberg, Wien, Austria, 1948.

[26] P. Egyedi and H. Obwegeser, "Zur operativen zungenverkleinerung," *Dtsch Zahn Mund Kieferheilk*, vol. 41, pp. 16–25, 1964.

[27] W. E. Morgan, E. M. Friedman, N. O. Duncan, and M. Sulek, "Surgical management of macroglossia in children," *Archives of Otolaryngology*, vol. 122, no. 3, pp. 326–329, 1996.

[28] J. Wang, N. M. Goodger, and M. A. Pogrel, "The role of tongue reduction," *Oral Surgery, Oral Medicine, Oral Pathology, Oral Radiology, and Endodontics*, vol. 95, no. 3, pp. 269–273, 2003.

[29] K. Fröhlich, B. Ingervall, and R. Schmoker, "Influence of surgical tongue reduction on pressure from the tongue on the teeth," *Angle Orthodontist*, vol. 63, no. 3, pp. 191–198, 1993.

# 21

# Peripheral Ossifying Fibroma

**Meenakshi Bhasin,[1,2] Vinny Bhasin,[3] and Abhilasha Bhasin[4]**

[1] *Department of Oral Medicine, Mansarovar Dental College, Bhopal, Madhya Pradesh 462042, India*
[2] *Department of Oral Medicine & Radiology, 153 Adarsh Nagar, Narmada Road, Jabalpur, Madhya Pradesh 482002, India*
[3] *Department of Orthodontia, Mansarovar Dental College, Bhopal, Madhya Pradesh 462042, India*
[4] *Department of Prosthodontics, Hithkarni Dental College, Jabalpur, Madhya Pradesh 482002, India*

Correspondence should be addressed to Meenakshi Bhasin; meenakshibhasin85@yahoo.com

Academic Editors: L. Junquera and M. A. D. A. M. Machado

Intraoral ossifying fibromas have been described in the literature since the late 1940s. Peripheral ossifying fibroma (POF) is usually a fibroma of the gingival which shows areas of calcification or ossification. It is a nonneoplastic enlargement of gingiva. Due to its clinical and histopathological similarities, some POFs are believed to develop initially as a pyogenic granuloma that undergoes fibrous maturation and subsequent calcification. It has been suggested that POF represents a separate clinical entity rather than a transitional form of pyogenic granuloma or irritation fibroma. This paper describes a case report of a 60-year-old female patient reported with growth on gingiva in the upper left front region of mouth three years ago.

## 1. Introduction

Many types of localized reactive lesions are seen on the gingiva, including focal fibrous hyperplasia, pyogenic granuloma, peripheral giant cell granuloma, and peripheral ossifying fibroma (POF) [1–3]. Synonyms of POF are peripheral cementifying fibroma, calcifying or ossifying fibroid epulis, and peripheral fibroma with calcification. These lesions may arise as a result of irritants such as trauma, microorganisms, plaque, calculus, faulty restorations, and dental appliances [2, 3]. It is typically seen as a gingival growth on interdental papilla and comprises about 9% of all gingival growths [1]. Females are more commonly affected, and anterior maxilla is the most prevalent location [1]. POFs are usually less than 1.5 cm in diameter, and diagnosis can be made by clinical inspection and biopsy [4]. It has not been clarified whether POF is a tumor or represents proliferation of a reactive nature. POF shows a clinically benign behavior [5]. Incidences of recurrence have been put at 16–20% [6]. The reasons for recurrence include incomplete removal of lesion, failure to eliminate local irritants, and difficulty in access during surgical manipulation due to intricate location of POF being present usually at interdental areas. Deep excisions have been preferred for recurrences [6].

## 2. Case Report

A 60-year-old female patient reported with the chief complaint of painless growth on the gingiva in the upper left front region of mouth three years ago. It had progressed gradually to increase in size and attained the present size. Growth was associated with bleeding on brushing occasionally. The patient did not give any history of trauma.

Intraoral examination revealed a solitary, sessile growth present on the residual ridge of the missing 23 in the interdental space between 22 and 24, extending mesiodistally from the distal aspect of 22 up to mesial aspect of the 24 region (Figure 1).

Superoinferiorly extending superiorly from marginal gingiva of 22 and 24 and inferiorly from 1-2 cm below the incisor line (Figure 2). Antero-posteriorly extending from inner aspect of upper lip to 3 cm towards hard palate (Figure 3).

It was of the same color of the adjacent gingiva with the mesial half being more reddish in color. The growth was oval in shape and approximately 2.5 × 3 cm in size in greatest dimensions with well-defined borders. The surface of the growth was lobulated.

No secondary changes were seen related to ulceration and fungation. The growth was firm and nontender on palpation.

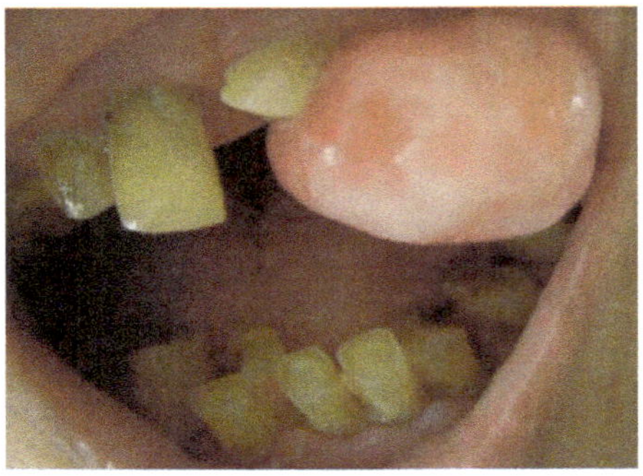

Figure 1

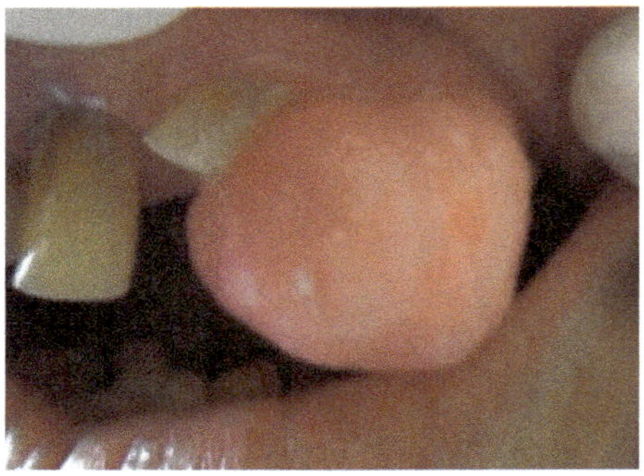

Figure 2

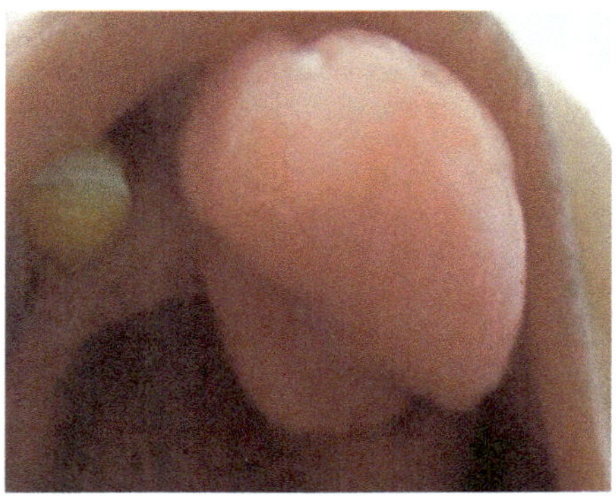

Figure 3

It was nonfluctuant, nonreducible, and noncompressible with mild bleeding on probing.

The clinical differential diagnoses for the growth were pyogenic granuloma, traumatic fibroma, peripheral giant cell granuloma, and peripheral ossifying fibroma, and provisional diagnosis of pyogenic granuloma with respect to the 22, 23, and 24 regions was made for the gingival growth.

Radiological investigations—intraoral periapical radiograph of left maxillary anterior region revealed the presence of 22 and 24 and missing 23. Evidence of faint, irregular radiopacity was noticed in the missing 23 region, suggestive of soft tissue mass, and mesial tipping of 22 and distal tipping of 24 were noticed (Figure 4).

Maxillary occlusal radiograph reveals the presence of 11, 12, 22, 24, and 25. Irregular radiopacity is seen interspersed in

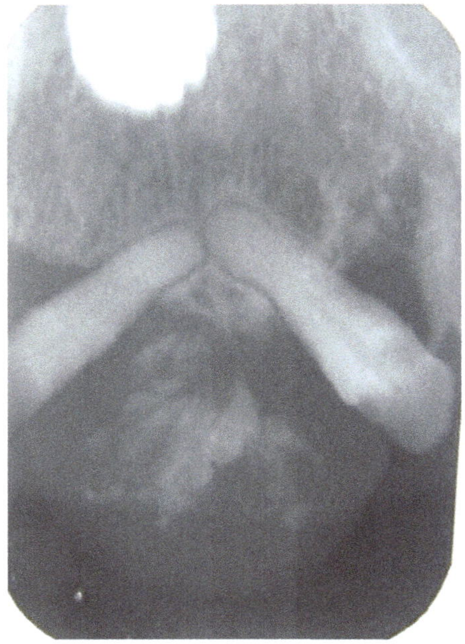

Figure 4

the soft tissue shadow. The density of which is almost similar to the bone, signifying the presence of ossification (Figure 5).

## 3. Treatment

Growth was excised conservatively. The excised tissue was oval, 2.5 × 3 cm in size, pale white in color, and firm in consistency. Tissue was sent for histopathological examination. Adjacent teeth were scaled to remove the local irritants. The patient was recalled after one week for review (Figure 6).

Histologically, the specimen showed parakeratinized stratifie squamous epithelium overlying the connective tissue stroma. Epithelium showed hyperplasia in some areas. Connective tissue stroma consisted of highly cellular mass of proliferating fibroblasts intermingled with fibrillar tissue. Fibrous connective tissue also consisted of large and small trabeculae of bone and some dystrophic calcifications. Based on history, clinical presentation, and radiological and histopathological examination, final diagnosis of peripheral ossifying fibroma with respect to the 22, 23, and 24 regions was put forth.

## 4. Discussion

Menzel first described the lesion ossifying fibroma in 1872, but its terminology was given by Montgomery in 1927 [7]. Peripheral ossifying fibroma occurs mostly in craniofacial bones and categorized into two types central and peripheral. The central type of ossifying fibroma arises from the endosteum or the periodontal ligament (PDL) adjacent to the root apex and expands from the medullary cavity of the bone, and the peripheral type occurs on the soft tissues overlying the alveolar process [8]. POF is a solitary, slow growing nodular

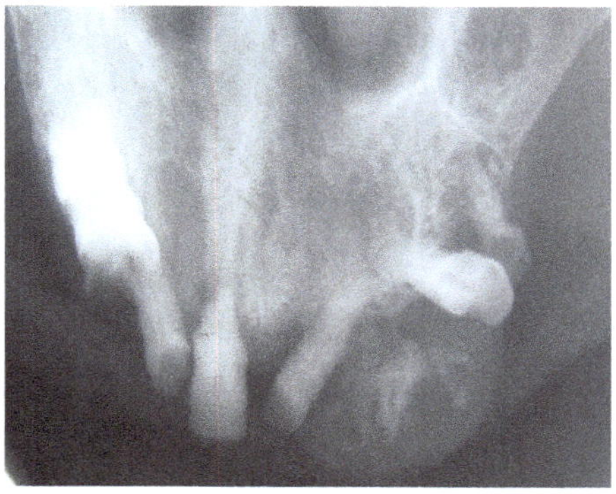

Figure 5

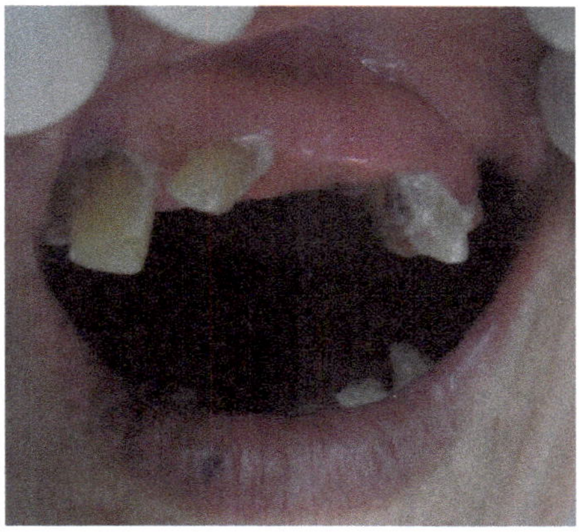

Figure 6

mass that is either pedunculated or sessile. Most often it is located in the gingival papilla between adjacent teeth [2].

Though the etiopathogenesis of POF is uncertain, origin from cells of periodontal ligament has been suggested. The reasons for considering periodontal ligament origin include excessive occurrence of POF in the gingival interdental papilla, the proximity of the gingival to periodontal ligament, the presence of oxytalan fibres within the mineralized matrix of some lesion, and the fibrocellular response in periodontal ligament [2, 8]. Migration of teeth with interdental bone destruction has been reported in some of the cases [9].

In vast majority of cases, there is no apparent underlying bone involvement visible on the roentgenogram. However, superficial erosion of bone is noted occasionally [2, 8, 9].

Peripheral ossifying fibroma has to be differentiated from traumatic fibroma, peripheral giant cell granuloma, pyogenic granuloma, and peripheral odontogenic fibroma.

Peripheral odontogenic fibroma is an uncommon neoplasm that is believed to arise from odontogenic epithelial rests in periodontal ligament or attached gingiva itself. Traumatic fibroma occur on buccal mucosa along the bite line. Pyogenic granuloma presents as soft, friable nodule, small in size that bleeds with tendency to hemorrhage and may or may not occasionally or do not show calcifications but tooth displacement and resorption of alveolar bone are not observed. Peripheral giant cell granuloma has clinical features similar to POF however POF lacks the purple or blue discoloration commonly associated with peripheral giant cell granuloma and radiographically shows flecks of calcification [10].

It is possible to histologically differentiate PGCG and peripheral odontogenic fibroma from POF as PGCG contains giant cells, whereas peripheral odontogenic fibroma contains odontogenic epithelium and dysplastic dentine; all the features are not seen in POF [11].

Treatment includes local surgical excision and oral prophylaxis [12]. Followup is essential because of the recurrence rates. Recurrence is due to incomplete excision and/or due to persistence of local factors [2].

## 5. Conclusion

POF being one of the commonest solitary swelling in the oral cavity is many times clinically diagnosed as pyogenic granuloma. Radiological and histopathological examination is required for confirmation of diagnosis.

## References


[1] S. N. Bhaskar and J. R. Jacoway, "Peripheral fibroma and peripheral fibroma with calcification: report of 376 cases," *The Journal of the American Dental Association*, vol. 73, no. 6, pp. 1312–1320, 1966.

[2] L. R. Eversole and S. Rovin, "Reactive lesions of the gingiva," *Journal of oral pathology*, vol. 1, no. 1, pp. 30–38, 1972.

[3] D. G. Gardner, "The peripheral odontogenic fibroma: an attempt at clarification," *Oral Surgery Oral Medicine and Oral Pathology*, vol. 54, no. 1, pp. 40–48, 1982.

[4] Z. E. S. Cuisia and R. B. Brannon, "Peripheral ossifying fibroma-a clinical evaluation of 134 pediatric cases," *Pediatric Dentistry*, vol. 23, no. 3, pp. 245–248, 2001.

[5] S. Chhina, A. Rathore, and A. Puneet, "Peripheral ossifying fibroma of gingiva: a case report," *International Journal of Case Reports and Images*, vol. 2, no. 11, pp. 21–24, 2011.

[6] D. C. Shetty, A. B. Urs, P. Ahuja, A. Sahu, A. Manchanda, and Y. Sirohi, "Mineralized components and their interpretation in the histogenesis of peripheral ossifying fibroma," *Indian Journal of Dental Research*, vol. 22, no. 1, pp. 56–61, 2011.

[7] G. Sujatha, G. Sivakumar, J. Muruganandhan, J. Selvakumar, and M. Ramasamy, "Peripheral ossifying fibroma-report of a case," *Indian Journal of Multidisciplinary Dentistry*, vol. 2, no. 1, pp. 415–418, 2012.

[8] C. S. Miller, R. G. Henry, and D. D. Damm, "Proliferative mass found in the gingiva," *The Journal of the American Dental Association*, vol. 121, no. 4, pp. 559–560, 1990.

[9] C. K. Poon, P. C. Kwan, and S. Y. Chao, "Giant peripheral ossifying fibroma of the maxilla: report of a case," *Journal of Oral and Maxillofacial Surgery*, vol. 53, no. 6, pp. 695–698, 1995.

[10] B. W. Neville, D. D. Damm, C. M. Allen, and J. E. Bouquot, *Oral and Maxillofacial Pathology*, Saunders, Philadelphia, Pa, USA, 1995.

[11] D. Gardener, "The peripheral ossifying fibroma: an attempt at clarification," *Oral Surgery, Oral Medicine, Oral Pathology*, vol. 54, no. 1, pp. 40–48, 1982.

[12] T. Farquhar, J. MacLellan, H. Dyment, and R. D. Anderson, "Peripheral ossifying fibroma: a case report," *Journal of the Canadian Dental Association*, vol. 74, no. 9, pp. 809–812, 2008.

22

# Magnet-Retained Facial Prosthesis Combined with Maxillary Obturator

**Mahnaz Hatami,[1] Hamid Badrian,[2] Siamak Samanipoor,[3] and Marcelo Coelho Goiato[4]**

[1] *Department of Prosthodontics, School of Dentistry, Shahid Sadoughi University of Medical Sciences, Yazd, Iran*
[2] *Dental Implant Research Center, School of Dentistry, Isfahan, Iran*
[3] *Department of Endodontics, School of Dentistry, Shahid Bahonar University of Medical Sciences, Kerman, Iran*
[4] *Faculty of Dentistry of Araçatuba, University of the State of São Paulo, Jose Bonifacio 1193, 16015-050 Araçatuba, SP, Brazil*

Correspondence should be addressed to Marcelo Coelho Goiato; goiato@foa.unesp.br

Academic Editors: I. Anic, S. Anil, R. Crespi, M. A. Qudeimat, and M. J. Wahl

Prosthetic rehabilitation of the midfacial defects has always perplexed prosthodontists. These defects lead to functional and esthetic deficiencies. The purpose of this clinical case report was the presentation of the prosthetic rehabilitation of an extraoral-intraoral defect using two-piece prosthesis magnetically connected. This prosthesis has dramatically improved the patient's speech, mastication, swallowing, and esthetic.

## 1. Introduction

Acquired midfacial defects may affect patients' speech, mastication, quality of life, psychology, and social behavior [1–4]. Midfacial defects are defined as defects in the middle third of the face in horizontal plane that communicate with intraoral maxillary defects. These defects can be classified into two major categories of midline and lateral-midline midfacial defects. Midline midfacial defects include complete or partial involvement of either nose or upper lip that communicate with an intraoral maxillary defect while the lateral midfacial defects include complete or partial involvement of cheek and orbital contents that communicate with an intraoral maxillary defect [5].

Midfacial defect can result from trauma, burns, most tumors of paranasal sinus, palatal epithelium, minor salivary glands [6–8], congenital abnormalities like vascular malformations [6], and some of other lesions like lethal midline granuloma [9] that require partial or radical maxillectomy. One of the other causes of such defects is mucormycosis that is caused by a fungus of the order Mucorales that is one of the most rapid fatal fungal infections known to man. Rhinocerebral mucormycosis is the most common type, and its extension to the orbit and brain is quite usual. The location of mucormycosis on the palate is rare and of late occurrence [10].

Large midfacial defects are rarely rehabilitated by surgical reconstruction alone. They usually require a facial prosthesis to restore function and esthetic [11].

In addition, an intraoral prosthesis such as an obturator should restore speech and deglutition. Fabrication of a facial prosthesis challenges the artistic ability of prosthodontists. On the other hand, size and weight of facial prostheses endanger the retention of them. This clinical case report describes the prosthodontic rehabilitation of an edentulous patient with a large midfacial (intraoral-extraoral) defect. The main aim of this rehabilitation was to provide the esthetic

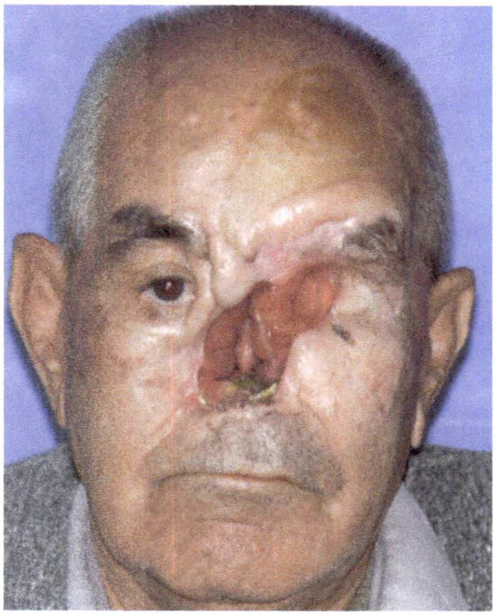

FIGURE 1: Midfacial defect after surgery.

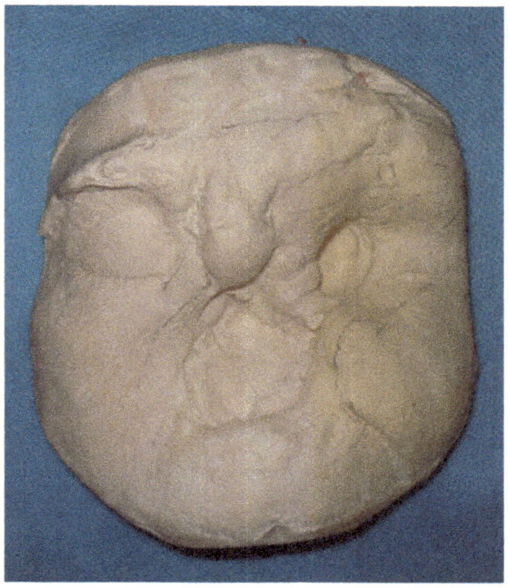

FIGURE 3: Working cast.

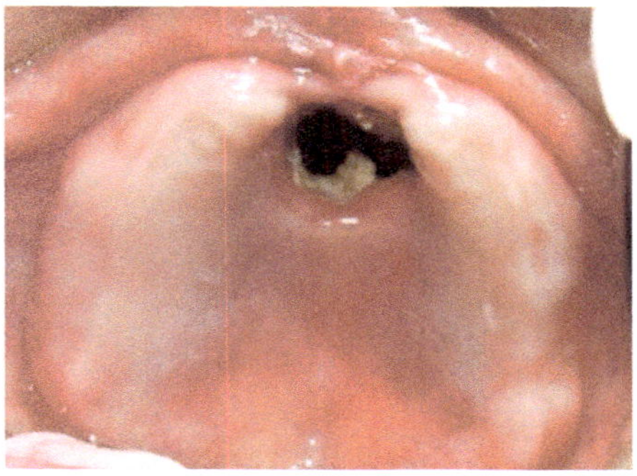

FIGURE 2: Intraoral view of maxillary defect.

needs of the patient and to improve the patient's quality of life.

## 2. Case Report

The patient was a 65-year-old edentulous male with a chief complaint of poor facial appearance and past medical history of diabetes mellitus. His facial tissues were affected by a fungal infection of rhinocerebral mucormycosis followed by diabetic ketoacidosis. For debridement and removal of necrotic tissues, ablative surgery has been done. Resected portions included anterior part of hard palate, nasal septum and conchae, left maxillary sinus, and orbital contents (Figures 1 and 2). Therefore, there was an open communication between the oral, nasal, and orbital cavities.

After precise evaluation of the case, the proposed treatment plan was to construct a complete denture with obturator, as well as a facial prosthesis which would be attached to the obturator with cobalt samarium magnets (Jobmasters, Randallstown, USA).

Treatment was started by the construction of a complete denture with obturator before facial prosthesis because anterior-posterior position of anterior denture teeth and labial flange has a basic role in lip support. The complete denture with obturator was made according to the procedure recommended by Zarb et al. [12] and Taylor [13].

The second stage was making an impression of the face defect and adjacent tissues using a thin layer of irreversible hydrocolloid (Hydrogum, Zhermack, Rovigo, Italy). The margin of impression was outlined on the face using the boxing wax (Kerr, Orange, CA, USA). Moist gauze was packed to prevent the flow of impression material into the undesired areas of the defect. The impression was reinforced with fast setting dental plaster (Ernst Hinrichs GMBH, Goslar, Germany) which has a thickness of 0.25 inch. The impression was boxed and poured in dental stone (Ernst Hinrichs GMBH, Goslar, Germany) (Figure 3).

Then working cast was trimmed, defect undercuts were blocked out, and tinfoil substitute was applied to the cast. The waxing up of the nose, orbit, some portions of check and upper lip was developed on a thin acrylic resin baseplate (Acropars, Marlic Co., Tehran, Iran) which adapted on the master cast. Before this step, ocular prosthesis had been made using paper iris disk technique [13]. The cuplike pattern of orbital defect made the basis for inserting the ocular prosthesis within the defect in the same frontal, sagittal, and horizontal planes as the normal eye. The ocular prosthesis was fabricated into a position that matches the gaze of another normal eye when the patient was directly staring at a point at eye level at least 6 feet away. Then eyelid aperture was reproduced by softening and placing two small strips of wax over the ocular section. The shape of the lid opening should make the opening of the other normal eye [13] (Figure 4).

Patient's previous photographs and the references from his first circle relatives were taken as a guide for shaping the wax pattern. The contour of final surface and skin texture was fabricated by carving in lines and wrinkles which observed, by pressing a wet gauze square into softened wax. In the next visit, trial placement of wax pattern was performed on

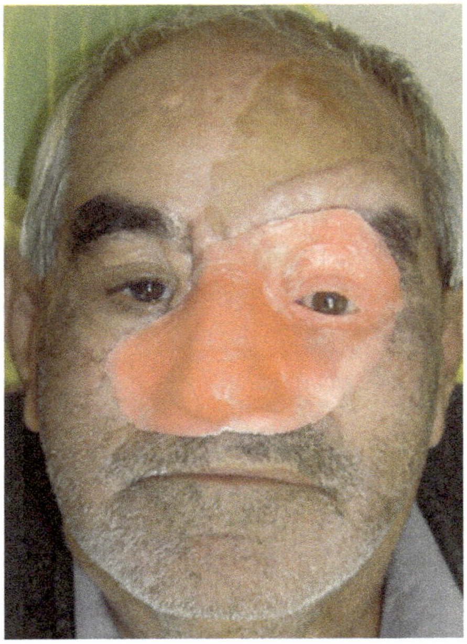

Figure 4: Wax pattern tryin.

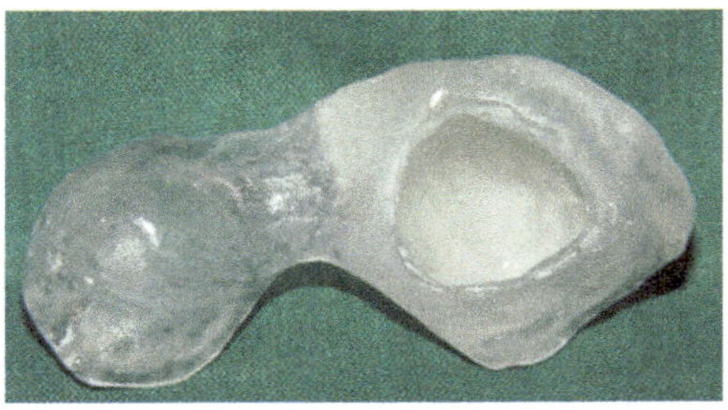

Figure 5: Hollow acrylic substructure.

the patient's face and marginal discrepancies were refitted by corrective wax (Kerr, Orange, CA, USA). Then a hollow acrylic resin framework was made in posterior aspect of wax pattern for decreasing weight of the prosthesis [14] (Figure 5).

The wax pattern was flask using die stone (Ernst Hinrichs GMBH, Goslar, Germany) to form a mold for packing the silicone. Wax elimination was performed in usual manner [15]. Then, the acrylic substructure was placed on the mold and was packed with a MDX4-4210-base silicone (Dow Corning Corp., Midland, USA). Laminar intrinsic staining was used in packing according to the patient's skin color [13]. The silicone was heated for 2 hours at 90°C, disinvested, trimmed, and cleaned. The prosthesis was trial fitted and extrinsically colored by medical adhesive type A (Dow corning, Midland, MI) and oil pigments (Factor II, Lakeside, USA).

Autopolymerizing resin (Acropars, Marlic Co., Tehran, Iran) was initially used to attach a magnet on the superior aspect of the obturator. Indelible pencil was drawn on the surface of the first magnet, and the facial prosthesis was positioned in its location to demarcate the area of most contact.

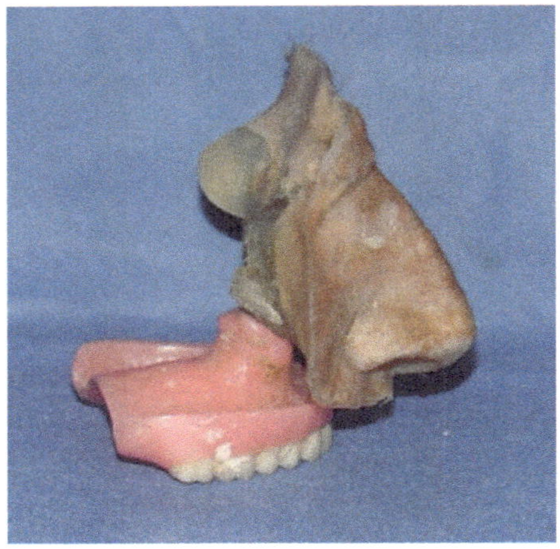

Figure 6: Attached intra and extraoral prostheses.

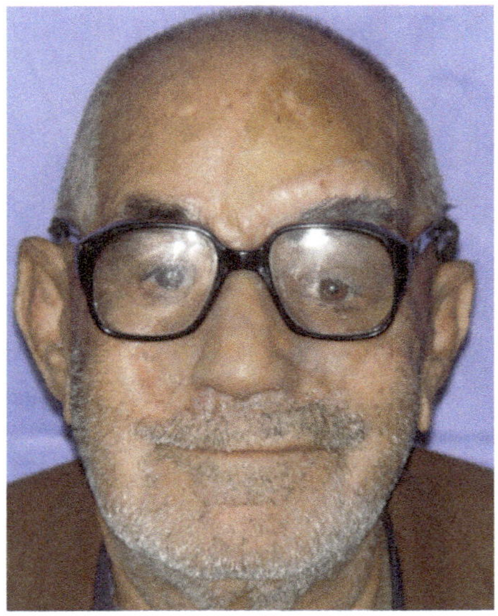

Figure 7: Completed facial prosthesis in place.

At the time of insertion of the facial prosthesis, the patient was instructed to close in maximum intercuspal position with obturator placed in the mouth.

On the demarcate area of the facial prosthesis extension (acrylic substructure), the second magnet was attached to self-curing acrylic resin. The extraoral prosthesis had adequate retention after using magnets and eyeglasses (Figures 6 and 7). Extra support for the glasses was gained by attaching an elastic band around the back of the head from one earpiece to another one.

The patient was given hygiene instructions for cleaning both prostheses. The patient attended recall visits every 4 to 5 months. During two years after prosthesis insertion, the prosthesis was still serviceable and the patient was pleased.

An esthetic improvement, intelligible speaking, andimproved deglutition and mastication were achieved for the patient by this prosthetic reconstruction.

## 3. Discussion

Restoration of midfacial defects can be accomplished surgically or prosthetically or by using a combination of both methods. Selection of each method depends on many factors including size, location of the defect, and age of patient [13].

Acceptable esthetic results usually can be obtained by a facial prosthesis. However, retention of a large prosthesis can be challenging.

Various methods of auxiliary retention for facial prosthesis have been described in the literature; they include eyeglasses [16], denture extensions that engage tissue undercuts [16, 17], magnets [16, 18], facial prosthetic adhesives [16], or combination of the above [16, 17, 19], and craniofacial implants [16, 17, 20, 21]. Respiratory epithelium is easily traumatized by frictional contact with prosthesis and limits the use of anatomic undercuts [22]. Soft tissues around defects may not always be ideal for adhesive retention because movements that occur during smiling compromise adaptation of prosthesis margins [23, 24].

For the first time, Nadeau [25] described the use of combination of extra- and intraoral prostheses connected by magnets. Durability of surface coatings of the long-term magnets is a major concern; hence, it is advised to use the magnets with strong surface coatings.

Connecting these prostheses often results in movement of facial prosthesis during mastication [26, 27]. The use of eyeglasses alone for retaining a nasal prosthesis has been well documented [28–30]. Although craniofacial implants may provide the most reliable prosthesis retention, additional surgeries, expenses, inadequate quantity or quality of the bone, and prior radiation to the area may contraindicate this type of treatment [31, 32].

A hollow acrylic resin framework used for facial prosthesis is advantageous as there is no need to fabricate the whole prosthesis again in case of discoloration or damage of the silicone layer because the outer silicon layer can be removed and repacked with the new silicon on the acrylic resin framework if the mold is preserved.

The advantages of this prosthesis are that the technique is noninvasive, cost effective, tissue tolerant, esthetic, comfortable to use, and easy to clean. The difficulty in maxillofacial rehabilitation of large defects often involves the compromise of functional adequacy versus esthetic.

## 4. Conclusion

Satisfactory functional and esthetic results are achievable in patients with a large lateral midfacial defect using a hollow acrylic resin framework for silicon facial prosthesis. Retention of facial prosthesis can be satisfactorily achieved with the use of strong magnets provided that the facial prosthesis is light in weight.

## Consent

Informed consent for medical photographs was obtained from the patient.

## Conflict of Interests

The authors report no conflict of interests.

## References


[1] J. B. Ludlow, L. E. Davies-Ludlow, S. L. Brooks, and W. B. Howerton, "Dosimetry of 3 CBCT devices for oral and maxillofacial radiology: CB Mercuray, NewTom 3G and i-CAT," *Dentomaxillofacial Radiology*, vol. 35, no. 4, pp. 219–226, 2006.

[2] "The glossary of prosthodontic terms," *The Journal of Prosthetic Dentistry*, vol. 94, no. 1, pp. 10–92, 2005.

[3] C. A. Lascala, J. Panella, and M. M. Marques, "Analysis of the accuracy of linear measurements obtained by cone beam computed tomography (CBCT-NewTom)," *Dentomaxillofacial Radiology*, vol. 33, no. 5, pp. 291–294, 2004.

[4] D. M. Hecker, J. P. Wiens, T. R. Cowper et al., "Can we assess quality of life in patients with head and neck cancer? A preliminary report from the American Academy of Maxillofacial Prosthetics," *Journal of Prosthetic Dentistry*, vol. 88, no. 3, pp. 344–351, 2002.

[5] M. T. Marunick, R. Harrison, and J. Beumer, "Prosthodontic rehabilitation of midfacial defects," *The Journal of Prosthetic Dentistry*, vol. 54, no. 4, pp. 553–560, 1985.

[6] D. M. Hecker, "Maxillofacial rehabilitation of a large facial defect resulting from an arteriovenous malformation utilizing a two-piece prosthesis," *Journal of Prosthetic Dentistry*, vol. 89, no. 2, pp. 109–113, 2003.

[7] S. Jain, K. Maru, J. Shukla, A. Vyas, R. Pillai, and P. Jain, "Nasal prosthesis rehabilitation: a case report," *The Journal of Indian Prosthodontic Society*, vol. 11, no. 4, pp. 265–269, 2011.

[8] H. Kurunmäki, R. Kantola, M. M. Hatamleh, D. C. Watts, and P. K. Vallittu, "A fiber-reinforced composite prosthesis restoring a lateral midfacial defect: a clinical report," *Journal of Prosthetic Dentistry*, vol. 100, no. 5, pp. 348–352, 2008.

[9] S. S. Guttal, N. P. Patil, and A. D. Shetye, "Prosthetic rehabilitation of a midfacial defect resulting from lethal midline granuloma—a clinical report," *Journal of Oral Rehabilitation*, vol. 33, no. 11, pp. 863–867, 2006.

[10] D. E. Kyrmizakis, P. G. Doxas, J. K. Hajiioannou, and C. E. Papadakis, "Palate ulcer due to mucormycosis," *Journal of Laryngology and Otology*, vol. 116, no. 2, pp. 146–147, 2002.

[11] R. Brignoni and J. T. Dominici, "An intraoral-extraoral combination prosthesis using an intermediate framework and magnets: a clinical report," *Journal of Prosthetic Dentistry*, vol. 85, no. 1, pp. 7–11, 2001.

[12] G. A. Zarb, C. L. Bolender, S. E. Eckert, R. Jacob, A. Fenton, and R. Mericske-Stern, *Prosthodontic Treatment for Edentulous Patients*, Mosby, St. Louis, Mo, USA, 2004.

[13] T. D. Taylor, *Clinical Maxillofacial Prosthetics*, Quintessence, Carol Stream, Ill, USA, 2000.

[14] P. G. Patil, "Modified technique to fabricate a hollow lightweight facial prosthesis for lateral midfacial defect: a clinical report," *The Journal of Advanced Prosthodontics*, vol. 2, no. 3, pp. 65–70, 2010.

[15] K. D. Rudd, R. M. Morrow, and J. E. Rhoads, *Dental Laboratory Procedures: Fixed Partial Dentures*, Mosby, 1986.

[16] K. F. Thomas, J. Penchas, and M. Sela, "Prosthetic rehabilitation," *Implant Dentistry*, vol. 3, no. 3, p. 198, 1994.

[17] J. B. Ludlow and M. Ivanovic, "Comparative dosimetry of dental CBCT devices and 64-slice CT for oral and maxillofacial

radiology," *Oral Surgery, Oral Medicine, Oral Pathology, Oral Radiology and Endodontology*, vol. 106, no. 1, pp. 106–114, 2008.

[18] H. B. Dumbrigue and A. Fylerb, "Minimizing prosthesis movement in a midfacial defect: a clinical report," *Journal of Prosthetic Dentistry*, vol. 78, no. 4, pp. 341–345, 1997.

[19] Y. Yang, E. Schreibmann, T. Li, C. Wang, and L. Xing, "Evaluation of on-board kV cone beam CT (CBCT)-based dose calculation," *Physics in Medicine and Biology*, vol. 52, no. 3, pp. 685–705, 2007.

[20] H. Menneking, M. Klein, B. Hell, and J. Bier, "Prosthetic restoration of nasal defects: indications for two different osseointegrated implant systems," *Journal of Facial and Somato Prosthetics*, vol. 4, no. 1, pp. 29–33, 1998.

[21] J. Tulasne, P. Worthington, and P. Branemark, *Advanced Osseointegration Surgery, Applications in the Maxillofacial Region. Advanced Osseointegration Surgery, Applications in the Maxillofacial Region*, 1992.

[22] A. Udagama and G. E. King, "Mechanically retained facial prostheses: helpful or harmful?" *The Journal of Prosthetic Dentistry*, vol. 49, no. 1, pp. 85–86, 1983.

[23] A. Shifman, "Selective-pressure impression technique for nasal prostheses," *The Journal of Prosthetic Dentistry*, vol. 58, no. 3, pp. 349–351, 1987.

[24] A. L. Martone, "Anatomy of facial expression and its prosthodontic significance," *The Journal of Prosthetic Dentistry*, vol. 12, no. 6, pp. 1020–1042, 1962.

[25] J. Nadeau, "Maxillofacial prosthesis with magnetic stabilizers," *The Journal of Prosthetic Dentistry*, vol. 6, no. 1, pp. 114–119, 1956.

[26] J. Nadeau, "Special prostheses," *The Journal of Prosthetic Dentistry*, vol. 20, no. 1, pp. 62–76, 1968.

[27] S. Birnbach and G. L. Herman, "Coordinated intraoral and extraoral prostheses in the rehabilitation of the orofacial cancer patient," *The Journal of Prosthetic Dentistry*, vol. 58, no. 3, pp. 343–348, 1987.

[28] M. F. Gomes, R. Teixeira, G. Plens, M. M. Silva, E. M. Pontes, and J. C. da Rocha, "Naso-orbicular tissue necrosis by Streptococcus parasanguis in a patient with Fanconi anemia: clinical and laboratory aspects," *Quintessence International*, vol. 35, no. 7, pp. 572–576, 2004.

[29] A. C. Cheng, D. Morrison, and A. G. Wee, "Immediate maxillofacial prosthodontic rehabilitation after radical mid-face tumor resection," *Journal of Prosthodontics*, vol. 6, no. 4, pp. 265–267, 1997.

[30] S. Rodrigues, V. K. Shenoy, and K. Shenoy, "Prosthetic rehabilitation of a patient after partial rhinectomy: a clinical report," *Journal of Prosthetic Dentistry*, vol. 93, no. 2, pp. 125–128, 2005.

[31] M. R. Arcuri, W. E. LaVelle, E. Fyler, and R. Jons, "Prosthetic complications of extraoral implants," *The Journal of Prosthetic Dentistry*, vol. 69, no. 3, pp. 289–292, 1993.

[32] E. Roumanas, R. Nishimura, J. Beumer, P. Moy, J. Weinlander, and J. Lorant, "Craniofacial defects and osseointegrated implants: six-year follow-up report on the success rates of craniofacial implants at UCLA," *International Journal of Oral and Maxillofacial Implants*, vol. 9, no. 5, pp. 579–585, 1994.

# 23

# Heterotopic Ossification: An Unusual Presentation

**Satish G. Patil,[1] Aisha Siddiqua,[1] Udupi Krishna Joshi,[1] Pallavi K. Deshmukh,[2] Bindu S. Patil,[3] and Anand Mangalgi[1]**

[1] *Department of Oral and Maxillofacial Surgery, S. Nijalingappa Institute of Dental Sciences and Research, Gulbarga, Karnataka 585105, India*
[2] *Department of Oral Medicine and Radiology, S. Nijalingappa Institute of Dental Sciences and Research, Gulbarga, Karnataka 585105, India*
[3] *Department of Periodontics, S. Nijalingappa Institute of Dental Sciences and Research, Gulbarga, Karnataka 585105, India*

Correspondence should be addressed to Satish G. Patil, zeal215@gmail.com

Academic Editors: M. A. Chinelatti, M. W. Roberts, and P. R. Warren

Heterotopic ossification (HO) is usually seen after-trauma, following traumatic injuries, surgeries involving major joints, neurogenic injury, and burns; however, atraumatic cases have also been reported. HO tends to cause pain, swelling, and limitation of joint movements. HO has been reported in adults as well as in pediatric cases, however, our search in the English literature has not revealed a single case in the infratemporal region, especially in children of developing age, where HO tends to affect the development and growth of adjacent bones. We are reporting a case of HO in close proximity to TMJ affecting the development of mandible and maxilla.

## 1. Introduction

Heterotopic ossification is the formation of mature lamellar bone in soft tissues outside the joint capsule and periosteum. HO usually occurs secondary to trauma and has been frequently reported after hip arthroplasty and spinal injury. It is usually symptomatic, and patient presents with pain and swelling. Cases showing limited range of motion, due to presence of HO in close proximity to joint, have been reported. However, literature has not revealed HO affecting the TMJ and its development. A case of one such patient, where HO occurred in close proximity to TMJ affecting its function and growth of maxilla and mandible, is reported. The incomplete development of maxilla and mandible resembles a mild case of Goldenhar syndrome. Until further evidence disproves this, this may be considered first such case of Goldenhar syndrome with HO.

## 2. Case Report

A four-year-old female child patient reported to the Department of Oral Surgery with her parents who complained of restricted mouth opening and asymmetry of face. History revealed that, the child was born with an apparently normal face and adequate mouth opening. Deviation of mouth and gradual reduction in mouth opening were noticed from the second year of life. Clinical examination revealed an obvious asymmetry of lower third of face (Figure 1). There was fullness of face on the right side as compared to the left side with a shallow groove in the left cheek at the junction of middle and lower one-third of the face, extending from the left angle of mandible and disappearing over the ramus. On opening of mouth, an obvious deviation of chin towards left side was noted. Preauricular skin tags were noticed on both sides, with the left one being more prominent.

Intraoral examination revealed a shift in midline towards left with the upper midline coinciding with the lower right canine with an overjet of 15 mm. Mouth opening was restricted to 2 cm (Figure 2). On palpation, a bony hard mass was felt in the posterosuperior part of the upper left buccal vestibule below the mucosa (Figures 3(a) and 3(b)). Boundaries could not be confirmed. The mass seemed to extend into the infratemporal region. Dimpling of the mucosa was present right below the mass and 1 cm × 1 cm

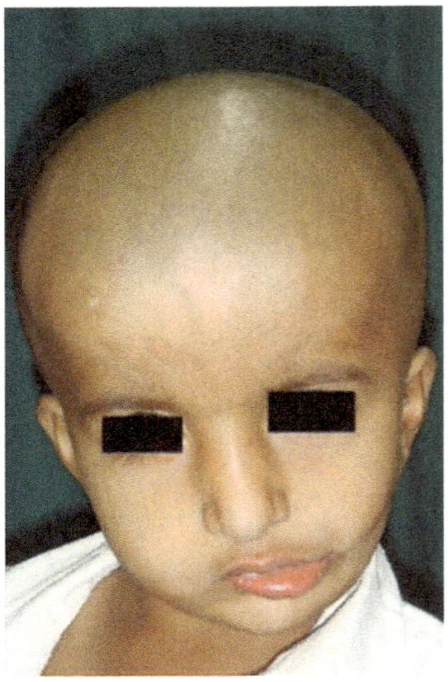

Figure 1: Preoperative frontal view.

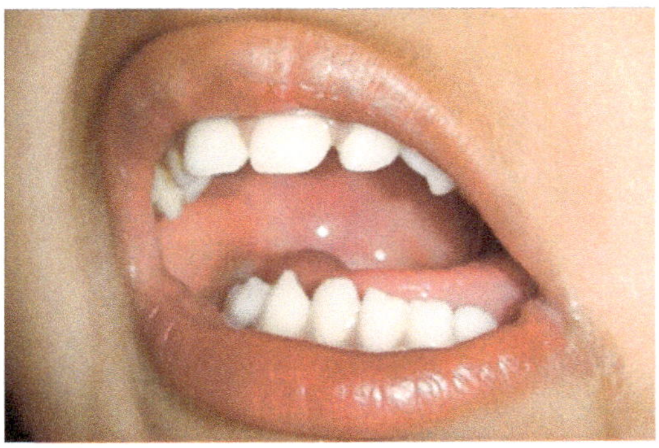

Figure 2: Deviated and restricted mouth opening.

of pale, and firm tissue could be palpated. History of trauma was not precise and could not be confirmed. There was no history of pain.

Computed tomography revealed a bony structure measuring 3 cms by 1.5 cms, roughly conical in shape in the infratemporal region, in front of the condyle and was overlying the coronoid process (Figures 4 and 5). The apex extended medial to the zygomatic arch. The bony mass was not attached to any of the adjacent. An abnormal development of the maxilla and mandible with a shift of the midline of the mandible to the left was seen. The anteroposterior growth of the right side of the mandible was more than that of the left side. The left coronoid was small representing stunted growth. The condyle seemed to be normal in structure. Based on the clinical and radiological findings a provisional diagnosis of heterotopic ossification was made.

Surgical procedure for excision of the bony mass was performed under general anesthesia. The bony mass was palpated, and a vertical mucosal incision was given over it. Blunt dissection was performed to expose the bony mass (Figure 6). The bony mass was easily separated from the surrounding tissues and removed in toto (Figure 7). The fibrous tissue adjacent to the mass was excised. Hemostasis was achieved, and site was closed with 3–0 vicryl. Postoperative period was uneventful. 3 years postoperatively patient showed adequate mouth opening (Figure 8). Histopathologic examination of the mass revealed presence of mature lamellar bone.

## 3. Discussion

Heterotopic ossification is the formation of mature lamellar bone in soft tissues. It forms outside the joint capsule and periosteum. It is usually symptomatic but can remain asymptomatic. When symptomatic, it causes pain, swelling and can present with functional impairment which is seen as limited range of motion when in proximity to a joint [1, 2]. Symptoms depend on the size and anatomical site.

The most common cause of HO is trauma [2], although, atraumatic HO has also been reported. Trauma could be in the form of musculoskeletal injury, surgical trauma, or warfare injuries. Other causes of HO are hereditary [3], burns [4], and neurogenic injury [2]. HO can occur in muscle, adipose tissue, and connective tissue.

Pathogenesis: although a precise pathophysiology of HO is yet to be made clear, a lot of studies indicate multifactorial process following trauma. Studies indicate role of various local and humoral factors [2, 5]. The role of BMP, osteogenic precursor cells, an appropriate environment that results following injury, is necessary for HO, with BMP induction causing the differentiation of precursor cells to osteoblasts. The precursor cells could be dormant osteoprogenitor cells [4], mesenchymal cells which are locally present or have migrated to the site of injury [5], or cells of vascular origin [2]. In neurogenic HO, studies suggest that BMP induction results in migration/release of osteogenic and other stem cells from the nerve [6].

Very few cases of HO have been previously reported in the literature in the maxillofacial region. Myositis ossificans has been reported in muscles of mastication [7]. A case of atraumatic HO in the scalp [8], HO following transposition of temporalis muscle in the cheek for the treatment of facial paralysis [9] and panniculitis ossificans in submental region [4], has been reported.

Our case is unique as she presents with HO at a very young age, at a very unusual site, and in connective tissue. As the child was in the growing age, the growth of both maxilla and mandible was affected on the involved side by the presence of bony mass. The mandible showed reduced anteroposterior growth of the body of the mandible and stunted growth of the coronoid on the affected side, resulting in asymmetrical mandible. Mild canting of the maxillary occlusal plane indicating reduced maxillary growth was noted.

In view of the presence of preauricular skin tags, first arch syndrome may be implicated. The features are consistent with the findings of Goldenhar syndrome. Goldenhar syndrome is a developmental anomaly of maxillofacial skeleton and hemifacial soft tissue. Characteristic features include facial asymmetry, hemifacial microsomia, microphthalmia, mandibular hypoplasia, unilateral ear deformity,

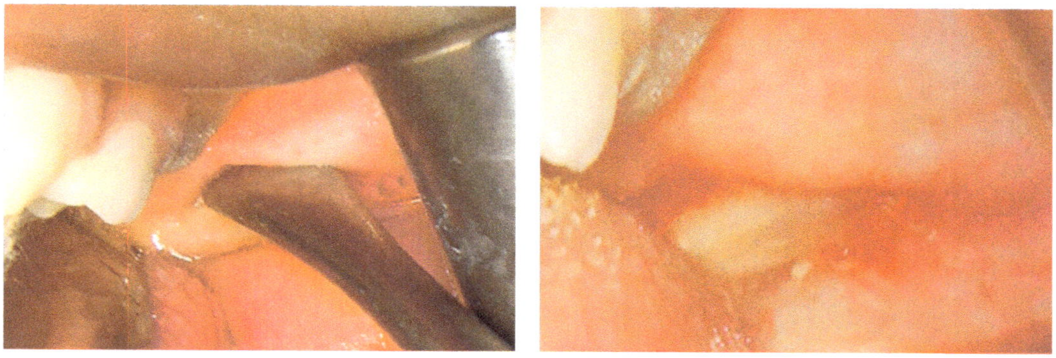

(a) (b)

FIGURE 3: (a) Intraoral photograph showing the mass, (b) irritational Fibroma.

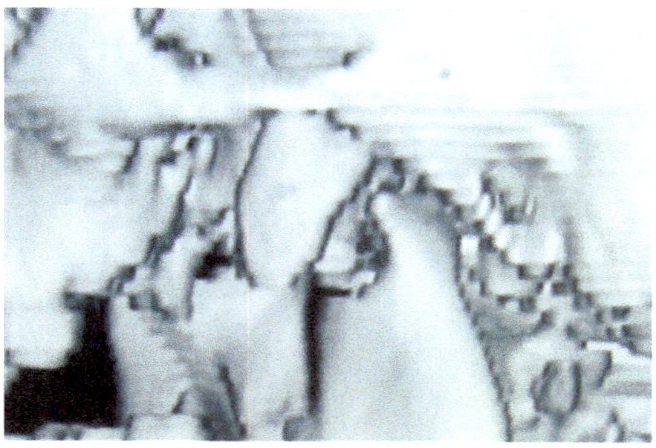

FIGURE 4: Computed tomography-lateral view.

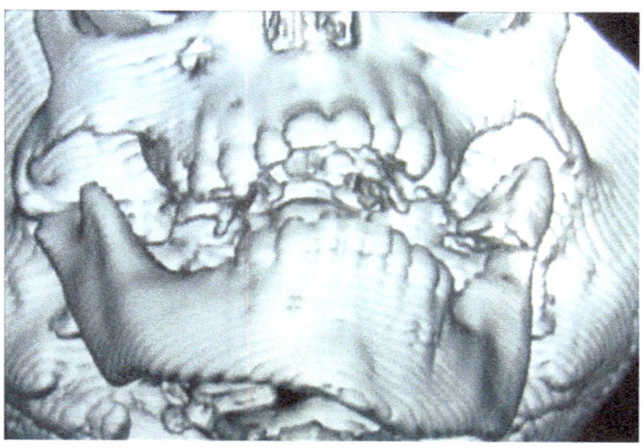

FIGURE 5: Computed tomography-frontal view.

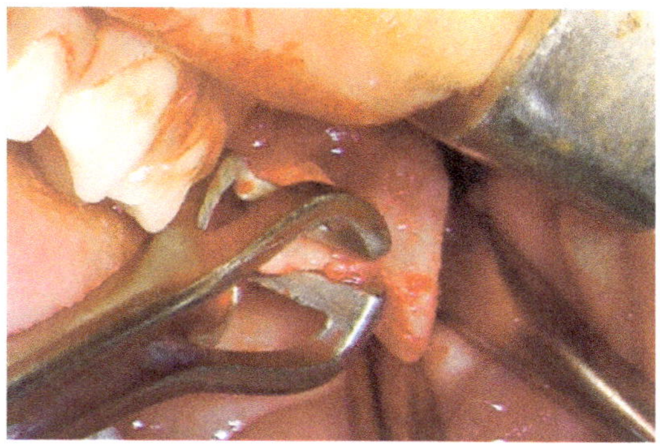

FIGURE 6: Intraoperative photograph showing excision of the lesion.

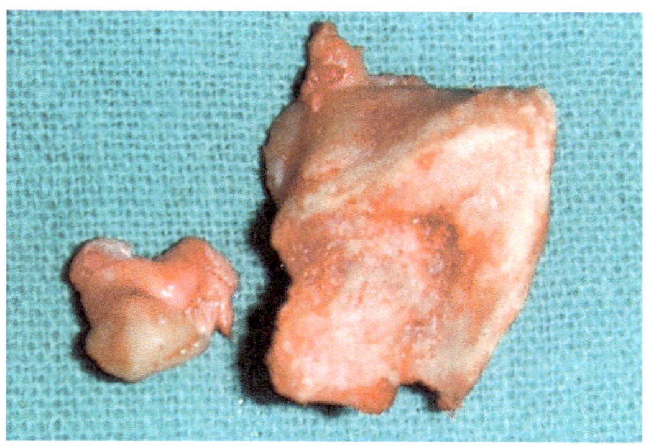

FIGURE 7: Excised osseous mass and soft tissue.

and preauricular tags or sinuses. The internal organs of the central nervous system, cardiovascular system, renal system, respiratory system, and the gastrointestinal system may also be underdeveloped or sometimes absent [10]. Our patient presents with an asymmetrical face with deviation of lower third of face to the left indicating deficient growth of the jaws on left side. No previous case of HO in Goldenhar syndrome or any developmental syndrome has been previously reported. This case can be considered a case of Goldenhar syndrome with mild representation and the first reported case of HO in Goldenhar syndrome.

Based on the clinical and radiological findings a differential diagnosis should include myositis ossificans circumscripta, myositis ossificans progressive, osteoma, nodular fasciitis, osteosarcoma, and chondrosarcoma. Slowly calcifying lesions synovial sarcoma, rhabdomyosarcoma, and malignant fibrous histiocytoma should also be included [7]. The most important pathology to be excluded is osteosarcoma. Histopathologic finding of mature lamellar bone confirms the diagnosis of HO.

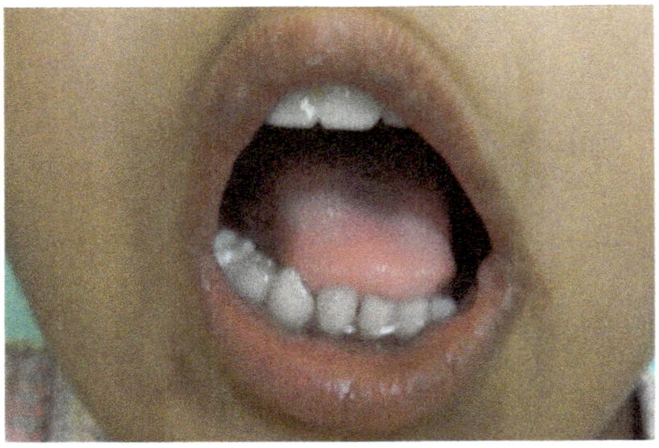

FIGURE 8: Adequate mouth opening postoperatively.

Postsurgically HO has been found to occur most frequently following total hip arthroplasty, hence various preventive modalities of HO have been discussed in the literature for such cases. Different modalities used include diphosphonates and NSAID's such as indomethacin and naproxen. Radiotherapy has also been used to reduce the incidence of HO in orthopedic management. Noggin, a BMP inhibitor, pulsed electromagnetic fields (PEMF), and free radical scavengers in the form of allopurinol and N-acetylcysteine are the three new methods being evaluated [11].

Patients present with various complaints as previously discussed. If radiographic examination and bone scanning reveal HO in formative stage, it is recommended to provide symptomatic treatment and wait for complete maturation of bone. Surgical excision is done thereafter. It has also been reported to either regress or stabilize.

## 4. Conclusion

HO can occur in pediatric age group in the maxillofacial region and affect the development and growth of the TMJ. History of trauma and symptoms like pain, swelling, and limited range of motion related to HO may or may not be present. When patient presents with facial asymmetry, restricted mouth opening, and improper development of jaws, HO and similar lesions like osteoma should be included in the provisional diagnosis. Early diagnosis and management can prevent the developmental abnormalities, which result in loss of function and esthetics.

## References


[1] K. Onder, B. Muhammed, U. Saime, and A. Haluk, "Post-traumatic heterotopic ossification of the crus: a case study," *Ortopedia Traumatologia Rehabilitacja*, vol. 13, no. 3, pp. 299–301, 2011.

[2] J. E. Hsu and M. A. Keenan, "Current review of heterotopic ossification," *Journal of Orthopaedics*, vol. 20, pp. 126–130, 2010.

[3] E. M. Shore and F. S. Kaplan, "Inherited human diseases of heterotopic bone formation," *Nature Reviews Rheumatology*, vol. 6, no. 9, pp. 518–527, 2010.

[4] G. A. E. Burke, D. Shah, and A. D. MacBean, "Panniculitis ossificans traumatica: an unusual presentation," *British Journal of Oral and Maxillofacial Surgery*, vol. 46, no. 7, pp. 596–598, 2008.

[5] N. Yildiz and F. Ardiç, "Pathophysiology and etiology of neurogenic heterotopic ossification," *Turkish Journal of Physical Medicine and Rehabilitation*, vol. 56, no. 2, pp. 81–87, 2010.

[6] E. Salisbury, E. Rodenberg, C. Sonnet et al., "Sensory nerve induced inflammation contributes to heterotopic ossification," *Journal of Cellular Biochemistry*, vol. 112, no. 10, pp. 2748–2758, 2011.

[7] S. Saussez, C. Blaivie, M. Lemort, and G. Chantrain, "Non-traumatic myositis ossificans in the paraspinal muscles," *European Archives of Oto-Rhino-Laryngology*, vol. 263, no. 4, pp. 331–335, 2006.

[8] C. S. L. Müller, K. Rass, and W. Tilgen, "Panniculitis ossificans non-traumatica of the scalp," *Journal of Cutaneous Pathology*, vol. 37, no. 6, pp. 703–704, 2010.

[9] N. Adler and B. Yaffe, "Ectopic bone formation following temporalis muscle transposition for facial paralysis: a rare complication?" *Annals of Plastic Surgery*, vol. 55, no. 4, p. 442, 2005.

[10] A. Castriota-Scanderbeg and B. Dallapiccola, *Abnormal Skeletal Phenotypes: from Simple Signs to Complex Diagnosis*, part 2, Springer, Heidelberg, Germany, 2005.

[11] E. O. Baird and Q. K. Kang, "Prophylaxis of heterotopic ossification-an updated review," *Journal of Orthopaedic Surgery and Research*, vol. 4, no. 1, article no. 12, 2009.

# Pseudoxanthoma Elasticum of the Skin with Involvement of the Oral Cavity

**Flávia Sayuri Matsuo,[1] Alceu Luiz Camargo Villela Berbert,[2] Sônia Antunes de Oliveira Mantese,[2] Adriano Mota Loyola,[3] Sérgio Vitorino Cardoso,[3] and Paulo Rogério de Faria[1]**

[1] *Department of Morphology, Laboratory of Histology, Institute of Biomedical Science, Federal University of Uberlândia, Avenue Pará 1720, Block 2B, Room 2B-256, 38405-320 Uberlândia, Minas Gerais, Brazil*

[2] *Department of Dermatology, School of Medicine, Federal University of Uberlândia, Avenue Pará 1720, Block 2U, Room 23, 38405-302 Uberlândia, Minas Gerais, Brazil*

[3] *Department of Oral Pathology, School of Dentistry, Federal University of Uberlândia, Avenue Pará 1720, University Hospital, Room 2K07, 38405-302 Uberlândia, Minas Gerais, Brazil*

Correspondence should be addressed to Paulo Rogério de Faria; paulorfaria@icbim.ufu.br

Academic Editors: J. Asaumi, J. H. Campbell, A. Kasaj, C. Ledesma-Montes, T. Lombardi, and G. Schierano

Pseudoxanthoma elasticum (PXE) is an inherited multisystemic disease of elastic fibers that primarily affects the skin and retina. A case of primary PXE of the skin with late involvement of the upper lip is reported. A 55-year-old woman with a previous diagnosis of PXE affecting her skin developed a lesion on her lower lip. An oral examination identified a yellowish macule of undefined limits. A biopsy from her lip was taken and both light and transmission electron microscopies confirmed the presence of fragmented elastic fibers and calcifications on her mucosa, which was compatible with the diagnosis of oral PXE. Since the manifestation of oral PXE is rare in this region, dental practitioners must be aware that this systemic condition may produce oral lesions, which sometimes may mimic other benign diseases of the oral cavity like Fordyce granules. So, the establishment of an appropriate diagnosis is necessary to provide adequate information and attention to the patient.

## 1. Introduction

Pseudoxanthoma elasticum (PXE) is a multisystemic heritable disease characterized by fragmentation and calcification of elastic fibers [1]. It has been associated with ABCC6-mutation gene, which is responsible for encoding an ATP-dependent transmembrane transporter especially in liver and kidneys [2]. However, the exact mechanism governing its occurrence is heretofore unknown [3, 4]. Classical manifestations include cutaneous yellow papules "pseudoxanthomas [*sic*]", loss of visual acuity, and atherosclerosis, with considerable morbidity and occasional mortality [1, 5]. The prevalence of PXE is estimated range from 1 : 25,000 to 1 : 100,000. However, the real number of cases may be much higher due to the difficulty of accurately establishing its diagnosis [3, 5]. Early PXE detection is extremely important to prevent systemic complications, especially as those seen in the cardiovascular system [6]. Involvement of the oral mucosa has been described in the literature and is potentially useful to the diagnosis of the disease, but little attention has been given in respect to the clinicopathological features of this manifestation in this region [1, 7–9].

To the best of our knowledge only six reported cases of oral PXE have been found in the English literature [7, 8, 10–12]. In this sense, it is worth reporting this case, especially to help dental practitioners in recognition of oral PXE lesions and in establishing an early and correct diagnosis of this life-threatening condition. So, this study describes a case of PXE affecting a woman who developed lesions in the oral mucosa during the progression of the disease and also presents detailed information about clinical, microscopic and ultrastructural aspects of the oral and skin lesions.

## 2. Case Report

A 55-year-old woman presented to our Dermatologic Service informing a previous diagnosis of PXE and looking for treatment for her condition. During the anamnesis, she reported that her condition appeared when she was 16-year old. According to her, at that time, progressive, coalescent yellow papules appeared first on the axillae and after on flexural sites including elbows, neck, and groin (Figures 1(a), 1(b), 1(c), and 1(d)). In respect to the PXE diagnosis, the patient also reported that it was made by a general practitioner. However, no other detailed information was gotten from her during the anamnesis. Moreover, we could not have access to her medical records to confirm all information foregoing. Neither visual loss nor gastrointestinal alterations were noticed by her, except for arterial systemic hypertension, and dyslipidemia, which have been treated by using specific medication. The patient's family history was unremarkable with none of her siblings and first- and second-degree relatives affected by the disease. Clinically, the skin lesions revealed yellowish plaques on the flexural locations including axillary and neck regions. Likewise, oral examination also revealed a yellowish macula on the inner aspect of her lower lip (Figure 1(a)). After dermatological and oral examinations, fragments from the skin and lower lip were taken, routinely processed, and stained with hematoxylin and eosin to confirm the PXE diagnosis. Also, a small piece of the lip lesion was cut out to be analyzed by transmission electron microscopy trying to identify ultrastructural changes in the connective tissue that could suggest PXE.

As the microscopic features of the skin lesion were similar to the oral one, we will describe herein only those seen in the oral lesion. Microscopically, the lip lesion showed a well-circumscribed, noncapsulated lesion composed of scattered deposits of fragmented and basophilic fibers among collagenous fibers of the connective tissue (Figures 2(a) and 2(b)). Neither inflammation nor signals of any causative agent were observed. Orcein and Von Kossa staining revealed a large amount of shortened, fragmented elastic fibers and deposits of black bodies throughout the lesion, confirming the presence of calcium and phosphorus (Figures 2(c) and 2(d)).

In addition, by using transmission electron microscopy, numerous aggregates usually large, but sometimes small, electron-dense calcified bodies in the cores of the elastic fibers were identified, resulting in the rupture of some elastic fibers (Figures 3(a) and 3(b)). Based on the clinical features and histopathological and ultrastructural aspects, a diagnosis of oral PXE was carried out.

Next, the patient was referred to the ophthalmologic department at our institution to be submitted to a funduscopic examination, which in turn revealed the formation of angioid streaks without visual loss. She was also sent to the cardiology and gastroenterology departments to be systemically evaluated, but no abnormalities were found. After that, it was explained to the patient about the nature and expected evolution of her condition, as well as the impossibility of curative treatment. She was also advised to be monitored regularly in an effort to detect early signals of the loss of acuity or secondary choroidal neovascularization (another severe ocular complication), as also to prevent other complications that are likely to develop over the progression of the disease, especially those affecting the gastrointestinal and cardiovascular systems. After three years of followup, both skin and oral lesions have remained stable, as also her ophthalmic condition. Additionally, cardiovascular and gastrointestinal monitoring has not revealed any alterations so far.

## 3. Discussion

PXE, first reported in the literature as a sporadic disease, is nowadays considered to be an inherited genodermatosis disorder of fiber elastics that present an estimated prevalence ranging from 1 : 25,000 to 1 : 100,000 [13]. Women are affected more often than men at ratio of 2 : 1 [6, 8, 14–16]. This disease can affect different populations worldwide, but present a much higher prevalence in Afrikaners living in South Africa [3]. Although PXE can be an inherited disorder as either an autosomal recessive or dominant inheritance, a rare pseudodominance inheritance has also been described in two families [2, 3]. Because of this, PXE is characterized by huge clinical heterogeneity in terms of the onset of the disease, the extent, and the degree of involvement of organ systems [2, 17]. However, even being a genetic disorder, the lack of familial history of PXE cannot be used to exclude the diagnosis of this condition [18]. Most of the patients develop clinical manifestations in early childhood, but cases becoming evident in late adulthood have been reported in the literature [19]. Here, our patient developed the first lesions at about the age of 16 years and none of her parents and relatives have manifested the condition until now. Although it is now believed that all cases of PXE present a familial genetic background, it is possible to speculate that PXE may also arise after a sporadic mutation, therefore culminating with the manifestation of the disease.

In respect to the pathogenesis of the disease, it has been associated with the presence of mutation in the *ABCC6* gene [2]. *ABCC6* gene belongs to the subfamily C of ATP-binding cassette (ABC) genes that encode a multidrug resistance-associated protein normally expressed in liver and kidneys [2]. The mutation detection varies from one study to another and has been estimated between 66 and 97% [17]. The functional association between mutated-*ABCC6* gene and PXE development is still completed unknown, especially because it was believed that the primary mutation would involve genes associated with elastic fibers synthesis, instead of a gene directly linked to a transmembrane transporter [2, 20, 21]. Otherwise, it was recently proposed that the absence of ABCC6 protein activity may lead to a reduction of inhibitors of aberrant mineralization in the peripheral tissues, which in turn are normally secreted by the liver [22].

The current classification system to support a definitive PXE diagnosis is based on the following three major criteria: (1) detectable yellowish lesions on flexural regions, (2) identification of shortened, fragmented elastic fibers as well as calcification deposits in the connective tissue on microscopic view, and (3) presence of ocular diseases, as

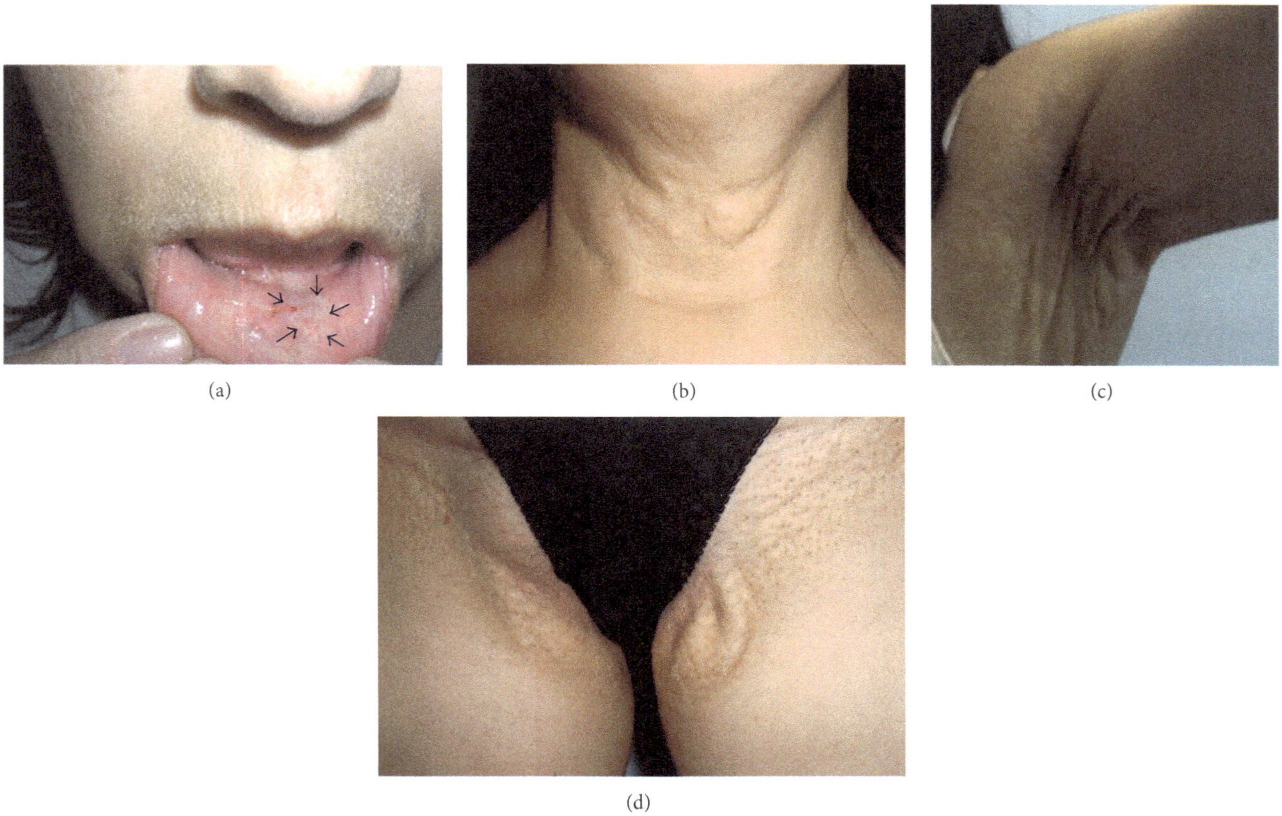


FIGURE 1: Clinical signs of the lesions. (a) White macule on the lower lip (arrows). (b) Skin lesion in the neck. (c) Skin lesion in the axillary region. (d) Skin lesion in the inguinal region.

angioid streaks, in individuals older than 20 years of old [23]. However, even considering that the majority of the cases meet all the criteria, there are reports showing PXE-affected patients who did not fulfill all the three conditions aforementioned [2, 17, 24]. For these cases, the detection of *ABCC6*-mutation gene may be useful to make a definitive diagnosis, as suggested in the literature, especially because similar alterations can be seen in other conditions, like elastosis, beta thalassemia, and Paget's disease, and a properly differential diagnosis must be made [2, 17]. Here, as our patient met all the major criteria that have been employed to confirm the PXE diagnosis, no mutational investigation of the *ABCC6* gene was performed.

Systemic abnormalities associated with PXE are often observed in locations in which elastic fibers are the main constituent, such as the eyes and blood vessels [6, 14]. Ocular manifestations are mainly characterized by the presence of angioid streaks that may lead to central visual loss although most lesions remain stationary even over the course of the disease [2]. Several life-threatening cardiovascular conditions may affect patients with PXE including angina pectoris, arterial hypertension, and cardiac failure [2, 20]. Moreover, peripheral vessel calcification and other vascular changes may lead to gastrointestinal bleeding with the risk of death. In the present case, the patient had been previously diagnosed with PXE and had already developed chronic hypertension by the time of her initial visit to our department, and it may be associated with the disease. Angioid streaks were also detected after an ophthalmological examination, but any loss of acuity has not yet been noticed. Additionally, no other systemic abnormalities have developed during the course of the disease even more than 30 years after diagnosing. In fact, it has been reported in the literature that, due to the pattern of inheritance in PXE, it is impossible to predict the phenotype of affected patients even among members of the same family [2].

The involvement of the oral mucosa in PXE patients has been reported in the literature [7]. In an extensive review of the literature, we could find only six case reports of PXE with oral involvement, with our case representing the seventh one published until now (Table 1). Although the exact prevalence of oral lesions needs to be determined, in a French study 83% of the patients presented involvement of oral mucosa, which may be considered high when compared to another study that reported an incidence of oral lesions of only 21% [1, 9]. In the oral cavity, the lesions commonly arise inside the lower lip, but other parts, including palate and cheeks, can also be affected [25]. Because of this location, they may be misdiagnosed as Fordyce granules [7, 15]. Clinically, oral lesions appear as yellowish-white macules or papules that may have a reticular growth pattern [1]. Our patient did not develop papules on her lip but a yellowish macule,

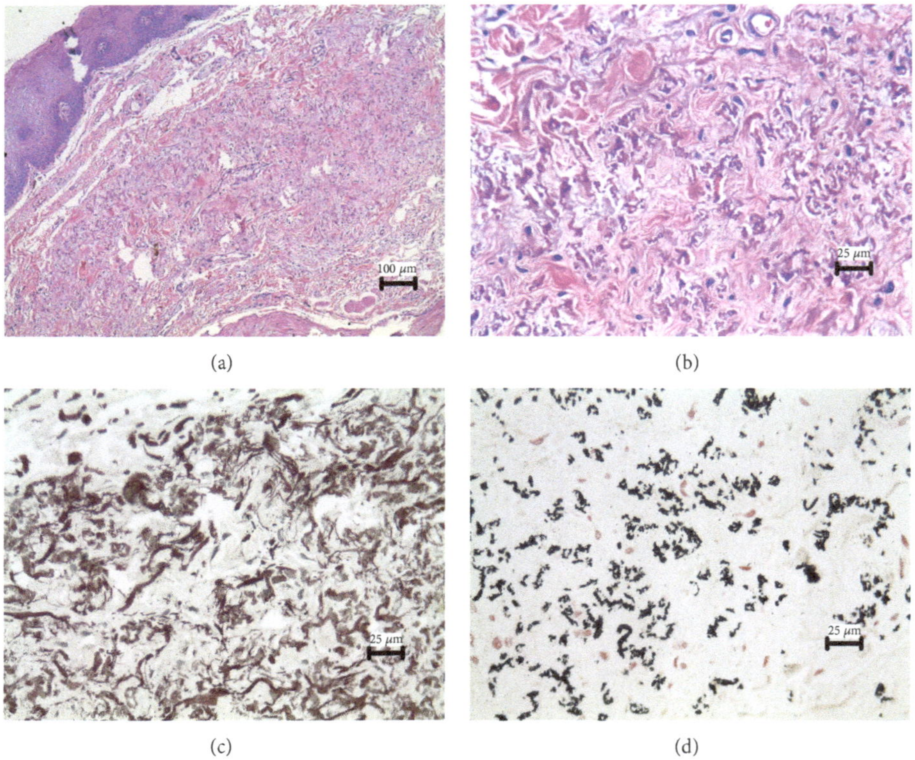


FIGURE 2: Histopathological aspects of the lesion. (a) Presence of a noncapsulated lesion in the connective tissue (H&E, original magnification ×100). (b) An aggregation of fragmented and basophilic fibers dispersed along with collagen fibers (H&E, original magnification ×400). (c) Orcein staining showing an increased amount of fragmented elastic fibers (original magnification ×400). (d) Von Kossa staining confirming the presence of calcium deposits inside the lesion (original magnification ×400).

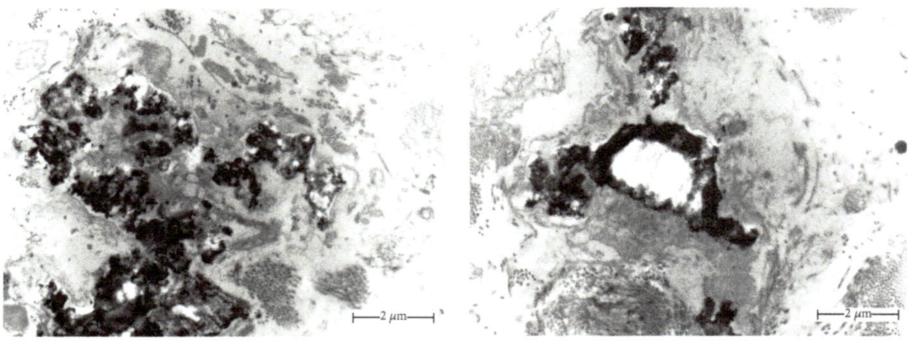


(a) (b)

FIGURE 3: An ultrastructural view of the lesion obtained from the oral cavity. (a) Note the presence of electron-dense calcified bodies in the core of the elastic fibers with some calcifications resulting in ruptures. (b) Observe the presence of calcified material in the center of an elastic fiber.

which had only appeared recently. Based on the patient's clinical signs, a biopsy was taken to confirm the condition. Light microscopy revealed a lesion composed of fragmented, granular, and calcified elastic fibers surrounded by normal connective tissue, which were histochemically confirmed by using Orcein and von Kossa stains, as described in the literature [2, 3, 16]. Although the pathogenesis of these lesions is still unknown, it has been suggested that an accentuated accumulation of proteoglycan in the PXE lesions may be involved by disturbing the assembly of the extracellular matrix and elastic fiber formation [16, 17]. The ultrastructural findings revealed electron-dense bodies deposited in the core of the elastic fibers, which can result in elastic fiber ruptures as a result of calcification or during tissue manipulation [3, 19]. All of these signs were observed in the patient's lesion and led us to confirm that her oral condition was a result of PXE.

In conclusion, considering that PXE is a heritable multisystem disease that may be associated with a certain degree

TABLE 1: Case reports of PXE with oral manifestation.

| Author's case | Sex | Age at presentation | Oral manifestations | Location |
|---|---|---|---|---|
| Matsuo et al. 2013 (present case) | Female | 55 years | Yellow patches | Labial mucosa |
| Velazquez-Cayon et al. 2012 [8] | Female | 30 years | Dental impactions | Maxilla and mandible |
| Morrier et al. 2008 [10] | Female | 10 years | Amelogenesis imperfecta | Maxilla and mandible |
| Sayin et al. 2007 [11] | Female | 19 years | Oligodontia, dental agenesis, and yellow patches | Maxilla, mandible, and oral mucosa |
| Goette and Carpenter 1981 [7] | Male | 62 years | Yellow patches | Labial mucosa |
| Danielsen and Kobayasi 1974* [12] | ? | ? | ? | ? |

*Without access to the article (cited by Goette and Carpenter 1981 [7]).

of morbidity and mortality, it is extremely important to the diagnosis of this disorder early in its course to establish a protocol for patient followup and to prevent cardiovascular, ocular, and gastrointestinal complications that may be life threatening. It is important that all PXE patients are evaluated for oral lesions. Additionally, the conditions of patients without a PXE diagnosis presenting with a yellow or white spot on the lips should not be underestimated by dental practitioners, and PXE must be considered even in the absence of skin lesions.

## Acknowledgments

The authors would like to acknowledge the Research Supporting Foundation of Minas Gerais (FAPEMIG) for financial support.

## References

[1] A. Utani, M. Tanioka, Y. Yamamoto et al., "Relationship between the distribution of pseudoxanthoma elasticum skin and mucous membrane lesions and cardiovascular involvement," *Journal of Dermatology*, vol. 37, no. 2, pp. 130–136, 2010.

[2] R. P. Finger, P. Charbel Issa, M. S. Ladewig et al., "Pseudoxanthoma elasticum: genetics, clinical manifestations and therapeutic approaches," *Survey of Ophthalmology*, vol. 54, no. 2, pp. 272–285, 2009.

[3] N. Chassaing, L. Martin, P. Calvas, M. le Bert, and A. Hovnanian, "Pseudoxanthoma elasticum: a clinical, pathophysiological and genetic update including 11 novel ABCC6 mutations," *Journal of Medical Genetics*, vol. 42, no. 12, pp. 881–892, 2005.

[4] F. Ringpfeil, L. Pulkkinen, and J. Uitto, "Molecular genetics of pseudoxanthoma elasticum," *Experimental Dermatology*, vol. 10, no. 4, pp. 221–228, 2001.

[5] J. Uitto, L. Bercovitch, S. F. Terry, and P. F. Terry, "Pseudoxanthoma elasticum: progress in diagnostics and research towards treatment: summary of the 2010 PXE International Research Meeting," *American Journal of Medical Genetics, Part A*, vol. 155, no. 7, pp. 1517–1526, 2011.

[6] S. Laube and C. Moss, "Pseudoxanthoma elasticum," *Archives of Disease in Childhood*, vol. 90, no. 7, pp. 754–756, 2005.

[7] D. K. Goette and W. M. Carpenter, "The mucocutaneous marker of pseudoxanthoma elasticum," *Oral Surgery Oral Medicine and Oral Pathology*, vol. 51, no. 1, pp. 68–72, 1981.

[8] R. T. Velazquez-Cayon, D. Torres-Lagares, R. M. Yanez-Vico et al., "Dental impactions related to pseudoxanthoma elasticum," *Journal of Oral and Maxillofacial Surgery*, vol. 70, no. 3, pp. e214–e216, 2012.

[9] L. Nozzi, D. Grenier de Cardenal, F. El Alamy, T. Duyninh, and L. Martin, "Prevalence of involvement of the oral mucosa and periodontal tissue in pseudoxanthoma elasticum," *Annales de Dermatologie et de Venereologie*, vol. 135, no. 3, pp. 183–186, 2008.

[10] J. J. Morrier, A. Romeas, E. Lacan, and J. C. Farges, "A clinical and histological study of dental defects in a 10-year-old girl with pseudoxanthoma elasticum and amelogenesis imperfecta," *International Journal of Paediatric Dentistry*, vol. 18, no. 5, pp. 389–395, 2008.

[11] M. O. Sayin, A. O. Atilla, E. Esenlik, T. Özen, and N. Karahan, "Oligodontia in pseudoxanthoma elasticum," *Oral Surgery, Oral Medicine, Oral Pathology, Oral Radiology and Endodontology*, vol. 103, no. 5, pp. e60–e64, 2007.

[12] L. Danielsen and T. Kobayasi, "Pseudoxanthoma elasticum. An ultrastructural study of oral lesions," *Acta Dermato-Venereologica*, vol. 54, no. 3, pp. 173–176, 1974.

[13] S. J. Brown, S. J. Talks, S. J. Needham, and A. E. M. Taylor, "Pseudoxanthoma elasticum: biopsy of clinically normal skin in the investigation of patients with angioid streaks," *British Journal of Dermatology*, vol. 157, no. 4, pp. 748–751, 2007.

[14] J. Uitto, Q. Li, and Q. Jiang, "Pseudoxanthoma elasticum: molecular genetics and putative pathomechanisms," *Journal of Investigative Dermatology*, vol. 130, no. 3, pp. 661–670, 2010.

[15] D. W. Sherer, A. N. Sapadin, and M. G. Lebwohl, "Pseudoxanthoma elasticum: an update," *Dermatology*, vol. 199, no. 1, pp. 3–7, 1999.

[16] K. Miki, T. Yuri, N. Takeda, K. Takehana, T. Iwasaka, and A. Tsubura, "An autopsy case of pseudoxanthoma elasticum: histochemical characteristics," *Medical Molecular Morphology*, vol. 40, no. 3, pp. 172–177, 2007.

[17] A. S. Plomp, A. A. B. Bergen, R. J. Florijn et al., "Pseudoxanthoma elasticum: wide phenotypic variation in homozygotes and no signs in heterozygotes for the c.3775delT mutation in ABCC6," *Genetics in Medicine*, vol. 11, no. 12, pp. 852–858, 2009.

[18] H. Akram, M. D. Sewell, and L. H. H. Cheng, "Pseudoxanthoma elasticum," *British Journal of Oral and Maxillofacial Surgery*, vol. 46, no. 3, pp. 237–238, 2008.

[19] E. Buteică, I. Stoicescu, F. Burada et al., "Pseudoxanthoma elasticum," *Romanian Journal of Morphology and Embryology*, vol. 49, no. 4, pp. 563–567, 2008.

[20] I. Georgalas, I. Tservakis, D. Papaconstaninou, M. Kardara, C. Koutsandrea, and I. Ladas, "Pseudoxanthoma elasticum, ocular manifestations, complications and treatment," *Clinical and Experimental Optometry*, vol. 94, no. 2, pp. 169–180, 2011.

[21] A. Iliás, Z. Urbán, T. L. Seidl et al., "Loss of ATP-dependent transport activity in pseudoxanthoma elasticum-associated mutants of human ABCC6 (MRP6)," *Journal of Biological Chemistry*, vol. 277, no. 19, pp. 16860–16867, 2002.

[22] Q. Li, Q. Jiang, E. Pfendner, A. Váradi, and J. Uitto, "Pseudoxanthoma elasticum: clinical phenotypes, molecular genetics and putative pathomechanisms," *Experimental Dermatology*, vol. 18, no. 1, pp. 1–11, 2009.

[23] M. Lebwohl, K. Neldner, F. M. Pope et al., "Classification of pseudoxanthoma elasticum: report of a consensus conference," *Journal of the American Academy of Dermatology*, vol. 30, no. 1, pp. 103–107, 1994.

[24] M. Lebwohl, R. G. Phelps, L. Yannuzzi, S. Chang, I. Schwartz, and W. Fuchs, "Diagnosis of pseudoxanthoma elasticum by scar biopsy in patients without characteristic skin lesions," *The New England Journal of Medicine*, vol. 317, no. 6, pp. 347–350, 1987.

[25] G. Spinzi, E. Strocchi, G. Imperiali, A. Sangiovanni, V. Terruzzi, and G. Minoli, "Pseudoxanthoma elasticum: a rare cause of gastrointestinal bleeding," *American Journal of Gastroenterology*, vol. 91, no. 8, pp. 1631–1634, 1996.

# 25

# Periodontal Management of Sturge-Weber Syndrome

**Butchibabu Kalakonda, Koppolu Pradeep, Ashank Mishra, Krishnanjaneya Reddy, Tupili Muralikrishna, Vijaya Lakshmi, and Radhika Challa**

*Department of Periodontics, Sri Sai College of Dental Surgery, Vikarabad 501101, India*

Correspondence should be addressed to Ashank Mishra; drashankmishra@gmail.com

Academic Editors: A. Epivatianos and M. B. D. Gaviao

Sturge-Weber syndrome (SWS) is a sporadic disorder and is frequent among the neurocutaneous syndromes specifically with vascular predominance. This syndrome consists of constellation of clinical features like facial nevus, seizures, hemiparesis, intracranial calcifications, and mental retardation. It is characterized by focal port-wine stain, ocular abnormalities (glaucoma), and choroidal hemangioma and leptomeningeal angioma most often involving occipital and parietal lobes. The present paper reports three cases of SWS with oral manifestations and periodontal management, which included thorough scaling and root planing followed by gingivectomy with scalpel and laser in cases 1 and 3 consecutively to treat the gingival enlargement. However, the treatment in case 2 was deferred as the patient was not a candidate for periodontal surgery.

## 1. Introduction

Sturge-Weber syndrome (SWS) is a sporadic disorder that occurs with frequency of 1 : 50,000 births [1]. Inspite of being rare, it is the most frequent disease among the neurocutaneous syndromes specifically with vascular predominance [2]. It is sporadic neurocutaneous disease characterized by focal port-wine stain, ocular abnormalities (glaucoma), and choroidal hemangioma and leptomeningeal angioma most often involving occipital and parietal lobes [3]. This syndrome consists of constellation of clinical features like facial nevus, seizures, hemiparesis, intracranial calcifications, and mental retardation [4].

Encephalofacial angiomatosis and encephalotrigeminal angiomatosis are used as synonyms of this syndrome as angiomas involve the leptomeninges and skin of face typically in ophthalmic and maxillary distributions of trigeminal nerve. SWS was initially described by Schirmer in 1860 and named by William Allen Sturge (1879) and Fredrick Parkes Weber (1929) [5].

Sturge associated the dermatological and ophthalmic changes with diseases of neurological manifestations, and Weber demonstrated gyriform intracranial calcifications and termed them "tramline," "tram-trac," or "trolley track" calcifications.

The present paper reports three cases of Sturge-Weber syndrome with oral manifestations and management.

## 2. Case Presentation

*Case 1.* A 23-year-old male patient came to the Department of Periodontics, Sri Sai College of Dental Surgery at Vikarabad, with a chief complaint of swelling in upper front region for 4 years which was gradually increasing in size with associated bleeding gums while eating or sometimes spontaneously. He gave no history of convulsions or glaucoma and no relevant family history.

Extraoral examination revealed the port-wine stain or nevus flammeus on the left side of the face.

The patient's mother had informed us that this stain was present on the face since his birth. Intraoral examination (Figures 1 and 2) reveals severe gingival overgrowth which was discrete, pedunculated, reddish-pink in relation to 11, 21, 22, 23, 24, and 25 involving marginal and attached gingiva and was suggestive of an inflammatory gingival overgrowth. The overgrowth extended palatally too in relation to 11, 21, 22, 23, and 24. Loss of Knife edge contour and bulbous papillae are seen in relation to 11 to 24 both labially and palatally. There was slight blanching of the gingival enlargement on pressure raising concerns that it might be an angiomatous (vascular)

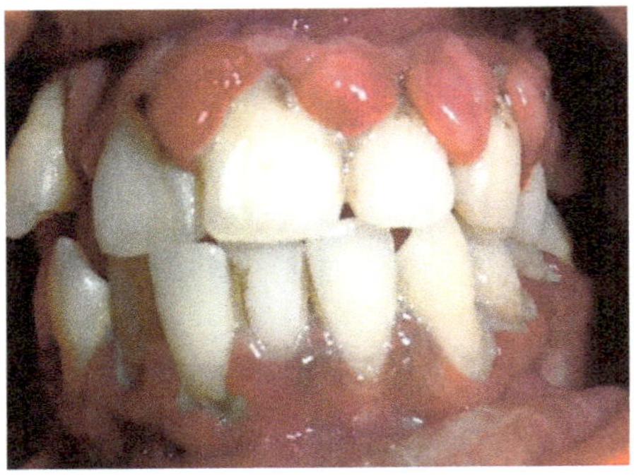

FIGURE 1: Intraoral view showing unilateral labial overgrowth.

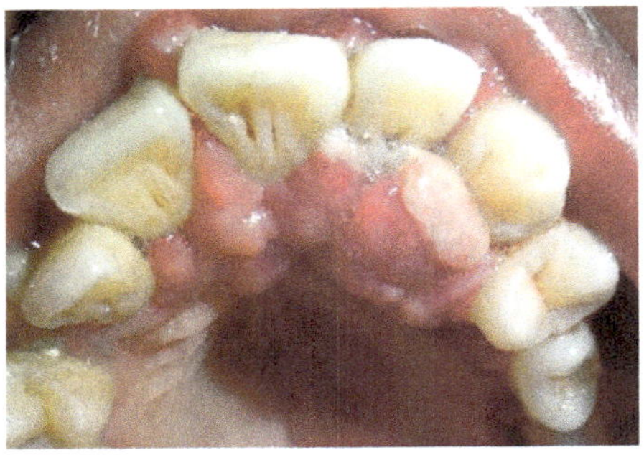

FIGURE 2: Intraoral view showing unilateral palatal overgrowth.

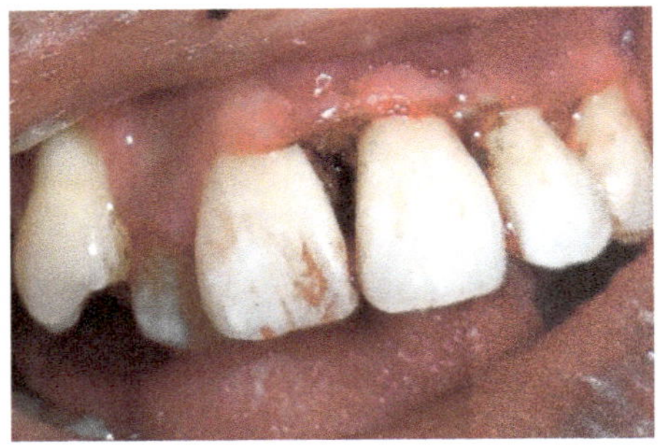

FIGURE 3: Immediate postoperative photograph.

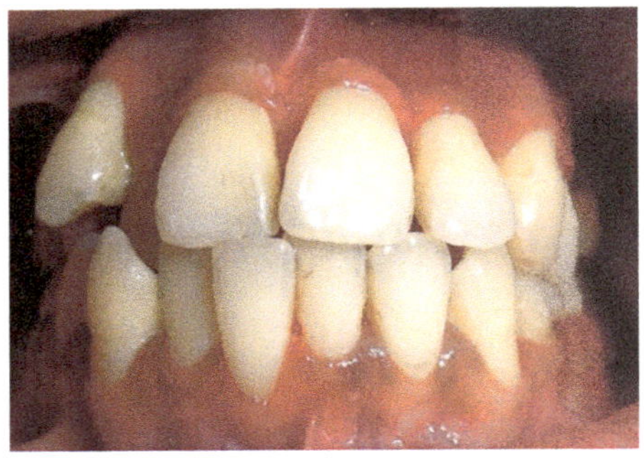

FIGURE 4: 3 months postoperative photograph.

nature of gingival enlargement. Radiographic and blood investigations were carried out which revealed no abnormality. Histopathological examination was suggestive of inflammatory fibroepithelial hyperplasia with vascular proliferation. Detailed clinical examination, history, and investigation confirmed the diagnosis of Sturge-Weber syndrome.

*Periodontal Management.* The complete treatment procedure was explained to the patient before proceeding with the treatment, a written consent was obtained from him, and a medical consent was obtained from the general physician.

2% lidocaine containing 1 : 80,000 adrenaline infiltration was given on the labial side in the maxillary anterior region and nasopalatine region. The swelling in relation to 11, 21–25 was excised at marginal gingiva, interdental papilla and attached gingiva with diode laser (Picasa 810 nm 1.8 W continuous mode) (Figure 3). The excised tissue was kept in formalin (10%) and sent for histopathologic examination. The patient was advised to use 0.2% chlorhexidine mouth rinse for 2 weeks postoperatively and analgesics as and when required. The patient was asked to return on postoperative day 7. The healing was progressing satisfactorily without any overt complications. At 3 months postoperatively (Figure 4) the healing was uneventful and no recurrence of gingival overgrowth was observed.

*Case 2.* A 32-year-old male patient was referred to the Department of Periodontics, Sri Sai College of Dental Surgery, with chief complaint of swelling in the left upper region for 2 years which was gradually increasing and associated bleeding from the gums while eating or sometimes spontaneously. He gave no history of convulsions or glaucoma. On further elaborated questioning regarding his medical history he revealed liver cirrhosis caused by hepatitis B. Family history was noncontributory for similar findings in his immediate or distant relatives.

Extraoral examination revealed a unilateral port-wine stain or nevus flammeus along multiple segments of trigeminal nerve on the left of the face (Figure 5). This lesion was present on the face since birth. There was noticeable facial asymmetry on the left side of the face with noticeable swelling of the left side of the upper lip (ipsilateral labial angioma). Intraoral examination (Figure 6) reveals gingival overgrowth which was highly inconsistent with the amount of plaque present. The gingival overgrowth was reddish-pink irt 24–27 involving marginal and interdental papilla of 24-25 with diffuse enlargement in relation to 26-27. The enlargement extended palatally too in relation to 25–27. Bleeding was present on slight provocation. Radiographic, blood investigations and liver function tests were carried out. Detailed clinical examination, history, and investigation confirmed the diagnosis of Sturge-Weber syndrome.

*Periodontal Management.* Nonsurgical periodontal therapy was done under strict aseptic conditions. The surgical treatment in this case was deferred as the patient was not a candidate for periodontal surgery as the patient is diagnosed with liver cirrhosis.

*Case 3.* A 12-year-old female patient came to the Department of Periodontics, Sri Sai College of Dental Surgery at

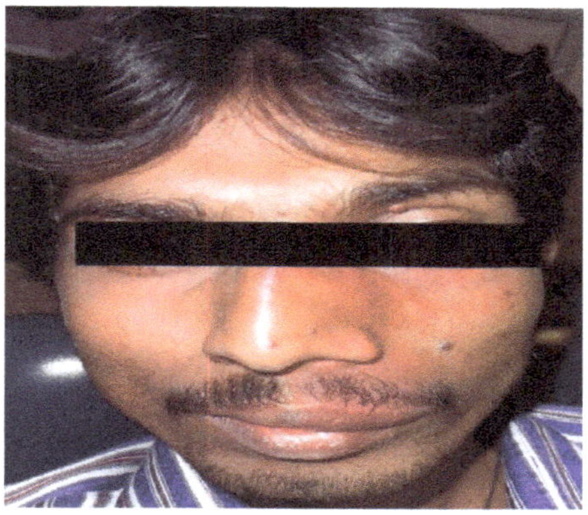

FIGURE 5: Extraoral view showing port-wine stain on the left side of the face.

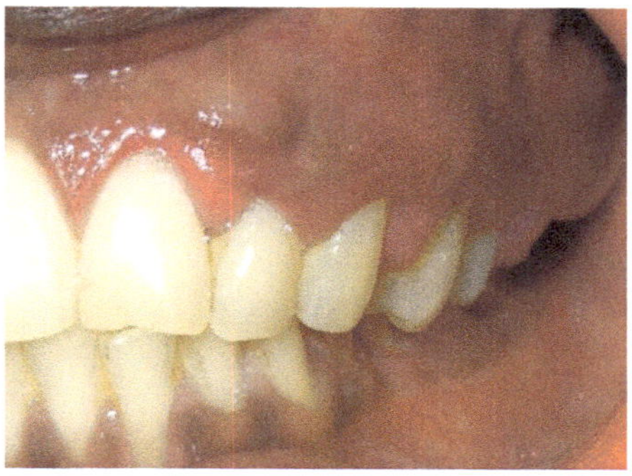

FIGURE 6: Intraoral view showing gingival overgrowth.

Vikarabad, with a chief complaint of swelling in the upper front region for 1 year which was gradually increasing in size with associated gum bleeding while eating or sometimes spontaneously. She gave no history of convulsions or glaucoma. She revealed no relevant family history.

Extraoral examination revealed the port-wine stain or nevus flammeus along multiple segments of trigeminal nerve on the right side of the face since birth (Figure 7). Reddish discoloration of the sclera of the right eye was seen. Intraoral examination (Figure 8) revealed discrete, sessile, reddish-pink gingival overgrowth in relation to 11 and 21 involving labial and palatal gingiva. Loss of Knife edge contour and bulbous papillae are seen in relation to 11 to 24 both labially and palatally. There was slight blanching of the gingival enlargement on pressure raising concerns that it might be an angiomatous (vascular) nature of gingival enlargement. Bleeding was present on slight provocation. Radiographic and blood investigations were carried out which revealed no abnormality. Histopathological examination (Figure 11) was suggestive of inflammatory fibroepithelial hyperplasia with vascular proliferation. Detailed clinical examination, history, and investigation confirmed the diagnosis of Sturge-Weber syndrome.

*Periodontal Management*. The complete treatment procedure was explained to the patient and her parents before proceeding with the treatment, a consent form was obtained from her

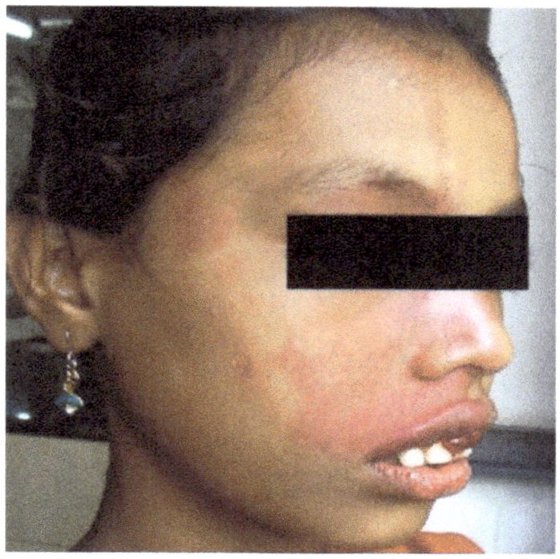

FIGURE 7: Extraoral view showing port-wine stain on the right side of the face.

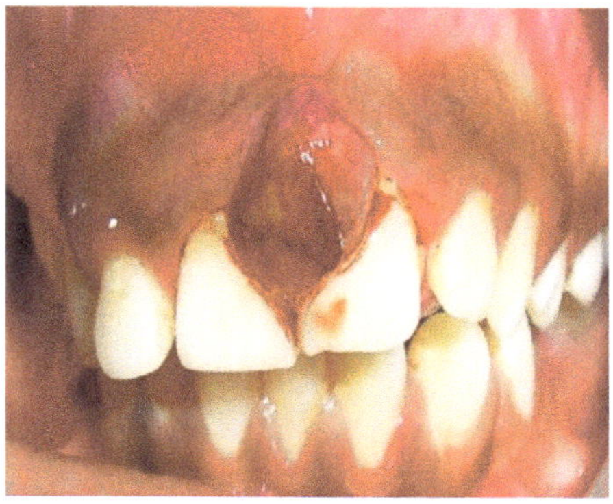

FIGURE 8: Intraoral view showing unilateral overgrowth.

parents, and a medical consent was obtained from the general physician. Cause-related therapy was done before the surgical intervention.

2% lidocaine containing 1 : 80,000 adrenaline infiltration was given on the buccal side in the maxillary anterior region and nasopalatine region. The pedunculated swelling irt 11 and 21 was excised initially followed by an external bevel gingivectomy performed irt 12, 13, and 14 with a Bard parker no. 15 surgical blade by excising the marginal gingiva, interdental papilla, and attached gingiva. After the excision (Figure 9) of the gingival enlargement, the bleeding points were cauterized with electrocautery. The bleeding was controlled with pressure packs. The excised tissue was kept in formalin (10%) and sent for histopathologic examination. The patient was kept under close observation for 24 hours for any postoperative complications. The patient was advised to take antibiotic and analgesic regimen (amoxicillin 250 mg, three times a day; Ibugesic kid, two times a day) for 3 days and use 0.2% chlorhexidine mouth rinse for 2 weeks postoperatively. The patient was discharged on postoperative day 2 and was asked to return on postoperative day 7 (Figure 10). The healing was progressing satisfactorily without any overt complications. The patient was asked to return after 15 days for postoperative checkup.

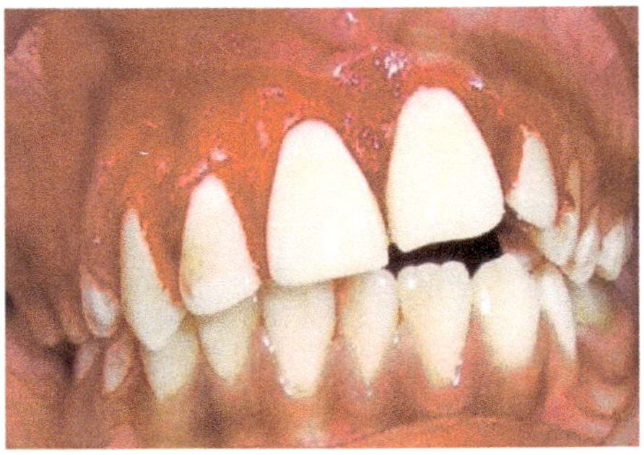

FIGURE 9: Immediate postoperative photograph.

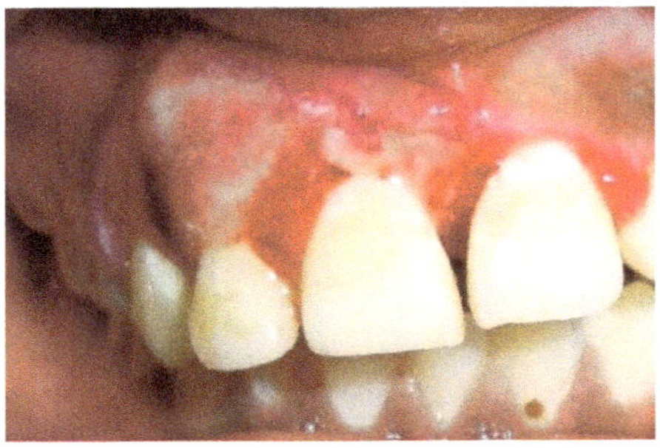

FIGURE 10: 1-week postoperative photograph.

## 3. Discussion

SWS has extremely varied clinical features, and its diagnosis can be characterized by port-wine stain on the face followed by other signs such as glaucoma, epilepsy, and mental retardation.

According to Inan and Marcus [6], the port-wine nevus is localized in the face, especially on the right side of the face, and detected in 87–90% of the cases. The lesion extension over the midline is observed in 50% of the patients and bilateral involvement in 33% of the cases. In case 3, the patient showed nevus flammeus only on the right side without extension over the middle line. Cases 1 and 2 showed nevus flammeus on the left side of the face. Inspite of the absence of neurological disorders, the distribution and extension of the skin angioma were suggestive of SWS in all the three cases. Case 3 was referred to as incomplete SWS and based on Roach scale, this patient was classified Type II SWS as only facial angiomas alone without CNS involvement.

Case 2 was referred to as incomplete SWS and based on Roach scale, this patient was classified Type II SWS as only facial angiomas alone without CNS involvement.

Case 1 was referred to as incomplete SWS and based on Roach scale, this patient was classified Type II SWS. In this case, laser [7] proved advantageous in improving surgical site visibility, bloodless field, and reducing the time of surgery, compared to conventional procedure. No noticeable postsurgical bleeding and discomfort were noted.

The treatment of SWS is variable and depends on the nature or intensity of its clinical features. Usually the port-wine stain may be improved by laser therapy or cosmetics [8], anticonvulsants for epilepsy, and glaucoma treatment to reduce intraocular pressure. One of the most important

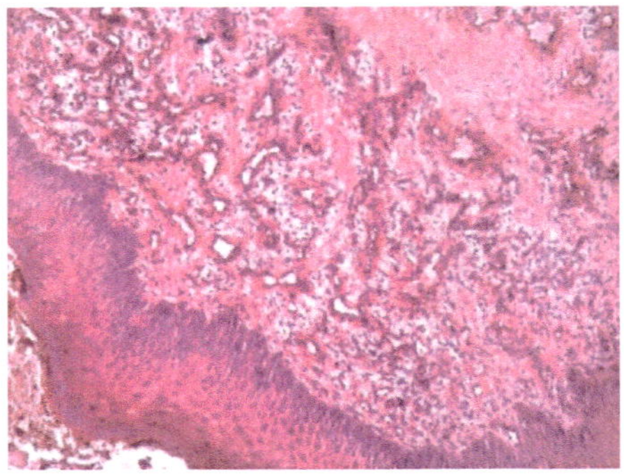

FIGURE 11: Histopathological view of overgrowth.

aspects of the treatment of SWS patients is psychological counselling of patients as well as parents.

## 4. Conclusion

The great frequency of oral manifestations of SWS demands dentists knowledge of this syndrome clinical features and treatment modalities. The consultations from various medical specialists are needed for proper treatment along with professional counselling which benefits the patient and the family to overcome their difficulties and improve the prognosis. Periodic systemic and oral examinations are recommended to prevent any cranial and oral complications. Laser, with its good haemostatic properties, is the best alternative in the surgical treatment of patients at great risk of haemorrhage, such as patients with SWS.

## References


[1] K. A. Thomas-Sohl, D. F. Vaslow, and B. L. Maria, "Sturge-Weber syndrome: a review," *Pediatric Neurology*, vol. 30, no. 5, pp. 303–310, 2004.

[2] P. Godge, S. Sharma, M. Yadav, P. Patil, and S. Kulkarni, "Sturge Weber syndrome: a case report," *Revista Odonto Ciência*, vol. 26, no. 4, pp. 366–369, 2011.

[3] H. I. Khan, M. F. Afzal, F. Anjum, and T. Javed, "Sturge-Weber syndrome. A case report," *Journal of Pakistan Association of Dermatologists*, vol. 16, no. 2, pp. 120–122, 2006.

[4] M. Chitlangia, P. Parakh, S. Yadav, G. S. Shah, and O. P. Mishra, "Sturge Weber syndrome with bilateral port-wine nevus," *Journal of Clinical Case Reports*, vol. 2, p. 12, 2012.

[5] K. Mandeep, "Orofacial manifestation of Sturge-Weber syndrome: a case report with review," *Journal of Orofacial Sciences*, vol. 4, no. 1, pp. 70–74, 2012.

[6] C. Inan and J. Marcus, "Sturge-Weber syndrome: report of an unusual cutaneous distribution," *Brain and Development*, vol. 21, no. 1, pp. 68–70, 1999.

[7] M. De Benedittis, M. Petruzzi, L. Pastore, F. Inchingolo, and R. Serpico, "Nd:YAG laser for gingivectomy in Sturge-Weber syndrome," *Journal of Oral and Maxillofacial Surgery*, vol. 65, no. 2, pp. 314–316, 2007.

[8] P. S. Yamauchi, T. T. Soriano, and G. P. Lask, "Treatment of port wine stains using the pulsed-dye laser at 55 nm with the dynamic cooling device," *Journal of Cosmetic and Laser Therapy*, vol. 2, no. 1, pp. 33–36, 2000.

# 26

# The Autosomal Recessive Inheritance of Hereditary Gingival Fibromatosis

**Poulami Majumder,[1] Vineet Nair,[2] Malancha Mukherjee,[2] Sujoy Ghosh,[3] and Subrata Kumar Dey[1]**

[1] *Department of Biotechnology, Centre for Genetic Studies, School of Biotechnology and Biological Sciences, West Bengal University of Technology, BF-142, Sector I, Salt Lake City, Kolkata, West Bengal 700064, India*
[2] *Department of Periodontics & Oral Implantology, Dr. R. Ahmed Dental College & Hospital, Kolkata, West Bengal 700014, India*
[3] *Department of Zoology, University of Calcutta, 35 Ballygunge Circular Road, Kolkata, West Bengal 700019, India*

Correspondence should be addressed to Poulami Majumder; plm.majumder@gmail.com

Academic Editors: R. S. Brown, J. A. Jayatilake, and G. Spagnuolo

Hereditary gingival fibromatosis (HGF) is a rare condition which is marked by enlargement of gingival tissue that covers teeth to various extents leading to aesthetic disfigurement. This study presents a case of a 28-year-old female patient and 18-year-old male who belong to the same family suffering from HGF with chief complaint of overgrowing swelling gingiva. The presence of enlarged gingiva with the same eruption was found in their other family members with no concomitant drug or medical history, and the occurrence of HGF has been found in one generation of this family which may indicate the autosomal recessive inheritance pattern of HGF. Hereditary gingival fibromatosis is an idiopathic condition as its etiology is unknown and it was found to recur in some cases even after surgical treatment. Both patients underwent thorough oral prophylaxis and later surgical therapy to correct the deformity.

## 1. Introduction

Hereditary gingival fibromatosis (HGF) is a clinical condition defined as an overgrowth of gingiva [1]. This is an important and very rare dental case (1 in 750,000) which is also referred to as idiopathic gingival hyperplasia in medical history [1, 2]. The maxillary and mandibular tissues of both arches are affected by slow enlargement of gingiva. This is considered as a benign condition, that is, associated with various factors like inflammation, hormonal imbalance, neoplasia, and some unknown causes [3, 4]. Healthy gingival tissue is characterized as pink, firm, fleshy, and made up of connective tissue covered by mucous membrane surrounding the neck of the teeth in a collar-like fashion on the jaw. However the HGF present in most of the anatomic crown of teeth causes abnormally shaped teeth, abnormal tooth movement, speech disorders, and other dental and oral problems [5].

It has been reported that both males and females are equally affected, with the phenotype and genotype frequency of HGF being 1 : 175,000 and 1 : 350,000, respectively [4]. HGF is more commonly associated with an autosomal dominant gene [5, 6]. According to various studies the pedigree analyses of HGF families confirm the autosomal dominant inheritance of HGF trait, although autosomal recessive or even as X-linked inherited cases have also been reported in some literature [7, 8]. Mutation in SOS-1 or son-of-sevenless gene is responsible for this disease; this has been reported by several authors [5, 9–11]. It is a guanine nucleotide-exchange factor that functions in the transduction of signals that control cell growth and differentiation [11]. Chromosomes numbers 2, 4, and 5 are found with their specific genetic loci including 2p21-p22 (GINGF), 2p13-p16, 2p22.3-23 (GINGF3), 5q13-q22 (GINGF2), 4q21, and 4q in association with HGF that enables mutations, duplications, deletions, and other genetic anomalies to take place. Other genetic loci like 8, 14q, 19p, 19q, and Xq are also related to various syndromes associated with hereditary gingival fibromatosis [11]. In current literatures it has been reported that a mutation in the son-of-sevenless-1 (SOS1) gene, which results in a single nucleotide insertion, causes hereditary gingival fibromatosis [11].

## 2. Case Presentation

There were two patients of 28 years and 18 years who were reported from Dr. R. Ahmed Dental College & Hospital, Kolkata, West Bengal, with the chief complaint of overgrowing gingiva surrounding all of their teeth. Those patients were referred for chromosomal diagnosis at our laboratory in Centre for Genetic Studies, West Bengal University of Technology.

*2.1. Family History.* The family history of affected persons was determined by questioning of the index case and it was confirmed that there were other family members who also had the symptoms of gingival overgrowth and that was subsequently confirmed by clinical examination of most of them. Among them two were females and the rest were male and they were siblings of the same parents.

A 28-year-old female patient was reported to the Department of Periodontics & Oral Implantology, Dr. R. Ahmed Dental College & Hospital, with the chief complaint of swelling in the gingiva for four years (Figure 1). Her 18-year-old brother was also reported with the same complaint but in milder form (Figure 2). According to the information provided by index cases, swelling of gingiva arose on approximately 3 to 4 years earlier and caused difficulties in speaking and eating but they had no history of oral pain. The female patient was married for 10 years and she had three children within the age range of 3–8 years and none of them were affected. The other members of their family like their parents and their other two brothers were unaffected. The family history of three generations was available and it was understood that the trait of gingival fibromatosis followed autosomal recessive pattern of inheritance in this family (Figure 3).

*2.2. Medical History.* Patients' medical history was normal. There was no history of taking long-term medicine for any particular disease. There was also no record of mental retardation or hypertrichosis and no other sign of clinical symptoms that could be associated with gingival enlargement.

*2.3. Clinical Diagnosis.* This enlargement affects the attached gingiva, as well as the gingival margin and interdental papilla, in contrast to phenytoin induced enlargement, which is often limited to the gingival margin and interdental papillae. The facial and lingual surfaces of the mandible and maxilla are generally affected, but the involvement may be limited to either jaw. The enlarged gingiva is pink, firm, and almost leathery in consistency and has a characteristic minutely pebbled surface. In severe cases teeth are almost completely covered, and the enlargement projects into the oral vestibule. The jaws appear distorted because of the bulbous enlargement of the gingiva. Secondary inflammatory changes are common at the marginal gingiva.

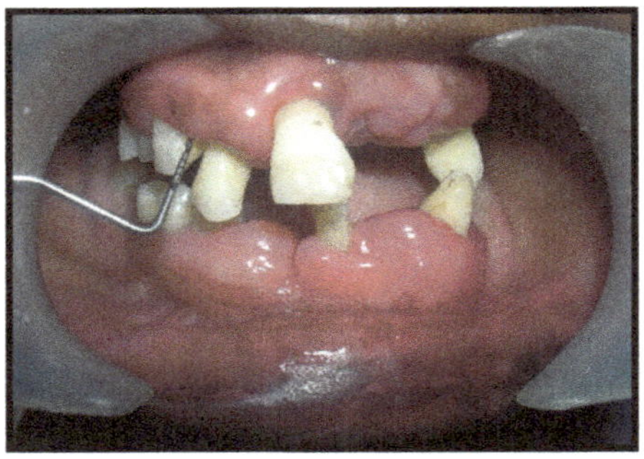

FIGURE 1: Female patient with gingival enlargement (preoperative view).

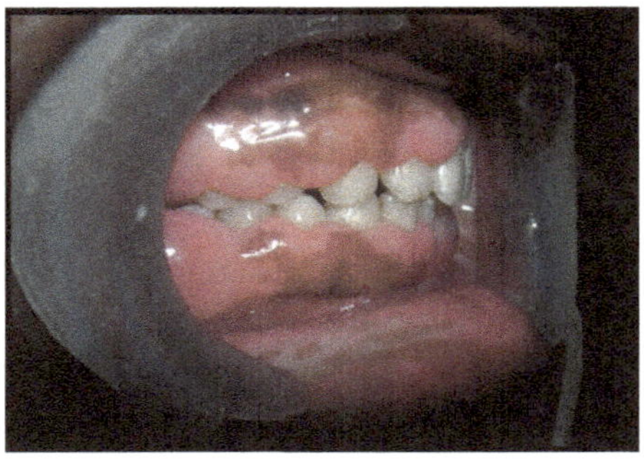

FIGURE 2: Male patient with gingival enlargement in milder form (preoperative view).

## 3. Treatment and Surgical Procedure

There is no such particular treatment or medicine for complete prevention of gingival fibromatosis but surgical procedure may cure this problem to some extent provided oral hygiene is thoroughly maintained. After local anesthesia bleeding points were marked on the gums of patients with the help of pocket marker (Figure 4). The excess tissue was removed by performing an internal bevel gingivectomy or undisplaced flap (Figures 5 and 6). Gingivoplasty was performed and continuous sling sutures were placed and periodontal dressing was applied (Figure 7). After 7 days sutures were removed and after 4 weeks they were recalled for further evaluation (Figure 8). Reevaluation was done after six months but no recurrence was observed (Figure 9). As the female patient was heavily affected, the ratio of cure was less than her brothers. Her left side gingival enlargement was cured but the right side is under observation.

## 4. Discussion

Here, we report a rare case of hereditary gingival fibromatosis which was not found in the last four years in Kolkata and is transmitted as an autosomal recessive inheritance. In this family, another female sibling who is 15 years old possesses similar clinical features which we may consider as the early symptoms of gingival fibromatosis. So it has been noticed that there is a tendency of sudden appearance of swelling gums around teeth at around 15 to 16 years of age, although

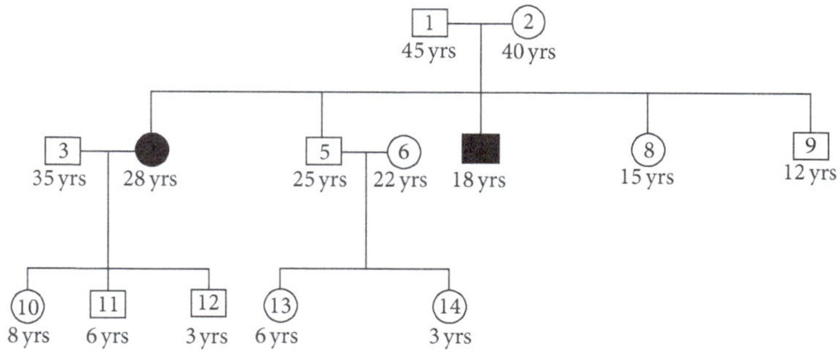


FIGURE 3: Pedigree of patient's family.

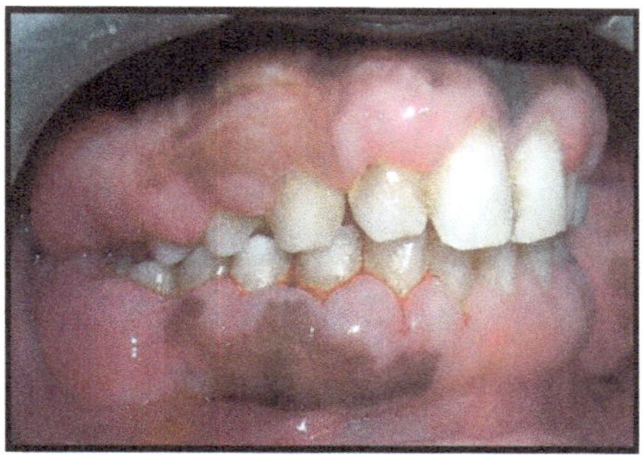

FIGURE 4: Pocket marker marked the bleeding points that denoted the excess portions of gum of male patient.

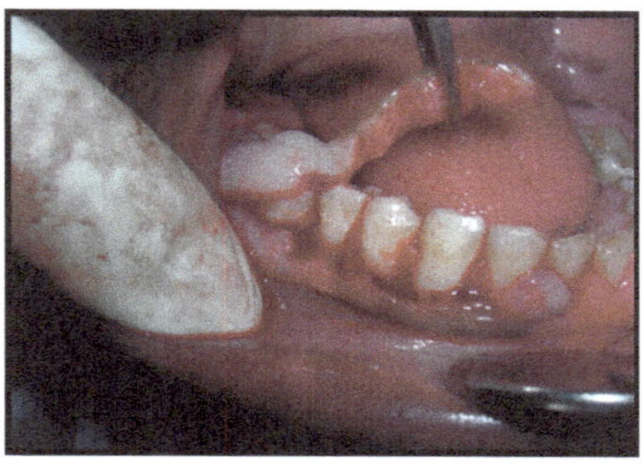

FIGURE 5: Internal bevel gingivectomy was done to remove the excess tissue of the male patient.

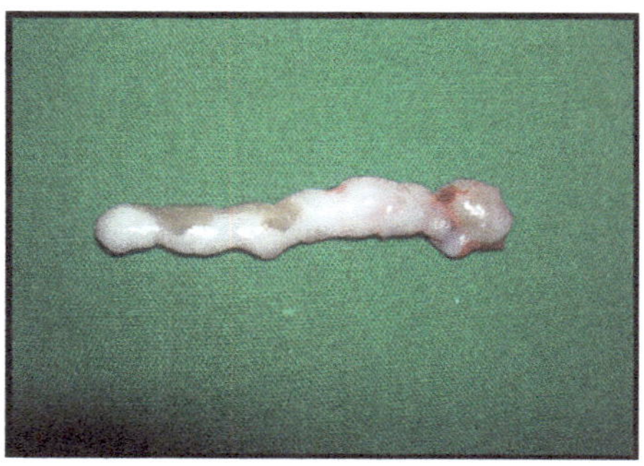

FIGURE 6: Surgically removed excess tissue.

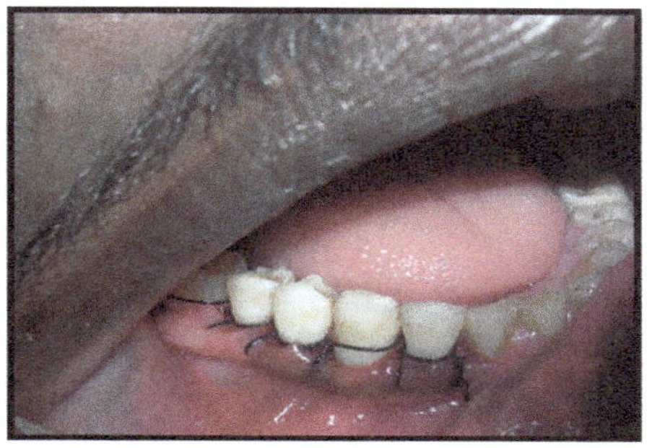

FIGURE 7: Gingivoplasty was done and continuous sling sutures were placed.

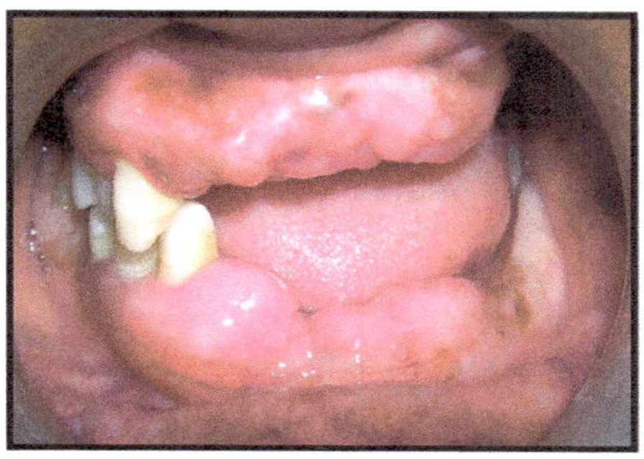

FIGURE 8: Postoperative view of female patient. It was shown that the left side gingival enlargement was cured.

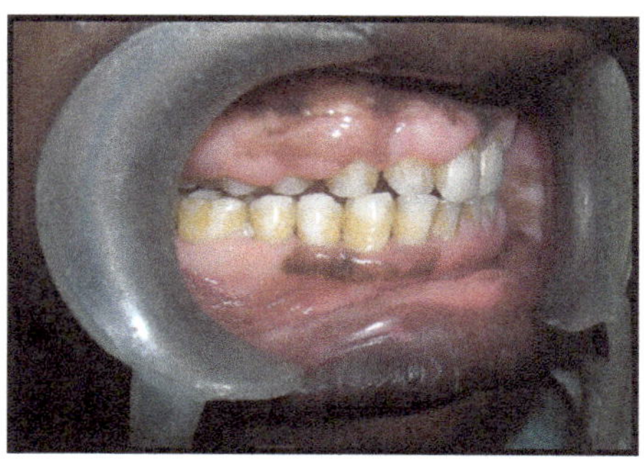

FIGURE 9: Postoperative view of male patient after six months.

some other studies report the occurrence of HGF also found in early age as well as juvenile state [12, 13]. Consequent to this there is compromised chewing efficiency and increasing mobility of teeth which may eventually lead to loss of teeth. The patients reported one month after they had undergone the surgical procedure and were again reviewed six months later. They were found to be in a stable condition though recurrence of HGF cannot be ruled out in the future. Generally surgical intervention after scaling and root planing of teeth and sufficient oral homecare is sufficient to alleviate the symptoms [3, 4]. In some literatures, various associated disorders of gingival enlargement had been discussed that include Zimmermann Laband syndrome (ear, nose, bone, and nail defects with hepatosplenomegaly), Rutherford syndrome (oculodental syndrome), Jones syndrome (progressive deafness), Cross syndrome (microphthalmia, mental retardation, athetosis, and hypopigmentation), Murray-Puretic Drescher syndrome (juvenile hyaline fibromas), and Ramon syndrome reasons, [9, 14–16], that is, why HGF is considered as part and parcel of multisystem syndrome [2, 10]. However, in this case, a thorough evaluation of the patients revealed that there was no association of HGF with any of the above syndromes.

## 5. Conclusion

Hereditary gingival fibromatosis stands apart from other gingival enlargements in the varied treatment options available and the nature of recurrence posttreatment. There is no consensus among authors related to the mode of treatment. Here, in this present case report, we highlight the autosomal inheritance patterns and the surgical treatment found in HGF cases.

## Conflict of Interests

The authors declare that there is no conflict of interests regarding the publication of this paper.

## Acknowledgment

The work was financially supported by DBT (Department of Biotechnology), India.

## References

[1] J. P. Fletcher, "Gingival abnormalities of genetic origin: preliminary communication with special reference to hereditary gingival fibromatosis," *Journal of Dental Research*, vol. 45, no. 3, pp. 597–612, 1966.

[2] T. Ramakrishnan and M. Kaur, "Multispeciality approach in the management of patient with hereditary gingival fibromatosis: 1-year followup: a case report," *International Journal of Dentistry*, vol. 2010, Article ID 575979, 5 pages, 2010.

[3] U. Khan, S. Mustafa, Z. Saleem, A. Azam, and Z. A. Khan, "Hreditary gingival fibromatosis diagnosis and treatment," *Pakistan Oral and Dental Journal*, vol. 32, no. 2, pp. 226–231, 2012.

[4] K. B. Butchi, K. Pavankumar, B. R. Anuradha, and N. Arora, "Hereditary gingival fibromatosis—a case report and management using a novel surgical technique," *Revista Sul-Brasileira de Odontologia*, vol. 8, no. 4, pp. 453–458, 2011.

[5] S. DeAngelo, J. Murphy, L. Claman, J. Kalmar, and B. Leblebicioglu, "Hereditary gingival fibromatosis—a review," *Compendium of Continuing Education in Dentistry*, vol. 28, no. 3, pp. 138–143, 2007.

[6] L. Bozzo, O. P. de Almeida, C. Scully, and M. J. Aldred, "Hereditary gingival fibromatosis. Report of an extensive four-generation pedigree," *Oral Surgery, Oral Medicine, Oral Pathology*, vol. 78, no. 4, pp. 452–454, 1994.

[7] R. D. Coletta and E. Graner, "Hereditary gingival fibromatosis: a systematic review," *Journal of Periodontology*, vol. 77, no. 5, pp. 753–764, 2006.

[8] S. L. Singer, J. Goldblatt, L. A. Hallam, and J. C. Winters, "Hereditary gingival fibromatosis with a recessive mode of inheritance. Case reports," *Australian Dental Journal*, vol. 38, no. 6, pp. 427–432, 1993.

[9] R. J. Jorgenson and M. E. Cocker, "Variation in the inheritance and expression of gingival fibromatosis," *Journal of Periodontology*, vol. 45, no. 7, pp. 472–477, 1974.

[10] T. C. Hart, Y. Zhang, M. C. Gorry et al., "A mutation in the SOS1 gene causes hereditary gingival fibromatosis type 1," *The American Journal of Human Genetics*, vol. 70, no. 4, pp. 943–954, 2002.

[11] A. Poulopoulos, D. Kittas, and A. Sarigelou, "Current concepts on gingival fibromatosis-related syndromes," *Journal of Investigative and Clinical Dentistry*, vol. 2, no. 3, pp. 156–161, 2011.

[12] L. P. Bittencourt, V. Campos, L. F. M. Moliterno, D. P. B. Ribeiro, and R. K. Sampaio, "Hereditary gingival fibromatosis: review of the literature and a case report," *Quintessence International*, vol. 31, no. 6, pp. 415–418, 2000.

[13] Y. Ramon, W. Berman, and J. J. Bubis, "Gingival fibromatosis combined with cherubism," *Oral Surgery, Oral Medicine, Oral Pathology*, vol. 24, no. 4, pp. 435–448, 1967.

[14] A. Piattelli, A. Scarano, A. Di Bellucci, and S. Matarasso, "Juvenile hyaline fibromatosis of gingiva: a case report," *Journal of Periodontology*, vol. 67, no. 4, pp. 451–453, 1996.

[15] I. B. Houston and N. Shotts, "Ruthurfurd's syndrome: a familial oculo-dental disorder. A clinical and electrophysiologic study," *Acta Paediatrica Scandinavica*, vol. 55, no. 2, pp. 233–238, 1966.

[16] M. Holzhausen, D. Gonçalves, F. de Oliveira Bello Corrêa, L. C. Spolidorio, V. C. Rodrigues, and S. R. P. Orrico, "A case of Zimmermann-Laband syndrome with supernumerary teeth," *Journal of Periodontology*, vol. 74, no. 8, pp. 1225–1230, 2003.

# Ameloblastomatous CCOT: A Case Report of a Rare Variant of CCOT with a Review of the Literature on Its Diverse Histopathologic Presentation

**Shailesh Menat,[1] Shylaja MD,[2] Kailash Attur,[3] and Kaushal Goyal[1]**

[1] *Department of Oral and Maxillofacial Surgery, Narsinhbhai Patel Dental College and Hospital, Visnagar, Gujarat 384315, India*
[2] *Department of Oral Pathology and Microbiology, Narsinhbhai Patel Dental College and Hospital, Visnagar, Gujarat 384315, India*
[3] *Department of Conservative and Endodontics, Narsinhbhai Patel Dental College and Hospital, Visnagar, Gujarat 384315, India*

Correspondence should be addressed to Shylaja MD; shylajamd@gmail.com

Academic Editors: M. H. K. Motamedi and M. O. Sayin

Calcifying odontogenic cyst is considered as a rare lesion and accounts for 1% of jaw cysts. It represents a heterogeneous group of lesions which exhibit a variety of clinicopathologic and behavioral features. It has been categorized as cyst and neoplasm. Even after several classification and subclassification, COC remains an enigma. WHO classification 2005 has reclassified the lesion as calcifying cystic odontogenic tumor (CCOT). Ameloblastomatous COC is a rare variant which is not much described in the literature. This report describes one such case which was large multicystic, involved the coronoid and condylar process of the mandible, and treated by subhemimandibulectomy. The case was recurrence free even after 1 year of followup.

## 1. Introduction

Calcifying odontogenic cyst (COC) was first described by Gorlin et al. (1962, 1964); hence, the eponym of "Gorlin cyst" is frequently used. The lesion has been widely occurring both peripherally and centrally in the jaws [1]. Although it was recognized as a distinct pathologic entity at first, COC shows extreme diversity in its clinical and histopathological features as well as its biological behavior [2].

COC was considered as a developmental odontogenic cyst with diverse origin [3]. It is a rare odontogenic pathology and constitutes to about from 0.37% to 2.1% of all odontogenic tumors [4] and about 1% of the jaw cysts reported [5]. A majority of COC are cystic in architecture and appear to be nonneoplastic, but they sometimes appear as a solid lesion; at least some of the solid lesions are neoplastic in nature [2].

According to the new WHO classification in 2005, COC has now been reclassified as calcifying cystic odontogenic tumor (CCOT) [6]. It often occurs in association with other odontogenic tumors such as ameloblastoma and complex odontoma [7]. The classification advocated by Hong et al. has two categories for CCOT associated with ameloblastoma: the ameloblastomatous cystic and the neoplastic variants associated with ameloblastoma.

Herewith, we are reporting a case of ameloblastomatous CCOT which will add one more rare case to the literature which might help in understanding the biologic behavior of this type of lesion.

## 2. Case Report

A 20-year-old male patient visited the department of oral and maxillofacial surgery with a chief complaint of swelling on lower left 1/3 of face and disfigurement of face for 2 years.

Swelling which started gradually increased to attain the present size.

Extraoral examination revealed a swelling in the lower left back tooth region of the jaw and on the angle of the mandible (Figure 1(a)). Anteroposteriorly, the swelling extended from 2 cms distal to the angle of mouth to the ramus of mandible.

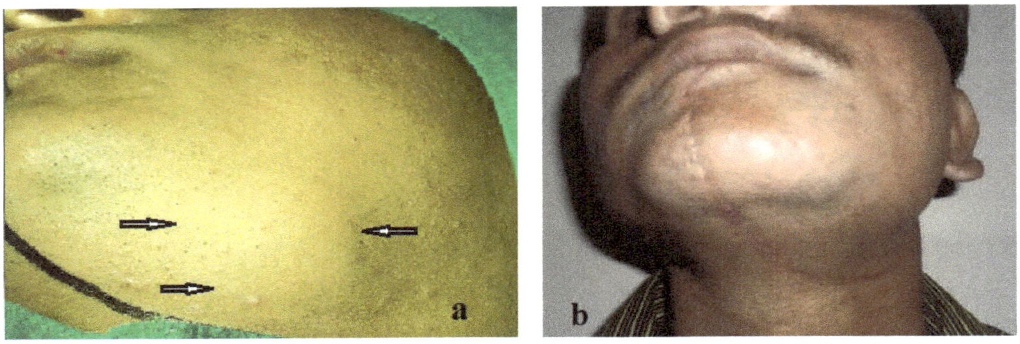


(a) (b)

FIGURE 1: (a) Extraoral picture of the patient showing swelling in the left submandibular region. (b) Extraoral picture after 1 year of followup.

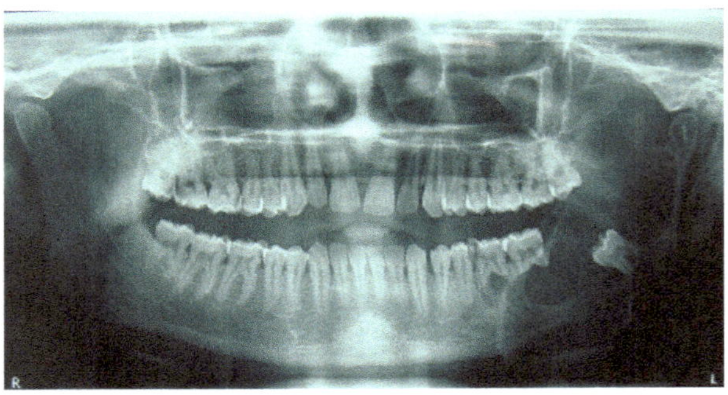


FIGURE 2: OPG showing multilocular radiolucency in relation to left third molar involving the angle, ramus, and coronoid process of the mandible. Root resorption is evident in mandibular I, II, and III molar.

Supero-inferiorly, it extends from 3 cms below the zygomatic arch to 1 cm beyond the lower border of the mandible.

Intraoral examination revealed a large swelling extending from mandibular left first molar to the ramus of the mandible, obliterating buccal vestibule and causing buccolingual expansion of the bone. Mucosa overlying the lesion was intact.

The orthopantomograph revealed a multilocular radiolucency on the left side of the mandible extending from molar upto the condyle and coronoid area (Figure 2). The lesion contained the unerupted third molar dislocated inferiorly at the angle of mandible. Root resorption of second molar was evident.

CT scan showed a multiloculated, large cystic, and expansile lesion involving left ramus of mandible with significant cortical thinning. The solid tumor measured about 2.6 × 3.6 cm in axial plane with craniocaudal extension measuring 7.3 cm (Figure 3).

Based on history clinical feature and radiographic appearance, a provisional diagnosis of ameloblastoma or odontogenic keratocyst was made. An incisional biopsy was obtained from the left retromolar area to establish final diagnosis. Histopathologic examination revealed follicles with peripheral palisading cells with reverse polarity of nucleus and central stellate reticulum-like cells. Cystic degeneration within the follicles was also evident, suggestive of cystic ameloblastoma.

The patient was taken for surgery under general anaesthesia, and the lesion was reached through lip split submandibular incision. Hemimandibulectomy with disarticulation was performed, and condylar reconstructive plate was fixed in the area (Figures 4(a) and 4(b)). The resected specimen was sent for histopathological examination.

The hemimandibulectomy specimen showed the resection margin till the mandibular left second premolar (Figures 5(a) and 5(b)). The bony margin was cut and taken for decalcification to know the adequacy of the surgery. Tissues were taken from multiple areas. The specimen was grossly cystic, but solid areas were seen on the lingual portion of the resected specimen. Bony tissues were taken for decalcification with 5% nitric acid. Soft tissues and decalcified tissue were routinely processed, and 4 $\mu$ thick sections were cut and stained with Hematoxylin and Eosin.

The section showed a cystic lining overlying fibrous stroma. The lining epithelium had flat to cuboidal basal cells with stellate superficial cells. Few areas showed tall columnar basal cells with reverse polarity of nucleus. In few areas, the stellate cells showed squamous differentiation. Few large eosinophilic, anucleated cells were seen with indistinct cell membrane suggestive of ghost cells (Figure 6). Few ghost cells showed features of calcification. Epithelium budding into the connective tissue was evident in many areas.

Stroma showed thick bundles of collagen fibers with spindle fibroblasts. Juxta-epithelial hyalinization was seen suggestive of dysplastic dentin (Figures 6(a) and 6(b)). Proliferative odontogenic islands with ghost cells were also seen in the connective tissue capsule (Figure 7). Daughter cysts with ghost cells were also evident. Few areas showed dysplastic dentin in and around some odotogenic islands.

The resected bony margin was clear and free of any infiltration.

With the above histopathologic features, a diagnosis of ameloblastomatous CCOT was made.

The patient has been under regular followup and has not exhibited any signs of recurrence after 1 yr of followup (Figure 1(b), Figure 8).

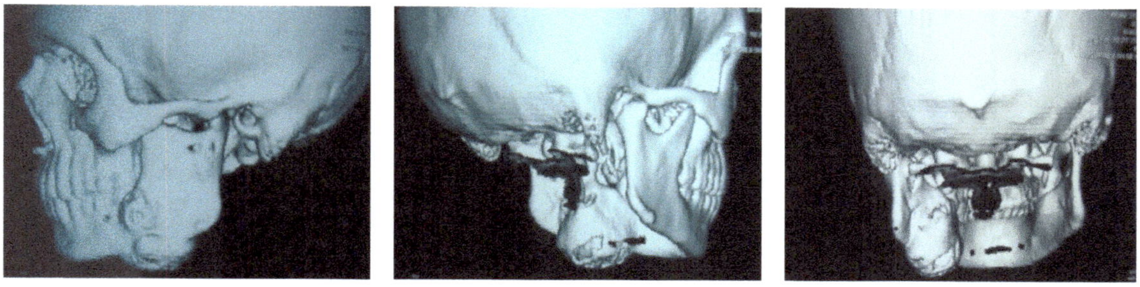

(a) (b) (c)

FIGURE 3: 3D CT image showing the lesion in the body and ramus of the mandible, (a) left lateral surface, (b) lingual surface of left mandible, and (c) lingual surface of mandible from the posterior view.

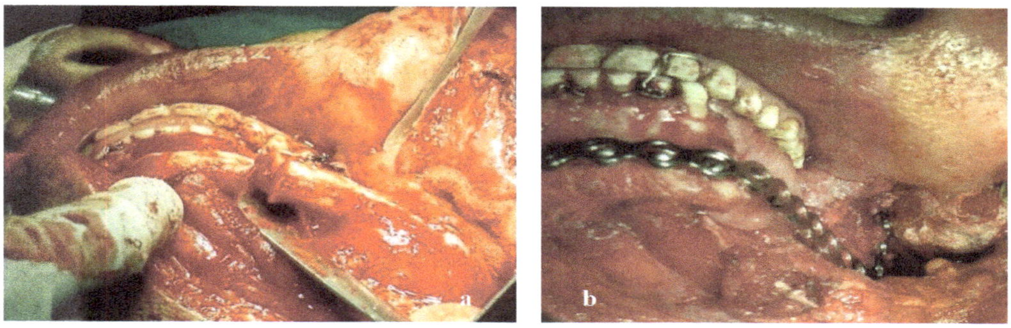

(a) (b)

FIGURE 4: (a) Surgical photograph showing hemimandibulectomy and (b) condylar reconstruction plate.

## 3. Discussion

CCOT was first described in 1932 by Rywkind who reported a lesion of the jaw which resembled cholesteatoma of the ear and thereafter called it as cholesteatoma of the jaw. In 1946, Thoma and Goldman described a lesion which they called a strange variant of ameloblastoma [7]. It was in 1962 that Gorlin first described it.

In recent classification of the World Health Organization (2005), the term calcifying cystic odontogenic tumor (CCOT) has been replaced with calcifying odontogenic cyst (COC) that constitutes a benign cystic neoplasia that presents an epithelium with ghost cells which may display calcification in it [8].

CCOT is common in the second decade of life. Buchner and Pretorius have drawn attention to a bimodal age distribution with a second peak in the 6-7th decade of life. The youngest recorded patient was a 1 year old, the oldest an 82 years old [1]. There is a distinct peak in the second decade [9]. There are no particular predilections for either the maxilla or mandible, although the cases in the maxilla are more often in older patients. This lesion tends to occur in the canine-incisor portion in both jaws, but those in the maxilla occur more often at the anterior portion than those in the mandible [10]. Freedman et al. (1975) pointed out that 70% of their sample occurring in patients before the age of 41 were in the maxilla, whereas 80% in patients older than 41 were in the mandible [1].

According to Shamaskin et al., central COCs occur more commonly than peripheral lesions by a 3 : 1 ratio, and they are usually diagnosed in the second decade of life, while the peripheral ones are usually noted after 50 years [11]. Coinciding with all these reports, our patient was a 20-year-old male, with the lesion presenting in the mandibular third molar region.

CCOT are generally a unilocular lesion, while in 5–13% of cases they are multilocular [12]. Some have a regular outline with well-demarcated margins. Others may be quite irregular and may have poorly defined margins. Early in their development, they will appear completely radiolucent. As they mature, they develop calcifications that produce a well-circumscribed, mixed radiolucent-radiopaque appearance. Three general patterns of radiopacity are seen. One is a salt and pepper pattern of flecks, the second is a fluffy cloud-like pattern throughout, and the third is a crescent-shaped pattern on one side of the radiolucency in a "new moon"-like configuration [4].

CCOT is usually intraosseous (70%) and extraosseous, accounts to 16–22%, and seen in individuals over 50 years of age [12]. About 50% of CCOT have been reported as being associated with an unerupted tooth. Displacement of teeth is often seen. Resorption of the roots of adjacent teeth is a frequent finding and is regarded as an important radiological feature [9]. Local expansion sometimes occurs, and perforation of the cortical plate, when present, may be radiologically demonstrable [1]. The present case report

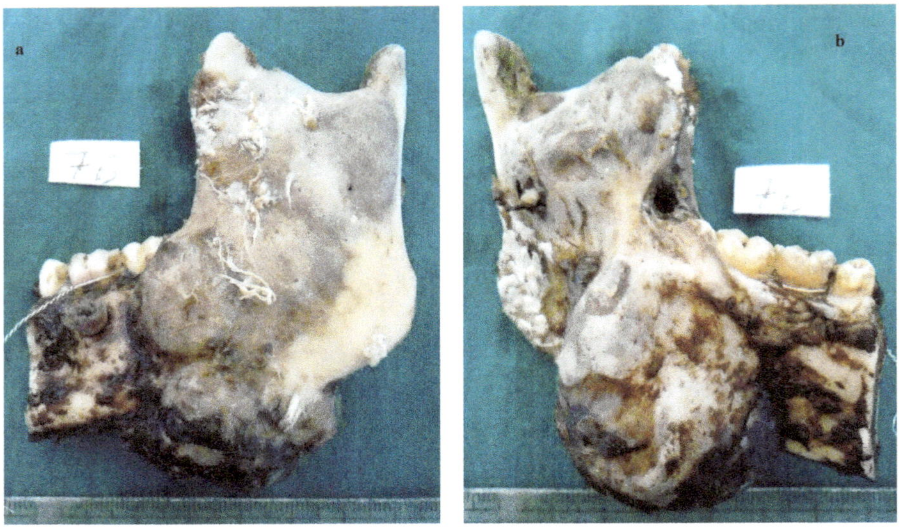


(a) (b)

Figure 5: Resected mandible sent for histopathologic examination, (a) lateral surface, and (b) medial surface of the mandible.

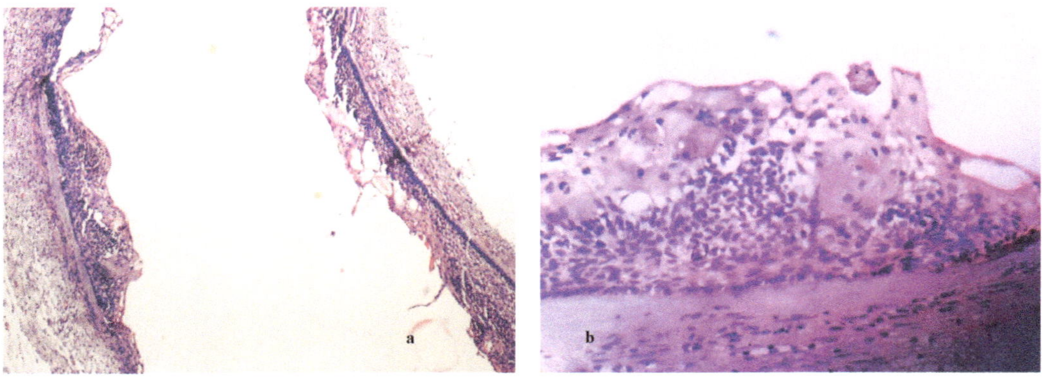


(a) (b)

Figure 6: H & E stained section showing cystic lining with ghost cells and stroma with dysplastic dentin, (a) magnification ×40, (b) magnification ×400.

showed multilocular radiolucent lesion associated with an impacted 38 which was displaced into the ramus of the mandible, and root resorption was noted in 36 and 37. In the mandible, several cases have crossed the midline, but this is less usual in the maxilla [4, 9]. Most of the peripheral lesions were located in the maxillary or mandibular gingiva or alveolar mucosa anterior to the first molar [1].

The epithelial lining of CCOT has characteristic odontogenic features. The most remarkable feature is the presence of ghost cells. Budding from the basal layer into the adjacent connective tissue and epithelial proliferations into the lumen are frequently seen. In the fibrous wall, there are usually strands and islands of odontogenic epithelium, either in direct contact with the epithelium or separately in the connective tissue. These vary from a few strands to extensive proliferations.

Takeda et al. stated that the cysts arise *de novo,* and Prætorius et al. concluded from their study that substantial evidence existed that the tumor developed from the wall of the cyst [1]. Hence, CCOT often coexist with other odontogenic tumors, such as odontoma, ameloblastoma, ameloblastic fibroma, ameloblastic fibroodontoma, and adenomatoid odontogenic tumor [10, 13]. Central CCOT has been reported with odontoma in 24–35% of cases and with an impacted tooth in 35% of cases, mostly canine [12].

Freedman et al. proposed that the neoplastic cells originated from well-differentiated ameloblasts, and its neural crest origin confers to this cell a pluripotential capacity to undergo terminal differentiation. Starting from this postulate that ameloblasts are stem cells, terminal differentiation is not necessarily required to originate the CCOT neoplastic cell. Praetorious et al. and Buchner et al. believe that CCOT cystic epithelium originates from the reduced enamel organ, from islands of odontogenic epithelium within the tooth follicle, or from the remnants of the odontogenic epithelium in the bone or gingival tissue [14].

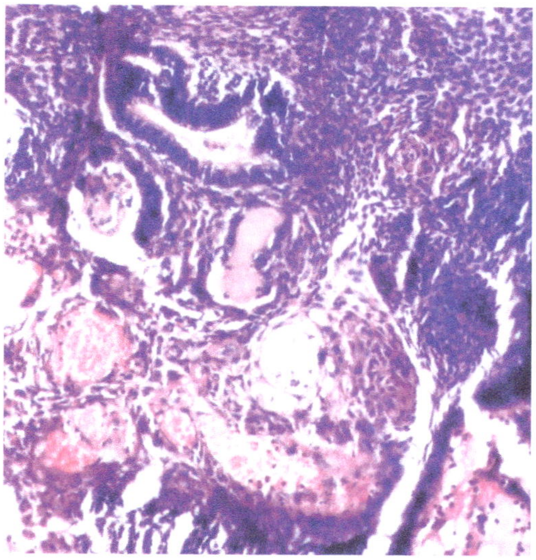

Figure 7: Odontogenic island in the stroma showing ghost cells.

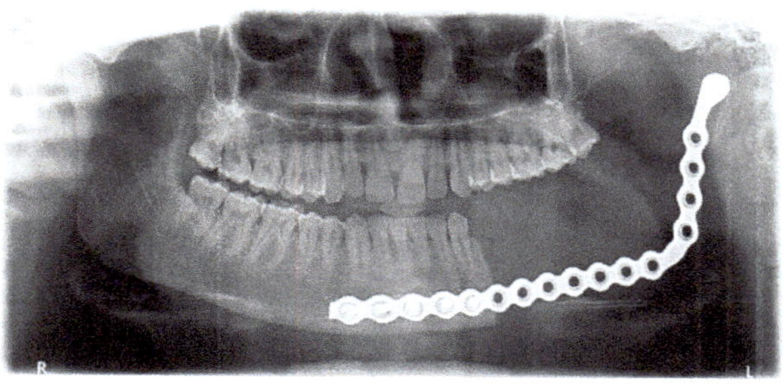

Figure 8: Posttreatment OPG after 1 year.

Toida classified CCOT into cyst and a neoplasm. Neoplasm is divided into benign and malignant types, and the terminology calcifying ghost cell odontogenic tumor (CGCOT) is used for benign neoplasm. The cyst or non-neoplastic variant accounts to 80–98% of cases. The solid and neoplastic type accounts to 11.5% of cases [12].

Pretorious et al. (2006) suggested classification of the odontogenic ghost cell lesions as Group 1 ("simple" cysts), Group 2 (cysts associated with odontogenic hamartomas or benign neoplasms), Group 3 (solid benign odontogenic neoplasms with similar cell morphology to that in the COC, and with dentinoid formation, dentinogenic ghost cell tumor), and Group 4 (malignant odontogenic neoplasms with features similar to those of the dentinogenic ghost cell tumor, ghost cell odontogenic carcinoma) [1].

The histologic variation of COC has led to different terminologies such as calcifying ghost cell odontogenic tumor (Fejerskov and Krogh, 1972), dentinogenic ghost cell tumor (Preatorius et al., 1981), epithelial odontogenic ghost cell tumor (Ellis and Shmookler, 1986), and odontogenic ghost cell tumor (Colmenero et al., 1990) [2, 10].

Gorlin et al., Ebling and Wagner, Gold, Bhasker, Komiya et al., and Regezi et al. all believed that ghost cells represent normal or abnormal keratinization. Levy suggested that they represent squamous metaplasia with subsequent calcification caused by ischemia. Sedano and Pindborg thought that the ghost cells represented different stages of normal and aberrant keratin formation and that they were derived from the metaplastic transformation of odontogenic epithelium. Other investigators suggested or implied that ghost cells may represent the product of abortive enamel matrix in odontogenic epithelium [4, 9].

The classification advocated by Hong et al. has two categories for COC associated with ameloblastoma: the ameloblastomatous cystic variant and the neoplastic variant associated with ameloblastoma. The former is characterized by a unicystic structure in which the lining epithelium shows unifocal or multifocal intraluminal proliferative activity that resembles ameloblastoma, although it also contains isolated or clustered ghost cells and calcifications. The ghost cells and dystrophic calcifications are within the proliferative epithelium, which lacks histopathologic criteria as suggested by Vickers and Gorlin and is confined to the cyst lumen. Ameloblastomatous COC occurs only intraosseously. The latter is called ameloblastoma arising from COC (ameloblastoma ex COC). It is characterized histopathologically as comprising few or no ghost cells with calcifications observed in the transformed ameloblastomatous epithelial portion, while the cyst lining of the epithelium contains a considerable number of ghost cells and calcifications [9, 13, 15].

The present report showed the cystic lining containing ghost cells and few areas showed juxta-epithelial hyalinization suggestive of dysplastic dentin. Proliferative odontogenic islands were seen in the connective tissue which also showed some ghost cells. Satellite cysts containing ghost cells were also noted.

Takeda et al. (1990) had performed a histological study of satellite cysts and odontogenic epithelial islands in the connective tissue and grouped them into the same three histological types described by Prætorius et al. (1981), but these did not always coincide with the typing of the mother cyst [1].

Gorlin et al. considered the appearance of dentinoid material in CCOT to represent an inflammatory response of the body tissue in response to ghost cells. Abraham and Howell further stated that masses of ghost cells induced granulation tissue to lay down juxta-epithelial osteoid which may calcify. Contrary to this interception, Sauk stated that the juxta-epithelial osteoid and dentinoid are frequently found in areas free of either granulation tissue or ghost cells and postulated that it might be an inductive phenomenon. To date, it still remains to be clarified that dentinoid is an inductive phenomenon or metaplastic change in connective tissue [14].

Melanin deposits are sometimes present in the epithelial linings. One case, recorded by Gorlin et al. (1964), was found in the parotid salivary gland [1]. CCOT was seen associated with an orthokeratinized odontogenic cyst [6].

## References

[1] M. Shear and P. M. Speight, *Cysts of Oral and Maxillofacial Regions*, Blackwell Munksgaard, Oxford, UK, 4th edition, 2007.

[2] M. Toida, "So-called calcifying odontogenic cyst: review and discussion on the terminology and classification," *Journal of Oral Pathology and Medicine*, vol. 27, no. 2, pp. 49–52, 1998.

[3] N. Eshghyar, N. Jalayer-Nadery, and R. Ashery, "Calcifying odontogenic cyst: an analysis of thirty-six cases," *Acta Medica Iranica*, vol. 44, no. 1, pp. 59–62, 2006.

[4] A. Sonone, V. S. Sabane, and R. Desai, "Calcifying ghost cell Odontogenic cyst: report of a case and review of literature," *Case Reports in Dentistry*, vol. 2011, Article ID 328743, 5 pages, 2011.

[5] D. Aithal, B. S. Reddy, S. Mahajan, K. Boaz, and M. Kamboj, "Ameloblastomatous calcifying odontogenic cyst: a rare histologic variant," *Journal of Oral Pathology and Medicine*, vol. 32, no. 6, pp. 376–378, 2003.

[6] V. F. Bernardes, J. C. T. de Lacerda, M. C. F. de Aguiar, and R. S. Gomez, "Calcifying odontogenic cyst associated with an orthokeratinized odontogenic cyst," *Head and Neck Pathology*, vol. 2, no. 4, pp. 324–327, 2008.

[7] N. Gupta and S. Gupta, "Ameloblastomatous calcifying odontogenic cyst: a rare clinicopathologic entity," *International Journal of Head and Neck Surgery*, vol. 2, no. 2, pp. 115–118, 2011.

[8] F. A. Mashhadi Abbas, M. A. Moshref, S. A. Sargolzaie, and N. A. Kargahi, "Ameloblastomatous calcifying cystic odontogenic tumor: a rare histologic variant," *Journal of Dentistry*, vol. 9, no. 1, pp. 45–48, 2009.

[9] H. P. Singh, M. Yadav, A. Nayar, C. Verma, P. Aggarwal, and S. K. Bains, "Ameloblastomatous calcifying ghost cell odontontogenic cyst—a rare variant of a rare entity," *Annali Di Stomatologia*, vol. 4, no. 1, pp. 156–160, 2013.

[10] S. Iida, T. Ueda, T. Aikawa, M. Kishino, M. Okura, and M. Kogo, "Ameloblastomatous calcifying odontogenic cyst in the mandible," *Dentomaxillofacial Radiology*, vol. 33, no. 6, pp. 409–412, 2004.

[11] N. Eshghyar, N. Jalayer-Nadery, and R. Ashery, "Calcifying odontogenic cyst: an analysis of thirty-six cases," *Acta Medica Iranica*, vol. 44, no. 1, pp. 59–62, 2006.

[12] K. Rajkumar, K. Kamal, M. R. Satish, and S. Leena, "Calcifying odontogenic cyst," *Journal of Oral and Maxillofacial Pathology*, vol. 8, no. 2, pp. 99–103, 2004.

[13] K. Nosrati and M. Seyedmajidi, "Ameloblastomatous calcifying odontogenic cyst: a case report of a rare histologic variant," *Archives of Iranian Medicine*, vol. 12, no. 4, pp. 417–420, 2009.

[14] M. Kamboj and M. Juneja, "Ameloblastomatous Gorlin's cyst," *Journal of Oral Science*, vol. 49, no. 4, pp. 319–323, 2007.

[15] K. Shikha, S. Palaskar, V. Prakashshetty, and A. Bhusha, "Intraosseous calcifying cystic odontogenic tumor," *Journal of Oral and Maxillofacial Pathology*, vol. 13, no. 1, pp. 27–29, 2009.

# 28

# Generalised versus Regional Odontodysplasia: Diagnosis, Transitional Management, and Long-Term Followup—A Report of 2 Cases

**Mostafa Ibrahim Mostafa,[1] Nehad Samir Taha,[2] and Mennat Allah Ismail Mehrez[1]**

[1] *Department of Oro-Dental Genetics, National Research Centre, 33 Tahrir Street, Dokki, Cairo 12311, Egypt*
[2] *Oral Histopathology Department, Misr International University (MIU), Cairo, Egypt*

Correspondence should be addressed to Mostafa Ibrahim Mostafa; mostafanrc@yahoo.com

Academic Editors: S. S. De Rossi and L. N. De Souza

*Background.* Odontodysplasia is an uncommon condition. It can be localised or generalised, isolated or part of a syndrome. *Case Report.* We first report the case of an 8.5-year-old boy who presented with abnormally shaped teeth and multiple intraoral abscesses. Findings of clinical and radiographic examinations were consistent with those of generalised odontodysplasia. A 2-step, conservative treatment plan was executed with a 10-year followup. Step 1 was root canal treatment of nonvital teeth. Step 2 was crowning without preparation of new vital, erupted, and malformed teeth. The second case is that of a 12-year-old girl who presented with lack of teeth in the upper-left quadrant. The impacted teeth were exposed surgically, and fixed restoration was performed for temporary aesthetic improvement. *Conclusion.* Instead of tooth extraction, an approach previously used in similar cases, conservative management is feasible and offers better prosthetic treatment options for the future.

## 1. Introduction

Odontodysplasia (OD) is an uncommon condition that affects the enamel and dentine of both primary and permanent dentitions. The cementum shows affection, but at a lower grade. The teeth are misshaped, pitted, and yellowish to brownish in colour, with excessive wear and underlying periapical abscesses. On radiographs, the enamel and dentine lack contrast, rendering the tooth a ghostlike appearance [1, 2].

This condition commonly presents as regional OD (ROD), wherein few teeth may be involved. Occasionally, an entire quadrant or more than 1 quadrant may be involved, but generalised involvement is extremely rare [3]. ROD may present as an isolated condition or as part of a syndrome such as oculodentodigital syndrome [OMIM:#164200] or epidermal nevus/Schimmelpenning-Feuerstein-Mims syndrome [OMIM: %163200] [4, 5].

The precise aetiology of OD is still unknown. Genetic predisposition has been proposed, but environmental causation has received greater support [1]. Previously employed treatment plans differed according to the degree of teeth involvement and the patient's age [6–8]. The treatment protocol advocated, provided that the patient is of proper age, is implant placement with a final fixed restoration [9].

In this paper, we present 2 cases, one of generalised OD and another with ROD, and propose a protocol for transitional management and long-term followup (10 and 5 years, resp.) of both types of cases.

## 2. Case 1: Generalised Odontodysplasia

An 8.5-year-old boy presented complaining of abnormally shaped teeth and multiple intraoral swellings. Oral examination revealed severe wear of the upper centrals, upper first molars, and the lower-right first molar, with no carious lesions. The lower-right first molar was mutilated beyond repair and was indicated for extraction. Abscesses and fistulas were related to upper-right and lower-left incisors. Microdontia was also evident (Figure 1(a)).

The patient reported that he had had delayed eruption and premature loss of the primary dentition and that the

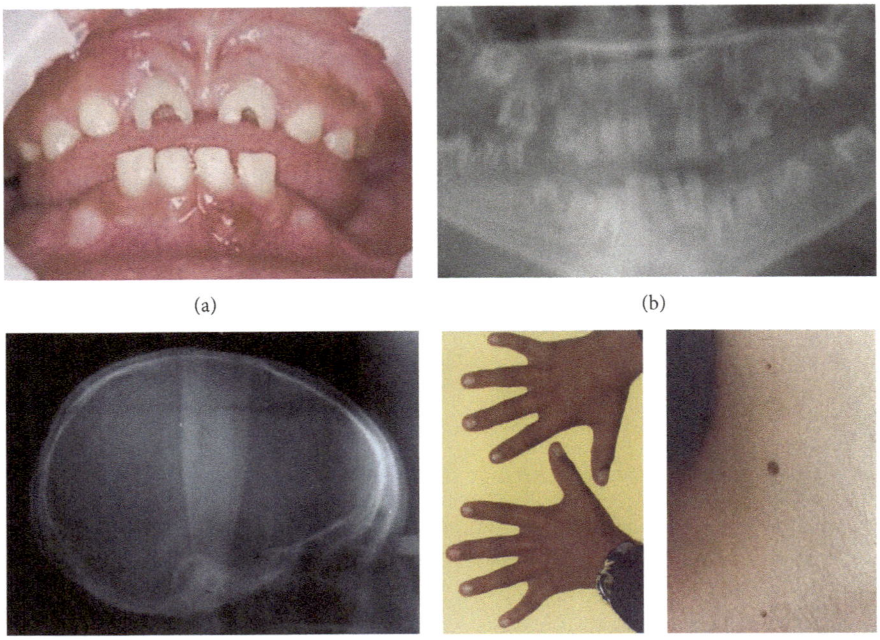

(a) (b) (c) (d) (e)

FIGURE 1: (a) Case 1. Oral condition of GOD at time of presentation. (b) Panoramic view showing ghost-shaped teeth, enlarged pulp chambers and root canals, and short roots and open apices. (c) Lateral cephalometric view depicting dolichocephaly. (d) Bilateral clinodactyly of the little fingers. (e) Multiple nevi on the neck.

lower-left first molar had been extracted. Vitality testing revealed that all incisors and the upper-right first and second molars were nonvital.

A panoramic radiograph showed ghost-shaped teeth. The roots had enlarged pulp chambers and root canals, short roots, and open apices (Figure 1(b)).

The patient was dolichocephalic (Figure 1(c)). He had clinodactyly and multiple nevi on both his neck and back (Figures 1(d) and 1(e)). Positive consanguinity was present with negative family history. Maternal pregnancy and delivery history were uneventful, and there was no evidence of any of the suggested causative factors.

Histopathologic examination of the extracted upper-right first molar revealed that the dentine had tortuous dentinal tubules and globular masses of dentine interrupting them (Figure 2(a)). Gingival biopsy examination, on the other hand, showed odontogenic tissue in the epithelium and intramesenchymal calcifications (Figure 2(b)).

The patient had normal levels of alkaline phosphatase and serum calcium and phosphorus. Based on the clinical and radiographic findings, generalised OD was diagnosed.

*Management.* Apexification of the upper centrals was first attempted over a period of 2 years but failed (Figure 2(c)). We formulated a conservative treatment plan to be carried out at the age of 12 years and over a period of 2.5 years. Step 1 was root canal treatment (RCT) of nonvital teeth, including those with open apices and abscesses underneath. Step 2 was crowning without preparation of the new vital, erupted, and malformed teeth, to protect them from the sequelae of poor development. Metal crowns fused to porcelain were used to meet aesthetic requirements, with gingival or subgingival metallic margins to minimise overhang.

We lost contact with the patient over the following year and a half. During this period, the lower-right second molar was extracted because of severe mutilation and abscess formation. This information was reported by the child's parents.

At the 10-year followup, the 7-year-old RCT was successful. Vitality of crowned teeth was preserved, and these teeth showed apex formation. The lower-left first premolar was still impacted. Radiolucency of the upper-right incisors and the lower-right lateral incisor persisted, although the radiolucent area was markedly smaller in the lower-right lateral incisor (Figures 2(d) and 2(e)).

## 3. Case 2: Regional Odontodysplasia

A 12-year-old girl presented to our clinic with lack of teeth in the upper-left quadrant. Examination revealed a canine and a root of a deciduous tooth. At the affected area, the gingiva was enlarged, fibrous, and tense (Figure 3(a)). The lower-right first molar was congenitally absent. Dolichocephaly was noted during the extraoral examination (Figure 3(c)), and there was no evidence of multiple nevi on the skin.

The maternal pregnancy and delivery history were unremarkable. There were no similar cases among the family, and there was no history of any of the suggested causative factors. Patient had osteopenia according to the DEXA scan.

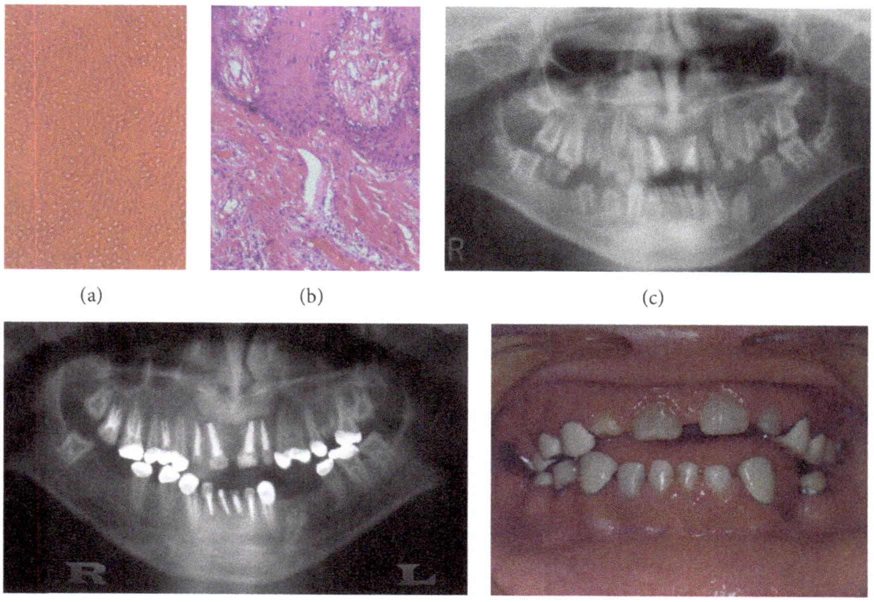

(a) (b) (c) (d) (e)

FIGURE 2: (a) Histological examination showing dentin having torturous dentinal tubules and globular masses of dentine interrupting them (original magnification 20x). (b) Gingival biopsy examination showing odontogenic tissue in the epithelium and intramesenchymal calcifications (original magnification 20x). (c) Panoramic view showing apexification trial. (d) RCT without crowning was done for incisors and upper-right second molar. RCT with crowning was performed for upper-right second premolar and first molar and upper-left first premolar. Crowning without RCT was done for the vital upper-left premolars, left second molar, lower left second premolar, lower left second molar, lower canines, right first premolar, and upper-right first molar. (e) Final oral condition at 18 years of age.

A panoramic radiograph revealed multiple impacted teeth in the upper-left quadrant and a missing lower-right first molar (Figure 3(b)). The patient had a twin brother whose teeth had erupted normally, except for the lower-first molar on the left side, which was congenitally absent (Figure 3(d)).

*Management.* The treatment plan was implant placement after completion of the growth period. Prevention of opposing overeruption was necessary, and a vacuum-formed tray was prepared for the lower jaw (Figure 4(a)).

After 2.5 years, a periapical abscess had developed at the canine, which had become loose. We extracted the canine but were in turn faced by another problem, the increased aesthetic demand of the now 14.5-year-old girl. A change in treatment strategy was mandatory. Surgical exposure of the impacted teeth was performed, followed by porcelain-fused-to-metal fixed restoration as a temporary aesthetic solution (Figure 4(b)).

Three years later, the gingiva at the restoration (as in Case 1) showed signs of inflammation, and a panoramic radiograph showed asymptomatic periapical radiolucency in the upper-left first premolar (Figures 4(c) and 4(d)). The patient was satisfied with the functional and aesthetic results.

## 4. Discussion

Early diagnosis of OD is critical. The diagnosis is based on clinical and radiographic examination, but extraoral features should not be neglected. Dentinogenesis imperfecta type III bears close resemblance to OD but can be excluded in the absence of opalescent dentine, bell-shaped crowns, and negative family history. Delayed eruption or failure of eruption and gingival enlargement occur only in OD [10].

Generalised OD in Case 1 showed some extraoral features of both oculodentodigital and epidermal nevus syndromes and could have been a mild variant of either syndrome. Dolichocephaly was present in both cases, while clinodactyly was only present in Case 1 (generalised OD). Dolichocephaly and clinodactyly could be associated with OD. Fanibunda and Soames (1996) reported a case of ROD associated with dolichocephaly and clinodactyly [11].

Several hypotheses have been proposed to explain the cause of OD. We agree with the hypothesis of local irritating factors during teeth development because the twin brother of the patient in Case 2 had only the missing premolar and was free from OD.

Our treatment plan was based on the theory of Gardner and Sapp (1973), who reported that the cause of pulpal necrosis and subsequent periapical abscess is bacterial invasion of the pulp through defective clefts in the enamel and dentine [12, 13]. This explains the completion of root formation and the lack of periapical pathosis in the newly erupted teeth after crowning in Case 1 (Figure 2(d)).

Since the teeth in these cases were not bell shaped, it was possible to crown them without preparation and with only a few fitting adjustments at the time of insertion. The upper

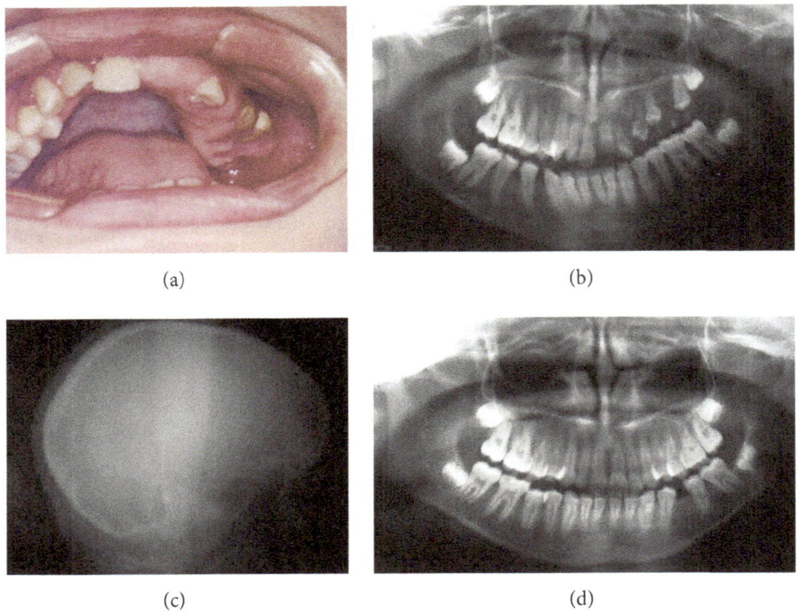

FIGURE 3: (a) Case 2. Oral condition of ROD of the upper-left quadrant at time of presentation. (b) Panoramic view of Case 2 showing multiple impacted teeth in the upper left quadrant and a missing lower right first premolar. (c) Lateral cephalometric view depicting dolichocephaly. (d) Panoramic view of Case 2 twin brother showing a missing lower left first premolar.

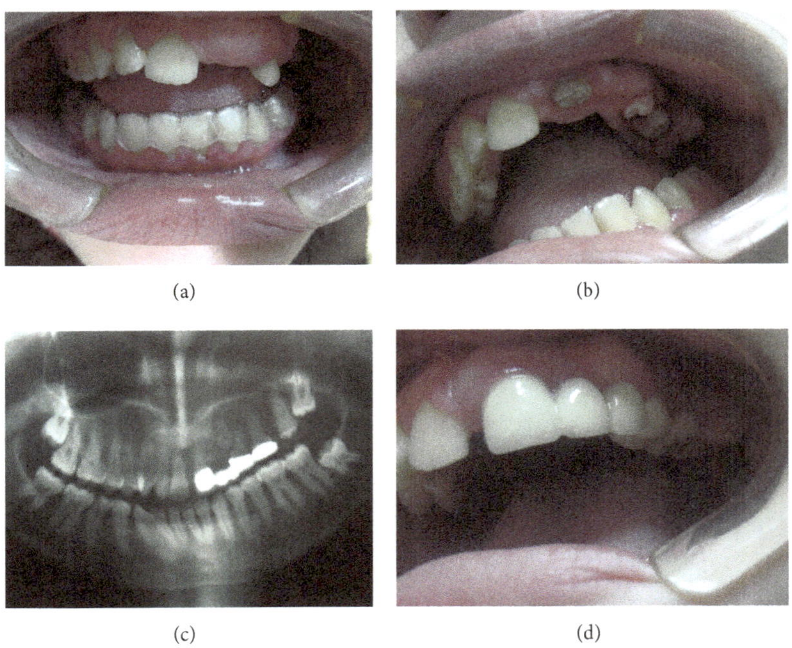

FIGURE 4: (a) Vacuum formed tray for the lower jaw to prevent overeruption of lower teeth. (b) Surgical exposure of the impacted teeth. (c) Panoramic view for the case after surgical exposure and placement of the porcelain fused to metal bridge. (d) Final oral condition at 17 years of age.

and lower incisors were not crowned because early failure was expected.

Regarding ROD in Case 2, the patient did not wear the vacuum tray, but the gingival enlargement acted as a stopper and achieved the purpose of the vacuum tray.

## 5. Conclusion

Maintenance of oral hygiene and periodic checkups are necessary in similar cases. In the authors' opinion, conservative treatment of these patients is preferable to extraction because it preserves optimum oral functionality and aesthetics until the end of the growth period. At that time, implants can be placed safely. Conservative treatment offers better prosthetic options for the future.

## Acknowledgments

This work was carried out under the annual research fund for the National Research Centre. The authors wish to thank Mr. M. Gomaa and his dental laboratory for their help with the cases' restorations. All authors have declared no conflict of interest.

## References

[1] M. A. Hamdan, F. A. Sawair, L. D. Rajab, A. M. Hamdan, and I. K. Al-Omari, "Regional odontodysplasia: a review of the literature and report of a case," *International Journal of Paediatric Dentistry*, vol. 14, no. 5, pp. 363–370, 2004.

[2] R. Carlos, E. Contreras-Vidaurre, O. P. De Almeida et al., "Regional odontodysplasia: morphological, ultrastructural, and immunohistochemical features of the affected teeth, connective tissue, and odontogenic remnants," *Journal of Dentistry for Children*, vol. 75, no. 2, pp. 144–150, 2008.

[3] N. Shah and Y. K. Gupta, "Generalized odontodysplasia—a case report," *Journal of Indian Society of Pedodontics and Preventive Dentistry*, vol. 16, pp. 40–43, 1998.

[4] A. Murakami, F. Skovby, J. O. Andreasen, M. M. Cohen Jr., B. L. Jensen, and S. Kreiborg, "Oral Manifestations of schimmelpenning syndrome: case report and review of literature," *Annals of the Academy of Medicine Singapore*, vol. 28, no. 5, pp. 744–748, 1999.

[5] V. A. McKusick, "Online Mendelian Inheritance in Man (OMIM)," 2012, http://www.ncbi.nlm.nih.gov/omim.

[6] Y. Melamed, J. Harnik, A. Becker, and J. Shapira, "Conservative multidisciplinary treatment approach in an unusual odontodysplasia," *ASDC Journal of Dentistry for Children*, vol. 61, no. 2, pp. 119–124, 1994.

[7] S. Y. Cho, "Conservative management of regional odontodysplasia: case report," *Journal of the Canadian Dental Association*, vol. 72, no. 8, pp. 735–738, 2006.

[8] B. Ozpinar, B. Gokce, G. Uzel, and M. E. Comlekoglu, "Prosthetic rehabilitation of segmental odontomaxillary dysplasia: seven-year follow up," *The Cleft Palate-Craniofacial Journal*, vol. 46, pp. 103–107, 2009.

[9] M. R. Bagherpoor, H. Siadat, S. Nokar, and M. Alikhasi, "Step-by-Step oral rehabilitation of a generalized odontodysplastic patient with implant-supported prostheses: a clinical report," *Implant Dentistry*, vol. 19, no. 2, pp. 122–127, 2010.

[10] M. J. Barron, S. T. McDonnell, I. MacKie, and M. J. Dixon, "Hereditary dentine disorders: dentinogenesis imperfecta and dentine dysplasia," *Orphanet Journal of Rare Diseases*, vol. 3, no. 1, article 31, 2008.

[11] K. B. Fanibunda and J. V. Soames, "Odontodysplasia, gingival manifestations, and accompanying abnormalities," *Oral Surgery, Oral Medicine, Oral Pathology, Oral Radiology, and Endodontics*, vol. 81, no. 1, pp. 84–88, 1996.

[12] D. G. Gardner and J. P. Sapp, "Regional odontodysplasia," *Oral Surgery, Oral Medicine, Oral Pathology*, vol. 35, no. 3, pp. 351–365, 1973.

[13] C. Armstrong, S. S. Napier, R. C. Boyd, and T. A. Gregg, "Histopathology of the teeth in segmental odontomaxillary dysplasia: new findings," *Journal of Oral Pathology and Medicine*, vol. 33, no. 4, pp. 146–148, 2004.

# 29

# Soft Tissue Management and Prosthetic Rehabilitation in a Tongue Cancer Patient

**Umberto Romeo, Marco Lollobrigida, Gaspare Palaia, Domenica Laurito, Riccardo Cugnetto, and Alberto De Biase**

*Division of Oral Surgery, Department of Oral and Maxillofacial Sciences, Sapienza University of Rome, Via Caserta 6, 00161 Rome, Italy*

Correspondence should be addressed to Alberto De Biase; alberto.debiase@uniroma1.it

Academic Editors: Y.-K. Chen, R. Crespi, and A. Kasaj

One major challenge in treating head and neck oncologic patients is to achieve an acceptable recovery of physiologic functions compatible with the complete tumor excision. However, after tumor resection, some patients present a surgically altered anatomy incompatible with prosthetic rehabilitation, unless some soft tissue correction is carried out. The aim of the present study is to describe the overall mandibular prosthetic rehabilitation of a postoncologic patient focusing on the possibility of soft tissue correction as a part of the treatment. A 72-year-old woman, who undergone a hemiglossectomy for squamous cell carcinoma several years before, was referred to our department needing a new prosthesis. The patient presented partial mandibular edentulism, defects in tongue mobility, and a bridge of scar tissue connecting one side of the tongue to the alveolar ridge. A diode laser (980 nm) was used to remove the fibrous scar tissue. After reestablishing a proper vestibular depth and soft tissue morphology, two implants were placed in the interforaminal region of the mandible to support an overdenture.

## 1. Introduction

Technical advances in head and neck cancer reconstructive surgery have led surgeons not to consider the complete ablation of neoplasms alone as the focus of treatment planning but rather inseparably from the possibility to return patients, as close as possible, to their premorbid condition. This means the necessity to preserve or restore several essential functions like speech, mastication and deglutition [1, 2]. Dental rehabilitation is an important aspect of such comprehensive treatments, aiming to replace teeth that are missing as a consequence of tumor resection or that patients have already lost.

Oral implants offer many advantages in treating edentulous patients who undergone cancer resection when prosthesis has to fit to an altered anatomy [3]. In particular, implant supported overdentures were demonstrated to be a predictable solution for edentulous patients with excellent long-term prognosis, assuring better retention and stability than conventional dentures [4]. While there is no doubt for postoncologic patients about the benefits of an implant supported rehabilitation in terms of stability and retention [5], some questions still remain about the opportunity of placing implants in those patients who received radiation therapy following the surgical treatment due to the possibility of soft tissue complications and low rates of osseointegration reported in the literature [6]. However, if the first decades of the modern implant era were characterized by an extremely cautious approach with regard to irradiated patients [7], nowadays, also considering the higher survival rates of cancer patients, oral implants are indicated for selected preirradiated patients too.

Another concern regards the relationship between prosthesis and soft tissue. Although many efforts are undertaken by surgeons to limit the degree of anatomical deformities during surgical resections of neoplasms, minor preprosthetic correction of the soft tissue may be helpful in some cases (like the one here presented) to eliminate unacceptable interferences of residual scar tissue with the prosthesis. The reconstruction of oral cavity defects always represents a difficult challenge depending on disease staging and patient condition [8]. Due to this unique and complex three-dimensional anatomical environment, the outcomes of reconstructive procedures are often a compromise that implies functional morbidity and, furthermore, may limit the possibility of an adequate prosthetic rehabilitation. In this regard, some laser systems may be useful to perform soft tissue surgery as an alternative to conventional techniques [9–12].

In this report, the overall mandibular prosthetic rehabilitation of a postoncologic patient is presented.

## 2. Case Presentation

The case refers to a 72-year-old Caucasian woman, diagnosed in 1995 (at the age of 58) with a squamous cell carcinoma (SCC) of the left lateral border of the tongue (Figure 1). The patient underwent hemiglossectomy associated with an en bloc resection of the corresponding lateral floor of the mouth and conservative neck dissection. Postoperative microscopic examination of the specimen revealed a multifocal low grade carcinoma and one lymph node metastasis (pT1pN1pMx G1). The resulting tissue defect was primarily closed with local flaps, and a 6-week postoperative radiotherapy (60 Gy) was delivered. Five months after the primary surgery the patient noted a swelling in the right lateral neck. A submandibular fine-needle aspiration was performed confirming the diagnosis of "metastatic carcinoma." The patient was then treated with a right conservative neck dissection associated with resection of the submandibular gland. After this second intervention, no signs of recurrent disease were observed, and the patient was rehabilitated with a resin removable partial prosthesis anchored to the remaining teeth. During the following years, the patient lived healthy but lost her teeth due to periodontal disease with the resultant impossibility to wear the prosthesis.

The patient was then referred to our department needing a new prosthesis. At the time of observation, medical history was significant for controlled hypertension and no other systemic diseases. Physical exam revealed defects and limitation in tongue mobility and a bridge of scar tissue connecting one side of the tongue to the alveolar ridge (Figures 2 and 3). The patient was referred for having suffered from limitation in tongue mobility since the surgical excision of the tumour, having difficulties in speech intelligibility and mastication.

After evaluating bone volume with a computed tomography scan and considering patient's complaints about the ability to chew and move the tongue, it was proposed to perform a soft tissue correction before proceeding with the extraction of the only residual tooth and the placement of two endosseous implants to support an overdenture. The aim of the proposed surgical procedure was to reestablish a suitable anatomy eliminating the fibrous scar resulting from the cancer resection, improving tongue mobility, and contextually deepening the sublingual sulcus and vestibular fornix for the receipt of the prosthesis.

It was used a diode laser (Wiser, Doctor Smile, Brendola, Italy) with a wavelength of 980 nm and 2 W power, operating in continuous-wave mode (CW), an optical fiber of 320 $\mu$m, and a fluence of 2488 J/cm$^2$. The radiation of this device is selectively adsorbed by hemoglobin, causing a thermal effect that allows a precise surgical cut. After local infiltration of anesthesia (without vasoconstrictor just to enhance hemoglobin light absorption), an incision was made transversally to the ridge involving both the vestibule and the floor of the mouth, dissecting tissues almost till the periosteum and muscles (Figure 4). After simple dissection, no more surgical manipulations were necessary. At the end of the procedure, it was acceptable to allow the laser wound to heal by secondarily epithelialization, and no sutures were applied. The patient was then instructed and informed about the importance of doing tongue exercises (like lifting and protruding) to avoid the formation of new scars. Although

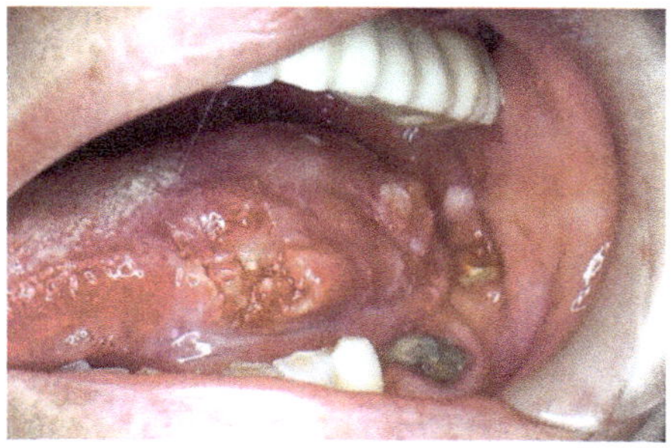

FIGURE 1: SCC of the left lateral border of the tongue at the time of the primary surgery.

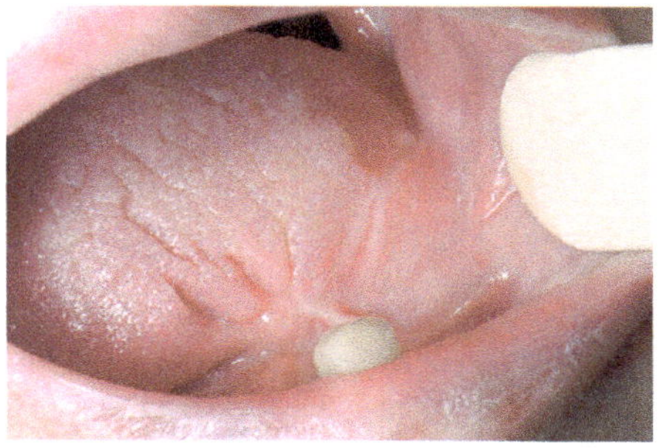

FIGURE 2: Clinical photograph of the patient's oral cavity as it was presented to the observation. The defect resulting from the hemiglossectomy was primarily closed with local flaps using the left buccal mucosa.

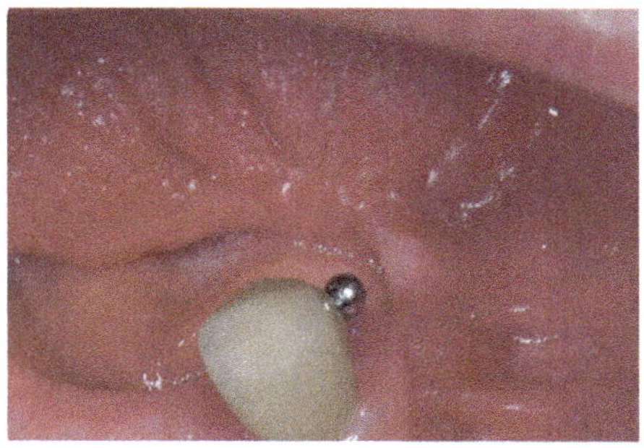

FIGURE 3: Fibrous scar tissue connecting the tongue to the alveolar ridge mucosa. Scar tissue was responsible for limitation in anterior tongue mobility and speech articulation.

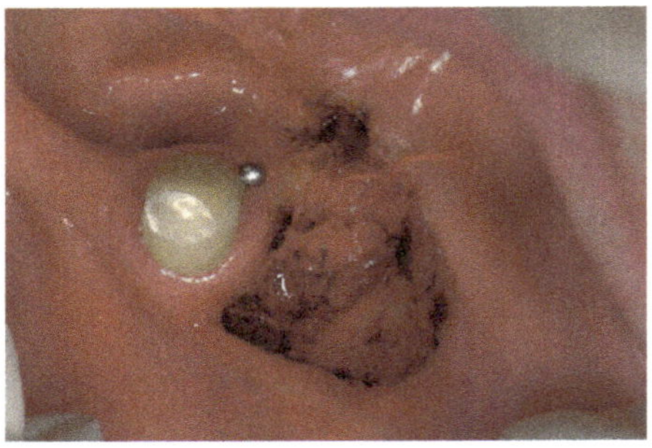

FIGURE 4: Intraoperatory picture. Tissues were dissected till the mandibular periosteum. Laser thermal effects assured a good visibility during the entire procedure.

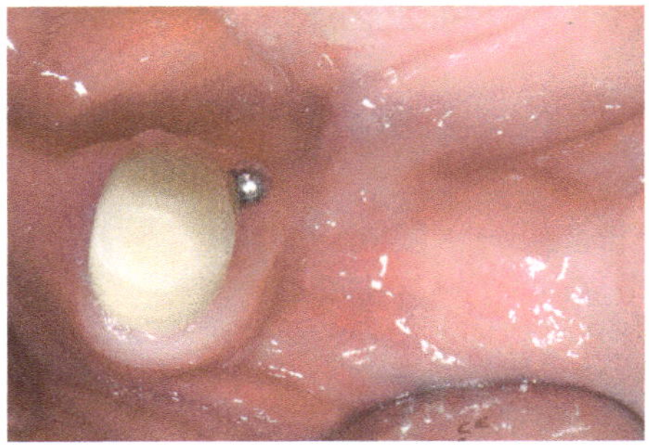

FIGURE 5: Clinical aspect 28 days after the laser dissection. The wound presented a complete reepithelization, and no scar tissue has formed.

no vasoconstrictor had been used, laser-induced coagulation guaranteed an adequate bleeding control during the surgery with good visibility. The procedure was fast and well tolerated. Immediately after the procedure, the patient showed an improvement in both tongue mobility and speech articulation. Gradual reepithelialization and no signs of infection occurred during the following weeks. The patient reported no particular discomfort in the postoperative period, and no scar tissue has formed. At 28 days, the defect was completely closed (Figure 5).

Six months after laser correction and extraction of the residual canine, two implants of 4.1 mm diameter and 13.0 mm length (ExFeel, Megagen Implant Co., Republic of Korea) were placed in the parasymphyseal region of the mandible under the guidance of a surgical template and submerged (Figure 6). At the time of implant placement, primary stability was obtained, and no signs of bone alterations were clinically observed during the healing period.

Six months later, an overdenture retained with two free-standing attachments was delivered to the patient. After an early period of adaptation, the patient reported an improved masticatory function in relation to her new diet regimen and defined herself as satisfied (Figures 7(a) and 7(b)).

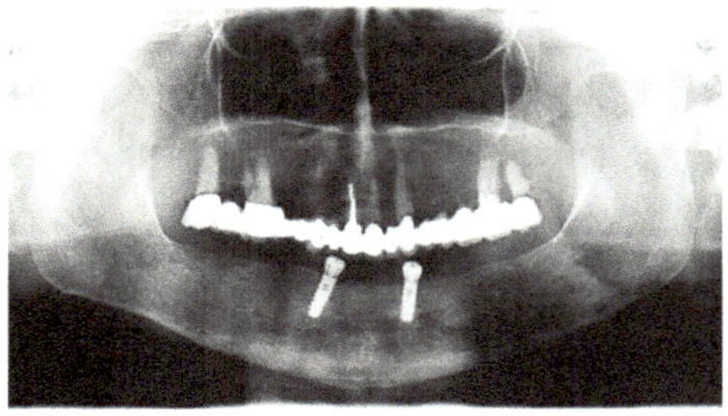

FIGURE 6: Panoramic radiograph showing the implants placed in the parasymphyseal region of the mandible. Implant supported prosthesis are particularly indicated in postoncologic patients with an altered oral anatomy.

## 3. Discussion

According to the international literature data, oral cancer represents the eighth most common cancer worldwide, with a constantly higher incidence among men [13]. Oral cancer patients often require a multidisciplinary approach, including surgical resection of the tumor and a series of complementary therapies aiming to a full rehabilitation of the patients.

Functional rehabilitation represents a fundamental concern in treating head and neck cancer patients, especially when important functions for social life are involved. Missing teeth, which are not replaced with prosthesis, clearly result in a poor quality of life (QOL) for both healthy and oncologic patients. In the latter ones, prosthetic rehabilitation often presents a variety of problems due to the unfavorable anatomy that clinicians may encounter as the result of using various types of flaps to correct large tissue defects of the oral cavity [14]. Implant supported prosthesis may represent a valid solution to overcome such anatomic restrictions. Implant supported overdentures have been proposed as the first choice for treating inferior edentulism [15]. Other authors recommend implant treatment only for those patients who complain about conventional prosthesis [16]. However, it is a fact that patients treated with implant supported overdenture present an improvement in the QOL and, generally, a good level of satisfaction [17, 18]. Furthermore, good long-term results confirm the efficacy and predictability of this prosthetic solution [19].

The patient referred to our observation, also after the soft tissue correction, still presented mouth conditions incompatible with a traditional prosthesis (complete denture), as the posterior vestibular depth was totally missing. The absence of any residual tooth and the particular anatomical environment meant that the implant solution was the only possible choice. However, the foremost objective of the treatment was indeed to improve patient's masticatory function and speech articulation, being aware of the impossibility of getting the patient back to her precancer condition. Despite that, the final result was more than acceptable.

Dealing with oncologic patients and dental implants, another important issue that must always be considered is the opportunity of placing implants in those patients who underwent radiotherapy. The suitability of implant placement in irradiated jaws depends on several factors like radiation dose [20], anatomic site [21], and time interval between bone radiation exposure and the implant placement [22]. The main current opinion is that dental implants should be placed in irradiated patients at least 1 year after the radiotherapy [23],

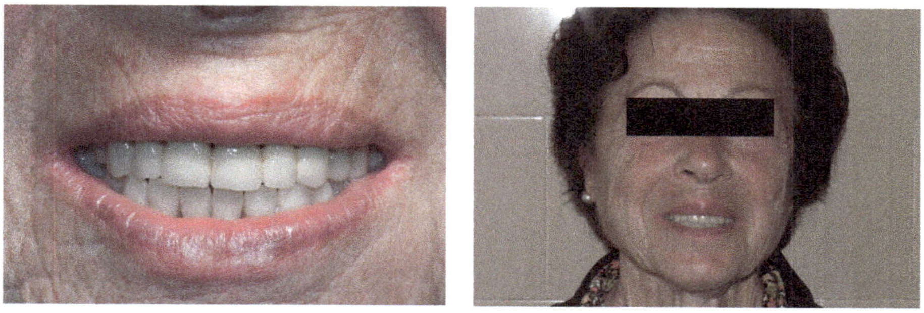

(a) (b)

FIGURE 7: ((a)-(b)) Patient's final appearance after the delivery of the prosthesis.

offering a stable bone environment to implants [24]. In the case presented, the patient received a radiation therapy a very long time before the secondary implant placement (17 years) and the radiation-related risk of bone complications and/or osseointegration failure was practically absent or, anyway, very low.

Finally, despite the above-mentioned advantages derived from the use of endosseous implants, in some postoncologic patients, it is unavoidable to perform a surgical management of the soft tissue before fabricating an adequate prosthesis. In the case presented, all the well-documented effects of laser surgery were desirable and have been confirmed. The decision to use a diode laser also was derived from the peculiar necessity to cut tissues already manipulated and whose vascularization was unknown by the operators. Taking this into account, laser features were particularly convenient. Fortunately, no hemorrhage or bleeding occurred during the procedure. However, simultaneous cutting and coagulation, allowing an adequate bleeding control and visibility, represent a very useful feature in preprosthetic procedures, particularly in oncologic patients with an altered anatomy. Reduction of postoperative pain and a relatively fast healing process without the necessity of sutures also make laser surgery well accepted by patients. The effects of the soft tissue correction were immediately observable, and the improvement in tongue mobility was clearly noticed by the patient. As result of the soft tissue modification, it was possible to fabricate a suitable inferior overdenture, fully satisfactory for retention, relationship with soft tissue, and aesthetics.

It is notable that morphology and oral structures arrangement are of primary importance for function and that even little changes in the anatomy may result in significant dysfunctions. This notion guides the reconstructive surgeons in their practice, attempting to limit the degree of permanent impairments resulting from cancer resections. Current multidisciplinary approaches have opened new horizons for cancer patients, aiming not only to eliminate the disease and improve disease-free survival rates but also to "rehabilitate" patients, focusing on an improvement of the QOL [25].

As an integral part of these comprehensive treatments, implant supported prosthesis represent a valid and sometimes the only possible solution to restore mastication and aesthetics in oral cancer patients.

## Conflict of Interests

The authors declare that there is no conflict of interests regarding the publication of this paper.

## References

[1] J. A. Logemann, B. R. Pauloski, A. W. Rademaker, and L. A. Colangelo, "Speech and swallowing rehabilitation for head and neck cancer patients," *Oncology*, vol. 11, no. 5, pp. 651–659, 1997.

[2] F. M. S. McConnel, B. R. Pauloski, J. A. Logemann et al., "Functional results of primary closure vs flaps in oropharyngeal reconstruction: a prospective study of speech and swallowing," *Archives of Otolaryngology—Head and Neck Surgery*, vol. 124, no. 6, pp. 625–630, 1998.

[3] R. A. Barrowman, P. R. Wilson, and D. Wiesenfeld, "Oral rehabilitation with dental implants after cancer treatment," *Australian Dental Journal*, vol. 56, no. 2, pp. 160–165, 2011.

[4] D. Laurito, L. Lamazza, M. J. Spink, and A. de Biase, "Tissue-supported dental implant prosthesis (overdenture): the search for the ideal protocol. A literature review," *Annali di Stomatologia*, vol. 3, no. 1, pp. 2–10, 2012.

[5] M. F. W.-Y. Chan, J. P. Hayter, J. I. Cawood, and R. A. Howell, "Oral rehabilitation with implant-retained prostheses following ablative surgery and reconstruction with free flaps," *International Journal of Oral and Maxillofacial Implants*, vol. 12, no. 6, pp. 820–827, 1997.

[6] G. Granström, "Osseointegration in irradiated cancer patients: an analysis with respect to implant failures," *Journal of Oral and Maxillofacial Surgery*, vol. 63, no. 5, pp. 579–585, 2005.

[7] NIH Consensus Development Program, *Dental Implants*, National Institutes of Health Consensus Development Conference Statement, 1988.

[8] P. C. Neligan, P. J. Gullane, and R. W. Gilbert, "Functional reconstruction of the oral cavity," *World Journal of Surgery*, vol. 27, no. 7, pp. 856–862, 2003.

[9] G. Romanos and G.-H. Nentwig, "Diode laser (980 nm) in oral and maxillofacial surgical procedures: clinical observations based on clinical applications," *Journal of Clinical Laser Medicine and Surgery*, vol. 17, no. 5, pp. 193–197, 1999.

[10] M. A. Pogrel, "The carbon dioxide laser in soft tissue preprosthetic surgery," *The Journal of Prosthetic Dentistry*, vol. 61, no. 2, pp. 203–208, 1989.

[11] U. Romeo, G. Palaia, A. del Vecchio et al., "Effects of KTP laser on oral soft tissues. An in vitro study," *Lasers in Medical Science*, vol. 25, no. 4, pp. 539–543, 2010.

[12] G. Palaia, G. Gaimari, R. L. Giudice, A. Galanakis, G. Tenore, and U. Romeo, "Excision of an oral angiolipoma by KTP laser: a case report," *Annali di Stomatologia*, vol. 2, no. 1-2, pp. 28–31, 2011.

[13] P. E. Petersen, "Oral cancer prevention and control—the approach of the World Health Organization," *Oral Oncology*, vol. 45, no. 4-5, pp. 454–460, 2009.

[14] K. Z. Siddall, S. N. Rogers, and C. J. Butterworth, "The prosthodontic pathway of the oral cancer patient," *Dental Update*, vol. 39, no. 2, pp. 98–106, 2012.

[15] J. S. Feine, G. E. Carlsson, M. A. Awad et al., "The McGill consensus statement on overdentures. Mandibular two-implant overdentures as first choice standard of care for edentulous patients," *Gerodontology*, vol. 19, no. 1, pp. 3–4, 2002.

[16] E. Emami, G. Heydecke, P. H. Rompré, P. de Grandmont, and J. S. Feine, "Impact of implant support for mandibular dentures on satisfaction, oral and general health-related quality of life: a meta-analysis of randomized- controlled trials," *Clinical Oral Implants Research*, vol. 20, no. 6, pp. 533–544, 2009.

[17] W. Att and C. Stappert, "Implant therapy to improve quality of life," *Quintessence International*, vol. 34, no. 8, pp. 573–581, 2003.

[18] J. M. Thomason, "The use of mandibular implant-retained overdentures improve patient satisfaction and quality of life," *Journal of Evidence-Based Dental Practice*, vol. 10, no. 1, pp. 61–63, 2010.

[19] T. Ueda, U. Kremer, J. Katsoulis, and R. Mericske-Stern, "Long-term results of mandibular implants supporting an overdenture: implant survival, failures, and crestal bone level changes," *The International Journal of Oral & Maxillofacial Implants*, vol. 26, no. 2, pp. 365–372, 2011.

[20] G. Granström, "Placement of dental implants in irradiated bone: the case for using hyperbaric oxygen," *Journal of Oral and Maxillofacial Surgery*, vol. 64, no. 5, pp. 812–818, 2006.

[21] A. Buddula, D. Assad, T. Salinas, and Y. Garces, "Survival of dental implants in native and grafted bone in irradiated head and neck cancer patients: a retrospective analysis," *Indian Journal of Dental Research*, vol. 22, no. 5, pp. 644–648, 2011.

[22] M. P. Claudy, S. A. Miguens Jr., R. K. Celeste, R. Camara Parente, P. A. Hernandez, and A. N. da Silva Jr., "Time interval after radiotherapy and dental implant failure: systematic review of observational studies and meta-analysis," *Clinical Implant Dentistry and Related Research*, 2013.

[23] K. C. Yerit, M. Posch, M. Seemann et al., "Implant survival in mandibles of irradiated oral cancer patients," *Clinical Oral Implants Research*, vol. 17, no. 3, pp. 337–344, 2006.

[24] R. B. Donoff, "Treatment of the irradiated patient with dental implants: the case against hyperbaric oxygen treatment," *Journal of Oral and Maxillofacial Surgery*, vol. 64, no. 5, pp. 819–822, 2006.

[25] K. Guru, U. K. Manoor, and S. S. Supe, "A comprehensive review of head and neck cancer rehabilitation: physical therapy perspectives," *The Indian Journal of Palliative Care*, vol. 18, no. 2, pp. 87–97, 2012.

# Maxillary First Molars with Six Canals Diagnosed with the Aid of Cone Beam Computed Tomography: A Report of Two Cases

**Mamta Kaushik and Neha Mehra**

*Department of Conservative Dentistry and Endodontics, Army College of Dental Sciences, Jai Jawahar Nagar, Secunderabad, Andhra Pradesh 500094, India*

Correspondence should be addressed to Mamta Kaushik; mamkaushik@gmail.com

Academic Editors: J. C. de la Macorra and M. H. K. Motamedi

The case reports present the endodontic management of two maxillary first molars with six canals. The diagnosis of morphology of multiple canal systems was identified under magnification of the dental operating microscope and was confirmed with the help of cone beam computed tomography. This paper discusses the variations in the canal morphology and the use of the latest adjuncts in successfully diagnosing and treating unusual canal anatomy.

## 1. Introduction

A thorough knowledge of the root canal anatomy, its variations, the presence of additional roots, and unusual root canal morphology is essential, as it determines the successful outcome of endodontic treatment [1]. To ensure the long-term success of root canal treatment, it is essential to access, clean, and fill all of the canal spaces. However, the anatomic complexities and variations are constant challenges for successful endodontic therapy [2].

The morphology of the maxillary first molar has been extensively studied and reported in the literature. Traditionally the maxillary first molar exhibits three roots and three canals. The occurrence of a fourth canal ranges from 50.4% to 95% [3–7] and a fifth canal 2.25% [8], and a few authors have also reported cases with 6 canals [9, 10].

The occurrence of 2 canals in distobuccal root has been less frequent and has been reported in 3.6% of maxillary molars [4, 10, 11]. Palatine root canal variations were well established by Christie et al. [8, 12], who reported the endodontic treatment of maxillary molars with 2 palatine roots and classified these teeth as types I, II, and III, according to root degree of divergence. Others reported cases of maxillary first molar with two canals in each of the three roots [9, 10, 13–15].

The present cases report the successful management of maxillary first molars with three roots and six canals. The clinical findings were confirmed with the help of operating microscope and cone beam computed tomography (CBCT).

## 2. Case Report 1

A 43-year-old female patient presented with the chief complaint of pain in the left upper back tooth. The pain was continuous and aggravated on heat stimulation. The patient also complained of pain at night. The patient's medical history was noncontributory.

Clinical examination revealed the left maxillary first molar with a deep carious lesion which was tender on percussion. Electric pulp testing gave a premature response, indicative of inflammatory pulpal changes. The radiographic examination revealed a radiolucent lesion on the mesial aspect of the crown extending to the pulp (Figure 1(a)). After the clinical and radiographic examination, the left maxillary first molar was diagnosed with irreversible pulpitis and endodontic treatment was suggested to the patient.

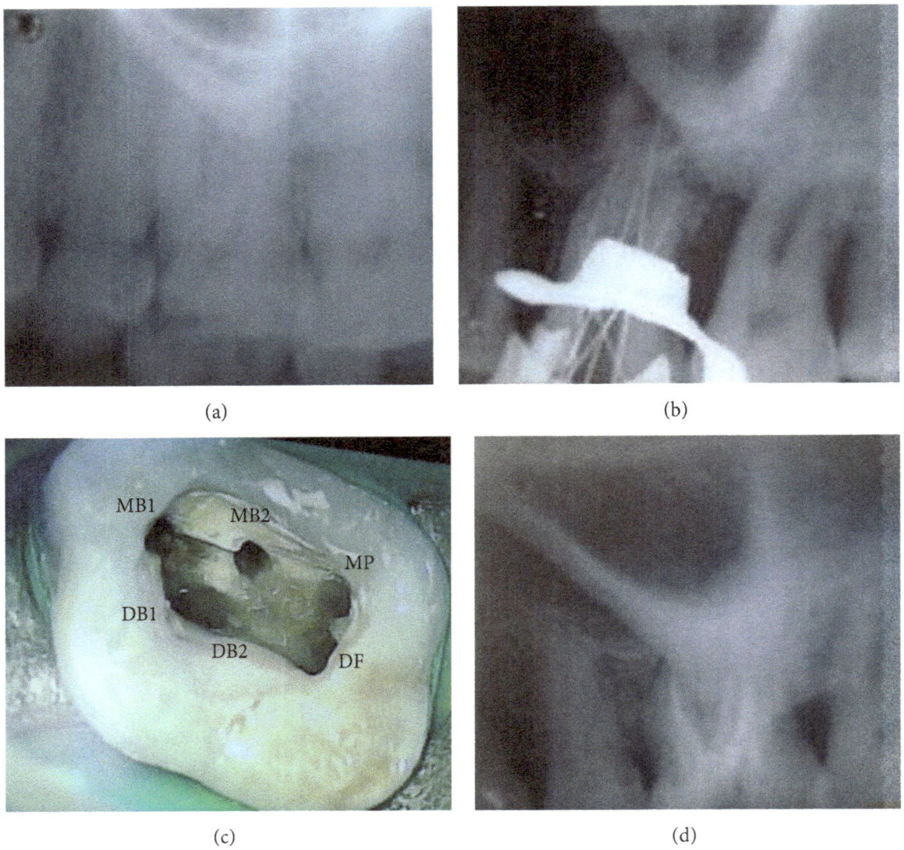


Figure 1: (a) Preoperative radiograph. (b) Working length radiograph showing multiple canals. (c) Access opening of the tooth showing multiple orifices. (d) Postobturation radiograph.

The tooth was anaesthetised with 1.8 mL of 2% lidocaine containing 1 : 80,000 epinephrine (Lignox 2%, Indoco Remedies Ltd., Mumbai, India) followed by rubber dam isolation. A conventional endodontic access cavity was prepared. Clinical evaluation of the internal anatomy revealed 3 principal root canal systems: mesiobuccal (MB), distobuccal (DB), and palatal. After probing with a DG 16 endodontic explorer, small hemorrhagic points were noted 2 mm palatal to the MB and DB canals. As the dentin that was occluding the orifice of the palatal canal was removed, a second palatal canal was also identified. This was further evaluated and verified by a Surgical Operating Microscope (Seiler, St. Louis, MO). There seemed to be 2 distinct orifices in all the roots (Figure 1(c)). A sterile cotton pellet and an interim restoration of Cavit (3 M Espe, Seefeld, Germany) were placed in the pulp chamber to seal the access cavity.

To confirm this unusual morphology and to ascertain the pattern of the canals in a 3-dimensional manner, a cone beam computed tomography (CBCT) imaging of the tooth was advised. An informed consent was obtained from the patient, and a multislice CBCT scan of the maxillary left side was performed (Kodak 9000 3D) with a tube voltage of 80 KV and a tube current of 8 mA. The involved tooth was focused and a 3D morphology was obtained.

The CBCT images confirmed the presence of six canals. The scans showed two mesiobuccal, two distobuccal, and two palatal canals (Figure 2). The mesiobuccal followed Vertucci's type IV classification. The distobuccal canals merged in the coronal third (2.4 mm from the orifice) and the palatal in the middle third (5.4 mm from the orifice) of the root to follow as a single canal (Vertucci's type II).

At the next visit, the working lengths of each canal were estimated by an electronic apex locator (Propex II, Dentsply) and confirmed with a radiograph (Figure 1(b)). The cleaning and shaping were performed using ProTaper nickel-titanium rotary instruments (Dentsply Maillefer, Switzerland). Irrigation between each instrument was done using 2.5% sodium hypochlorite solution and 17% EDTA. The canals were dried and obturation was performed using cold lateral compaction of gutta-percha (Dentsply Maillefer) and a resin-based sealer (AH Plus, Maillefer, Dentsply, Konstanz, Germany) (Figure 1(d)). The tooth was then restored with a posterior composite resin core (P60; 3 M Dental Products, St. Paul, MN). The patient was advised a full-coverage porcelain crown and was asymptomatic during the follow-up period.

## 3. Case Report 2

A 28-year-old female patient presented with the chief complaint of pain in the left upper back tooth. The pain was continuous and aggravated on heat stimulation. The patient's

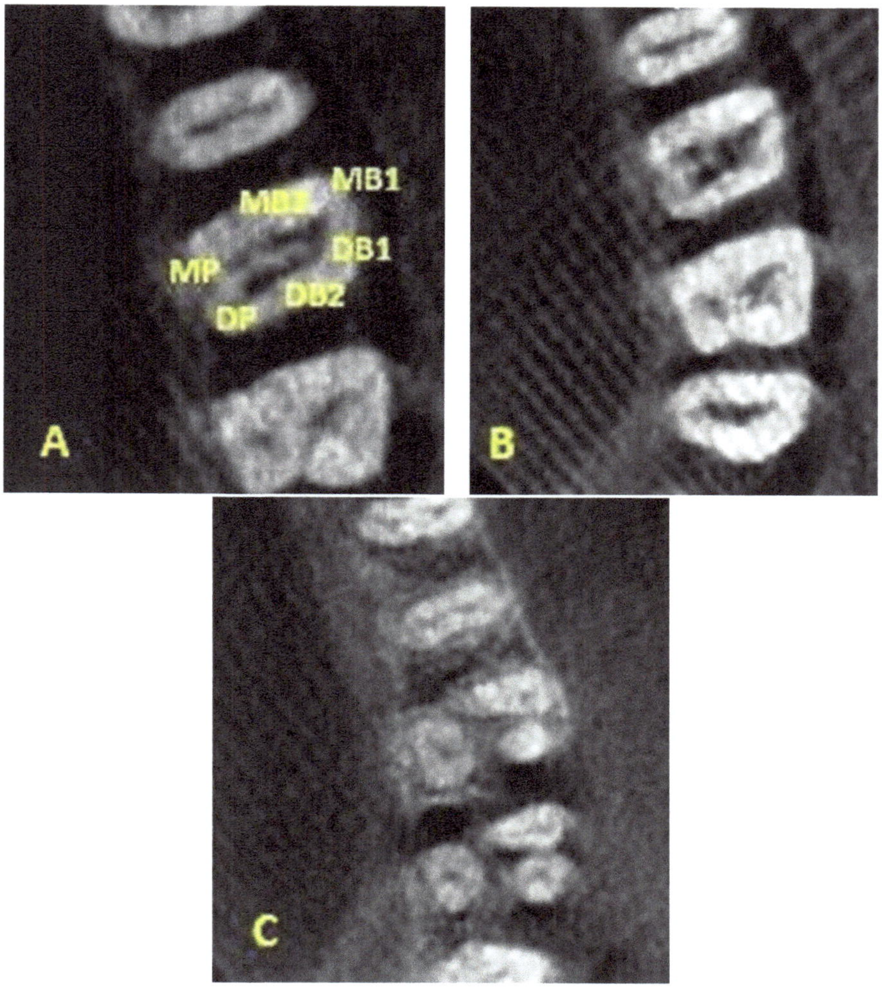


FIGURE 2: CBCT images showing 2 canals in each root.

medical history was noncontributory. Based on clinical and radiographic examination a diagnosis of irreversible pulpitis was made and endodontic treatment was suggested to the patient.

The tooth was anaesthetised with 2% lidocaine containing 1 : 80,000 epinephrine (Lignox 2%, Indoco Remedies Ltd., Mumbai, India). A conventional endodontic access cavity was prepared under rubber dam isolation. Clinical evaluation of the internal anatomy revealed 3 principal root canal systems: mesiobuccal (MB), distobuccal (DB), and palatal. After probing with a DG 16 endodontic explorer, small hemorrhagic points were noted palatal to the mesiobuccal canal. On evaluation MB2 and MB3 were identified. Further exploration led to the identification of a second palatal canal. The distobuccal orifice also seemed to be indicating multiple canal system (Figure 3(a)). This was evaluated and verified by a Surgical Operating Microscope (Seiler, St. Louis, MO). The access cavity was sealed with Cavit (3 M Espe, Seefeld, Germany).

For further evaluation of this unusual morphology, a CBCT imaging of the tooth was advised. An informed consent was obtained from the patient, and a multislice CBCT scan of the maxillary left side was performed (Kodak 9000 3D) with a tube voltage of 80 KV and a tube current of 8 mA.

The CBCT images confirmed the presence of six canals. The scans showed three mesiobuccal, two palatal, and an oblong distobuccal canal systems (Figure 4). The MB1 was an independent canal but the MB2 and MB3 merged (Vertucci's type II) to progress as one. The mesiopalatal and distopalatal canals (Vertucci's type II) merged in the middle third of the root to follow as a single canal.

At the next visit, the working lengths of each canal were estimated by an electronic apex locator (Propex II, Dentsply) and confirmed with a radiograph (Figure 3(b)). The cleaning and shaping were performed using ProTaper nickel-titanium rotary instruments (Dentsply Maillefer, Switzerland) with copious irrigation of 2.5% sodium hypochlorite solution and 17% EDTA. The canals were dried and obturation was performed using cold lateral compaction of gutta-percha (Dentsply Maillefer) and a resin-based sealer (AH Plus, Maillefer, Dentsply, Konstanz, Germany) (Figure 3(c)). The tooth was then restored with a posterior composite resin

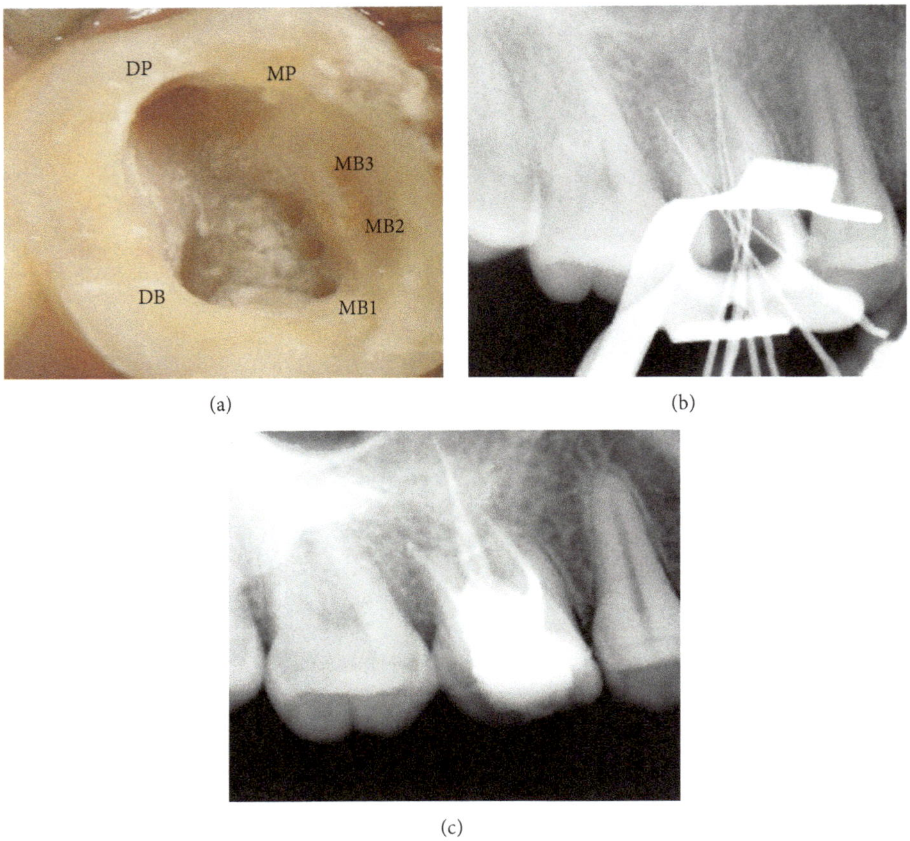


FIGURE 3: (a) Access opening showing three MB, two palatal, and one oblong distobuccal canal orifices. (b) Working length radiograph. (c) Postobturation radiograph.

core (P60; 3 M Dental Products, St. Paul, MN). The patient was advised a full-coverage porcelain crown and was asymptomatic during the follow-up period.

## 4. Discussion

Anatomical aberrations are commonly observed in maxillary first molar ranging from one to seven canals [4]. It is generally accepted that maxillary first molar has three roots and three canals with a fourth canal (MB2) seen in 50.4–91% of cases [3–6]. The simultaneous occurrence of double canal system in all roots of a maxillary molar is an unusual finding [8, 9, 14, 15]. Case 1 highlights the unusual anatomy of maxillary first molar with double canals in all three roots.

Prevalence of additional root canals has been reported and discussed by several authors [15, 16]. Case 2 displayed a highly unusual morphology of 3 mesiobuccal, 2 palatal, and an oblong distobuccal canal systems.

Proper access opening and modifying the shape of the access to approach all orifices is a key to success in identifying and negotiating unusual anatomy of root canals [14]. In the present case reports, the conventional triangular access was modified to trapezoidal to improve access to the additional canals.

Diagnostic measures such as multiple preoperative radiographs, examination of the pulp floor with a sharp explorer, troughing of grooves with ultrasonic tips, staining the chamber floor with 1% methylene blue dye, performing the hypochlorite champagne bubble test, and visualising canal bleeding points are important aids in locating root orifices [17]. In the presented cases, examination of the pulpal floor to follow the dentinal map and exploration of haemorrhagic points with the DG16 was the first indication to hint at presence of extra orifices and canals.

An important aid for locating root canals is the Surgical Operating Microscope (SOM). It brings minute details into clear view by enhancing lighting and visibility. Studies have demonstrated that magnification and illumination by the SOM increased the identification of MB2 canals tremendously [3, 18–20]. The use of magnification aids in verifying the presence of morphologic variations.

Radiographic examination is an essential component for management of endodontic problems. But they produce only a 2D image of a 3D object resulting in superimposition of images [21]. CBCT is a valuable method for initial identification and effective evaluation of internal morphology of teeth [3, 22–25]. Although conventional CT scans produce a high level of detail, it is essential that the radiation dosage is kept as low as reasonably possible [26].

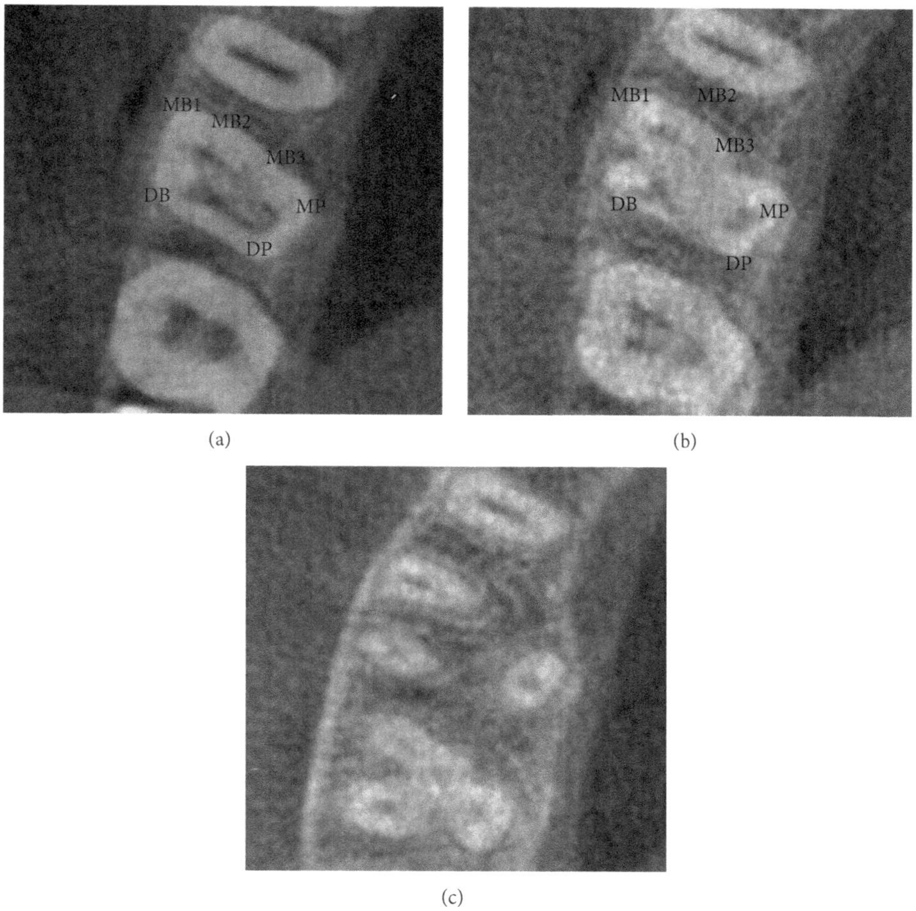


FIGURE 4: CBCT images showing distinct canal configuration.

In the present cases, CBCT scanning was used for a better understanding of the complex root anatomy. For case 1, the images confirmed the presence of double canal system in three roots. The images showed that the palatal and distobuccal canals present with a Vertucci type II pattern and the mesiobuccal canals follow a Vertucci type IV configuration. Similarly, for case 2, the images confirmed the occurrence of multiple canal systems. The mesiobuccal root showed a Sert and Bayirli [27] type XV canal configuration. MB1 was an independent canal and MB2 and MB3 joined at the middle third to exit from one apical foramen. The palatal canals showed Vertucci's type II pattern.

The simultaneous occurrence of double canal systems in all roots of maxillary first molar is an unusual finding, as is the occurrence of 3 mesiobuccal and 2 palatal canals in the same tooth. Thus, it is important to be conscious to variations from the expected and to use all the armamentaria available to locate and treat the entire root canal system.

## 5. Conclusion

Although the incidence of root variations is rare, their importance should not be underestimated. Careful examination of radiographs and the internal anatomy of teeth are essential. The present cases confirm the necessity for meticulous examination of the pulpal floor at high magnification under sufficient illumination of the operating microscope and emphasize the importance of newer imaging techniques like CBCT in preoperative assessment.

## Conflict of Interests

The authors deny any conflict of interests. they have no secondary interest as regards to any of the commercial identities used. The products used are the ones which are available in the department and the institute. They have no direct or indirect financial relation with the commercial identities mentioned in the paper.

## References

[1] V. Malagnino, L. Gallottini, and P. Passariello, "Some unusual clinical cases on root anatomy of permanent maxillary molars," *Journal of Endodontics*, vol. 23, no. 2, pp. 127–128, 1997.

[2] O. A. Peters, "Current challenges and concepts in the preparation of root canal systems: a review," *Journal of Endodontics*, vol. 30, no. 8, pp. 559–567, 2004.

[3] F. Baratto Filho, S. Zaitter, G. A. Haragushiku, E. A. de Campos, A. Abuabara, and G. M. Correr, "Analysis of the internal anatomy of maxillary first molars by using different methods," *Journal of Endodontics*, vol. 35, no. 3, pp. 337–342, 2009.

[4] B. M. Cleghorn, W. H. Christie, and C. C. S. Dong, "Root and root canal morphology of the human permanent maxillary first molar: a literature review," *Journal of Endodontics*, vol. 32, no. 9, pp. 813–821, 2006.

[5] R. P. Thomas, A. J. Moule, and R. Bryant, "Root canal morphology of maxillary permanent first molar teeth at various ages," *International Endodontic Journal*, vol. 26, no. 5, pp. 257–267, 1993.

[6] J. C. Kulid and D. D. Peters, "Incidence and configuration of canal systems in the mesiobuccal root of Maxillary first and second molars," *Journal of Endodontics*, vol. 16, no. 7, pp. 311–317, 1990.

[7] G. Hartwell, C. M. Appelstein, W. W. Lyons, and M. E. Guzek, "The incidence of four canals in maxillary first molars—a clinical determination," *Journal of the American Dental Association*, vol. 138, no. 10, pp. 1344–1346, 2007.

[8] H. M. Fogel, M. D. Peikoff, and W. H. Christie, "Canal configuration in the mesiobuccal root of the maxillary first molar: a clinical study," *Journal of Endodontics*, vol. 20, no. 3, pp. 135–137, 1994.

[9] A. Martínez-Berná and P. Ruiz-Badanelli, "Maxillary first molars with six canals," *Journal of Endodontics*, vol. 9, no. 9, pp. 375–381, 1983.

[10] J. L. Bond, G. Hartwell, and F. R. Portell, "Maxillary first molar with six canals," *Journal of Endodontics*, vol. 14, no. 5, pp. 258–260, 1988.

[11] L. H. Stone and W. F. Stroner, "Maxillary molars demonstrating more than one palatal root canal," *Oral Surgery Oral Medicine and Oral Pathology*, vol. 51, no. 6, pp. 649–652, 1981.

[12] W. H. Christie, M. D. Peikoff, and H. M. Fogel, "Maxillary molars with two palatal roots: a retrospective clinical study," *Journal of Endodontics*, vol. 17, no. 2, pp. 80–84, 1991.

[13] E. J. Neaverth, L. M. Kotler, and R. F. Kaltenbach, "Clinical investigation (In Vivo) of endodontically treated maxillary first molars," *Journal of Endodontics*, vol. 13, no. 10, pp. 506–512, 1987.

[14] Y.-Y. Lee, P.-Y. Yeh, S.-F. Pai, and S.-F. Yang, "Maxillary first molar with six canals," *Journal of Dental Sciences*, vol. 4, no. 4, pp. 198–201, 2009.

[15] K. Karthikeyan and S. Mahalaxmi, "New nomenclature for extra canals based on four reported cases of maxillary first molars with six canals," *Journal of Endodontics*, vol. 36, no. 6, pp. 1073–1078, 2010.

[16] J. Kottoor, N. Velmurugan, R. Sudha, and S. Hemamalathi, "Maxillary first molar with seven root canals diagnosed with cone-beam computed tomography scanning: a case report," *Journal of Endodontics*, vol. 36, no. 5, pp. 915–921, 2010.

[17] F. J. Vertucci, "Root canal morphology and its relationship to endodontic procedures," *Endodontic Topics*, vol. 10, pp. 3–29, 2005.

[18] L. A. Baldassari-Cruz, J. P. Lilly, and E. M. Rivera, "The influence of dental operating microscope in locating the mesiolingual canal orifice," *Oral Surgery, Oral Medicine, Oral Pathology, Oral Radiology, and Endodontics*, vol. 93, no. 2, pp. 190–194, 2002.

[19] M. C. Coelho De Carvalho and M. L. Zuolo, "Orifice locating with a microscope," *Journal of Endodontics*, vol. 26, no. 9, pp. 532–534, 2000.

[20] T. Schwarze, C. Baethge, T. Stecher, and W. Geurtsen, "Identification of second canals in the mesiobuccal root of maxillary first and second molars using magnifying loupes or an operating microscope," *Australian Endodontic Journal*, vol. 28, no. 2, pp. 57–60, 2002.

[21] S. Patel, A. Dawood, E. Whaites, and T. Pitt Ford, "New dimensions in endodontic imaging: part 1. Conventional and alternative radiographic systems," *International Endodontic Journal*, vol. 42, no. 6, pp. 447–462, 2009.

[22] M. K. Nair and U. P. Nair, "Digital and advanced imaging in endodontics: a review," *Journal of Endodontics*, vol. 33, no. 1, pp. 1–6, 2007.

[23] S. Patel, "New dimensions in endodontic imaging: part 2. Cone beam computed tomography," *International Endodontic Journal*, vol. 42, no. 6, pp. 463–475, 2009.

[24] T. P. Cotton, T. M. Geisler, D. T. Holden, S. A. Schwartz, and W. G. Schindler, "Endodontic applications of cone-beam volumetric tomography," *Journal of Endodontics*, vol. 33, no. 9, pp. 1121–1132, 2007.

[25] D. A. Tyndall and S. Rathore, "Cone-beam CT diagnostic applications: caries, periodontal bone assessment, and endodontic applications," *Dental Clinics of North America*, vol. 52, no. 4, pp. 825–841, 2008.

[26] C. G. Diederichs, W. G. H. Engelke, B. Richter, K.-P. Hermann, and J. W. Oestmann, "Must radiation dose for CT of the maxilla and mandible be higher than that for conventional panoramic radiography?" *American Journal of Neuroradiology*, vol. 17, no. 9, pp. 1758–1760, 1996.

[27] S. Sert and G. S. Bayirli, "Evaluation of the root canal configurations of the mandibular and maxillary permanent teeth by gender in the Turkish population," *Journal of Endodontics*, vol. 30, no. 6, pp. 391–398, 2004.

# Prosthetic Rehabilitation in Children: An Alternative Clinical Technique

**Nádia Carolina Teixeira Marques,[1] Carla Vecchione Gurgel,[1] Ana Paula Fernandes,[1] Marta Cunha Lima,[2] Maria Aparecida Andrade Moreira Machado,[1] Simone Soares,[3,4] and Thais Marchini Oliveira[1,4]**

[1] *Department of Pediatric Dentistry, Orthodontics and Public Health, Bauru School of Dentistry, University of São Paulo, Al. Octávio Pinheiro Brisolla 9-75, 17012-901, Bauru-SP 73, Brazil*
[2] *Matrix Dynamics Group, Faculty of Dentistry, University of Toronto, Toronto, ON, Canada*
[3] *Department of Prosthetic Dentistry, Bauru School of Dentistry, University of São Paulo, São Paulo, Bauru, Brazil*
[4] *Hospital for the Rehabilitation of Craniofacial Anomalies, University of São Paulo, São Paulo, SP, Brazil*

Correspondence should be addressed to Thais Marchini Oliveira; marchini@usp.br

Academic Editors: M. B. D. Gaviao and M. W. Roberts

Complete and partial removable dentures have been used successfully in numerous patients with oligodontia and/or anodontia. However, there is little information in the literature regarding the principles and guidelines to prosthetic rehabilitation for growing children. This case report describes the management of a young child with oligodontia as well as the treatment planning and the prosthetic rehabilitation technique.

## 1. Introduction

Prosthetic treatment can play an important role when treating children whose dentition fails to develop normally. The congenital absence of teeth is one of the most frequent reasons for the need of complete and partial dentures for young children [1]. Some genetic conditions, such as hypohidrotic ectodermal dysplasia and Papillon-Lefevre syndrome, may cause oligodontia or anodontia. Premature loss of primary teeth due to grossly caries may be another reason for the need of complete dentures for preschool children [2].

Treatment of patients with oligodontia can challenge the clinician not only because patients present a great number of congenitally missing teeth, or even anodontia, but also because of the age they are usually referred for rehabilitation [3]. Several treatment strategies have been reported for the management of patients suffering from anodontia, oligodontia, and malformed teeth. Conventional removable complete or partial dentures are usually the most frequent prosthetic treatment plan for these young patients [3–6].

Since alveolar bone development is dependent on the presence of teeth, children with oligodontia or anodontia have atrophy of the alveolar bone and consequently little or no bone ridge to support dentures [5, 7]. Indeed being edentulous has many consequences, speech impairment, deforming lingual habits, and a poor nutrition, due to the fact that mastication is difficult or impossible [8, 9]. Furthermore, primary teeth are necessary for the acquisition and maturation of diverse functions, which are important for normal growth [10]. Also, in these patients the poor appearance of the teeth can affect self-esteem, which challenges the clinician [5, 8].

Complete and partial removable dentures have been used successfully in numerous patients with oligodontia and/or anodontia. However, there is little information in the literature regarding the principles and guidelines to prosthetic rehabilitation for growing children. The rehabilitation of a child's dentition with a removable prosthesis is more complex and time consuming than in adults. All these factors should be considered during fabrication in order to provide a prosthesis that is functional, esthetic, and age appropriate [11].

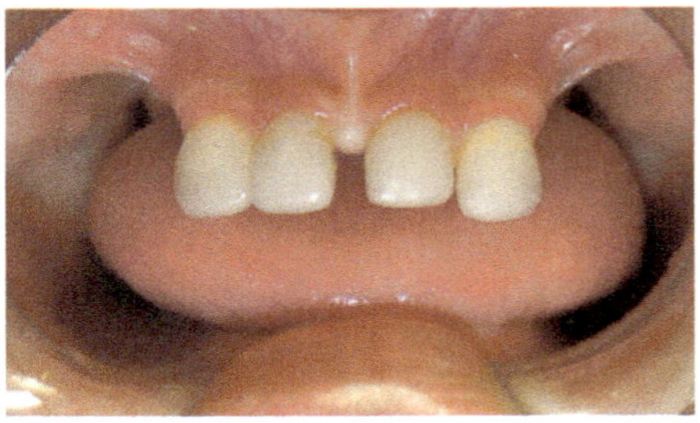

Figure 1: Initial intraoral view showing the maxillary incisors.

This case report describes the treatment planning of a young child with oligodontia as well as the prosthetic rehabilitation technique.

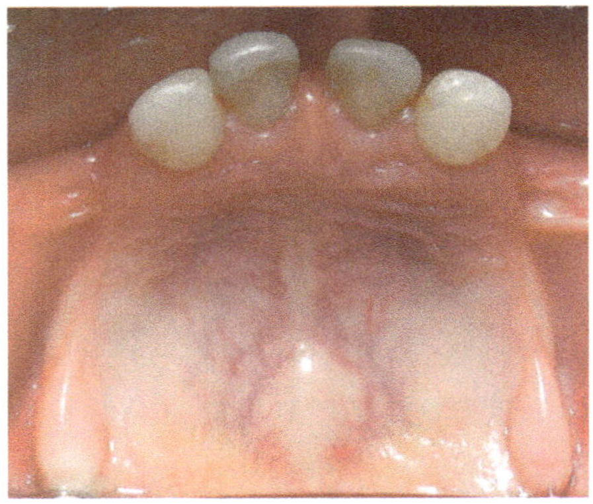

Figure 2: Occlusal view of the maxilla.

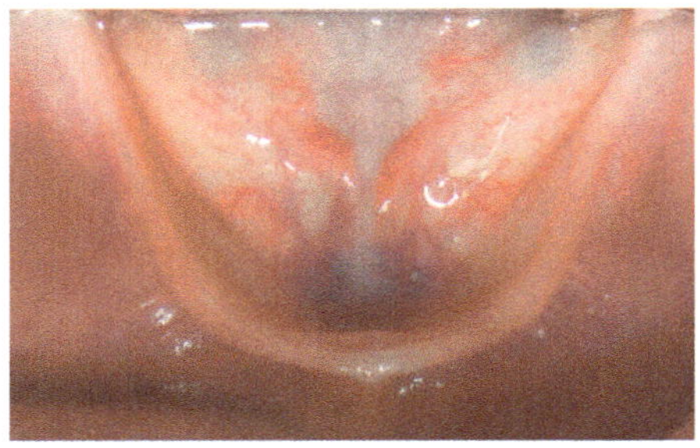

Figure 3: Occlusal view of the mandible.

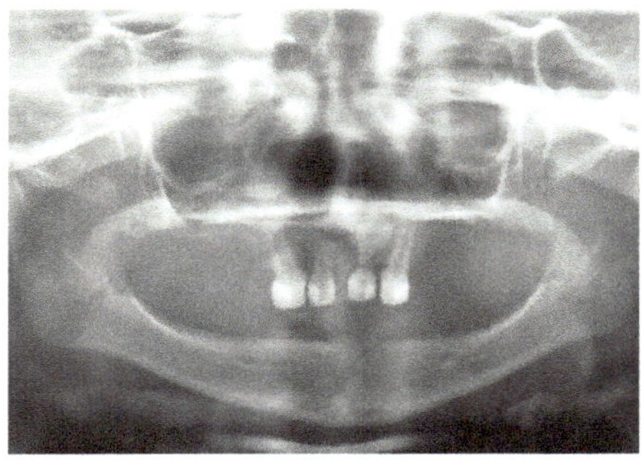

Figure 4: Panoramic radiograph showing oligodontia and lack of alveolar bone development.

## 2. Case Report

A 5-year-old boy presented to the Department of Pediatric Dentistry of our university due to the lack of teeth and problems with speech and mastication. The mother related that an evaluation by a pediatrician resulted in the diagnosis of hypohidrotic ectodermal dysplasia (HED).

The extraoral examination revealed the typical facial physiognomy of HED with prominent forehead and ears, protuberant and everted lips, and a sunken nasal bridge ("saddle nose"). The patient also presented with sparse scalp hair, missing eyelashes and eyebrows, and severe hypohidrosis. The skin appeared dry with hyperpigmentation around the eyes and the mouth. A diminished lower facial height contributed to a senile facial expression.

Clinical and radiographical examination revealed a partially edentulous maxilla and a completely edentulous mandible. In the maxilla only the primary maxillary central and lateral incisors were present. The primary maxillary central and lateral incisors had apparently been previously restored using resin strip crowns, because these teeth are often conical in shape in ectodermal dysplasia (Figures 1, 2, and 3). Both alveolar ridges were poorly developed with normal appearance of alveolar mucosa. The palate was shallow and the oral mucosa was healthy with a slight dry appearance. The tongue was relatively large, with no signs of macroglossia. Radiographic examination revealed the complete absence of permanent tooth germs, except the permanent maxillary left central incisor (Figure 4).

In order to improve the appearance, mastication, and speech, the treatment plan included a removable partial upper denture and a complete lower denture. The parents were informed about the procedures involved in the fabrication of the dental prostheses and the need for continuing reevaluation and remaking of the oral prostheses as the alveolar ridges and oral environment changed due to growth.

Behavioral management techniques, such as tell-show-do, were used throughout the procedures for construction of the dentures. The smallest stock tray was selected, due to limited mouth opening and developing swallowing mechanisms. First the mandibular impression was made and then the maxillary impression in order to decrease anxiety in the patient. Impressions were made in two stages but in the same session. We used trays and modeling with impression compound silicone putty (Express XT, 3M ESPE, são Paulo, SP, Brazil). The second modeling was made with silicone soft (Figure 5). The first impression was necessary to ensure that vestibular sulcus was properly printed with correct height and width.

During hardening of the material, the lips and cheeks were manipulated to shape the buccal and labial aspects of the impression. The child was asked to protrude the tongue to raise the floor of the mouth. The final casts were made in dental stone.

Shellac base plates were adapted on upper and lower casts, and wax occlusal rims were then fabricated. Maxillo-mandibular records were made by placing the occlusal rims in

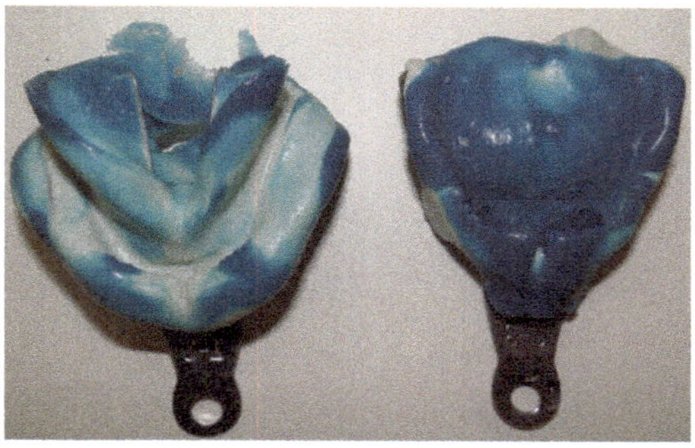

FIGURE 5: Silicone maxillary and mandibular impressions.

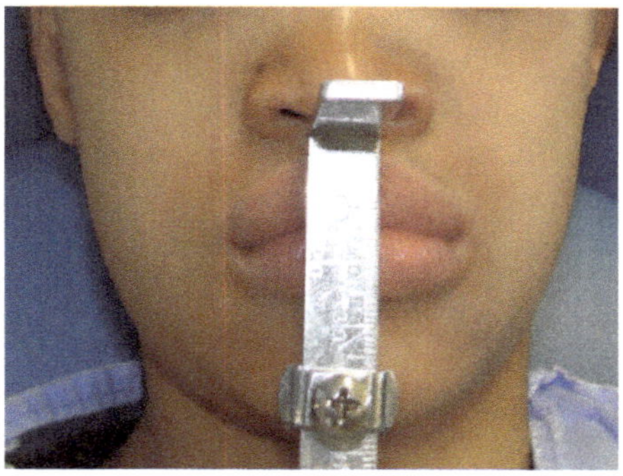

FIGURE 6: Initial frontal view of the patient. Note the diminished OVD.

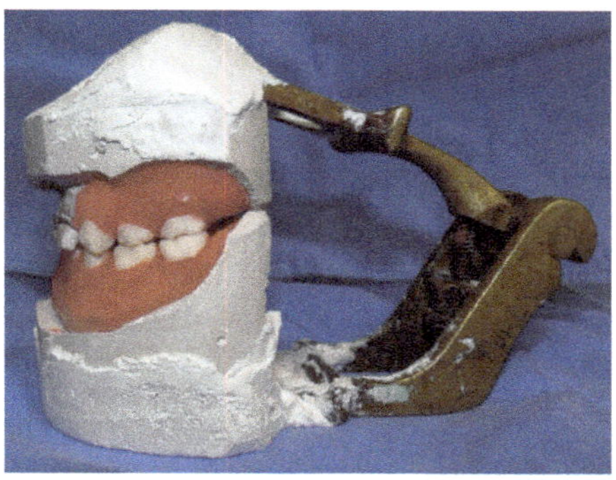

FIGURE 7: Working casts mounted in a simple articulator.

the oral cavity, with a freeway space of 2 mm, and using Willi's measurements (Figure 6). Using the interocclusal record, the working casts were mounted in a simple articulator to evaluate dentition and occlusal vertical dimension (OVD) (Figure 7).

The artificial teeth needed for the denture were fabricated at the lab with a suitable shade of heat cure acrylic resin (Figure 8). The teeth shaped as primary teeth were arranged on the wax occlusal rim with spacing to simulate the natural spacing expected for the patients' age. The artificial teeth were arranged in wax for trial evaluation. Tooth positions, occlusal relationships, and the necessary corrections were made before processing the dentures after the prosthesis wax try-in (Figure 9).

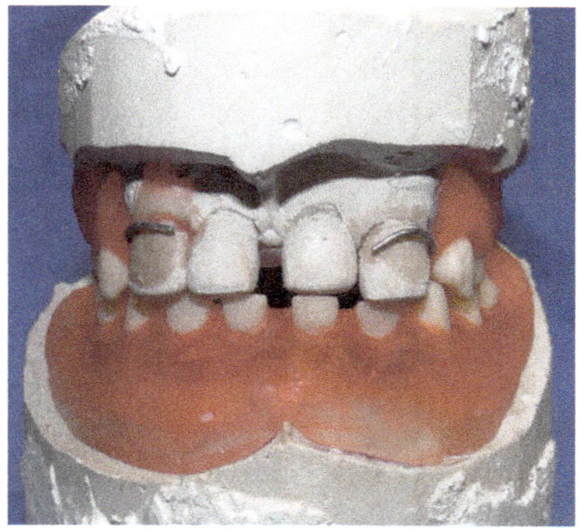

FIGURE 8: Frontal view of the casts mounted in a simple articulator with artificial teeth.

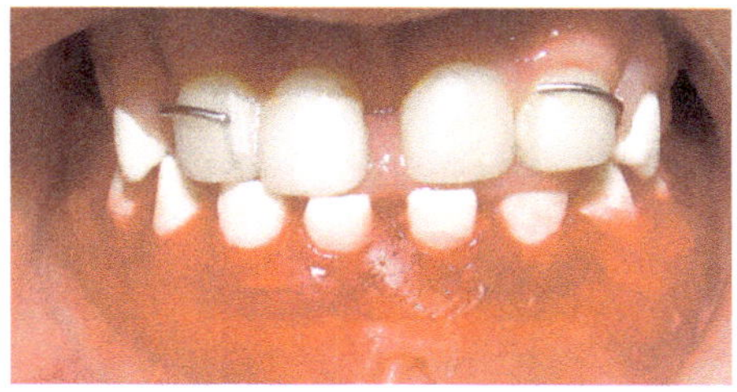

FIGURE 9: Wax try-in of the maxillary and mandibular dentures.

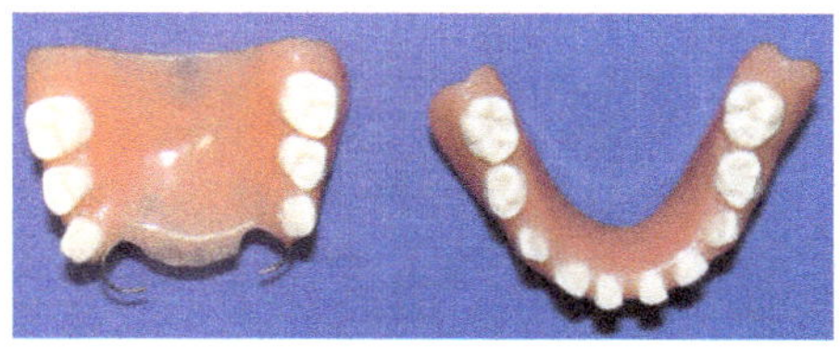

FIGURE 10: Artificial teeth in acrylic resin.

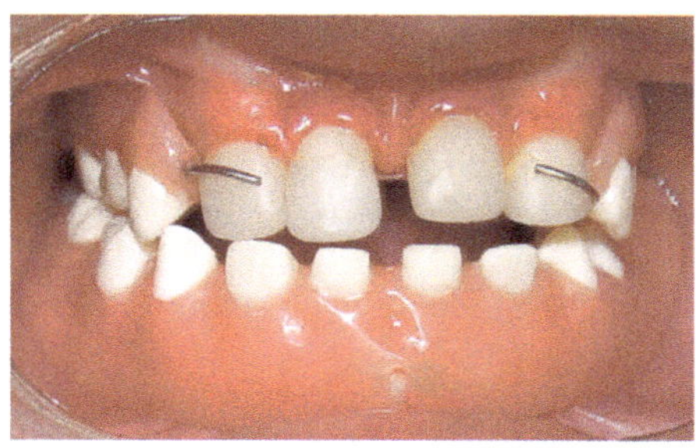

FIGURE 11: Maxillary and mandibular complete dentures in occlusion.

Later the dentures were processed with heat cure acrylic resin. The flashing errors were corrected after processing. On insertion of the denture, occlusal interferences were eliminated, and finishing and polishing of the final denture were done (Figures 10 and 11).

After the final insertion, the patient and parents were instructed in routine oral hygiene for dentures. At recall appointments, no pressure spots were noticed, and the static and dynamic occlusion showed no interferences. Retention was excellent, and the parents reported a significant improvement of his speech and mastication. The increased self-esteem improved the socialization skills of the boy. The patient has been followed up for 12 months in our institution, and when the denture does not fit properly, a new denture will replace this one, year-by-year, if necessary, until his development stops, and the treatment plan can be reassessed.

## 3. Discussion

Several treatment strategies have been reported for the management of patients suffering from anodontia and oligodontia. Conventional removable complete or partial dentures are usually the treatment of choice for these patients [2, 6]. Providing early prosthetic care for very young completely edentulous patients seems advisable. Early intervention with complete dentures in these patients may have a profound impact by providing masticatory efficiency, swallowing ability, good phonetics, as well as improvement in esthetics [5, 6, 8–10, 12]. Also, prosthetical rehabilitation is recommended to improve both the sagittal and vertical skeletal relationship during craniofacial growth and development [1]. Hence, the problems involved in attempting to restore function and appearance are greater than usual [5], because the children's face and jaws are constantly growing and undergoing changes in dentition [11].

While it is recognized that early intervention is necessary to support oral normal development, there is no consensus in the literature on the ideal age for the beginning of treatment [10, 13]. However, the necessity for a proper prosthetic treatment before school age has been reported by the majority of the authors because of functional, phonational, psychological, and esthetic needs [7, 10, 13]. Khazaie et al. [14] recommend that prosthetic treatment may be carried out as early as preschool years where young children usually adapt to their use. The majority of the authors agree that if the child is cooperative, prosthetic intervention in those as young as age 2 or 3 years can be successful [1, 11, 15]. Derbanne et al. [10], after treating more than 40 patients with anodontia and oligodontia with removable prosthesis, considered that the sooner the prosthetic rehabilitation begins, the better the results will be in terms of functions, social integration, and self-esteem of the patient. Early intervention affords the child the opportunity to develop normal forms of speech, chewing, and swallowing; normal facial support; and improved temporomandibular joint function [1, 13, 15]. The prosthodontic treatment enhances the tonus of the masticatory muscles and provides normal mastication, swallowing, and regular phonation [13]. Imirzalioglu et al. [15] described a clinical case of a child that, after 1 year of the complete dentures installed, had maxillary horizontal development as well as the condylar remodeling and posterior rotation of the mandible related to the improved vertical dimension.

The technique for denture construction is similar to that for adult patients, comprising stages of preliminary and final impressions, registration of occlusion, wax try-in, and insertion of the finished denture. However, in children some modifications of the accepted techniques are usually indicated and require special attention [2]. It is necessary to simplify the technique of fabricating complete dentures in children to promote better cooperation and ensure them a positive dental experience [11]. The fabrication of prosthesis for a child requires an extensive diagnostic process together with a detailed medical and dental history. All these factors should be considered during fabrication in order to provide a prosthesis that is not only functional but also esthetic and age appropriate [11]. Retention and stability of the prosthesis are also difficult to obtain during children's growth, particularly because of the insufficient bone support, typically amorphous tooth structure, and lack of sufficient undercut zones [11, 15]. When planning dentures in these patients, care should be taken to obtain a wide distribution of occlusal load fully extending the denture base [2].

Also, special attention must be paid to the impression technique; for complete dentures, support should not be limited to the denture base area but should also include the entire vestibular sulcus reflection for a retentive base construction with sealed border [1]. Irreversible hydrocolloid material with higher viscosity is the material suggested by the majority of the authors for primary impressions, probably because it sets faster, consequently helps prevent aspiration of the impression material, and ameliorates the patient's comfort [1, 14]. Accurate impressions with proper anatomic extensions are needed to fabricate a good custom tray, which will probably help make a superior final impression [11]. For final impressions, in the presented case report, the authors preferred silicone for border molding and as an impression material because these materials are cleaner and have the required accuracy, better working time, and a fast setting time. Some clinicians have used border molding techniques with a warm green stick compound prior to making the final impression. Due to insufficient evidence, it can be argued that this technique has limited advantages for children because of the requisite time, patient discomfort related to the procedure, and potential risk of thermal injury. Furthermore, there will be a future need for a relining or remaking of the prosthesis to accommodate jaw growth [11].

The implementation of special management and motivational techniques becomes essential to maintain a good level of cooperation from these patients [3]. Regular periodic recalls of young patients with complete dentures are usually necessary, because prosthesis adjustments or replacement will be needed as a result of continuing growth and development, until more definitive implant-assisted prostheses can be delivered [2, 5, 6, 14]. Imirzalioglu et al. [15] emphasize that the continuous jaw growth and the dentition changes of children must be closely monitored. Complete dentures require regular adjustments and should be relined, rebased, or replaced when a decreased vertical dimension of occlusion and an abnormal mandibular posture are detected due to growth [1]. Therefore, frequent (3–6-month recall intervals) follow-up examinations and denture adjustments are needed.

Oral prosthesis on patients at an early age represents a long-term commitment on the part of all who are involved in the process: clinician, patient, and parents [2]. Pediatric dentistry specialists form a part of the interdisciplinary team that treats these young people, providing successful clinical outcomes and proper emotional development [14].

## 4. Conclusion

Prosthetic rehabilitation in children must be performed at the earliest age possible in order to maintain the oral functions, provide normal development, and increase self-esteem improving socialization skills.

## Conflict of Interests

The authors declare that they have no conflict of interest.

## References

[1] I. Tarjan, K. Gabris, and N. Rozsa, "Early prosthetic treatment of patients with ectodermal dysplasia: a clinical report," *Journal of Prosthetic Dentistry*, vol. 93, no. 5, pp. 419–424, 2005.

[2] S. T. Paul, S. Tandon, and M. Kiran, "Prosthetic rehabilitation of a child with induced anodontia," *The Journal of Clinical Pediatric Dentistry*, vol. 20, no. 1, pp. 5–8, 1995.

[3] R. Mussa, S. J. Esposito, and T. R. Cowper, "The use of colored elastomeric "O"s as a motivational instrument for patients with anodontia: report of case," *Journal of Dentistry for Children*, vol. 66, no. 2, pp. 98–102, 1999.

[4] M. A. Pigno, R. B. Blackman, R. J. Cronin Jr., and E. Cavazos, "Prosthodontic management of ectodermal dysplasia: a review of the literature," *Journal of Prosthetic Dentistry*, vol. 76, no. 5, pp. 541–545, 1996.

[5] K. A. Vieira, M. S. Teixeira, C. G. Guirado, and M. B. D. Gavião, "Prosthodontic treatment of hypohidrotic ectodermal dysplasia with complete anodontia: case report," *Quintessence International*, vol. 38, no. 1, pp. 75–80, 2007.

[6] S. Pettit and P. R. Campbell, "Ectrodactyly-ectodermal dysplasia-clefting syndrome: the oral hygiene management of a patient with EEC," *Special Care in Dentistry*, vol. 30, no. 6, pp. 250–254, 2010.

[7] E. Paschos, K. C. Huth, and R. Hickel, "Clinical management of hypohidrotic ectodermal dysplasia with anodontia: case report," *The Journal of Clinical Pediatric Dentistry*, vol. 27, no. 1, pp. 5–8, 2002.

[8] H. A. Al-Ibrahim, S. M. Al-Hadlaq, T. S. Abduljabbar, K. S. Al-Hamdan, and H. A. Abdin, "Surgical and implant-supported fixed prosthetic treatment of a patient with ectodermal dysplasia: a case report," *Special Care in Dentistry*, vol. 32, no. 1, pp. 1–5, 2012.

[9] R. Kohli, S. Levy, C. M. Kummet, D. V. Dawson, and C. M. Stanford, "Comparison of perceptions of oral health-related quality of life in adolescents affected with ectodermal dysplasias relative to caregivers," *Special Care in Dentistry*, vol. 31, no. 3, pp. 88–94, 2011.

[10] M. A. Derbanne, M. C. Sitbon, M. M. Landru, and A. Naveau, "Case report: early prosthetic treatment in children with ectodermal dysplasia," *European Archives of Paediatric Dentistry*, vol. 11, no. 6, pp. 301–305, 2010.

[11] A. S. Bidra, J. W. Martin, and E. Feldman, "Complete denture prosthodontics in children with ectodermal dysplasia: review of principles and techniques," *Compendium of Continuing Education in Dentistry*, vol. 31, no. 6, pp. 426–444, 2010.

[12] A. A. Sholapurkar, S. Setty, and K. M. Pai, "Total anodontia in patient with hypohidrotic ectodermal dysplasia. Report of rare case of Christ-Siemens Touraine syndrome," *The New York State Dental Journal*, vol. 77, no. 1, pp. 36–39, 2011.

[13] A. Açikgöz, O. Kademoglu, S. Elekdag-Türk, and F. Karagöz, "Hypohidrotic ectodermal dysplasia with true anodontia of the primary dentition," *Quintessence International*, vol. 38, no. 10, pp. 853–858, 2007.

[14] R. Khazaie, E. M. Berroeta, C. Borrero, A. Torbati, and W. Chee, "Five-year follow-up treatment of an ectodermal dysplasia patient with maxillary anterior composites and mandibular denture: a clinical report," *Journal of Prosthodontics*, vol. 19, no. 4, pp. 294–298, 2010.

[15] P. Imirzalioglu, S. Uckan, and S. G. Haydar, "Surgical and prosthodontic treatment alternatives for children and adolescents with ectodermal dysplasia: a clinical report," *Journal of Prosthetic Dentistry*, vol. 88, no. 6, pp. 569–572, 2002.

# Porous Titanium Granules and Blood for Bone Regeneration around Dental Implants: Report of Four Cases and Review of the Literature

**Andreas Thor**

*Department of Plastic & Oral and Maxillofacial Surgery, Institute of Surgical Sciences, Uppsala University, 751 85 Uppsala, Sweden*

Correspondence should be addressed to Andreas Thor; andreas.thor@telia.com

Academic Editors: M. A. Chinelatti and S. Nammour

A regenerative procedure treating a local osseous defect around titanium dental implant using porous titanium granules is described in four patients. Porous titanium granules represent, for maxillofacial surgery, a new alternative in augmenting osseous defects. Its earliest application was in the field of orthopedics for stabilization of tibia plateau fractures and for reoperations in prosthetic fixation of femoral stems. There is emerging scientific evidence regarding titanium for its potential use in the maxillofacial area and porous titanium granules are now commercially available. The scientific background for the osteoconductive use of porous titanium granules is elucidated in this paper and the supporting literature is reviewed.

## 1. Introduction

Bone augmentation of the alveolar crest in implant dentistry has attracted a substantial interest in the maxillofacial literature [1, 2]. Bone substitutes represent an important contribution to this field as augmentation with autogenous bone has drawbacks such as morbidity for the patient as well as problems with various degrees of resorption of the grafted bone volume over time [3].

After installation of dental implants, multifactorial conditions may all contribute to a peri-implant state of disease, for example, poor oral hygiene and a history of periodontitis, diabetes, or smoking. The mucosal status of attached or free gingiva at the fixture site is also of importance for long time success [4]. This problem has recently been discussed extensively in the dental implant literature; soft tissue peri-implant mucositis may affect about 50% of the implant sites and bone-affecting peri-implantitis may be seen in as many as 12–40% of the implant sites according to a consensus report from a European group of workers [4]. Implantology offers huge possibilities for patients and the restorative team, but the potential problem that may arise around implants needs to be addressed and not neglected by the implant surgeon.

The candidates among bone substitutes have been many over the years and some have proven to be successful [5]. Porous titanium granule (PTG) represents a new alternative in augmenting osseous defects in maxillofacial surgery. Its earliest application was seen in orthopedics and used for stabilization of tibial plateau fractures and for prosthetic reoperations for femoral stem fixations. A case operated in 1995 where dental implants in a split-crest procedure were supported by PTG represents the earliest reported surgery in the literature [6–9]. There is emerging scientific evidence of this material regarding the potential use in the maxillofacial area and the material is now marketed commercially [10, 11]. The aim of this paper is to describe a procedure treating local osseous defects around titanium dental implants using porous titanium granules in four patients. The available literature, compiled through a search on PubMed, is also discussed.

## 2. Case Presentation

Four patients, three females and one male, were scheduled for peri-implant regenerative surgery. All presented with local

TABLE 1: Demographic data describing the four study subjects.

| Subject | Gender | Age | Implant position | Time of preop. prosthetic loading | Duration of followup |
|---|---|---|---|---|---|
| 1 | F | 37 | Upper right canine | 12 months | 26 months |
| 2 | M | 58 | Lower right premolar | 36 months | 12 months |
| 3 | F | 66 | Upper right molar | 84 months | 11 months |
| 4 | F | 64 | Lower right molar | 22 months | 9 months |

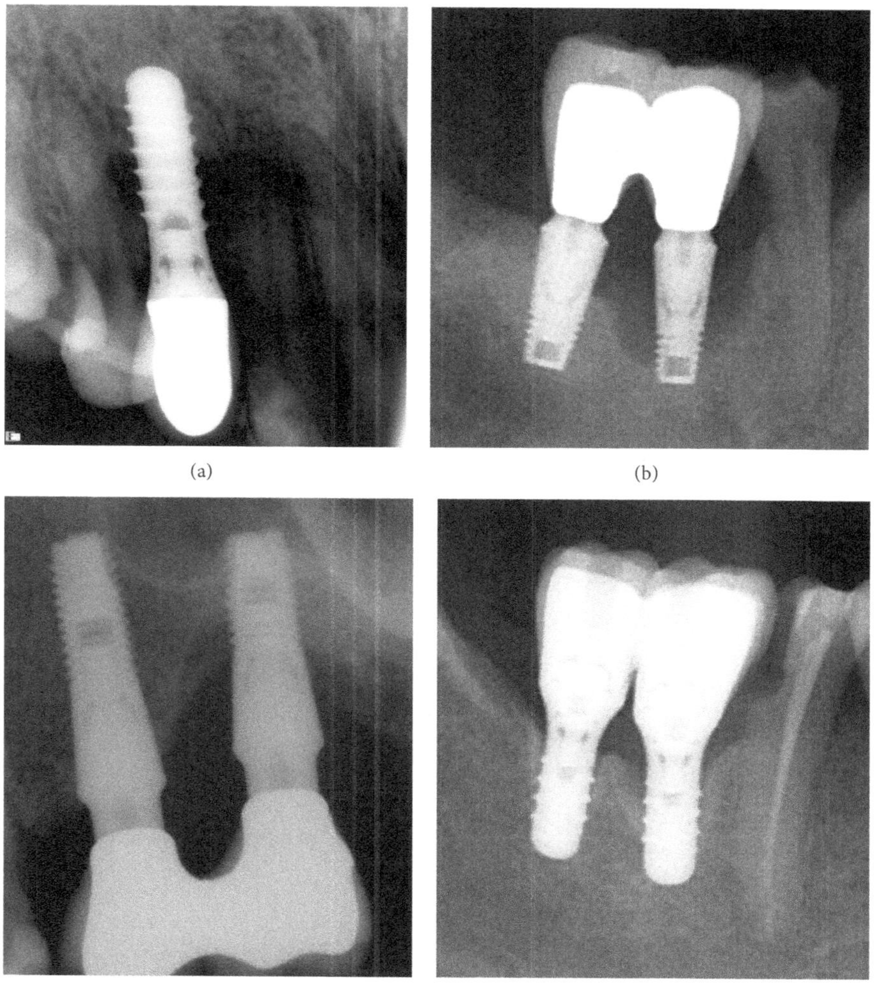

(a) (b) (c) (d)

FIGURE 1: Preoperative radiological situation in subjects 1–4.

defects around implants some time after prosthetic loading of the implants (Table 1). The male patient previously went through a periodontal surgical debridement for removal of granulation tissue around the affected two implants in the lower right premolar area, but bone destruction around the implants progressed. All four patients were preoperatively evaluated with clinical and radiological examination (Figure 1). Prosthetic overload was suspected as a contributing factor in three patients due to localized defects around implants and the occlusion was corrected accordingly in these patients prior to surgery. In two of the cases the defects were extensive and the procedure with PTG was considered as a salvage therapy for the implants that only displayed osseointegration in the most apical part.

Antibiotics were administered preoperatively (2-gram phenoxymethylpenicillin, Kåvepenin, Astra Zeneca, Södertälje, Sweden, and metronidazole, Flagyl, Sanofi-Aventis, Bromma, Sweden). Surgery was commenced in local anesthesia as flaps were raised in the area of the affected implants in order to augment the defects. Debridement of the surgical sites was performed. Granulation tissue in the defects as well as on the flaps was removed. After carefully cleaning the implants with scalers as well with a titanium brush (Tigran Brush No1, Tigran Technologies, Malmö, Sweden),

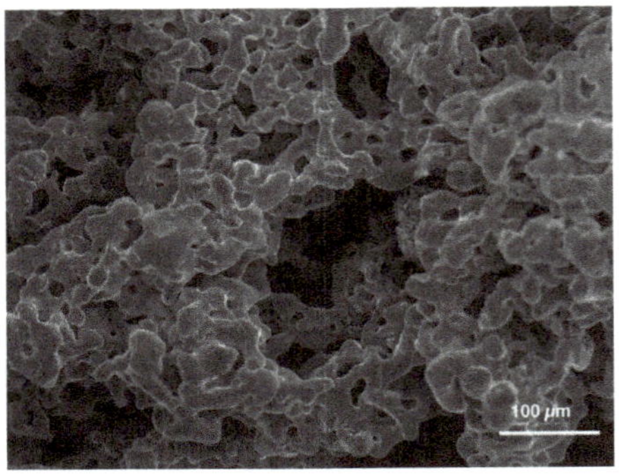


FIGURE 2: A porous titanium granule (PTG) seen with SEM. Particle size 500–1000 $\mu$m with a total porosity of approximately 80%.

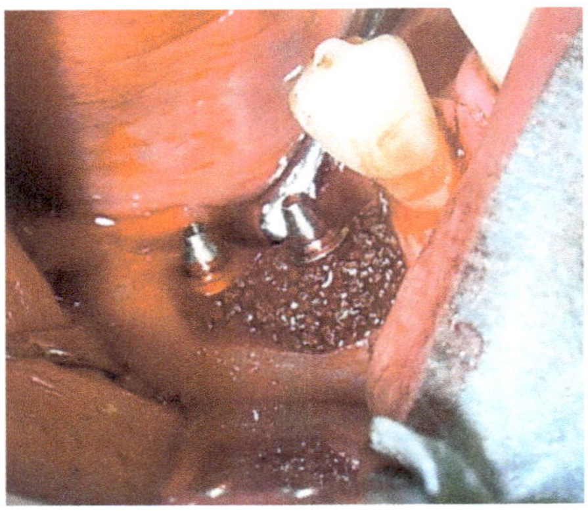

FIGURE 3: Clinical example of PTG implanted in marked vertical defect around implants in the lower right jaw of patient number 2.

rinsing of the surgical site with 3% hydrogen peroxide ($H_2O_2$) complemented by copious amounts of saline (NaCl), porous titanium granules (Tigran Technologies, Malmö, Sweden) were inserted in the defects and mixed with blood. The bony walls of the defects were prepared to stimulate small bleeding points with a small bur prior to insertion of the granules. Following the protocol supplied by the manufacturer, PTG (particle size 700–1000 $\mu$m, Figure 2) was gently condensed into the defects and around the fixtures up to the superior part of the implant, filling out the defects. In the three patients where overload of the implant retained bridge was suspected and the occlusion corrected preoperatively, the supraconstructions were temporarily removed during surgery for access to the surgical site and then replaced after suturing. The level of augmentation mimicked the original previous bone level at the installation of the fixtures (Figure 3). The granules connected well together in the clot forming a lightly moldable mass of the augmentative material. After the removal of visible granulation tissuefromthe flaps, they were repositioned with nonresorbable sutures around the restorations (the two-unit bridge in the three patients was repositioned at this time). In the fourth patient, who had a localized defect probably caused by a remaining minor tooth fragment in close contact with the installed implant eventually causing a defect in the bone, PTG was also densely

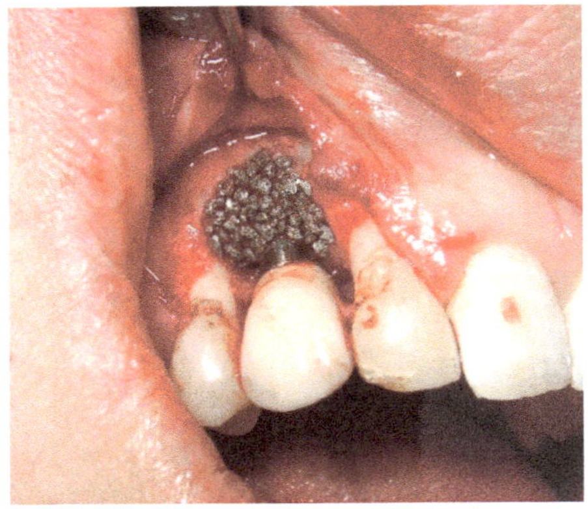

FIGURE 4: Clinical example of PTG implanted in bone defect around implant in position of upper right canine of patient number 1.

inserted into the defect (Figure 4) and the flap repositioned accordingly. Antibiotics (metronidazole starting preoperatively 3 days for the male patient due to a severe local bony destruction and pus formation around one of the fixtures; phenoxymethylpenicillin for the three female patients) were administered also postoperatively for all patients for one week. Chlorhexidine mouth rinse was used for the patients for two weeks postoperatively. Patients were advised not to clean the operated area mechanically with a brush for the first 10 days after augmentation. Sutures were removed one week postoperatively and all patients tolerated the procedure well with no adverse reactions recorded. Patients have now been followed between 9 to 26 months.

Clinical evaluation displayed a stable situation around the implant in two of the four patients with no loss of grafting material during followup. In the other two patients, the level of the marginal gingiva had been apically positioned and the loss of grafting material from the site of augmentation was progressively seen during the first month of followup, also reflected in the radiological examinations on followup (Figures 5 and 6). However, no visible inflammation or pus formation nor bleeding was seen around these implants. None of the implants have been lost in the followup and progression of bone loss appears to be halted.

## 3. Discussion

This paper reports on the results of four patients illustrating a rather novel technique for bone augmentation in the maxillofacial area using PTG. However not yet extensively explored regarding its use the biomaterial renders interest and is supported on the basis of innovative ideas that may be clinically important in the future. Bone substitutes represent an important area in reconstructive dental implantology and have been studied extensively [3, 12, 13]. The search for osteoinductive as well as osteoconductive materials has lead to the novel idea of using titanium in bone augmentations of the alveolar crest [10, 14]. The indications for the use of PTG in this area have so far been limited to recently reported sinus augmentations and for defects around dental

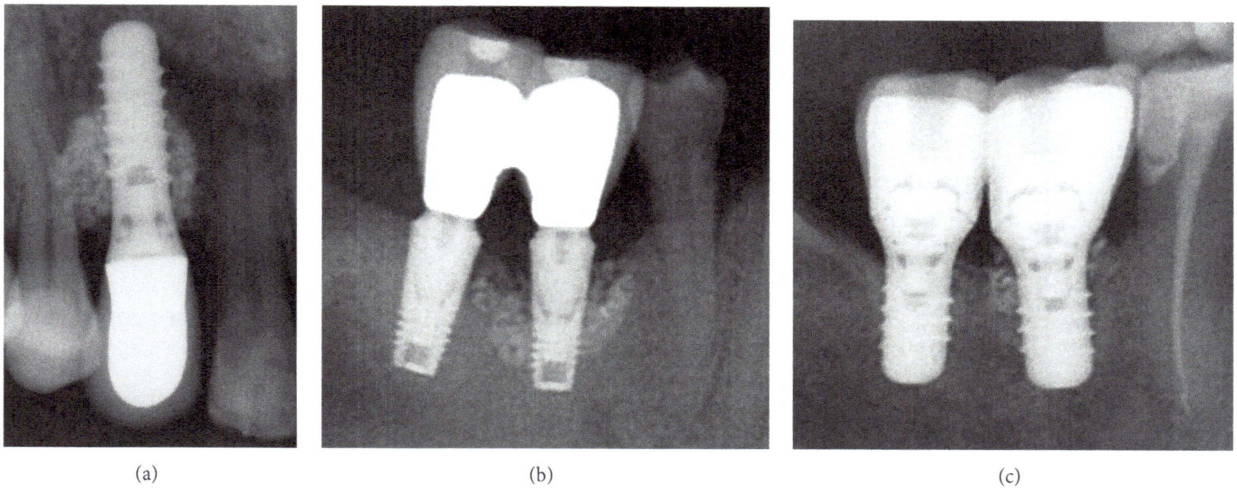

FIGURE 5: Radiological followup of patients 1, 2, and 4 after 26, 12, and 9 months, respectively, after surgery.

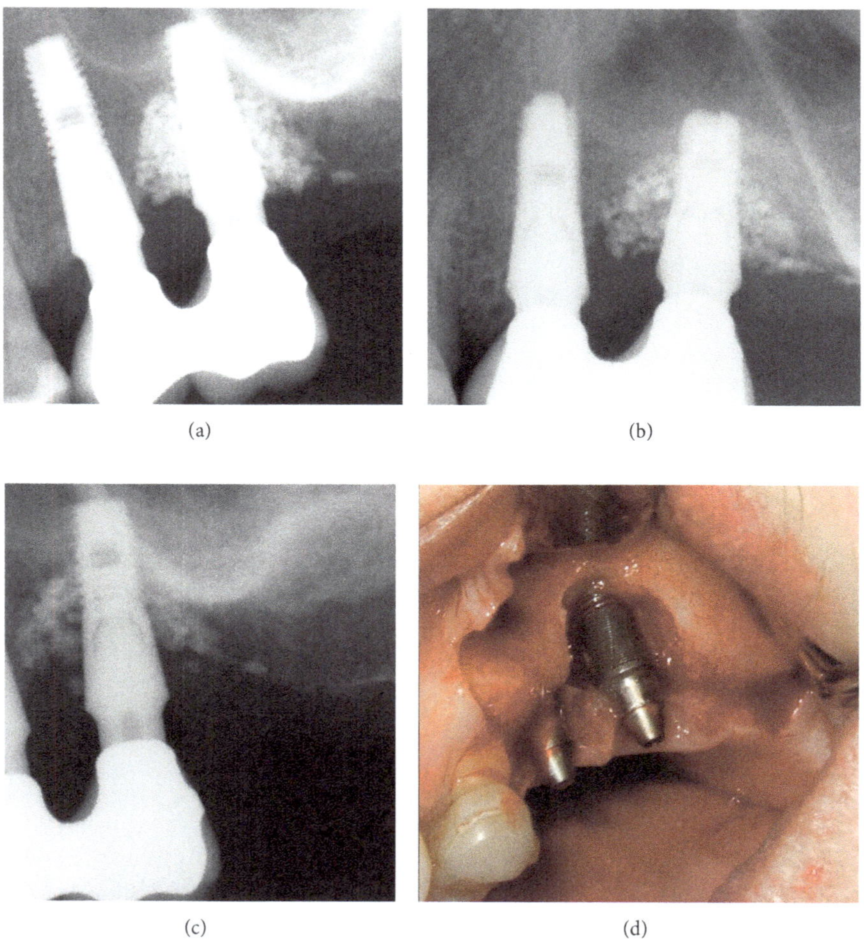

FIGURE 6: Illustration of sequence of radiological followup and clinical baseline status of patient number 3. Note the marked loss of grafting material in the defect (narrow crest). Extensive filling of defect with PTG at surgery resulted in loss of grafting material but with a gingival level that accordingly was positioned more apically without signs of marked inflammation or infection.

implants, even though the idea was first tried in a pilot case in 1995 [6, 11]. Just recently, Wohlfahrt et al. published a paper evaluating PTG in mandibular degree II furcation defects. The authors considered the material as safe in close proximity of root surface but found that the clinical result of the surgical treatment with PTG in 10 patients was diverging regarding the studied parameters. The values of probing depth and radiographic vertical furcation height were significantly reduced after one year, but no significant results were seen in clinical attachment levels or gingival recession [15]. Additionally, a clinical study where defects aroud implants were treated with PTG, surgical debridement, decontamination, and healing in a submerged fashion for six months, showed radiological improvement around implants but no significantly different clinical improvement compared to the same treatment without the use of PTG [16].

The overall experimental and clinical extent of the available literature so far is limited. PTG was initially used in orthopedics for stabilization of tibial plateau fractures and for reoperations in prosthetic fixation of femoral stems. Clinical results in a limited amount of patients in two case series reported satisfactory results on the materials ability to form a stable foundation for femoral stems and support for the elevation of condylar bone in depressed proximal tibia fractures [7, 8]. The material has also been evaluated in a clinical study of sinus augmentations where the main part of the included study subjects (12 patients) had implants simultaneously installed and PTG placed around them in the sinus floor in a one-stage procedure. Four patients had a delayed placement of implants due to insufficient primary stability at the time of augmentation. Three implant losses after an observation period of 12–36 months were seen and two of these were in the staged group. In the simultaneous placement group one implant was lost after one year of loading (after a history of postoperative sinus infection). The authors raised questions regarding the usage of the material in staged sinus lifts as well as further explore the risk of displacement of granules into the sinus during augmentation [11].

PTG has been subject to comparison with other grafting materials. A recent in vitro study with human primary mesenchymal stem cells comparing PTG with bovine bone (Bio-Oss, Geistlich Pharma AG, Wolhusen, Switzerland) and $\beta$-tricalcium phosphate (Bone Ceramic, Straumann AG, Basel Switzerland) reported better results for PTG regarding cell viability and proliferation as well as porosity, interconnectivity, open pore size, and surface area-to-volume ratio [17]. Additionally, Faria et al. explored the use of titanium in filling bone defects in a canine model with the purpose of comparing porous *titanium sponge rods* with synthetic hydroxyapatite. The titanium foam was constructed by mixing together titanium powder and space-holding particles and thereafter compacted and sintered: first to remove the space holding particles resulting in giving the titanium powder a porous structure [18]. In the humerus of six mongrel dogs, a total of 36 defects were randomly either filled with titanium foam in the shape of rods, particulate hydroxyapatite, or a blood clot serving as control. Healing times of two or four months were used and results displayed a higher density of grafting material in the test defects with titanium foam and less amount of newly formed bone accordingly compared to control defects with coagulum. Titanium foam and hydroxyapatite were comparable regarding new bone formation in both time intervals. Interestingly, the authors stated that the better contact between the marginal bone and the titanium material resulted in a better preservation of the marginal bone levels in the defects filled with titanium-foam compared to control. More mature bone was also seen around the titanium material. The titanium-foam, with a porosity of about 80% (same as in PTG used in the presented cases) and with good ingrowth properties for bone, was proposed as material for future use in bone augmentation [14].

One explanation for successfully maintaining the marginal bone levels in the defects in the previously mentioned study and for swift maturation of new bone may be the use of titanium in contact with whole blood which has been discussed and proposed in the literature as a relevant combination of materials for bony reconstruction [19, 20]. Blood can be regarded as the primary tissue in "gap" bony healing, as seen in fractures [21], distraction osteogenesis [22], or even in the maxillary sinus floor when using the sinus elevation technique for simultaneous installation of implants without the use of bone grafts or bone substitutes [23, 24]. However, initially the search for a biocompatible material to be used in the human vascular system or for blood contact medical devices (e.g., stents, vascular grafts and catheters) led to the recommendation of avoiding the use of titanium, as the material was found to be very potent regarding activation of the coagulation system with unwanted thrombus formation as a result of blood contact. Thrombus formation and inflammation involve the activation of both the coagulation and the complement system: the initiation of these systems causes plasma protein adsorption on the surface followed by the activation and adhesion of platelets and leukocytes [25]. The use of titanium as well as tantalum and indium in an in vitro study was found to display pronounced thrombogenic properties. Aluminium, nickel, and especially iridium were regarded as nonthrombogenic [26]. The opposite potential positive effect for the use of titanium in bone was therefore introduced, where the thrombogenic activity of the material could be useful for the onset of a rapid start of the healing process in healing of bone [23, 27].

Modifications of the titanium surface of a dental implant regarding topography, structure, surface chemistry, charge, and wettability have been proven to alter the osseointegration [28]. As an example, a surface modification of titanium that was titanium dioxide blasted and etched with hydrofluoric acid displayed the ability to enhance the onset of coagulation and caused a stronger release of growth factors in contact with blood [20]. Another titanium surface was chemically modified (hydroxylated/hydrated) resulting in increased hydrophilic properties and displayed superior results compared to control smooth titanium surfaces regarding influence on cell differentiation and growth factor release as well as improving soft and hard tissue integration [29]. Recently, a lot of focus has been directed to the fact that surface modifications result in a nanotopography of the implant surface and investigations continue to be published in the literature. Nanotopography in the form of $TiO_2$

nanotubes resulted experimentally in better proliferation and adhesion of osteoblasts resulting and improved bone-bonding strength as compared to $TiO_2$-gritblasted surfaces [30]. The importance of this nanotexture was confirmed as nanoporous alumina membranes with pore diameters of 20 and 200 nm were shown to activate platelets differently. Platelet microparticle generation, as a marker of procoagulant activity, was shown to be higher in pore size of 200 nm. As smooth alumina earlier was shown to be nonthrombogenic, these studies indicate that there may be a direct influence on thrombogenicity from the size of nanopores. The optimal pore size is still to be explored [26, 31, 32]. Smooth, machined titanium as well as modified titanium surfaces has proven to be efficient in the activation of the coagulation cascade in blood contact and one may therefore argue its value as a material used for regeneration in defects with new bone formation. Furthermore, the porous titanium granules are hollow in their total volume to 80 percent. The capillary action on blood to fill these pores in the granules parallel to the supposed strong initiation of coagulation and release of growth factors and clot formation results clinically in the formation of a moldable mass that can be placed in peri-implant defects. The results of the cases presented in this paper show however that the use must be with moderation; bone formation outside the skeletal envelope, or as in these two cases reported herein where loss of grafting material was rather extensive, is not easily achieved. The affected *implants* were not covered by the flaps after the defects were augmented with the scaffold of PTG. Submerging the implants may have resulted in a better outcome and less loss of material in two of the four cases where the initial crest was narrow. Coverage of the graft with a membrane may also increase the level of outcome. Overloaded supraconstructions may have added to the bony defect progression around the implants in these two specific cases. The reasons for progression for defects around implants must be widely investigated. Another issue is the availability of attached gingival around implants, something that may be a commonly encountered problem in situations of long-standing edentulism, for example, in the lower jaw premolar area.

In conclusion, further clinical and experimental studies on the use of porous titanium granules as a bone augmentation material are needed, even though there are some studies published on the material to support its use.

## References


[1] M. Esposito, M. G. Grusovin, P. Coulthard, and H. V. Worthington, "The efficacy of various bone augmentation procedures for dental implants: a Cochrane systematic review of randomized controlled clinical trials," *International Journal of Oral and Maxillofacial Implants*, vol. 21, no. 5, pp. 696–710, 2006.

[2] M. Chiapasco, P. Casentini, and M. Zaniboni, "Bone augmentation procedures in implant dentistry," *International Journal of Oral and Maxillofacial Implants*, vol. 24, supplement, pp. 237–259, 2009.

[3] M. Hallman and A. Thor, "Bone substitutes and growth factors as an alternative/complement to autogenous bone for grafting in implant dentistry," *Periodontology 2000*, vol. 47, no. 1, pp. 172–192, 2008.

[4] J. Lindhe and J. Meyle, "Peri-implant diseases: consensus report of the sixth European workshop on Periodontology," *Journal of Clinical Periodontology*, vol. 35, no. 8, pp. 282–285, 2008.

[5] M. Esposito, M. G. Grusovin, H. V. Worthington, and P. Coulthard, "Interventions for replacing missing teeth: bone augmentation techniques for dental implant treatment," *Cochrane Database of Systematic Reviews*, no. 3, Article ID CD003607, 2006.

[6] L. Holmberg, L. Forsgren, and L. Kristerson, "Porous titanium granules for implant stability and bone regeneration—a case followed for 12 years," *Upsala Journal of Medical Sciences*, vol. 113, no. 2, pp. 217–220, 2008.

[7] T. M. Turner, R. M. Urban, D. J. Hall, and G. B. J. Andersson, "Bone ingrowth through porous titanium granulate around a femoral stem: histological assessment in a six-month canine hemiarthroplasty model," *Upsala Journal of Medical Sciences*, vol. 112, no. 2, pp. 191–197, 2007.

[8] P. A. Alffram, L. Bruce, L. M. Bjursten, R. M. Urban, and G. B. J. Andersson, "Implantation of the femoral stem into a bed of titanium granules using vibration: a pilot study of a new method for prosthetic fixation in 5 patients followed for up to 15 years," *Upsala Journal of Medical Sciences*, vol. 112, no. 2, pp. 183–189, 2007.

[9] B. Jónsson and B. Mjöberg, "Surgical treatment of depression fractures of the lateral tibial plateau using porous titanium granules," *Upsala Journal of Medical Sciences*, vol. 114, no. 1, pp. 52–54, 2009.

[10] J. C. Wohlfahrt, M. Monjo, H. J. Rønold, A. M. Aass, J. E. Ellingsen, and S. P. Lyngstadaas, "Porous titanium granules promote bone healing and growth in rabbit tibia peri-implant osseous defects," *Clinical Oral Implants Research*, vol. 21, no. 2, pp. 165–173, 2010.

[11] H. Bystedt and L. Rasmusson, "Porous titanium granules used as osteoconductive material for sinus floor augmentation: a clinical pilot study," *Clinical Implant Dentistry and Related Research*, vol. 11, no. 2, pp. 101–105, 2009.

[12] S. S. Jensen and H. Terheyden, "Bone augmentation procedures in localized defects in the alveolar ridge: clinical results with different bone grafts and bone-substitute materials," *International Journal of Oral and Maxillofacial Implants*, vol. 24, supplement, pp. 218–236, 2009.

[13] I. Darby, S. T. Chen, and D. Buser, "Ridge preservation techniques for implant therapy," *International Journal of Oral and Maxillofacial Implants*, vol. 24, supplement, pp. 260–271, 2009.

[14] C. E. Wen, Y. Yamada, K. Shimojima, Y. Chino, T. Asahina, and M. Mabuchi, "Processing and mechanical properties of autogenous titanium implant materials," *Journal of Materials Science*, vol. 13, no. 4, pp. 397–401, 2002.

[15] J. C. Wohlfahrt, S. P. Lyngstadaas, L. Heijl, and A. M. Aass, "Porous titanium granules in the treatment of mandibular class ii furcation defects: a consecutive case series," *Journal of Periodontology*, vol. 83, no. 1, pp. 61–69, 2012.

[16] J. C. Wohlfahrt, S. P. Lyngstadaas, H. J. Rønold, E. Saxegaard, J. E. Ellingsen, and S. Karlsson, "Porous titanium granules in the surgical treatment of peri-implant osseous defects: a randomized clinical trial," *International Journal of Oral and Maxillofacial Implants*, vol. 27, no. 2, pp. 401–410, 2012.

[17] R. Sabetrasekh, H. Tiainen, S. P. Lyngstadaas, J. Reseland, and H. Haugen, "A novel ultra-porous titanium dioxide ceramic with

excellent biocompatibility," *Journal of Biomaterials Applications*, vol. 25, no. 6, pp. 559–580, 2011.

[18] P. E. P. Faria, A. L. Carvalho, D. N. B. Felipucci, C. Wen, L. Sennerby, and L. A. Salata, "Bone formation following implantation of titanium sponge rods into humeral osteotomies in dogs: a histological and histometrical study," *Clinical Implant Dentistry and Related Research*, vol. 12, no. 1, pp. 72–79, 2010.

[19] J. Hong, K. Nilsson Ekdahl, H. Reynolds, R. Larsson, and B. Nilsson, "A new in vitro model to study interaction between whole blood and biomaterials. Studies of platelet and coagulation activation and the effect of aspirin," *Biomaterials*, vol. 20, no. 7, pp. 603–611, 1999.

[20] A. Thor, L. Rasmusson, A. Wennerberg et al., "The role of whole blood in thrombin generation in contact with various titanium surfaces," *Biomaterials*, vol. 28, no. 6, pp. 966–974, 2007.

[21] J. E. Davies and M. M. Hosseini, *Histodynamics of Endosseous Wound Healing*, EM Squared incorporated, Toronto, Canada, 2000.

[22] J. B. Cope and M. L. Samchukov, "Mineralization dynamics of regenerate bone during mandibular osteodistraction," *International Journal of Oral and Maxillofacial Surgery*, vol. 30, no. 3, pp. 234–242, 2001.

[23] A. Thor, L. Sennerby, J. M. Hirsch, and L. Rasmusson, "Bone formation at the maxillary sinus floor following simultaneous elevation of the mucosal lining and implant installation without graft material: an evaluation of 20 patients treated with 44 Astra Tech implants," *Journal of Oral and Maxillofacial Surgery*, vol. 65, no. 7, supplement, pp. 64–72, 2007.

[24] S. Lundgren, S. Andersson, F. Gualini, and L. Sennerby, "Bone reformation with sinus membrane elevation: a new surgical technique for maxillary sinus floor augmentation," *Clinical Implant Dentistry and Related Research*, vol. 6, no. 3, pp. 165–173, 2004.

[25] M. B. Gorbet and M. V. Sefton, "Biomaterial-associated thrombosis: roles of coagulation factors, complement, platelets and leukocytes," *Biomaterials*, vol. 25, no. 26, pp. 5681–5703, 2004.

[26] J. Hong, A. Azens, K. N. Ekdahl, C. G. Granqvist, and B. Nilsson, "Material-specific thrombin generation following contact between metal surfaces and whole blood," *Biomaterials*, vol. 26, no. 12, pp. 1397–1403, 2005.

[27] J. Hong, J. Andersson, K. N. Ekdahl et al., "Titanium is a highly thrombogenic biomaterial: possible implications for osteogenesis," *Thrombosis and Haemostasis*, vol. 82, no. 1, pp. 58–64, 1999.

[28] J. E. Ellingsen, P. Thomsen, and S. P. Lyngstadaas, "Advances in dental implant materials and tissue regeneration," *Periodontology 2000*, vol. 41, no. 1, pp. 136–156, 2006.

[29] F. Schwarz, M. Herten, M. Sager, M. Wieland, M. Dard, and J. Becker, "Bone regeneration in dehiscence-type defects at chemically modified (SLActive) and conventional SLA titanium implants: a pilot study in dogs," *Journal of Clinical Periodontology*, vol. 34, no. 1, pp. 78–86, 2007.

[30] L. M. Bjursten, L. Rasmusson, S. Oh, G. C. Smith, K. S. Brammer, and S. Jin, "Titanium dioxide nanotubes enhance bone bonding *in vivo*," *Journal of Biomedical Materials Research Part A*, vol. 92, no. 3, pp. 1218–1224, 2010.

[31] N. Ferraz, J. Carlsson, J. Hong, and M. K. Ott, "Influence of nanoporesize on platelet adhesion and activation," *Journal of Materials Science*, vol. 19, no. 9, pp. 3115–3121, 2008.

[32] N. Ferraz, J. Hong, and M. Karlsson Ott, "Procoagulant behavior and platelet microparticle generation on nanoporous alumina," *Journal of Biomaterials Applications*, vol. 24, no. 8, pp. 675–692, 2010.

# Management of Unilateral Masseter Hypertrophy and Hypertrophic Scar—A Case Report

**Naresh Shetty,[1] Rajanikanth K. Malaviya,[2] and M. K. Gupta[3]**

[1] *Department of Oral & Maxillofacial Surgery, Faculty of Dentistry, Melaka Manipal Medical College, 75150 Melaka, Malaysia*
[2] *Department of Oral & Maxillofacial Surgery, Sharad Pawar Dental College, Wardha 442005, India*
[3] *Department of Oral & Maxillofacial Surgery, Peoples Dental Academy, Bhopal 462010, India*

Correspondence should be addressed to Naresh Shetty, shetty.naresh1@gmail.com

Academic Editors: R. S. Brown, A. C. B. Delbem, and I. El-Hakim

Masseter muscle hypertrophy is a rare condition of idiopathic cause. It clinically presents as an enlargement of one or both masseter muscles. Most patients complain of facial asymmetry; however, symptoms such as trismus, protrusion, and bruxism may also occur. Several treatment options reported for masseter hypertrophy are present, which range from simple pharmacotherapy to more invasive surgical reduction. Keloid scar with unilateral masseter hypertrophy is a rarely seen in clinical practice. This paper reports a case of unilateral masseter hypertrophy with keloid scar in the angle of the mandible for which surgical treatment was rendered to the patient by using a single approach.

## 1. Introduction

Masseter hypertrophy is usually an asymptomatic enlargement of one or both masseter muscles. In majority of the cases, the etiology is idiopathic. The highest incidence for this condition is in the second and third decades of life, with no gender predilection. A congenital variety also exists, but acquired masseter hypertrophy is more common. Unilateral occurrence can be seen when patients chew or clench primarily on one side. Muscle function may also be impaired, thus causing conditions such as trismus, protrusion, and bruxism. Numerous factors such as malocclusion, bruxism, clenching, or temporomandibular joint disorders, have been cited. The accurate diagnosis is more difficult in unilateral cases. A hypertrophied masseter will alter facial lines, cause generating discomfort, and negative cosmetic impacts in many patients. Masseter hypertrophy leads to the prominent mandibular angle which is aesthetically unacceptable to the patient. The differential diagnosis includes parotid tumor, lipoma, benign or malignant muscle tumors, and vascular tumors.

## 2. Case Report

A 28-year-old male patient reported to the department of oral and maxillofacial surgery at people's dental academy complaining of asymmetry of the face and scar in the mandibular angle region on the left side since 3 years. The patient gave a history that he had tripped and fallen down 3 years back and he had a laceration on the left side of the face that developed in to a scar. The patient's chief complaint was left side facial growth without pain. The patient had no history of systemic diseases. Extraoral examination showed an obvious unilateral swelling centered over the mandibular angle. Palpation indicated that the swollen tissue was normal in tone and nontender. Mandibular movements were in the normal range. When the patient was asked to clench, the swelling became more prominent and firm. The patient said that he uses the left side of the jaw more while chewing food. There was no history of temporomandibular joint clicking, and no family history of masseter hypertrophy. Physical examination revealed that the patient had unilateral masseter muscle bulging, with a prominent mandibular angle at the

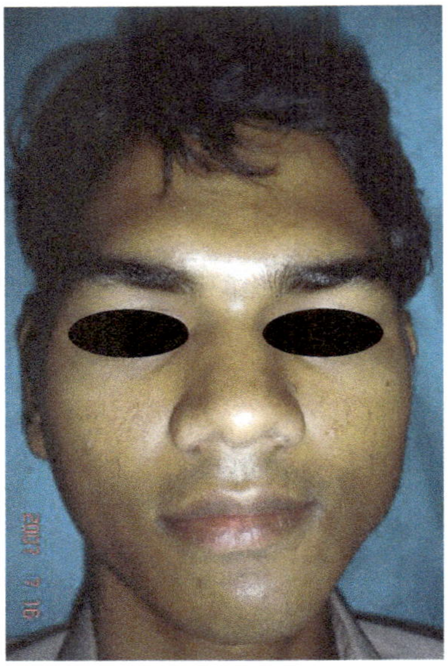

Figure 1: Pre-op frontal view.

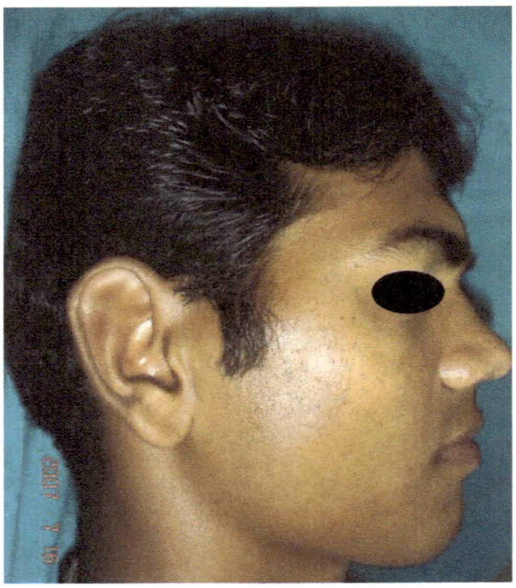

Figure 2: Pre-op right lateral view.

lower border. Intraoral examination revealed distoangularly impacted 38 and 48. OPG showed a prominent mandibular angle. Data from clinical and radiographic examination led to the diagnosis of unilateral masseter muscle hypertrophy (Figures 1, 2, 3, 4, 5, and 6). Nonsurgical options such as botox therapy and the advantages and disadvantages of both surgery and botox treatment were discussed with the patient. The patient opted for surgical option as he wanted to get rid of the scar immediately and we told him that we can do the correction of masseter hypertrophy and scar revision through one incisional approach only. A combined reduction of the mandibular angle and shaving of the masseter muscle was planned. The surgery was done under general anesthesia with nasotracheal intubation. Xylocaine 2% with adrenalin

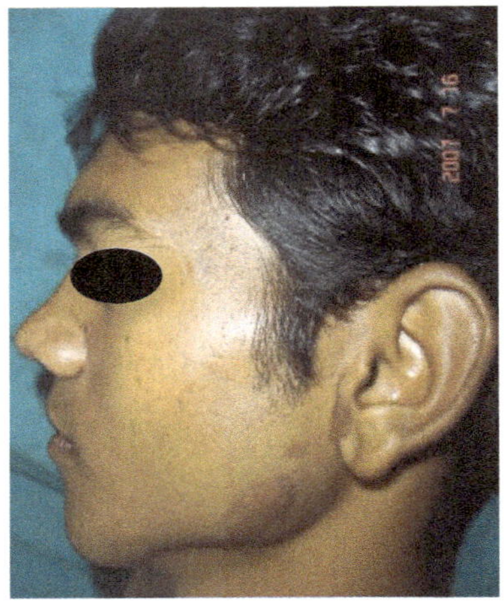

Figure 3: Pre-op left lateral view.

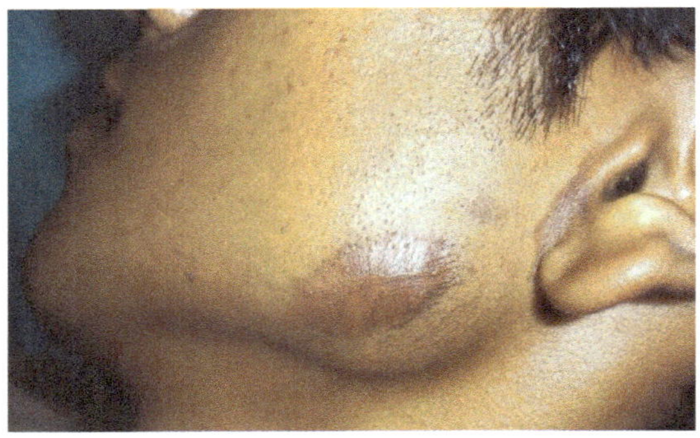

Figure 4: Pre-op left close-up view.

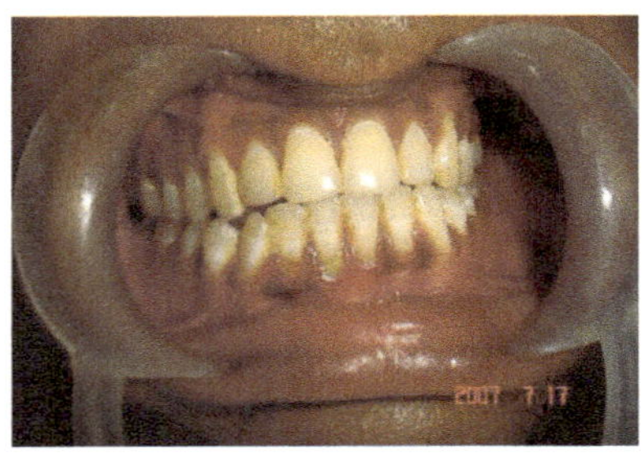

Figure 5: Pre-op occlusion.

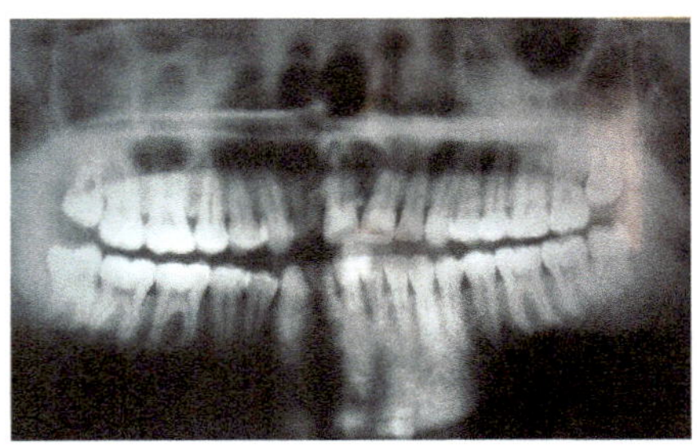

Figure 6: Pre-op OPG.

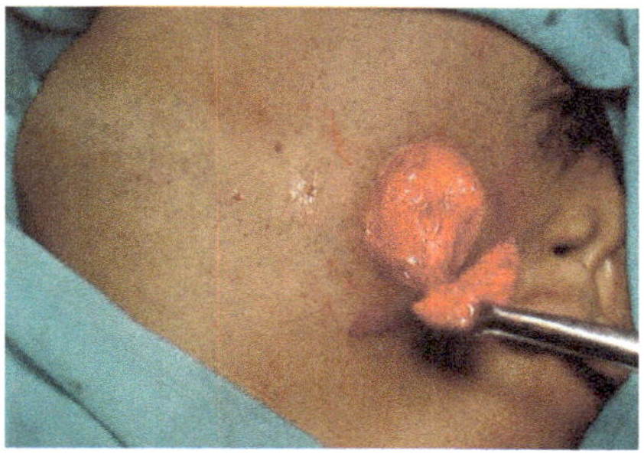

FIGURE 7: Intraoperative view.

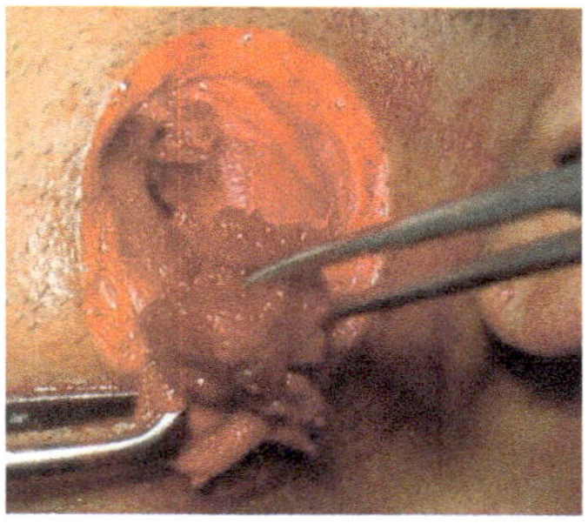

FIGURE 8: Hypertrophic muscle removed.

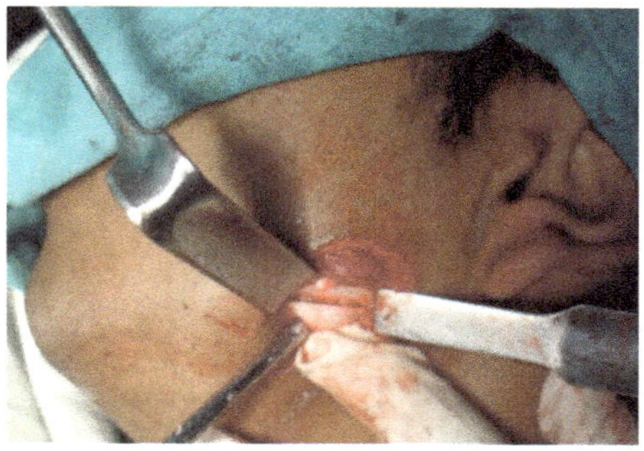

FIGURE 9: Bony excess resected at angle.

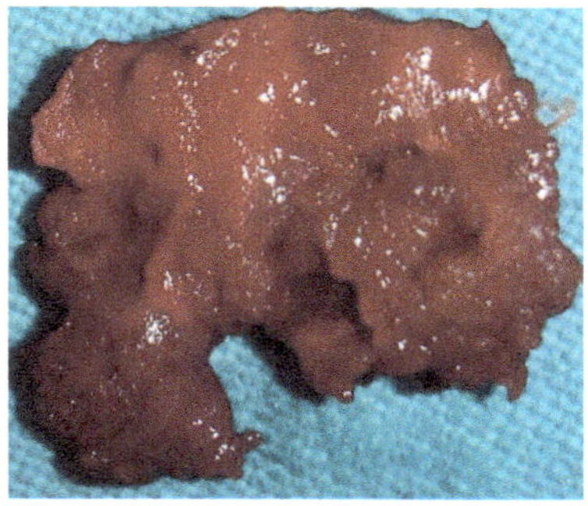

FIGURE 10: Resected masseter muscle.

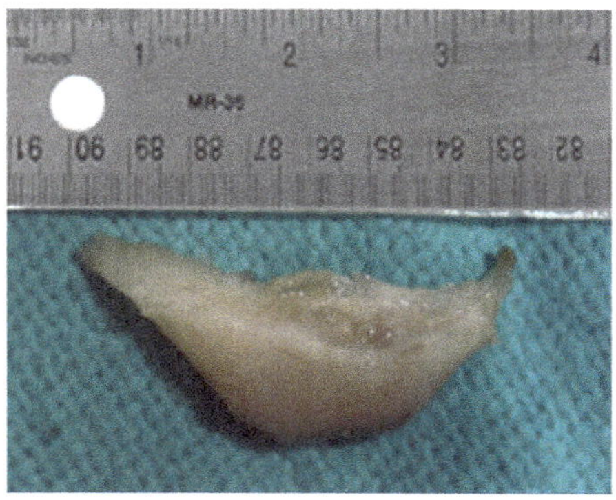

FIGURE 11: Resected angle.

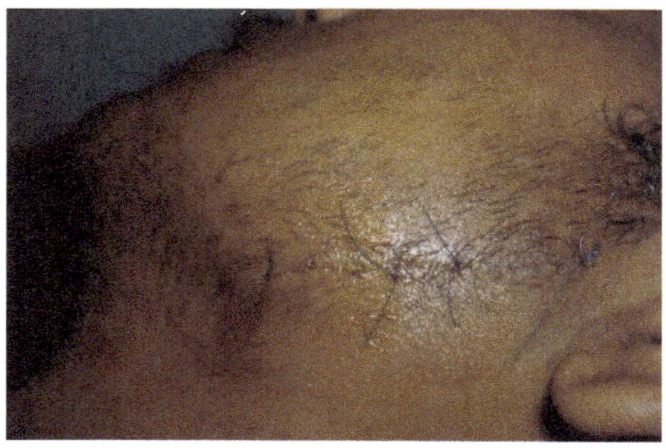

FIGURE 12: Sutures placed.

was infiltrated in the angle of the mandible. An elliptical incision was placed around the hypertrophic scar and the scar was removed (Figure 7). The marginal mandibular nerve was identified and protected. Debulking of the masseter muscle was performed as the patient was very worried about the asymmetry of the face (Figure 8). The muscle was incised approximately 5 mm above the mandibular basilar. The entire ascending portion of the masseter muscle was detached, and a vertical internal muscle band equivalent to two third of the thickness of the muscle was resected. After the muscle was resected, the remaining external third was sutured to its site of origin onto the muscle stump inserted in the mandibular basilar. The bony deformity was trimmed and removed in the angle of the mandible with surgical bur (Figure 9). Sharp margins were trimmed with a bone file. The shaved masseter muscle and the resected excess mandibular angle was sent to oral pathology department in 10% formalin (Figures 10 and 11). Primary closure was done with 5-0 prolene suture (Figure 12). After 1 week, the prolene sutures were removed and the wound healed uneventfully.

## 3. Discussion

The masseter muscle is essential for adequate mastication and is located laterally to the mandibular ramus and thus plays an important role in facial esthetics. Diagnosis of masseter hypertrophy can be achieved from clinical examination, history, panoramic X-ray, and muscle palpation. The best diagnostic test is to palpate the masseter muscle with fingers, while the patient clenches his/her teeth so the muscle is more prominent during contraction. With the muscle is relaxed and the patient's mouth is slightly open, extraoral palpation with both hands will pinpoint the intramuscular location of the hypertrophy. Upon relaxation, the jaw angle may reveal irregularities that on the X-ray image may appear to be a bone increase. Idiopathic masseter muscle hypertrophy was first described by Legg in 1880, reporting on the case of a 10-year-old girl with concurrent idiopathic temporalis muscle hypertrophy [1]. According to Teixeira et al., there are two types of masseter muscle hypertrophy: congenital or familial and acquired due to functional hypertrophy [2]. There are various treatment modalities for the management of masseter hypertrophy. This can be categorized into nonsurgical and surgical. Management of the idiopathic masseter hypertrophy is based on psychological counseling, use of mouth guards, -muscle relaxant, and anxiolytic drugs, analgesics, physical therapy, dental restorations, and occlusal adjustments to correct premature contacts. A good result can be achieved in the patients with mild hypertrophy but there is no reliable report on the literature on the success rates of isolated clinical therapy. Injection of botulinum toxin type A into the masseter muscle is generally considered a less invasive modality and has been advocated for cosmetic sculpting of the lower face. Injection of botulinum toxin type A into the masseter muscle was first introduced by Smyth, Moore, and Wood in 1994 and considered a less invasive modality for the treatment of muscle hypertrophy [3]. Local injection of very small doses of the toxin into a muscle produces local paralysis and therefore, individual muscles can be selectively weakened and atrophy of the muscle occurs. Botulinum toxin type A is a powerful neurotoxin which is produced by the anaerobic organism clostridium botulinum and when injected into a muscle causes interference with the neurotransmitter mechanism producing selective paralysis and subsequent atrophy of the muscle. Perhaps the biggest disadvantage of botulinum toxin therapy is that the treatment effect wears away and reverts to the original condition in 6 months [4]. The traditional method of treatment for masseter hypertrophy is the surgical partial excision of masseter muscle under general anesthesia. The surgical treatment is based on intra- and extraoral approaches. Both techniques revolve around the removal of excessive muscle fibers from the inner third of the masseter vertical muscle fibers. Reduction osteoplasty may be performed in cases of bony hyperplasia of the mandibular angle [5]. The remaining external bundle of the masseter should be attached to the mandibular periosteum to allow for adequate functional recovery. The choice between intra- and extraoral approaches is not related to cosmetic or functional outcomes or to the risk of introducing vascular and nerve injury, but to the skill and experience of the surgeon in performing surgery using either of the approaches. In the beginning, the extraoral approach was widely indicated, because it offered better visualization. The procedure is carried out through a submandibular incision, Risdon. Unlike surgical excision of muscle tissue that reduces the actual number of muscle cells, botulinum toxin type A only reduces muscle volume temporarily. Surgical treatment was proposed for the first time by Gurney in 1947 [6]. The procedure consists of a submandibular incision and the removal of three fourth to two third of all muscle tissue available from the muscle upper aponeurosis to the lower mandibular border. Removal of the masseter muscle insertion by means of a triangular incision was done by Martensson in a patient with history of bruxism and unilateral masseter muscle hypertrophy [7]. Beckers in 1977 surgically treated 17 patients using the intraoral approach in which internal muscle band was removed from the hypertrophied masseter. An internal muscle band was removed from the hypertrophied masseter from the upper insertion in the zygomatic arc to the lower insertion in the mandibular angle, thus avoiding the production of a visible scar on the patient's face and reducing the possibility of injuring branches of the facial nerve [8]. Another surgical technique is, in which the bony protuberance is removed from the mandibular angle without removing any parts of the masseter muscle [9]. Complications from surgical excision of masseter include hematoma formation, facial nerve paralysis, infection, mouth opening limitation and sequelae from general anesthesia [10]. Nonsurgical approaches such as botox therapy have both advantages and disadvantages to surgical approaches [11, 12].

## 4. Conclusion

The masseter hypertrophy was removed along with hypertrophic scar. With a single surgery treatment of masseteric hypertrophy and hypertrophic scar have been carried out which is probably the first time and long-term followup is required following the surgery.

## Acknowledgment

The authors are thankful to Dr. M. K. Gupta for being a constant source of support and encouragement.

## References

[1] W. Legg, "Enlargement of the temporal and masseter muscle in both sides," *Transactions of the Pathological Society of London*, vol. 63, no. 5, pp. 361–364, 1880.

[2] V. C. Teixeira, J. E. S. Mejia, and A. Estefano, "Tratamento cirúrgico da hipertrofia benigna do masseter por abordagem intra-oral," *Revista Brasileira de Cirurgia*, vol. 86, no. 4, pp. 165–170, 1996.

[3] B. Bab, B. Ozan, M. Muolali, and N. Celebi, "Treatment of masseteric hypertrophy with botulinum toxin: a report of two cases," *Medicina Oral Patología Oral Cirugia Bucal*, vol. 15, pp. 649–652, 2010.

[4] H. T. Al-Ahmad and M. A. Al-Qudah, "The treatment of masseter hypertrophy with botulinum toxin type A," *Saudi Medical Journal*, vol. 27, no. 3, pp. 397–400, 2006.

[5] L. A. Whitaker, "Prominent mandibular angle: preoperative management, operative technique and results in 42 patients (Discussion)," *Plastic and Reconstructive Surgery*, vol. 83, no. 2, article 279, 1989.

[6] C. E. Gurney, "Chronic bilateral benign hypertrophy of the masseter muscles," *The American Journal of Surgery*, vol. 73, no. 1, pp. 137–139, 1947.

[7] G. Martensson, "Hypertrophy of the masseter muscle," *Acta Otolaryngologica*, vol. 50, pp. 526–530, 1989.

[8] H. L. Beckers, "Masseteric muscle hypertrophy and its intraoral surgical correction," *Journal of Maxillofacial Surgery*, vol. 5, no. 1, pp. 28–35, 1977.

[9] M. J. Black and M. D. Schloss, "Masseteric muscle hypertrophy," *Journal of Otolaryngology*, vol. 14, no. 3, pp. 203–205, 1985.

[10] Z. R. Daniel, M. C. Paulo, L. P. Jose, R. F. Vinicius, K. M. Karina, and A. C. Marcela, "Benign masseter muscle hypertrophy," *Revista Brasileira de Otorrinolaringologia*, vol. 74, no. 5, pp. 790–793, 2008.

[11] G. Furdui-Carr and L. Mandel, "Unilateral masseteric hypertrophy: a case report," *New York State Dental Journal*, vol. 76, no. 4, pp. 46–48, 2010.

[12] R. Peretta, M. Melison, R. Meneghello et al., "Unilateral masseter muscle hypertrophy: morpholofunctional analysis of relapse after treatment with botulinum toxin: a case report," *The Journal of Craniomandibular Practice*, vol. 27, no. 3, pp. 200–210, 2009.

# Complete Maxillary Crossbite Correction with a Rapid Palatal Expansion in Mixed Dentition Followed by a Corrective Orthodontic Treatment

**Orlando Motohiro Tanaka,[1,2] Isabelle Adad Fornazari,[3] Ariane Ximenes Graciano Parra,[4] Bruno Borges de Castilhos,[4] and Ademir Franco[5,6]**

[1] *Graduate Dentistry Program in Orthodontics, Pontifícia Universidade Católica do Paraná, Rua Imaculada Conceição 1155, 80215-901 Curitiba, PR, Brazil*
[2] *Postdoctoral Fellowship at The Center for Advanced Dental Education, Saint Louis University, St. Louis, MO, USA*
[3] *Dentistry, Pontifícia Universidade Católica do Paraná, Curitiba, PR, Brazil*
[4] *Orthodontics, Pontifícia Universidade Católica do Paraná, Curitiba, PR, Brazil*
[5] *Department of Oral Health Sciences, Forensic Dentistry, KU Leuven and Dentistry, University Hospitals Leuven, Leuven, Belgium*
[6] *Stomatology, Pontifícia Universidade Católica do Paraná, Curitiba, PR, Brazil*

Correspondence should be addressed to Orlando Motohiro Tanaka; tanakaom@gmail.com

Academic Editor: Hüsamettin Oktay

This case report presents the interceptive orthodontic treatment of a boy, aged 8 years 4 months with a Class I malocclusion with severe transverse maxillary deficiency and complete maxillary crossbite and correction using Haas expansion and fixed appliance. The treatment goals were to correct the posterior crossbite and anterior crossbite and restore the normality of the dentition and occlusion. In phase I, the patient was treated with a modified Haas-type palatal expander, which provided a clinically significant palatal expansion and increased the maxillary arch perimeter with favorable conditions for orthodontic treatment with fixed appliances in phase II. The optimization of E-space and the use of intermaxillary Class III elastics helped to maintain the mandibular incisors upright. A removable wraparound type appliance and a bonded lingual canine-to-canine retainer were used as retention. Although the literature has reported a high rate of relapse after palatal expansion, after 2 years 9 months of posttreatment follow-up, the occlusal result was stable and no skeletal reversals could be detected.

## 1. Introduction

The posterior crossbite is one of the most frequent malocclusions in orthodontics [1], and its possible etiologies include prolonged retention or loss at an early age of deciduous teeth, crowding, cleft palate, genetic factors, tooth-size arch-length discrepancies, abnormalities in tooth morphology, eruption sequence, thumb sucking habits, and mouth breathing during critical growth periods [2].

The rapid palatal expansion (RPE) is often used to expand the maxilla in patients with mixed dentition positively impacting the treatment of related deficiencies [3, 4]. Specifically, this technique may be used to correct transverse and sagittal crossbite, generating space in the dental arch and, consequently, solving cases of borderline crowding [5].

The RPE is extremely useful for the treatment of Class III patients and cases of real and relative maxillary deficiencies [6]. Occlusal acrylic splints are considered the most effective devices for RPE in young patients because they produce therapeutic effects that are not only limited to the correction of crossbite or the increase in arch width [5, 7].

Posterior crossbite and anterior crossbite do not have a spontaneous correction and should be treated with maxillary expansion as early as possible, after an accurate diagnosis with the patient in centric relation [8] and treatment planning

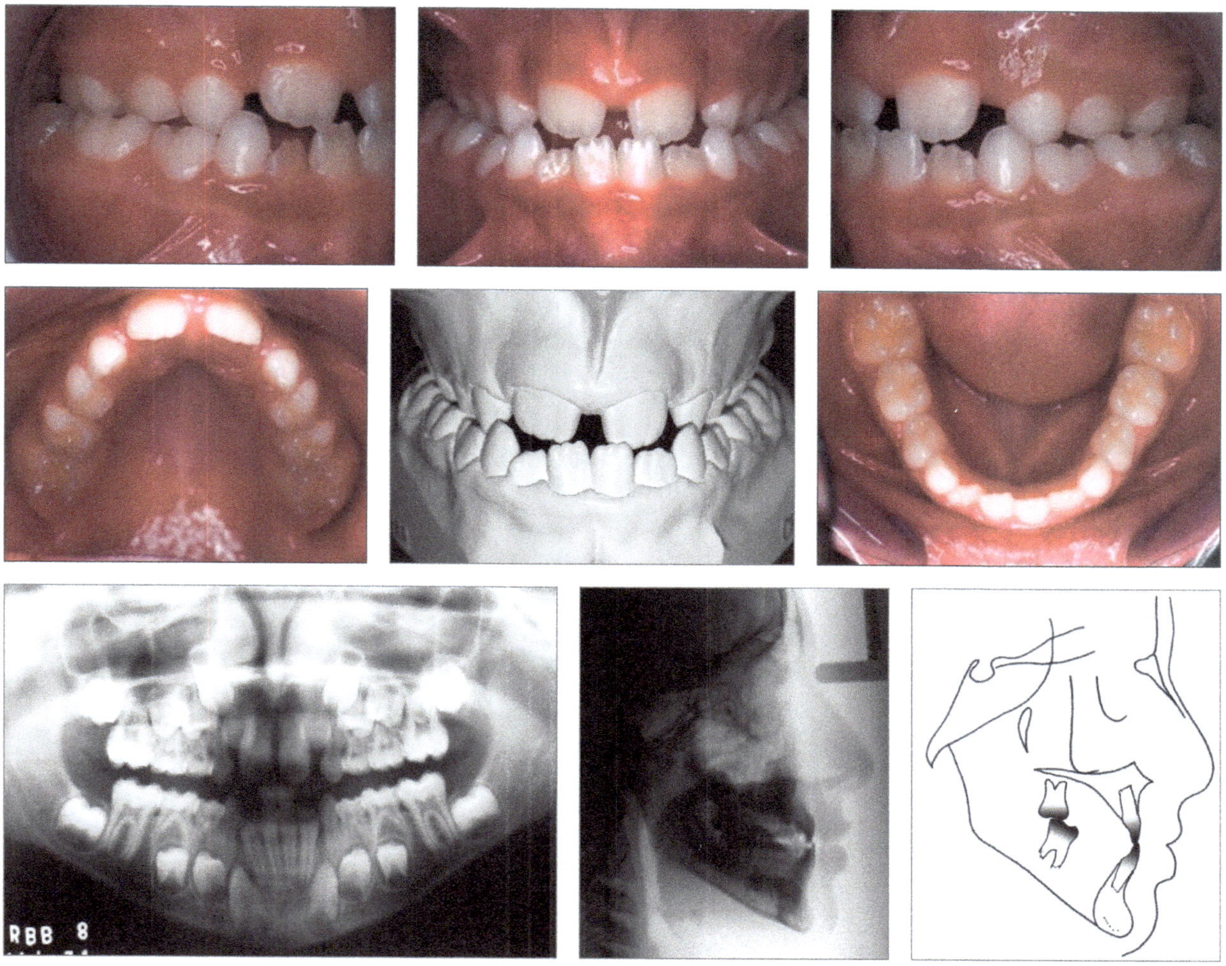


FIGURE 1: Pretreatment intraoral photographs, panoramic and cephalometric radiographs, and cephalometric tracing. Angle Class III malocclusion. Complete maxillary crossbite.

accomplished with the patient compliance in using the appliance.

This paper aims to describe the great palatal expansion obtained after RPE, in mixed dentition, with the modified Haas palatal expander in a patient with complete maxillary crossbite and, after 2 years 9 months of posttreatment follow-up, the occlusal result was stable and no skeletal relapse could be detected.

## 2. Case Report

An 8.4-year-old male patient was referred by his general practitioner. On examination, the following factors were revealed: diastema between the central incisors and lack of space for lateral incisors eruption. Radiographically, the correct sequence of eruption, skeletal Class I malocclusion (ANB = 1°), with a Class III tendency (Ao-Bo = −8 mm) and angle Class III malocclusion, vertical growth trend, and upright maxillary and mandibular incisors were noted (Figure 1 and Table 1).

*2.1. Treatment Objectives.* The purpose of phase I was to correct the complete crossbite and indirectly increase the maxillary arch perimeter. The maintenance of the E-space in the mandibular arch with a lingual holding arch was recommended. The patient and parents were instructed that an undesirable growth pattern could occur based on the cephalometric measurements (Table 1) and also due to the genetic component (his father is skeletal Class III).

*2.2. Treatment Alternatives.* In phase I, the promptly correction of complete crossbite was advised, since the patient complied with the placement, use of the expanders, and especially the oral hygiene. The Haas, HYRAX, quad-helix, and bonded expander types were explained to the patient and his father.

*2.3. Treatment Progress.* The choice was the Haas-type fixed palatal expander [3] with modification in the anterior region, due to the absence of premolars [6]. Both maxillary first permanent molars were banded and the expander was built

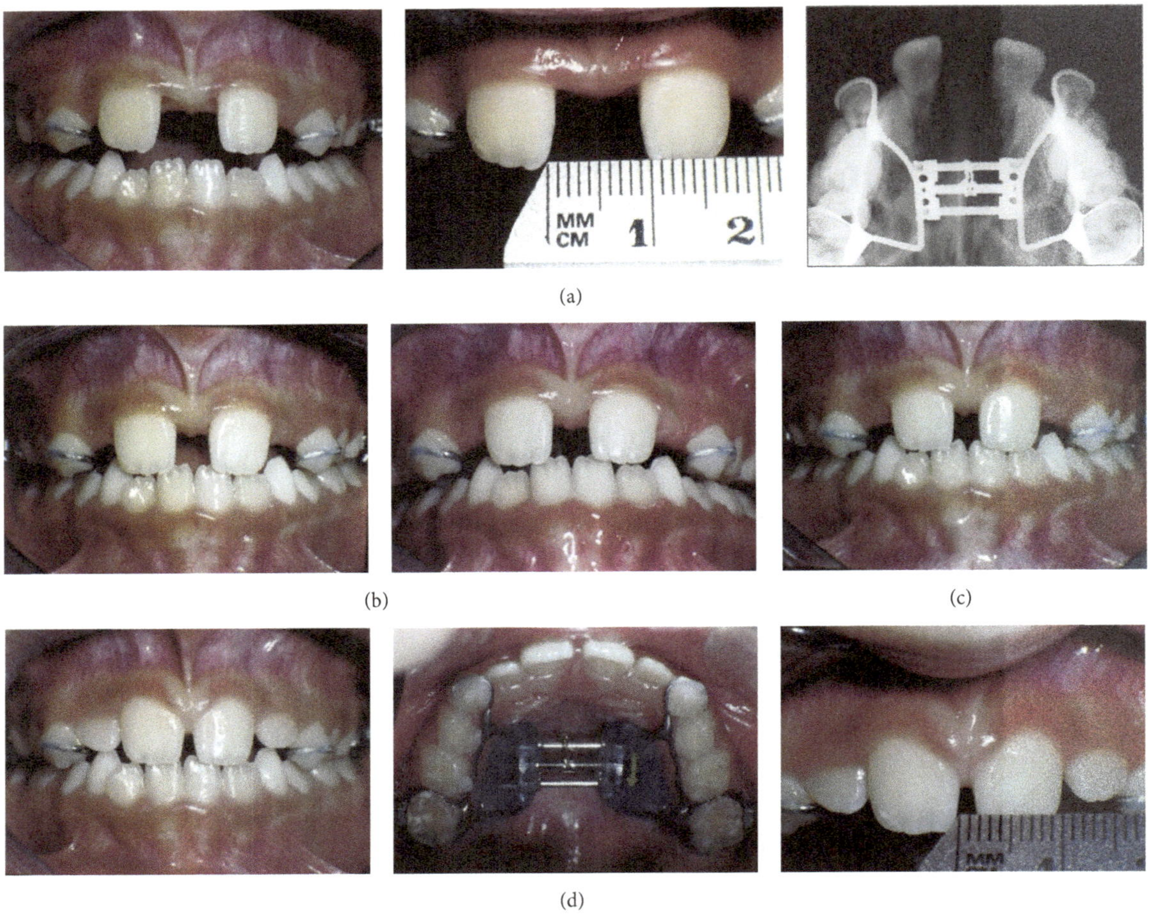


FIGURE 2: Midline diastema with clinical signs of the suture opening. Occlusal radiographs with real disjunction of the suture. (a) After three weeks and 52 screw activations. (b) 43 days and (c) and (d) 5 months and 6 months after retention. The diastema returned to the initial dimensions in the retention phase of the screw.

with the 110M series (044-001, Summit Orthodontics). The expander was cemented in the permanent molars and bonded to the deciduous molars and canines. The orientation about care (food, hygiene, and activation) was explained after the palatal expander had been fixed (Figure 2).

Activation of expansion was performed with 2-quarter turns (0.5 mm) per day until the desired overexpansion was achieved, evaluated by the diastema opening and posterior transverse relationship on clinical observation. There was a very clinically significant opening of the diastema between the maxillary central incisors of 10.0 mm after three weeks and 52 screw activations. The occlusal radiograph shows the real disjunction of the sutures. The diastema returned to the initial dimensions at the retention phase (Figure 2). The expander was maintained as a retainer for a period of 6 months. The use of the remaining E-space enabled the alignment of the anterior lower teeth (Figure 3).

*2.4. Treatment Results.* In phase I, the RPE made the correction of the posterior crossbite and, concomitantly, the anterior crossbite possible due to the proclination of the maxillary incisors and uprighting of the lower incisors. There was also a clinically significant space gain in the maxillary dental arch allowing the alignment of the lateral incisors into the occlusion line, while the perimeter of the lower arch was maintained with the lingual holding arch (Figure 3).

In phase II, at the age of 12 years 2 months, standard 0.022-in edgewise fixed appliance was recommended and the classic sequence of corrective treatment was applied with biomechanical control to minimize the proclination of the mandibular incisors. In the alignment and leveling stages, a Class III intermaxillary elastic on the left side and vertical elastics in the canine region on the right side were used to maintain and avoid canting the occlusal plane. The lingual arch was removed after the individual distalization of the premolars. Retraction and coordinated finishing arches were used. After removal of the fixed appliance, a removable wraparound type appliance in the maxillary arch and a wire segment were bonded lingually from canine to canine. The results of the alignment, leveling, and intercuspation are illustrated in Figure 4. Table 1 shows the maintenance of

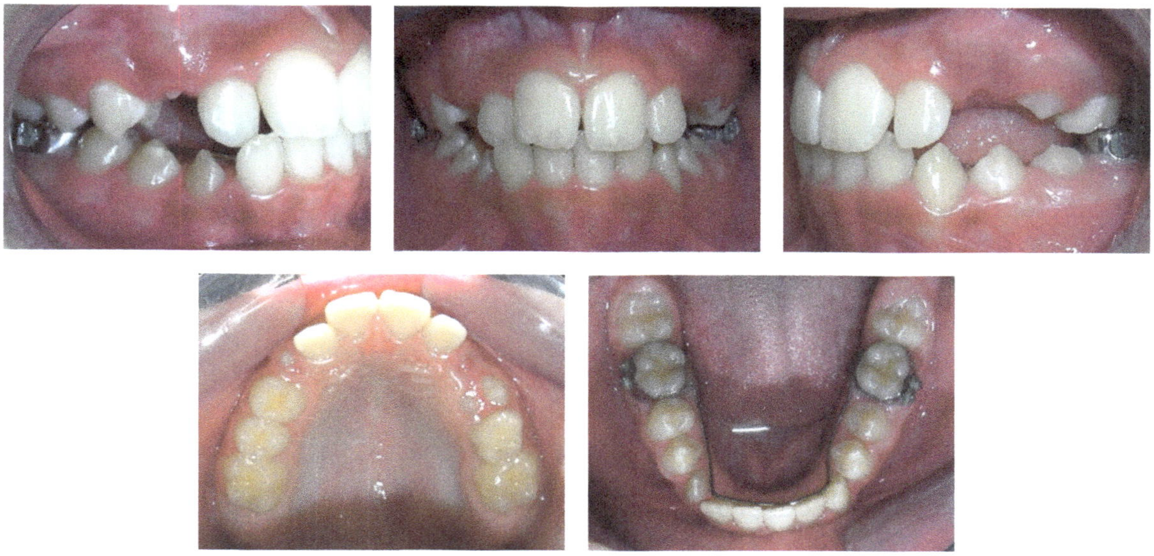

FIGURE 3: Lingual holding arch and the maintenance of the E-space.

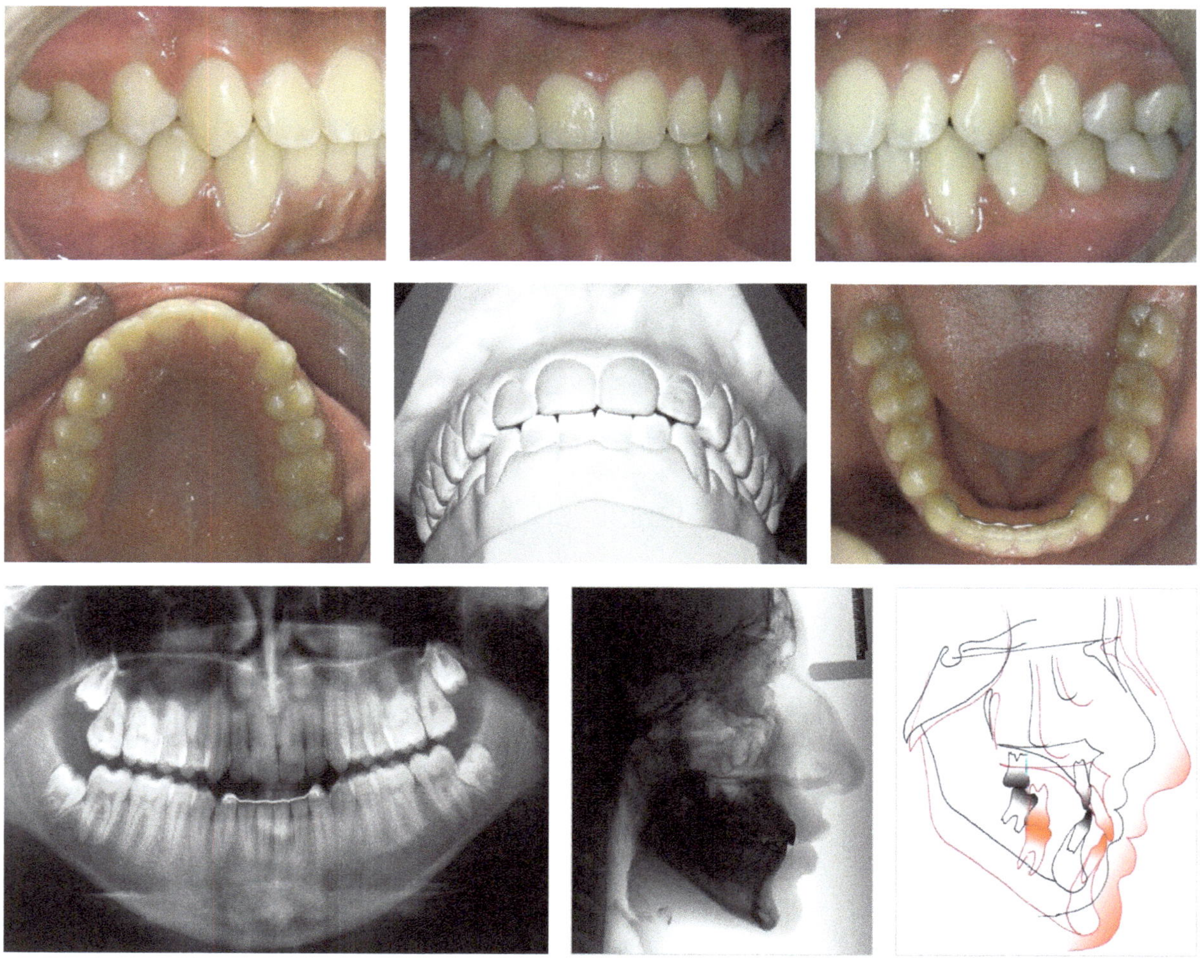

FIGURE 4: Posttreatment intraoral photographs. Good intercuspidation and adequate overjet and overbite. The skeletal and dental characteristics remained. Superimposition: pretreatment, black; posttreatment, red.

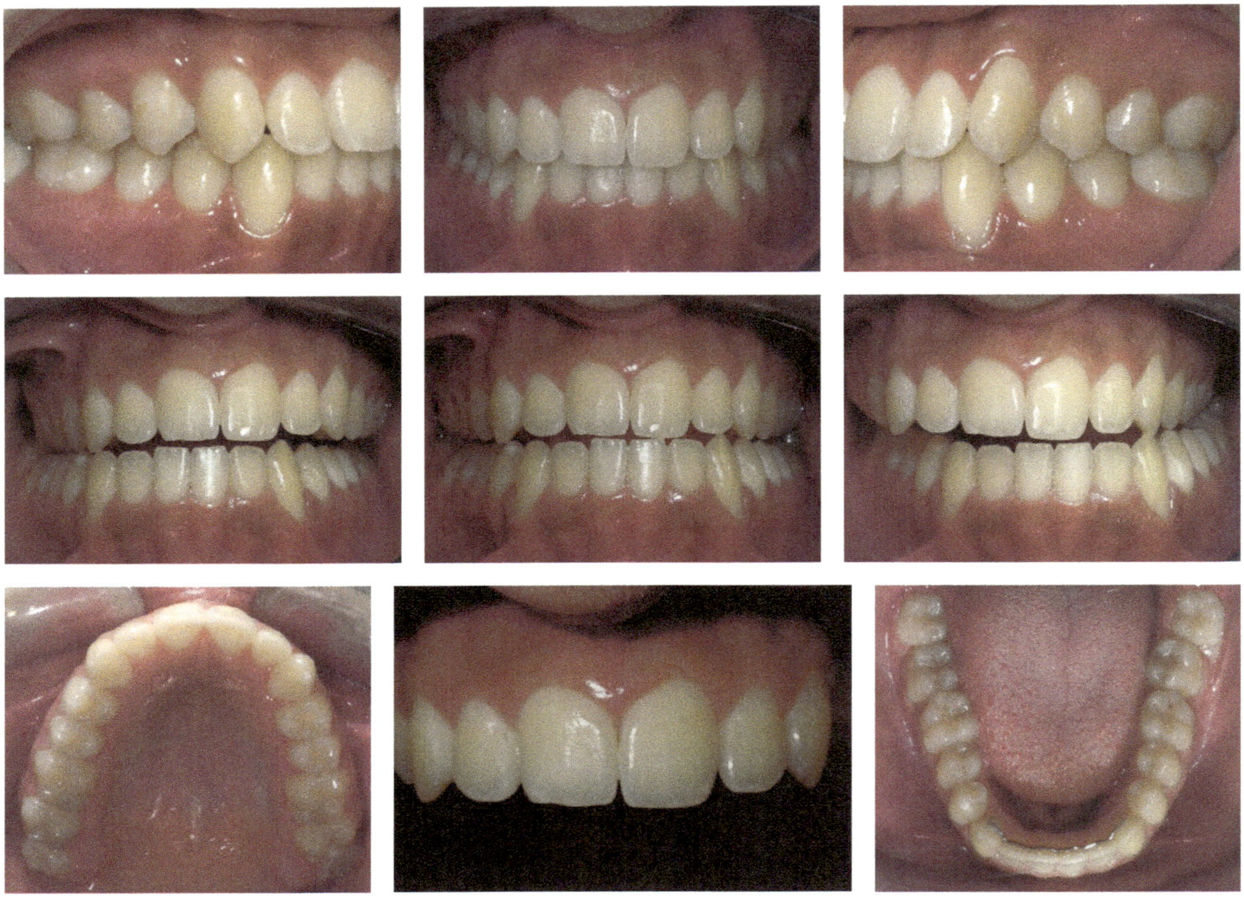

FIGURE 5: Two years nine months of posttreatment follow-up. Stability of the functional and occlusal results. Eruption of the third molars.

the skeletal pattern (ANB = 0°; Ao-Bo = −2 mm) and proclination of the maxillary incisor with the uprighting of the mandibular incisors. The patient had vertical growth favoring the stability of the occlusion.

The functional and occlusal results were fully maintained at 2 years 9 months of posttreatment follow-up. All third molars were fully erupted (Figure 5).

## 3. Discussion

In the present case report, the patient had bilateral skeletal posterior crossbite, and a modified Haas-type expansion appliance was indicated. Early correction of posterior crossbite has been recommended in order to prevent inadequate skeletal transversal growth.

This clinical case did not present any difference between centric relation and maximum intercuspation confirming the differential diagnosis of complete maxillary crossbite, so the modified Haas expansion appliance was appointed [6]. Early age correction of posterior crossbite is recommended in order to prevent improper skeletal growth and to ensure the stability of the results.

The RPE performed in this clinical case was carried out in mixed dentition and reached maximum expansion with stability of the transverse dimension. The RPE promoted skeletal and dental positive effects enabling the correction of a transverse maxillary deficiency. Indirectly, it also corrected the anterior crossbite as noted by Haas, 1961 [9], on the projection of point "A," with an increased SNA angle and an increased facial convexity angle, even if temporarily, causing the correction of the anterior crossbite. The choice of a great magnitude screw was another aspect of the clinically magnificent maxillary expansion. The maintenance of the Haas-type appliance as retention for 6 months can be considered as one of the stability factors as seen in this clinical case.

Although the correction of functional unilateral posterior crossbite can be achieved effectively at an early age with the quad-helix appliance [10] and treatment with the Haas-type expander, both are dependent on the cooperation of the patient and are in symbiosis with the diagnosis [11]. The success of the treatment is highly dependent on the degree of patient cooperation and motivation to accept unpleasant things, such as allowing adaptation, taking impressions, setting the expander, and properly brushing the teeth. They are also equally effective on the stability of the correction of posterior crossbite in increasing width and intermolar angulation [12].

Table 1: Cephalometric measurements.

| Measurements | Pretreatment 8.3 | Progress 9.7 | Posttreatment 17.2 |
|---|---|---|---|
| SNA angle (°) | 77 | 78 | 76 |
| SNB angle (°) | 76 | 78 | 76 |
| ANB angle (°) | 1 | 0 | 0 |
| Ao-Bo (mm) | −8 | −4 | −2 |
| Facial angle (°) | 86 | 88 | 87 |
| Convexity (°) | −3 | −5 | −7 |
| FMA (°) | 34 | 33 | 35 |
| GoGn-SN (°) | 43 | 40 | 41 |
| $y$-axis (°) | 61 | 59 | 61 |
| 1-NA (mm) | 2 | 5 | 8 |
| 1-NA (°) | 17 | 28 | 29 |
| 1-NB (mm) | 4 | 5 | 5 |
| 1-NB (°) | 22 | 14 | 18 |
| Interincisal angle (°) | 140 | 138 | 136 |
| $Z$-angle (°) | 71 | 71 | 75 |

In this clinical case, the activation was a 2-quarter turn a day. In theory, RPE applies a force on the posterior teeth, without giving enough time for the tooth movement to occur, so that the force is transferred to the sutures, resulting in a larger opening of the suture than teeth inclination [13]. The slow palatal expansion has advantages and disadvantages [14, 15]. Both, rapid and slow palatal expansion protocols cause buccal displacement of the first permanent maxillary molars, with more body displacement in the group with slow maxillary expansion, while more inclination in the group with RPE. Vertical and horizontal bone losses were noted in both groups; however, the slow expansion group had a great bone loss [14].

Despite the bonded expander and occlusal splint and the banded modified Haas type used in this clinical case, the response might be different. The vertical response of the posterior teeth appears to be greater in cases where the expansion was carried out without the occlusal stop [16]. This may also have favored the alignment and leveling of the lower teeth minimizing protruded maxillary incisors. The functional and esthetic results were fully achieved due to a combination of factors such as the significant arch-length perimeter, E-space optimization, vertical and sagittal proportional growth, and patient compliance.

## 4. Conclusion

The rapid palatal expansion using a modified Haas-type expander and the appropriate screw promotes positive skeletal (orthopedic) and dental (orthodontic) effects, affording, thus, the correction of a complete maxillary crossbite in mixed dentition. Favorable conditions have been provided for orthodontic treatment in permanent dentition with full braces obtaining function, facial and dental aesthetics, and the stability of the results.

## Competing Interests

The authors declare that they have no competing interests.

## References

[1] D. Allen, J. Rebellato, R. Sheats, and A. M. Ceron, "Skeletal and dental contributions to posterior crossbites," *Angle Orthodontist*, vol. 73, no. 5, pp. 515–524, 2003.

[2] G. Kutin and R. R. Hawes, "Posterior cross-bites in the deciduous and mixed dentitions," *American Journal of Orthodontics*, vol. 56, no. 5, pp. 491–504, 1969.

[3] A. J. Haas, "The treatment of maxillary deficiency by opening the midpalatal suture," *The Angle Orthodontist*, vol. 35, pp. 200–217, 1965.

[4] R. A. Wertz, "Skeletal and dental changes accompanying rapid midpalatal suture opening," *American Journal of Orthodontics*, vol. 58, no. 1, pp. 41–66, 1970.

[5] J. A. McNamara Jr., "Early intervention in the transverse dimension: is it worth the effort?" *American Journal of Orthodontics and Dentofacial Orthopedics*, vol. 121, no. 6, pp. 572–574, 2002.

[6] O. Tanaka, B. Orellana, and G. Ribeiro, "Singular aspects to operate rapid palatal expansion procedures," *Revista Dental Press de Ortodontia e Ortopedia Facial*, vol. 9, pp. 98–107, 2004.

[7] C. J. Vogel, "An interview with James A. McNamara Jr.," *Dental Press Journal of Orthodontics*, vol. 16, no. 3, pp. 32–53, 2011.

[8] F. V. Celenza, "The theory and clinical management of centric positions: II. Centric relation and centric relation occlusion," *The International Journal of Periodontics & Restorative Dentistry*, vol. 4, no. 6, pp. 62–86, 1984.

[9] A. J. Haas, "Rapid expansion of the maxillary dental arch and nasal cavity by opening the midpalatal suture," *The Angle Orthodontist*, vol. 31, no. 2, pp. 72–90, 1961.

[10] M. Figueiredo, D. Siqueira, S. Bommarito, and M. Scanavini, "The early orthodontic treatment of posterior crossbites with attachment Quad-helix," *Revista Clínica de Ortodontia Dental Press*, vol. 5, pp. 75–86, 2007.

[11] O. Tanaka, H. Maruo, and E. Camargo, "A intransponível grandeza do diagnóstico em Ortodontia," *Revista de Clínica e Pesquisa Odontológica*, vol. 1, article 3, 2004.

[12] T. Huynh, D. B. Kennedy, D. R. Joondeph, and A.-M. Bollen, "Treatment response and stability of slow maxillary expansion using Haas, hyrax, and quad-helix appliances: a retrospective study," *American Journal of Orthodontics and Dentofacial Orthopedics*, vol. 136, no. 3, pp. 331–339, 2009.

[13] A. J. Haas, "Long-term posttreatment evaluation of rapid palatal expansion," *Angle Orthodontist*, vol. 50, no. 3, pp. 189–217, 1980.

[14] M. Brunetto, J. Da Silva Pereira Andriani, G. L. U. Ribeiro, A. Locks, M. Correa, and L. R. Correa, "Three-dimensional assessment of buccal alveolar bone after rapid and slow maxillary expansion: a clinical trial study," *American Journal of Orthodontics and Dentofacial Orthopedics*, vol. 143, no. 5, pp. 633–644, 2013.

[15] R. M. A. Lima Filho and A. C. de Oliveira Ruellas, "Long-term maxillary changes in patients with skeletal Class II malocclusion treated with slow and rapid palatal expansion," *American Journal of Orthodontics and Dentofacial Orthopedics*, vol. 134, no. 3, pp. 383–388, 2008.

[16] C. L. Miller, E. A. Araújo, R. G. Behrents, D. R. Oliver, and O. M. Tanaka, "Mandibular arch dimensions following bonded and banded rapid maxillary expansion," *Journal of the World Federation of Orthodontists*, vol. 3, no. 3, pp. 119–123, 2014.

# 35

# Christ-Siemens-Touraine Syndrome: A Case Report and Review of the Literature

**Sepideh Mokhtari,[1] Saeedeh Mokhtari,[2] and Ali Lotfi[1]**

[1] *Department of Oral and Maxillofacial Pathology, Dental School of Shahid Beheshti University of Medical Sciences, Tehran 4739, Iran*
[2] *Department of of Pediatric Dentistry, Dental School of Shahid Beheshti University of Medical Sciences, Tehran 4739, Iran*

Correspondence should be addressed to Saeedeh Mokhtari, samo8889@yahoo.com

Academic Editors: W. L. Chai and S. S. De Rossi

Ectodermal dysplasia is a rare disorder with defects in two or more of the following structures: the teeth and the skin and its appendages including hair, nails, eccrine, and sebaceous glands. Anhidrotic ectodermal dysplasia is the most common type of disease. This rare disorder, also known as Christ-Siemens-Touraine syndrome, manifests as a triad of hypotrichosis, asteatosis, and anhidrosis. In view of the rarity of this entity, a classical case of anhidrotic ectodermal dysplasia is reported. We have also provided a review of recent investigations in the area of dental abnormalities in this syndrome.

## 1. Introduction

Ectodermal dysplasia (ED) is a genetic disorder that has congenital birth defects of two or more ectodermal structures. Ectodermal dysplasia is divided into two types based on the number and function of sweat glands: hidrotic ectodermal dysplasia (Clouston syndrome) and hypohidrotic (anhidrotic) ectodermal dysplasia (Christ-Siemens-Touraine syndrome) [1]. Hypohidrotic ectodermal dysplasia (HED) is an X-linked condition and is the most common form of ED. In this type of syndrome, there are no sweat glands or they are significantly decreased. HED (Christ-Siemens-Touraine syndrome) has characteristic triad of reduction in the amount of hair (hypotrichosis), absence of sebaceous glands (asteatosis), and absence of sweat glands (anhidrosis) [2]. Some cases are mild, whereas some others are severe.

Patients often show these manifestations in their appearance: depressed nasal bridge, protuberant lips, prominent supraorbital ridges, sunken cheeks, and wrinkled hyperpigmented skin around the eyes. The oral manifestations include conical or peg-shaped teeth, hypodontia or complete anodontia in both deciduous and permanent dentition, malformation of present teeth, generalized spacing, delayed eruption of permanent teeth, underdeveloped alveolar ridges, and high palatal arch or a cleft palate. Hypoplasia of salivary glands and the absence of oral accessory glands are also present and result in xerostomia and dry cracked lips [1, 3]. In view of the rarity of this syndrome, here, a classical case of anhidrotic ectodermal dysplasia is reported. We have also provided a review of recent investigations in the area of dental abnormalities in this syndrome.

## 2. Case Presentation

A 7-year old boy presented with the chief complaint of difficulty in mastication and lack of esthetics. On general examination, he had sparse, thin, light, blond hair over the scalp, scanty eyebrow and eyelashes, depressed nasal bridge, frontal bossing, and prominent supraorbital ridges. Lips were dry, everted, and prominent. The skin was dry and wrinkled. Hyper pigmentation was evident around the eyes (Figure 1), and plantar dyskeratosis was also present (Figure 2). Oral examination revealed partial anodontia, hypoplastic conical teeth, and delayed eruption of permanent dentition (Figure 3). Panoramic radiograph showed four cone-shaped crowns suggestive of primary canines. Maxillary primary molars and incisors were also present. There was some evidence of tooth formation in both jaws and eight tooth buds

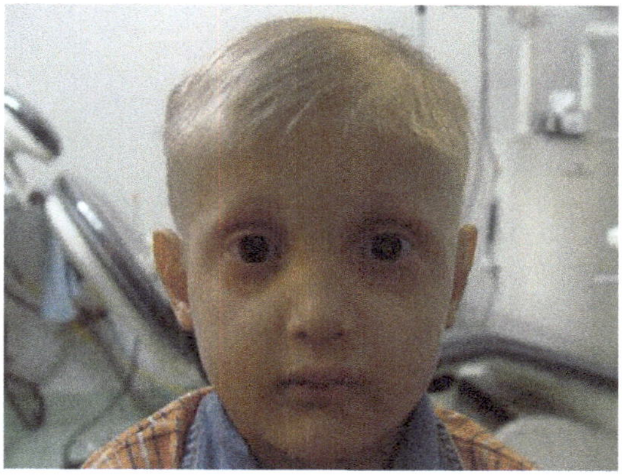

FIGURE 1: Clinical examination of the patient reveals fine sparse scalp hair, eyebrows, and eyelashes with wrinkled hyperpigmented skin around the eyes.

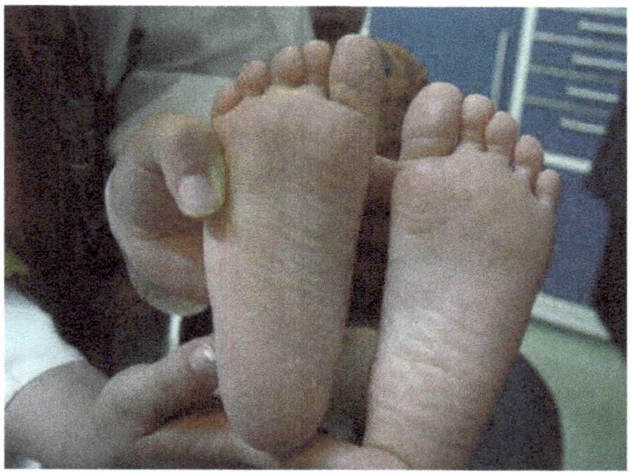

FIGURE 2: Plantar dyskeratosis is present.

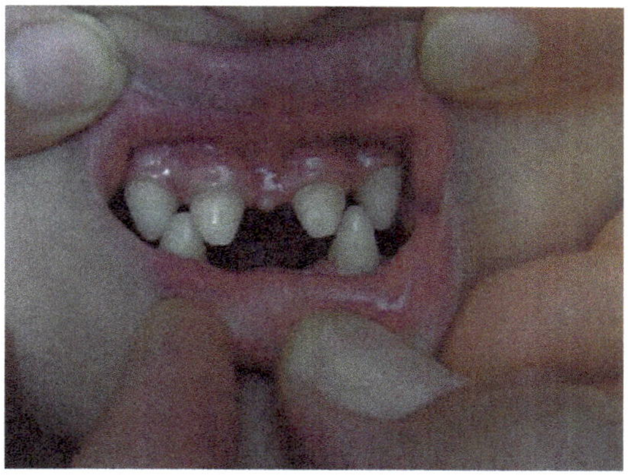

FIGURE 3: Teeth are reduced in number and are conical in shape.

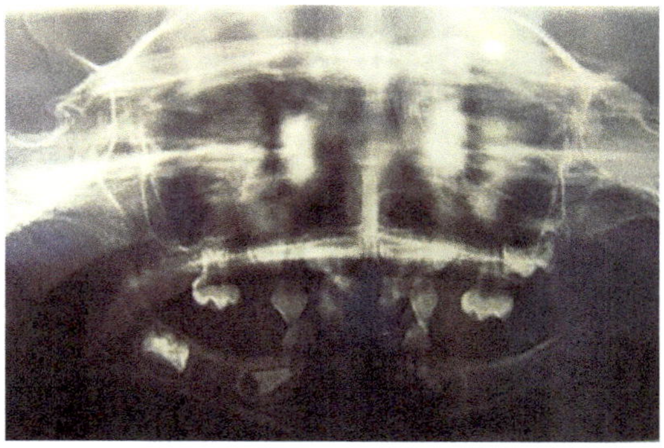

FIGURE 4: Panoramic radiograph shows eight erupted teeth of primary dentition and eight tooth buds.

probably related to the permanent canines, and first molars and maxillary incisors were present. However, hypodontia in the right and left side was asymmetric, and mandible had more missing teeth than maxilla (Figure 4). He had no nail dystrophy, and his intelligence was normal. His mother stated that her child had recurrent episodes of unexplained hyperpyrexia and thirst; he was not able to sweat, and she had to apply some precautions to protect him from overheating during physical exertion or warm weather. The child was born of nonconsanguineous marriage. Nobody in his family had similar presentations. The child was diagnosed as a case of Christ-Siemens-Touraine syndrome. However, he did not accept to undergo any genetic testing. We considered a removable partial denture as the best treatment option for the child, and so he was referred to a prosthodontist to receive professional prosthodontic procedures.

## 3. Discussion

This patient was a case of Christ-Siemens-Touraine syndrome with the typical presentation of disease in his face and oral cavity. Hypohidrotic ED (Christ-Siemens-Touraine syndrome) is the most frequent form of ectodermal dysplasia, and genetic defects in ectodysplasin signal transduction pathways are the basis of this syndrome. Epithelial cells in hair follicles, eccrine sweat glands, and developing teeth use this pathway during morphogenesis. Therefore, genetic defects result in aplasia, hypoplasia, or dysplasia of these structures. They also lead to disturbances in the enamel matrix and tooth buds and subsequent hypodontia and hypoplasia of teeth [2]. Mutations in the gene Ectodysplasin-A (EDA) underlie X-linked recessive inheritance, which is the most common form of HED. Mutations in the gene Ectodysplasin-A receptor (EDAR) and Ectodysplasin-A Receptor-Associated Adapter (EDARADD) are also responsible for the rare autosomal dominant and autosomal recessive forms [1, 2].

The X-linked recessive HED has full expression in males. Female carriers are more than affected men, but they have little or no signs of the condition and their clinical identification is difficult. However, some investigations have shown that the heterozygous females have a significantly high frequency of agenesis of permanent teeth. They also present an increased prevalence of tooth malformations and reduced tooth size, especially in the mesiodistal dimension [3].

Recently, Zhang et al. have described some correlations between the phenotypes and genotypes of X-linked HED and nonsyndromic hypodontia subjects. They suggested that nonsyndromic hypodontia is probably a variable expression of X-linked HED [4]. Significant differences in the number of primary missing teeth have been detected between X-Linked HED and autosomal recessive HED in recent investigations [5].

Congenital missing of third molars and maxillary lateral incisors is the most common missing. Complete anodontia of both deciduous and permanent dentition is rarely reported. Açikgöz et al. reported the absence of all primary and permanent teeth except the bilaterally unerupted maxillary permanent canines. This shows that the permanent tooth can develop in the absence of its predecessor [6]. Many HED patients also exhibit a relative enlargement of the pulp with various degrees of taurodontism [7].

Even in the case of complete anodontia, the general facial growth pattern is normal in these children. This implies that the development of the jaw does not depend to the presence of teeth. Nevertheless, the alveolar process does not develop in the absence of teeth, and the vertical dimension is reduced, which explains the protuberant everted appearance of lips in these patients [1]. In this case, missing teeth were more in the mandible than in the maxilla. Therefore, the underdevelopment of alveolar process in mandible was more evident in clinical and radiographic features.

Alterations in bone structure, such as hyperdensity of medullary bone, have been found in mandibular symphysis area and other jaw locations of these patients. Although changes in the alveolar bone can be related to oligodontia, changes in the bone structure seem to be tooth independent and suggest a direct effect of genetic defect on bone formation and/or remodeling in this syndrome [1].

If hypohidrosis is managed appropriately, the prognosis for most patients will be very good. Treatment of these children is protecting them from high temperature. In most cases, the preferred treatment option for dental disorders is a removable partial denture, which could also be associated with direct composite restorations. This allows the child to have adequate nutrition, normal appearance, and speech with significant psychosocial benefits. When child reaches teenage years, orthodontic treatment will prepare the mouth for a fixed partial denture or implants in future. In some patients, alveolar ridges are severely hypotrophic due to oligo- or anodontia. This can seriously affect a young person physically and psychologically. In these cases, augmentation of jaws by the use of bicortical corticocancellous bone blocks from hip and delayed implant placement seems to be a suitable treatment option [8]. Immediate loading has also been applied successfully in patients with ectodermal dysplasia [9]. Anesthetic problem is rarely reported in this syndrome [10].

Dentists are often the first who diagnose these patients. Therefore, they should be aware of the clinical manifestations of this syndrome. This will be helpful in proper diagnosis, early interventions, and appropriate therapies for these patients.

## Conflict of Interests

The authors confirm that there is no conflict of interests for this paper.

## References

[1] H. Lesot, F. Clauss, M. C. Manière, and M. Schmittbuhl, "Consequences of X-linked hypohidrotic ectodermal dysplasia for the human jaw bone," *Frontiers of Oral Biology*, vol. 13, pp. 93–99, 2009.

[2] G. Balci, S. Z. Baskan, and S. Akdenizi, "Ectodermal dysplasia: report of four cases and review of literature," *International Dental and Medical Disorders*, vol. 1, pp. 56–59, 2008.

[3] M. O. Lexner, A. Bardow, J. M. Hertz, L. A. Nielsen, and S. Kreiborg, "Anomalies of tooth formation in hypohidrotic ectodermal dysplasia," *International Journal of Paediatric Dentistry*, vol. 17, no. 1, pp. 10–18, 2007.

[4] J. Zhang, D. Han, S. Song et al., "Correlation between the phenotypes and genotypes of X-linked hypohidrotic ectodermal dysplasia and non-syndromic hypodontia caused by ectodysplasin-A mutations," *European Journal of Medical Genetics*, vol. 54, no. 4, pp. e377–e382, 2011.

[5] F. Clauss, N. Chassaing, A. Smahi et al., "X-linked and autosomal recessive hypohidrotic ectodermal dysplasia: genotypic-dental phenotypic findings," *Clinical Genetics*, vol. 78, no. 3, pp. 257–266, 2010.

[6] A. Açikgöz, O. Kademoglu, S. Elekdag-Türk, and F. Karagöz, "Hypohidrotic ectodermal dysplasia with true anodontia of the primary dentition," *Quintessence International*, vol. 38, no. 10, pp. 853–858, 2007.

[7] C. I. Gros, F. Clauss, F. Obry, M. C. Manière, and M. Schmittbuhl, "Quantification of taurodontism: interests in the early diagnosis of hypohidrotic ectodermal dysplasia," *Oral Diseases*, vol. 16, no. 3, pp. 292–298, 2010.

[8] R. Kirmeier, C. Gluhak, P. Marada, W. A. Wegscheider, A. Eskici, and N. Jakse, "Oral rehabilitation of adult twins with severe lack of bone due to hypohidrotic ectodermal dysplasia—a 12-month follow-up," *Journal of Oral and Maxillofacial Surgery*, vol. 67, no. 1, pp. 189–194, 2009.

[9] A. D'Ambrosio, A. Cioffi, A. Cirillo, and G. Sammartino, "Immediate loading in ectodermal dysplasia: clinical case," *Journal of Oral and Maxillofacial Surgery*, vol. 69, no. 9, pp. 2351–2356, 2011.

[10] R. Kuriakose and M. Balakrishnan, "Anesthetic problems in Christ Siemens Touraine syndrome—a case report," *Middle East Journal of Anesthesiology*, vol. 18, no. 3, pp. 647–650, 2005.

# 36

# Immediate Esthetic Rehabilitation of Periodontally Compromised Anterior Tooth Using Natural Tooth as Pontic

**K. Pavan Kumar, Surya Kumari Nujella, S. Sujatha Gopal, and K. Karthik Roy**

*Conservative Dentistry & Endodontics, MNR Dental College and Hospital, Sangareddy, Telangana 522094, India*

Correspondence should be addressed to K. Karthik Roy; kkarthikroy@gmail.com

Academic Editor: Andrea Scribante

For patients who require removal of anterior teeth and their replacement various treatment modalities are available. With advancement in technology and availability of glass/polyethylene fibres, use of natural tooth as pontic with fibre reinforced composite restorations offers the promising results. The present case report describes management of periodontally compromised mandibular anterior tooth using natural tooth pontic with fibre reinforcement. A 1-year follow-up showed that the bridge was intact with good esthetics and no problem was reported.

## 1. Introduction

Dentists occasionally face complex situations that warrant removal of teeth from high esthetic zone. Despite wide range of treatment options that can be provided to conserve the tooth, extraction of an single anterior tooth is inevitable in case of trauma, advanced periodontal disease, root resorption, or failed endodontic therapy [1]. Following loss of the anterior tooth, it is important that an immediate replacement is provided in order to avoid esthetic, masticatory, and phonetic difficulties and to maintain the edentulous space [2]. Also the missing anterior tooth will have serious psychological implications on the patients. The treatment options for such situations should include the immediate replacement of the missing tooth which has to fulfil the cosmetic demands and functional needs and should be conservative, minimally invasive, biocompatible with permitting of oral hygiene maintenance.

Conventionally, the solution to this clinical problem has been the provision of a single tooth, removable temporary acrylic prosthesis, implants, or resin bonded bridges [3, 4]. Each method has its own advantages, disadvantages with varying levels of patient acceptance. Using the natural tooth as a pontic in this scenario has advantages of being the right size, shape, and color with a high level of patient acceptance due to the positive psychological value of using his or her natural tooth [5]. However use of natural tooth as pontic is not new technique; it was described 35 years earlier [6]. Despite the advantages of this clinical approach, it does not seem to be widespread in daily dental practice due to the compromised results over long a period of time. With the utilisation of newly advent fibre reinforcement technique use of natural tooth as pontic provides promising results. The present case report describes using natural tooth as pontic with fibre reinforcement.

## 2. Case Report

A 30-year-old healthy male patient reported to the Department of Conservative Dentistry and Endodontics, MNR Dental College and Hospital, with a chief complaint of the mobility of mandibular leftcentral incisor. Upon clinical examination tooth was grade III mobile one with probing depth of 8 mm. Diagnostic radiograph of the tooth revealed bone loss around the mandibular left central incisor (Figure 1). The diagnosis was chronic localized periodontal disease. All the possible treatment modalities were explained to the patient. As the patient was highly concerned with esthetics, the possibility of using the clinical crown as a natural pontic was proposed.

The tooth was extracted under local anaesthesia atraumatically (Figures 2 and 3) and haemostasis was achieved. The length of the natural tooth pontic was determined by measuring the distance from incisal edge of central incisor

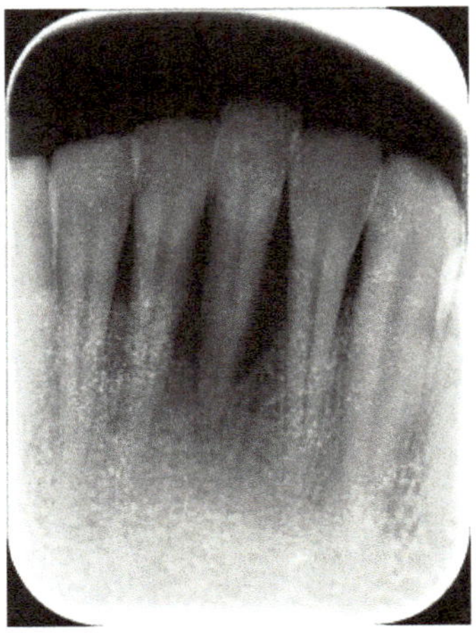

Figure 1: Preoperative radiograph.

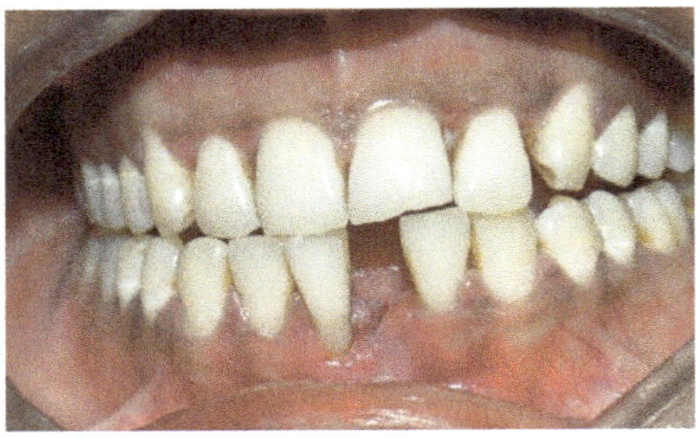

Figure 2: Atraumatic extraction.

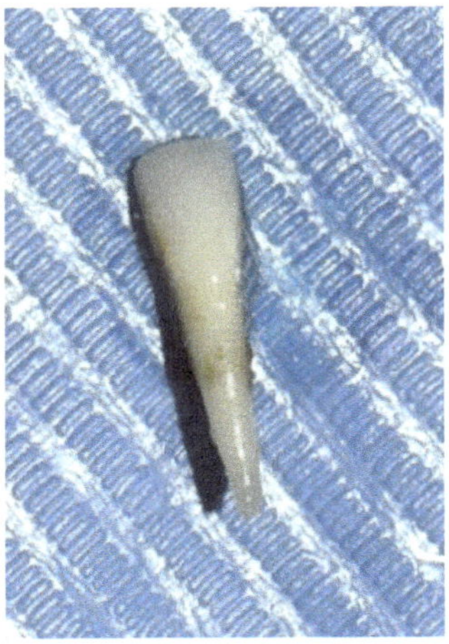

Figure 3: Extracted tooth.

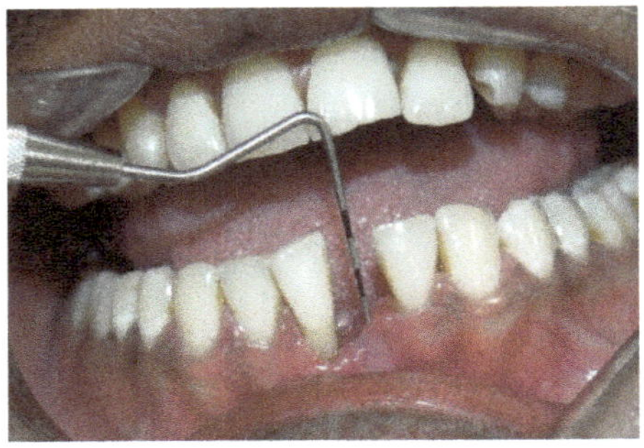

Figure 4: Space measurement for pontic.

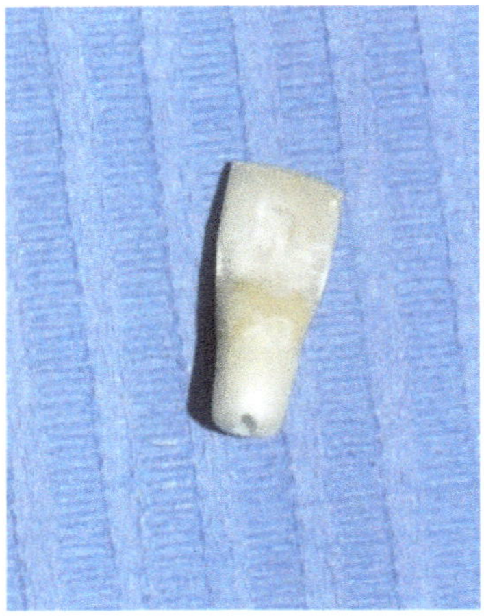

Figure 5: Pontic preparation.

to the extraction site with periodontal probe (Figure 4). An additional 2 mm length was added to the pontic to compensate for the gingival recession during healing phase. The tooth was sectioned (Figure 5) to the measured length and root canal was instrumented and debrided retrogradely. Copious irrigation with 5.25% of sodium hypochlorite was done to dissolve any pulpal remnants, if present. The canal was dried with the paper points and then sealed with flowable composite resin (G-ænial flo GC America). A modified ridge lap shape was given to the cervical area of the pontic as it provides both oral hygiene and esthetics [5].

The required length of fibre strip (everStick crown and bridge material, Stick Tech Ltd., Finland) was measured and cut. Recess grooves were prepared on the lingual surface of pontic and adjacent abutment teeth were roughened. The natural tooth pontic was stabilized with flowable composite resin (G-ænial Universal flo GC America) on the facial surface and the wedge was placed to preserve the interdental space. Prepared surface was acid etched; bonding agent was applied and cured. A thin layer of flowable composite (G-ænial Universal flo GC America) was placed across the grooves and abutment teeth. Precut fibre was then placed in position and pressed into the prepared grooves for its close adaptation and cured (Figure 6). A further layer of composite was dispensed on the surface of fibre and cured, ensuring that all of the fibre surface was covered by composite and not exposed directly to the oral cavity. Excess composite resin was removed and occlusal interferences were again checked in protrusion and lateral excursions. Finishing and polishing were done to remove any rough surface, if present which might result in plaque retention. Immediate postoperative radiograph (Figure 7) and photographs were taken (Figures 8 and 9). Patient was recalled after every 3 months for the postoperative evaluation. A 1-year evaluation showed that

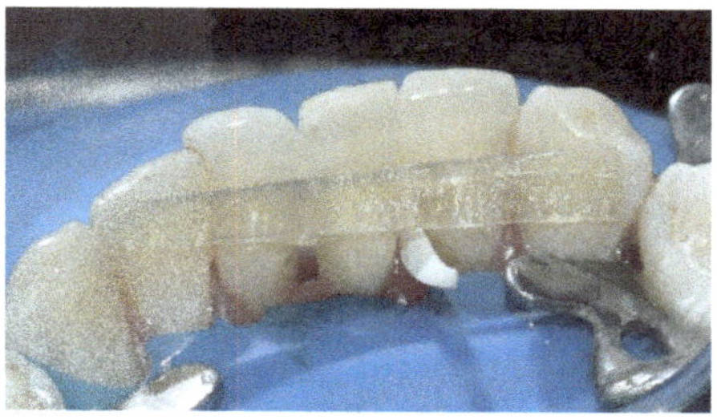

Figure 6: Trial placement of fibre.

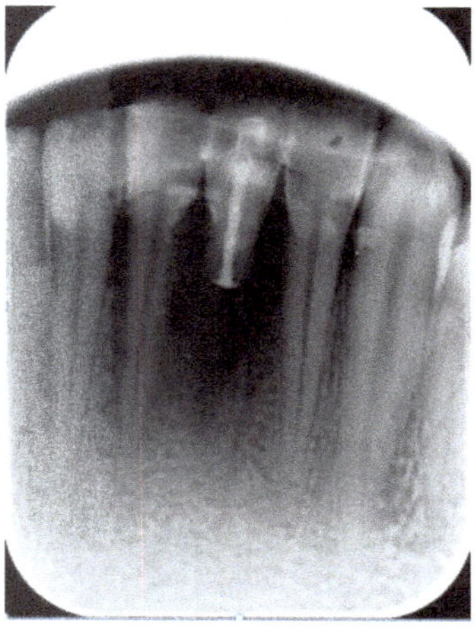

Figure 7: Postoperative radiograph.

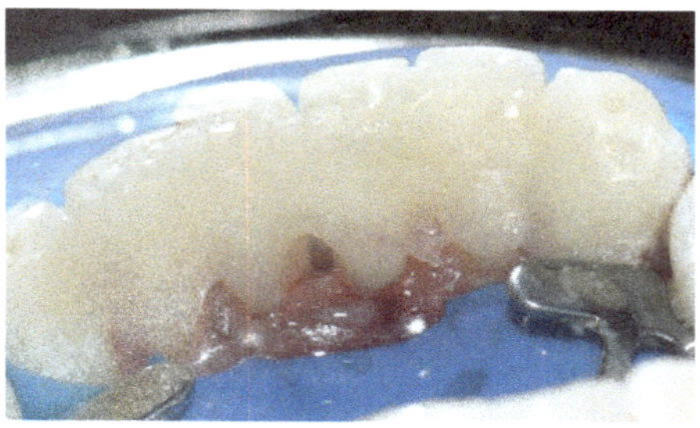

Figure 8: Postoperative palatal view.

the bridge was intact with good esthetics and no problem was reported (Figure 10).

## 3. Discussion

Various treatment options were available for the replacement of edentulous space created as a result of removal of single tooth in anterior esthetic zone. Each option has its own advantages and disadvantages. Acrylic removable partial dentures which can be placed immediately after the tooth are extracted. But they may be bulky, unesthetic, uncomfortable for the patient and inadequately preserve the extraction socket which may impede healing result in loss of soft and hard tissues [7]. The Fixed Partial Dentures (FPD) are widely proposed treatment option in such case due to their

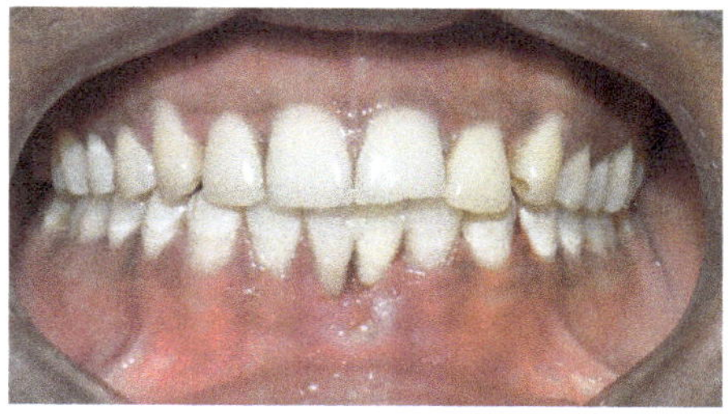

Figure 9: Immediate postoperative photograph.

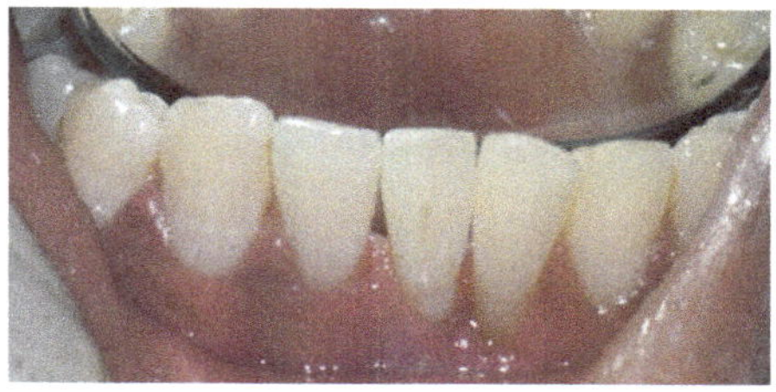

Figure 10: Recall visit, 1 year.

high strength and esthetic appearance compared to removal dentures. But they require aggressive tooth preparation of adjacent tooth for abudment, which may pose a high risk for pulp exposure especially in lower anterior teeth. Implant supported prostheses are more conservative in nature and first line of treatment. But they are more invasive, traumatic, and expensive. Moreover in this particular scenario compromised periodontal condition may compromise the long term prognosis and also does not match patients financial condition.

The use of natural tooth as a pontic was described in literature long back. However in those earlier days these pontics were connected to the adjacent teeth with adhesive composite resins, wire, metal mesh, nylon mesh, and cast metal frameworks bonded to the adjacent teeth. The inherent problems with these materials were their inability to be chemically incorporated into the composite resin and they could not support the repeated loading stresses placed on the bridge during normal and parafunction. When the thickness of composite resin used for bonding was increased it resulted in an increase in food and plaque retention subsequently poor oral hygiene [8]. Also due to low fracture strength of the bonded composite resin, if pontic debonds unexpectedly will results in an unpleasant social situation.

This challenge to place a thin but strong, bondable composite resin bridge was met with introduction of fibre reinforcement by creating a chemical bond between the strengthening fibre and composite [9, 10]. These materials have similar elasticity to dentin, thus distributing the mechanical stress concentrated within the connector to a wider area and diminishing the risk of failure.

EverStick crown and bridge fibre (Stick Tech Ltd., Finland) consist of individual silane glass fibres. The fibres are locked to each other with linear polymers (PMMA) and cross-linking monomers (bis-GMA) to form unique and patented Interpenetrating Polymer Network or IPN structure. IPN ensures both micromechanical and chemical bonding of everStick fibres to composites, adhesives, or composite cements. The bond strength is based on the ability of the polymer matrix to partially dissolve in the resin used for bonding. The significance of this is that surfaces can be reactivated even after final polymerisation. This reactivation dissolves linear polymers and forms new chemical bonds. The resin can also penetrate deeper into the fibre matrix which improves the micromechanical retention. With these crown and bridge fibres it was possible to produce a thin but strong, composite resin bonded bridge in a single visit. This prosthesis has been referred to as Resin Bonded Fibre Reinforced Composite Fixed Partial Denture or FRC FPD. These bridges show rigidity and flexural strength 7 times that of composite resin alone [11].

## 4. Conclusion

The use of fibre composite to bond natural tooth to adjacent teeth in case of isolated single tooth loss appears to be promising treatment option in immediate esthetic rehabilitation. The advantages of natural tooth pontic are its excellent shade matching, life-like translucency, and patients superior psychological acceptance.

## Conflict of Interests

The authors declare that there is no conflict of interests.

## References

[1] A. Parolia, K. M. Shenoy, M. S. Thomas, and M. Mohan, "Use of a natural tooth crown as a pontic following cervical root fracture: a case report," *Australian Endodontic Journal*, vol. 36, no. 1, pp. 35–38, 2010.

[2] A. T. Ulusoy and Z. C. Cehreli, "Provisional use of a natural tooth crown following failure of replantation: a case report," *Dental Traumatology*, vol. 24, no. 1, pp. 96–99, 2008.

[3] C. G. Daly and E. J. Wilkinson, "Use of patient's natural crown as the pontic in a composite resin-retained temporary bridge," *Australian Dental Journal*, vol. 28, no. 5, pp. 301–303, 1983.

[4] M. Ashley and V. Holden, "An immediate adhesive bridge using the natural tooth," *British Dental Journal*, vol. 184, no. 1, pp. 18–20, 1998.

[5] S. Bhargava, R. Namdev, S. Dutta, and R. Tiwari, "Immediate fixed temporization with a natural tooth crown pontic following failure of replantation," *Contemporary Clinical Dentistry*, vol. 2, no. 3, pp. 226–229, 2011.

[6] C. B. Jenkins, "Etch-retained anterior pontics. A 4-year study," *British Dental Journal*, vol. 144, no. 7, pp. 206–208, 1978.

[7] T. Tüzüner, A. Kuşgöz, and B. G. Nur, "Temporary management of permanent central incisors loss caused by trauma in primary dentition with natural crowns: a case report," *Dental Traumatology*, vol. 25, no. 5, pp. 522–526, 2009.

[8] R. P. Pollack, "Non-crown and bridge stabilization of severely mobile, periodontally involved teeth. A 25-year perspective," *Dental Clinics of North America*, vol. 43, no. 1, pp. 77–103, 1999.

[9] H. E. Strassler, D. Taler, and L. Sensi, *Single Visit Natural Tooth Pontic Bridge with Fiber Reinforcement Ribbon*, Oral Health, North York, Canada, 2007.

[10] A. Chafaie and R. Portier, "Anterior fiber-reinforced composite bridge," *Pediatric Dentistry*, vol. 26, pp. 530–534, 2004.

[11] A. J. Goldberg and M. A. Freilich, "An innovative Pre-impregnated glass fiber for reinforcing composites," *Dental Clinics of North America*, vol. 43, no. 1, pp. 127–133, 1999.

# Gingival Overgrowth Leading to the Diagnosis of Familial Tuberous Sclerosis Complex

**Parth Purwar,[1,2] Sagar Sareen,[1] Vaibhav Sheel,[1] Abhishek Gupta,[3] Uzma Ansari,[1] Patel Umeshbhai Becharbhai,[1] Manisha Dixit,[1] Amitesh Bhargava,[1] Rajiv Ratan Singh Yadav,[4] Utkarsh Bansal,[5] and Jaya Dixit[1]**

[1]*Department of Periodontology, Faculty of Dental Sciences, King George's Medical University, Lucknow, Uttar Pradesh, India*
[2]*Ankur Diagnostic Center, Lakhimpur Road, Gola Gokaran Nath, Kheri, Uttar Pradesh 262802, India*
[3]*Department of Community Medicine, Hind Institute of Medical Sciences, Barabanki, Uttar Pradesh, India*
[4]*Emergency Medicine, Dr. Ram Manohar Lohia Institute of Medical Sciences, Uttar Pradesh, India*
[5]*Department of Paediatrics, Hind Institute of Medical Sciences, Barabanki, Uttar Pradesh, India*

Correspondence should be addressed to Parth Purwar; parth_94151@yahoo.com

Academic Editor: Yuk-Kwan Chen

Tuberous sclerosis complex (TSC), a neurocutaneous syndrome, is characterized by the development of benign tumours affecting different body systems. We herein present a report of a 40-year-old female patient presenting with dental enamel pits and localized gingival overgrowth that eventually lead to the diagnosis of a case of familial TSC. Diagnosis of familial TSC by comprehensive oral examination and detection of oral manifestations proved to be inevitable as it resulted in institution of appropriate treatment strategies and genetic counselling of the affected family.

## 1. Introduction

Tuberous sclerosis complex (TSC) shows variable clinical expressivity with oral manifestations observed in less than 10% of the cases and familial inheritance pattern perceived in only 30% of the cases reported [1, 2]. The most commonly noted oral manifestations in TSC are presence of oral fibromas, gingival hyperplasia, and enamel hypoplasia in the form of dental enamel pitting. This case highlights the importance of oral manifestations in the diagnosis of a case of familial TSC.

## 2. Case Presentation

A 40-year-old female patient reported to the Department of Periodontology of King George's Medical University, Lucknow, in April 2015, with a chief complaint of painless gingival overgrowth in left upper posterior teeth region (Figure 1). On further elaboration of her complaint she revealed that initially the overgrowth was localized and freely movable. However, in last 6 months, the growth has progressively increased in size with involvement of multiple teeth leading to compromised aesthetics and poor masticatory efficiency.

On thorough physical examination the propositor did not show any signs or symptoms of cardiovascular, endocrine, respiratory, immune, or musculoskeletal disorders. On further elaboration of the medical history, the propositor's elder brother revealed occurrence of sporadic epileptic episodes since childhood with eventual reoccurrences occasionally which was treated with irregular use of antiseizure drugs. Upon extra oral examination some nodular lesions were also seen around the nasal and perinasal area. On intraoral examination a localized diffuse gingival overgrowth involving marginal, papillary, and attached labial gingiva was seen extending from the left maxillary premolar to left maxillary canine. The overlying gingiva was pink, nonerythematous, and of semifirm consistency with loss of stippling. Some form of enamel hypoplasia/pitting on vestibular surface of upper anterior teeth was also observed which further jeopardized her esthetics. The propositor's attendant also gave history

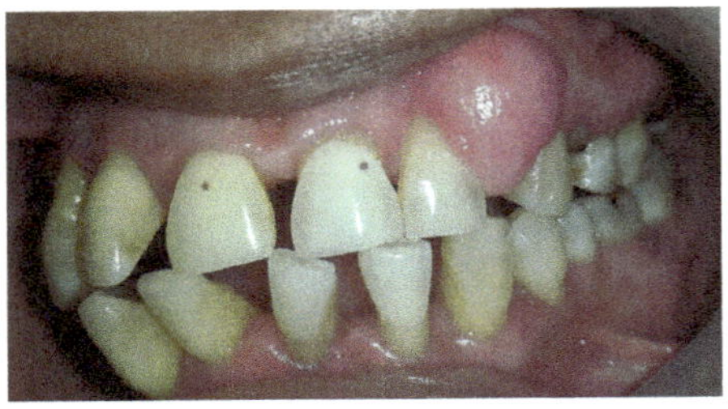

FIGURE 1: Preoperative facial view showing gingival overgrowth in upper left premolar region.

of delayed eruption of the permanent teeth. The propositor also disclosed that she had been a tobacco chewer since her teenage years. Based on the clinical presentation and history of intake of antiseizure drugs a provisional diagnosis of drug induced gingival overgrowth was made and a tailored treatment plan was constituted which included institution of oral hygiene instructions and initiation of phase I periodontal therapy. During second recall visit, on reviewing the patient history, the sporadic use of antisiezure drugs made us think on the lines of associated syndromic conditions.

On reexamining the patient, the comorbid appearance of small enamel pits (Figure 2) and gingival overgrowth indicated the possible clinical working hypothesis of tuberous sclerosis complex (TSC). Comprehensive dermatological examination was performed to look for the cutaneous manifestations, if any, to potentiate the clinical diagnosis of TSC. Examination by dermatologist revealed presence of nodular lesions in nasal and perinasal area which appeared in a characteristic butterfly fashion (Figure 3). Further questioning also revealed that other family members of the propositor had similar lesions on face and were later on invited to undergo oral and dermatological examination to confirm the familial nature of the disease. Six members of the family who were in direct blood relation including her father and brother showed ungual lesions, hypopigmented macules in perinasal area, and dental enamel pits on upper front teeth. The familial findings indicated an autosomal dominant inheritance pattern of the disease in the present case. To further affirm the diagnosis, the propositor was submitted to the imaging analysis. Ultrasonography of abdomen showed viscera to be normal; however both the kidneys were poorly visualized. Furthermore, computed tomography (CT) of whole abdomen showed that both the kidneys were totally replaced by heterogeneous mass lesion showing fat components and thick septations. The affection was found to be more prominent in the left kidney than in the right one. The renal lesion in left side measured approx 18 × 15 cm while right renal mass measured 9 × 7 cm. Only small renal parenchyma was appreciated at the lower pole of both the kidneys. A written informed consent for the photographs being used was taken from the patient.

Based on the clinical and radiological findings along with the familial inheritance pattern the diagnosis of autosomal dominant tuberous sclerosis complex (TSC) was established consisting of a triad of bilateral renal angiomyolipoma,

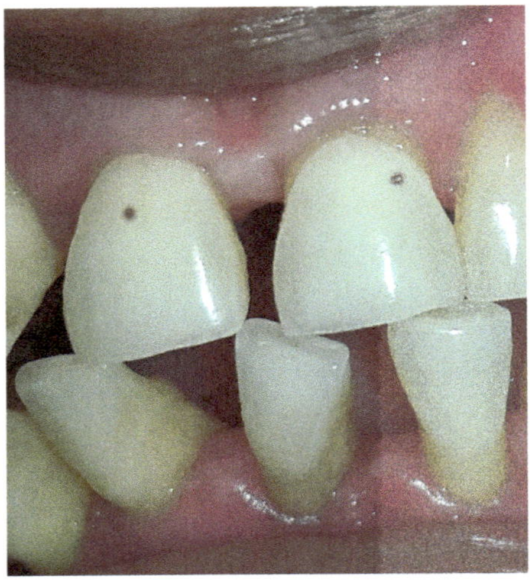

FIGURE 2: Enamel pitting in upper permanent central incisor region.

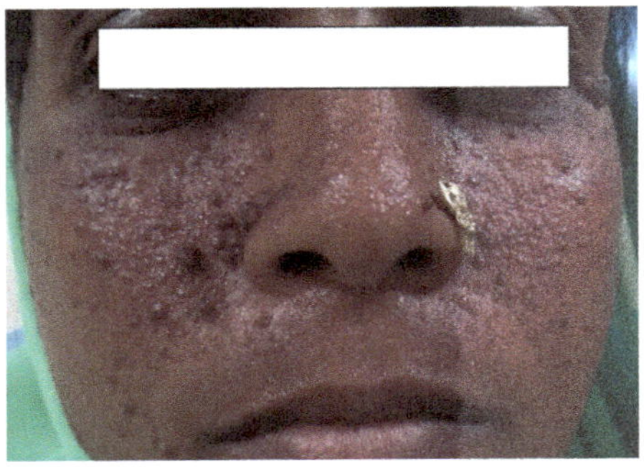

FIGURE 3: Multiple angiofibromas affecting the nasolabial folds and nose.

pancreatic angiomyolipoma, and skin angiofibroma along with intraoral findings as gingival overgrowth and enamel pits.

## 3. Investigations

Routine haematological investigations were conducted and were found to be within the reference range. Imaging analysis included USG and CT scan of whole abdomen. Kidney function test was normal and asymptomatic. The urine analysis did not reveal any significant finding. Echocardiography (ECG) and fundoscopy examinations were found to be nonsignificant. Magnetic resonance imaging (MRI) could not be performed due to financial constraints. Oral imaging revealed normal bone morphology as evident by orthopantamograms (Figure 4).

## 4. Differential Diagnosis

Other forms of neurocutaneous syndromes include type 1 and type 2 neurofibromatosis, Sturge-Weber syndrome, ataxia-telangiectasia and von Hippel Landau disease, and tuberous sclerosis complex [3, 4]. Facial and oral papules/nodules

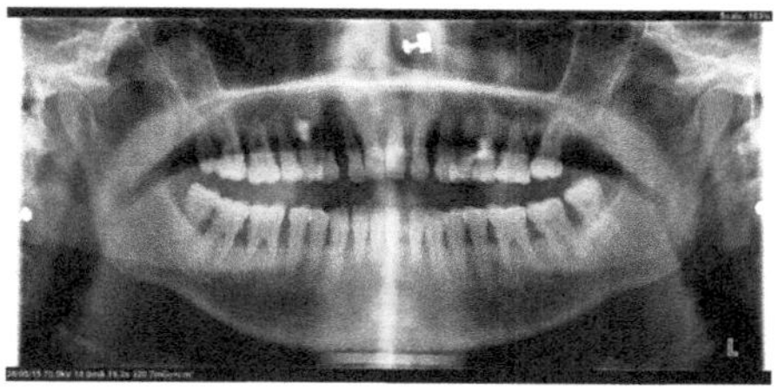

FIGURE 4: Orthopantomogram showing normal bone morphology.

can also be seen in Cowden syndrome, Birt-Hogg-Dube syndrome, and multiple endocrine neoplasia type-1 [3, 4]. Enamel pits can be associated with multiple conditions such as pitted hypoplastic amelogenesis imperfecta, vitamin-D dependent rickets, pseudohypoparathyroidism, and junctional epidermolysis bullosa [4].

## 5. Treatment

During initial treatment visit, gentle scaling and root planing were done along with institution of oral hygiene instructions. Plaque control measures lead to the improvement in the periodontal status but the lesion did not resolve completely on subsequent visits. For the same reason, complete excision till periosteum was planned with surgical scalpel under local anaesthesia. An informed written consent was taken from the propositor. Under local anesthesia full thickness mucoperiosteal flap was reflected involving permanent canine and premolars. Root planing and flap curettage were done and irrigated with saline. Flap was repositioned with figure of eight sutures and noneugenol surgical periodontal dressing was placed. Postoperative instructions as well as indicated medications were prescribed. The excised gingival tissue appeared pale pink and fibrous and did not differ from any usual enlarged gingival tissue. Also, the patient has been referred to the department of urology for laproscopic examination for diagnosing renal lesions. For hamartomatous lesions on face, cosmetic treatments have been advised ranging from cryosurgery to lasers.

## 6. Outcome and Follow-Up

The patient was recalled after 10 days for follow-up. The periodontal dressings were removed and healing took place uneventfully. Oral hygiene instructions were reinforced. No recurrence has been observed till now. The genetic counselling for the propositor and affected family members has been rendered from the Centre for Advanced Research, KGMU.

## 7. Discussion

There is a paucity of literature in which the diagnosis of tuberous sclerosis complex (TSC) was based on the oral findings; the aim of this case report is to emphasize oral manifestations for the diagnosis of familial case of TSC.

TSC or Bourneville's disease (MIM 191100) is an autosomal dominant inherited disorder affecting multiple organs such as skin, adnexa, CNS, heart, and kidneys [2–5]. TSC was first described by Von Recklinghausen and later by Pringle [6].

In this case report the propositor presented with findings of multiple angiofibromatous hamartomatous lesions distributed in a butterfly wing-like pattern around malar region, infrequent occurrence of seizures and renal and pancreatic angiomyolipomas along with enamel pitting, and localized gingival overgrowth. TSC has been associated with epilepsy in 90% of cases, with Koenen tumours in 15–20% and angiofibromas in 70% of cases, and with renal angiomyolipomas in 50% of the cases [7, 8]. The extraoral and intraoral findings herein presented are in agreement with the clinical diagnostic criteria of TSC (major and minor features) as described by Northrup and Krueger in 2013 [9]. However the genetic diagnostic criteria could not be confirmed due to financial constraints. The incidence of oral fibromas in TSC cases varies between 50 and 69% with an average diameter of 5 mm [10]. The aggressivity of such oral lesions depends upon the presence of local irritating factors. Herein, the gingival overgrowth was carefully excised with the help of scalpel after performing phase 1 periodontal therapy. No reoccurrence has been noted till 6 months follow-up owing to the effectiveness of the treatment. Although gingival overgrowth can also be caused by the use of antiseizure drugs as in the present case, the pattern of gingival overgrowth induced by antiseizure drug was not found in the present case was not found in the present case.

Angiofibromas in TSC have been frequently reported in upper anterior region and rarely on lip, tongue, and palate. Enamel pits seen in association with TSC may be associated with high risk of dental caries. Less frequent dental findings reported in association with TSC include high arched palate, bifid uvula, hare lip and/or cleft palate, delayed eruption of teeth, and presence of diastema [11]. The mutational analysis have also become an additional diagnostic tool for the diagnosis of cases of familial TSC. Two disease determining genes have been identified, namely, TSC-1 and TSC-2. TSC-1 protein product is hamartin and TSC-2 protein product is tuberin. Both of these proteins are involved in cell growth and differentiation [12]. Till date no studies have found an association between TSC and oral cancer; however TSC-2 overexpression may exert antitumor effect due to its oncosuppressor genes [13, 14]. In the present case the patient had a history of epilepsy and showed cutaneous fibromas but the identification of dental enamel pits and gingival overgrowth was fundamental in the diagnosis of TSC. The patient acceptance to the treatment was also assessed by a 3-point rating scale during the follow-up visit as described by Purwar et al. [15] and the patient rated it with a score of 3 (highly satisfied) on the grounds of presurgical, surgical, and postsurgical protocol and cost-effectiveness of the treatment.

This case report illustrates the importance of identification of intraoral findings in achieving early diagnosis of TSC which leads to appropriate screening examination, treatment, and genetic counselling.

## Learning Points

(i) Early and accurate diagnosis of oral lesions may be helpful in diagnosis of TSC.

(ii) TSC patients must adapt measures for careful oral and dental hygiene with regular dental visits in order to eliminate potential irritative factors.

(iii) Oral health care professional must request a detailed medical report on the condition of the patient.

(iv) Due to frequent pulmonary, cardiac, and renal involvement pre- and postmedication should be administered with caution.

## Consent

The patient described in the case report has given their informed consent for the case report to be published.

## Conflict of Interests

There is no conflict of interests among authors regarding the publication of this paper.

## References

[1] R. J. Gorlin, M. N. Cohen, and R. C. Hennekan, *Syndromes of Head and Neck*, Oxford University Press, New York, NY, USA, 4th edition, 2001.

[2] E. S. Roach and V. S. Miller, *Neurocutaneous Disorders*, Cambridge University Press, Cambridge, UK, 2004.

[3] L. De Jesus Araújo, L. Yamamoto De Almeida, J. Santos Lima, H. Martelli-Júnior, and P. R. Ferreti Bonan, "Evaluation of MMP-1, MMP-10, TIMP-1, a-SMA and TGF-b1 in angiofibromas of tuberous sclerosis," *Minerva Stomatologica*, vol. 60, no. 1-2, pp. 25–33, 2011.

[4] L. De Jesus Araujo, L. S. Lima, T. M. M. Alvarenga et al., "Oral and neurocutaneous phenotypes of familial tuberous sclerosis," *Oral Surgery, Oral Medicine, Oral Pathology, Oral Radiology and Endodontology*, vol. 111, no. 1, pp. 87–94, 2011.

[5] V. Narayanan, "Tuberous sclerosis complex: genetics to pathogenesis," *Pediatric Neurology*, vol. 29, no. 5, pp. 404–409, 2003.

[6] J. J. Pringle, "A case of congenital adenoma sebaceum," *British Journal of Dermatology*, vol. 2, pp. 1–14, 1890.

[7] R. A. Schwartz, G. Fernández, K. Kotulska, and S. Jóźwiak, "Tuberous sclerosis complex: advances in diagnosis, genetics, and management," *Journal of the American Academy of Dermatology*, vol. 57, no. 2, pp. 189–202, 2007.

[8] S. Gupta, R. Bhowate, and S. S. Degwekar, "Clinical and radiological findings related to tuberous sclerosis complex: a case report," *The Journal of Contemporary Dental Practice*, vol. 9, no. 4, pp. 85–91, 2008.

[9] H. Northrup and D. A. Krueger, "Tuberous sclerosis complex diagnostic criteria update: recommendations of the 2012 Iinternational Tuberous Sclerosis Complex Consensus Conference," *Pediatric Neurology*, vol. 49, no. 4, pp. 243–254, 2013.

[10] N. A. Lygidakis and R. H. Lindenbaum, "Oral fibromatosis in tuberous sclerosis," *Oral Surgery, Oral Medicine, Oral Pathology*, vol. 68, no. 6, pp. 725–728, 1989.

[11] L. D. J. Araújo, G. B. Muniz, E. Santos, J. P. V. Ladeia, H. M. Júnior, and P. R. F. Bonan, "Tuberous sclerosis complex diagnosed from oral lesions," *Sao Paulo Medical Journal*, vol. 131, no. 5, pp. 351–355, 2013.

[12] A. Apak, G. Haliloğlu, G. Köse, E. Yilmaz, B. Anlar, and S. Aysun, "Mutation analysis of TSC2 gene in 33 Turkish familial cases with tuberous sclerosis," *The Turkish Journal of Pediatrics*, vol. 45, no. 1, pp. 1–5, 2003.

[13] S. Kawaguchi, K. Harada, Suprianto, H. Yoshida, and M. Sato, "Overexpression of tuberous sclerosis complex 2 exerts antitumor effect on oral cancer cell lines," *Oral Oncology*, vol. 39, no. 8, pp. 836–841, 2003.

[14] P. Curatolo, R. Bombardieri, and S. Jozwiak, "Tuberous sclerosis," *The Lancet*, vol. 372, no. 9639, pp. 657–668, 2008.

[15] P. Purwar, J. Dixit, K. Bhartiya, and S. Sareen, "Conflation of gingival overgrowth and schwannoma," *BMJ Case Reports*, 2014.

# Oral Verruciform Xanthoma: A Case Report and Literature Review

**Akshay Shetty,[1] Kourosh Nakhaei,[2] Yogesh Lakkashetty,[3] Maryam Mohseni,[2] and Iman Mohebatzadeh[2]**

[1] *Department of Oral and Maxillofacial Surgery, Sri Rajiv Gandhi College of Dental Sciences and Hospital, Cholanagar, RT Nagar, Bangalore 560032, India*
[2] *Sri Rajiv Gandhi College of Dental Sciences and Hospital, Cholanagar, RT Nagar, Bangalore 560032, India*
[3] *Department of Oral and Maxillofacial Pathology, Sri Rajiv Gandhi College of Dental Sciences and Hospital, Cholanagar, RT Nagar, Bangalore 560032, India*

Correspondence should be addressed to Kourosh Nakhaei; koorosh_intheflesh@yahoo.com

Academic Editors: A. Ferri and A. Markopoulos

Verruciform xanthoma is a benign mucocutaneous, uncommon, nonsymptomatic lesion of uncertain etiopathology, which occurs mostly on the oral mucosa of middle-aged individuals. Histopathologically, VX is diagnosed by presence of lipid-laden foam cells in papillary region of connective tissue. A 60-year-old male patient presented with a painless growth on the left buccal mucosa. On clinical examination a yellowish white exophytic lesion, measuring 11 × 7 mm in size, was found, which was cauliflower-shaped on inspection and painless on palpation. Histopathological examination revealed varying degrees of surface parakeratosis and the accumulation of numerous foam cells in the connective tissue papillae among the uniformly elongated epithelial ridges. On immunohistochemical staining, there was a neutrophilic infiltrate of the epidermis with CD68 positive xanthoma cells restricted to the papillary dermis, mixed with other chronic inflammatory cells.

## 1. Introduction

Verruciform xanthoma (VX) is an uncommon benign mucocutaneous lesion that resembles virus-induced papilloma but has an unknown etiology and uncertain nature. It was first reported by Shafer in 1971. VX usually occurs in the oral mucosa of the middle-aged individuals. It most commonly presents with a verrucous appearance. However in some instances it may appear polypoid, papillomatous, or sessile. It occurs as a small (0.2–2 cm), solitary, asymptomatic, slow growing, white or yellowish red lesion with no sex predilection [1, 2].

Histologically VX is distinguished from other lesions by the presence of large numbers of foam cells in, and essentially limited to, the connective tissue papillae. The foam cells on ultrastructural studies have been concluded to be fat-laden macrophages [3, 4]. Other cell types, including Langerhans cells, intraepithelial neutrophilic infiltrate, and even fibroblasts, have been reported [1–3]. A variable degree of parakeratosis is observed which is present in the crypts between papillae which are of variable length and thickness, often extending close to the surface. The rete pegs are extremely elongated and uniform [2]. Almost every VX case is diagnosed on histological examination as the clinical appearance is not diagnostic. Differentiation from other lesions with foamy or granular cells is not difficult as the VX is the only lesion to have these cells confined to the papillae [4, 5].

Differential diagnosis includes erythroplasia of Queyrat (Bowen disease of the glans penis), seborrheic keratosis, verrucous carcinoma, verruca simplex, and condyloma acuminatum [6, 7]. The treatment of the VX lesion involves local surgical excision which is almost always curative, and recurrence is rare [2].

## 2. Case Presentation

A-60-year old male patient presented with the chief complaint of a painless growth on the left buccal mucosa (Figure 1). He had a habit of smoking for the past 10 years.

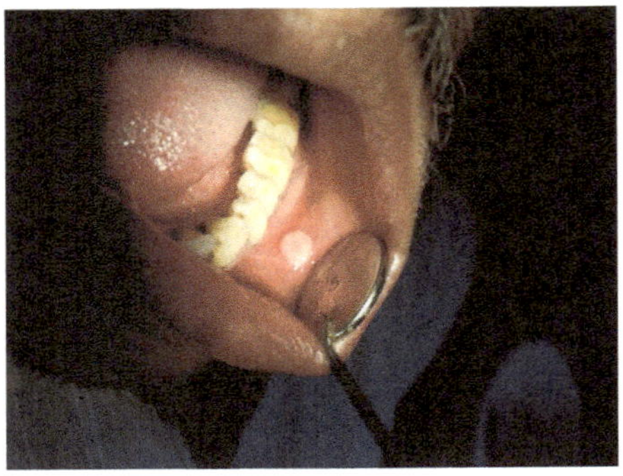

FIGURE 1: Clinical photograph showing the exophytic lesion on the left buccal mucosa.

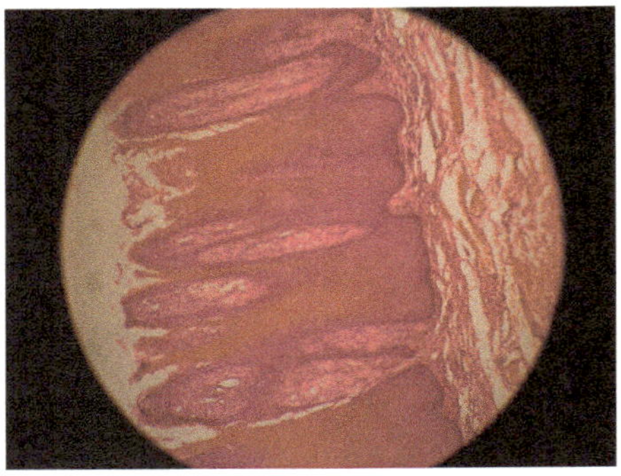

FIGURE 2: Showing epithelial hyperplasia with parakeratosis and elongated rete pegs. There is an abundance of foam cells in the connective tissue papilla (H&E stain 10x).

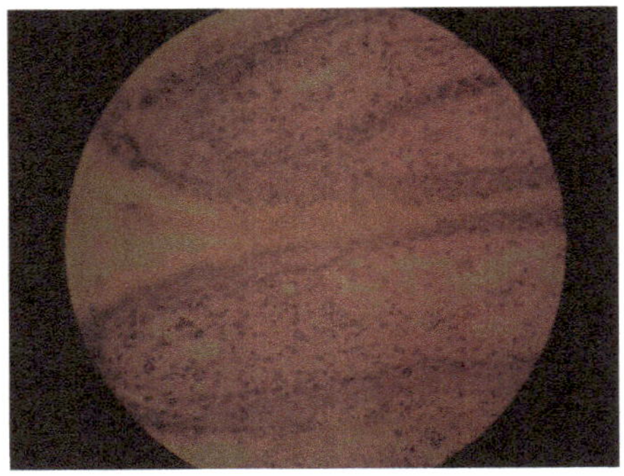

FIGURE 3: Presence of large numbers of lipid-laden foamy histiocytes confined to the connective tissue papillae (H&E stain 40x).

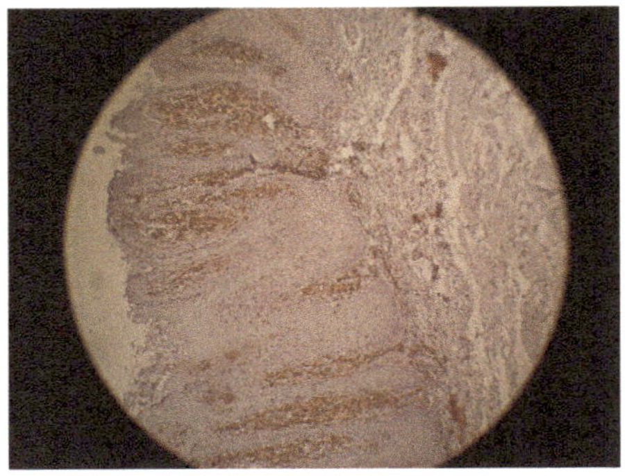

FIGURE 4: Showing foam cells with strong cytoplasmic CD68 immunostaining. The epithelial cells were negative (IHC stain 10x).

On clinical examination, a yellowish white exophytic lesion, measuring 11 × 7 mm in size, was found, which had a cauliflower shape on inspection. The lesion was asymptomatic and soft in consistency. Lymph nodes were not palpable. There were no systemic diseases and he was otherwise healthy. A provisional diagnosis of papilloma was made. After clinical examination an excisional biopsy was taken to rule out malignancy.

On histopathological examination, the hematoxylin and eosin (H&E) stained sections showed parakeratotic epithelium with columns of parakeratin plugging into it. Owing to the uniformly elongated rete pegs, deep connective tissue papillae were seen, some of which extended into overlying surface epithelium (Figures 2 and 3). Few neutrophils were also seen in the upper spinous layer. The papillary zone of lamina propria showed numerous lipid-laden foam cells. There was no evidence of dysplasia or malignancy. The fact that the foam cells were confined to the papillary region of connective tissue confirmed the diagnosis as VX.

The immunohistochemical staining for CD68 was positive for the foamy macrophages. All the foam cells were strongly stained with anti-macrophage antibodies (Figures 4 and 5).

The treatment was performed under local anesthesia. The whole lesion was excised in one piece during excisional biopsy (Figure 6). Postoperative check-up showed no sign of recurrence.

## 3. Discussion

Verruciform xanthoma is a rare lesion, accounting for 0.025–0.095% of all cases [3] with an unknown etiopathology. It can be because of the damage to the squamous cells due to trauma, irritation, or infection, which can cause increased epithelial turnover leading to the disease. The epithelial breakdown leads to an inflammatory response and a subsequent release of lipid material from the degenerated cells [2, 8–11]. Most of the cases occur in otherwise healthy individuals. Due to its clinical and histopathological resemblance to human papilloma virus-induced lesions, verruciform xanthoma was believed to be caused by HPV. However, most investigators have not found any evidence for the presence of HPV in these lesions [3]. However a few cases have been reported which were associated with inflammatory conditions such as pemphigus vulgaris, lichen planus, discoid lupus erythematosus, warty dyskeratoma, epidermal nevus/CHILD nevus, dystrophic epidermolysis bullosa, and seborrheic keratosis [12]. A few cases have also been reported to be associated with disorders of lipid metabolism [13]. On serological examination, our case had a normal serum lipid profile. The lesion is benign, nonsymptomatic, and slow growing and rarely exceeds 2 cm in size. It is sessile

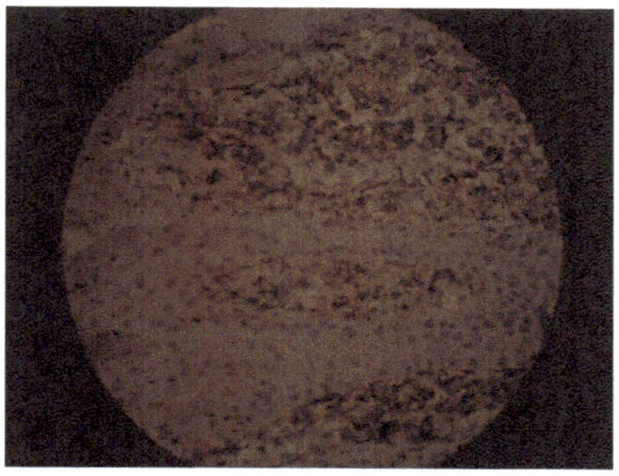

FIGURE 5: The infiltrated foam cells in the papillary dermis were CD68 positive (IHC stain 40x).

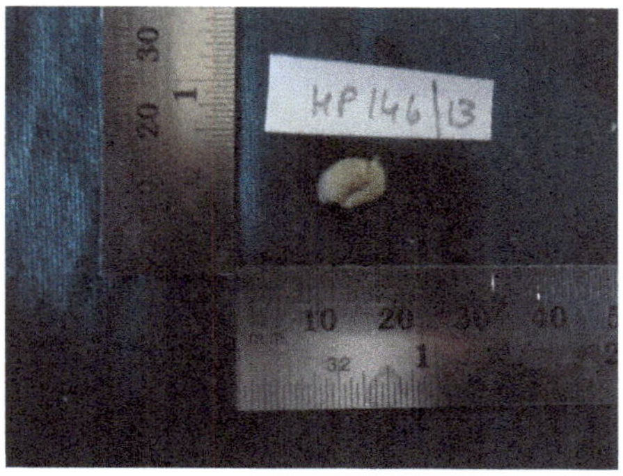

FIGURE 6: Showing the lesion after excision.

or pedunculated and can resemble leukoplakia or squamous papilloma. It occurs most commonly in 4th–6th decade of life with equal distribution between both sexes. However, it has been reported that there is a slight male predilection [1, 2, 14]. The lesion is usually present in the intraoral regions especially on alveolar ridge, gingiva, followed by buccal mucosa, palate, floor of the mouth, and lip. Extra oral sites include vulva, scrotum, penis, and skin of thigh and perineum, which are usually associated with other conditions like lymphedema, epidermal nevi, congenital hemidysplasia, and limb defect syndrome [6, 7, 15].

Histologically, VX shows three patterns: verrucous (most common), flat, and papillary (least common) [16, 17]. There is parakeratosis of the hyperplastic epithelium which is variable in extent and is usually more marked in the verrucous and papillary patterns. The rete pegs are elongated, uniform, and thin, with deep central keratinized clefts and keratin plugging. However, there is no evidence of dysplasia. The characteristic histological feature is the presence of xanthoma cells in the connective tissue [2, 18]. The lipid-laden foam cells are present in the superficial connective tissue. There is a controversy over the exact origin of these cells. They are said to be a lineage of monocytes/macrophages [19, 20]. The lipid found in the xanthoma cells is said to be the same as seen in other inflammatory reactions [12]. In our case, the foam cells showed strong CD68 immunoreactivity. CD68 is a cell marker confirming the possible role of macrophages in the formation of foam cells [12].

The treatment of choice is complete surgical excision which is very effective with no recurrence. However, a recurrent VX of the vulva has been reported in a 30-year-old woman, 8 years after the initial treatment [20]. Histopathological examination of the biopsies should be performed to distinguish VX from other verrucous lesions [2, 21].

## References

[1] S. K. Mohsin, M. W. Lee, M. B. Amin et al., "Cutaneous verruciform xanthoma: a report of five cases investigating the etiology and nature of xanthomatous cells," *The American Journal of Surgical Pathology*, vol. 22, no. 4, pp. 479–487, 1998.

[2] R. Rajendran, *Shafer's Textbook of Oral Pathology*, 6th edition, 2009.

[3] A. Buchner, L. S. Hansen, and P. W. Merrell, "Verruciform xanthoma of the oral mucosa: report of five cases and review of the literature," *Archives of Dermatology*, vol. 117, no. 9, pp. 563–565, 1981.

[4] W. G. Shafer, "Verruciform xanthoma," *Oral Surgery, Oral Medicine, Oral Pathology*, vol. 31, no. 6, pp. 784–789, 1971.

[5] T. Xia, G. Li, I. S. Jun, Y. N. Yinglu Guo, and M. K. Chung, "Verruciform xanthoma of the penis," *Korean Journal of Urology*, vol. 45, pp. 297–298, 2004.

[6] O. Reich and S. Regauer, "Recurrent verruciform xanthoma of the vulva," *International Journal of Gynecological Pathology*, vol. 23, no. 1, pp. 75–77, 2004.

[7] S. S. Farahani, N. S. Treister, Z. Khan, and S.-B. Woo, "Oral verruciform xanthoma associated with chronic graft-versus-host disease: a report of five cases and a review of the literature," *Head and Neck Pathology*, vol. 5, no. 2, pp. 193–198, 2011.

[8] N. M. Khaskhely, H. Uezato, T. Kamiyama et al., "Association of human papillomavirus type 6 with a verruciform xanthoma," *The American Journal of Dermatopathology*, vol. 22, no. 5, pp. 447–452, 2000.

[9] S. K. Mohsin, M. W. Lee, M. B. Amin et al., "Cutaneous verruciform xanthomna: a report of five cases investigating the etiology and nature of xanthomatous cells," *The American Journal of Surgical Pathology*, vol. 22, pp. 479–487, 1998.

[10] S. Y. Rawal, J. R. Kalmar, and D. N. Tatakis, "Verruciform xanthoma: immunohistochemical characterization of xanthoma cell phenotypes," *Journal of Periodontology*, vol. 78, no. 3, pp. 504–509, 2007.

[11] H. P. Philipsen, P. A. Reichart, T. Takata, and I. Ogawa, "Verruciform xanthoma: biological profile of 282 oral lesions based on a literature survey with nine new cases from Japan," *Oral Oncology*, vol. 39, no. 4, pp. 325–336, 2003.

[12] S. S. Farahani, N. S. Treister, Z. Khan, and S.-B. Woo, "Oral verruciform xanthoma associated with chronic graft-versus-host disease: a report of five cases and a review of the literature," *Head and Neck Pathology*, vol. 5, no. 2, pp. 193–198, 2011.

[13] D. J. Zegarelli, E. C. Zegarelli Schmidt, and E. V. Zegarelli, "Verruciform xanthoma: further light and electron microscopic studies, with the addition of a third case," *Oral Surgery Oral Medicine and Oral Pathology*, vol. 40, no. 2, pp. 246–256, 1975.

[14] V. Raphael, H. Das, R. Sarma, and B. Shunyu, "Oral verruciform xanthoma: a case report," *International Journal of Oral and Maxillofacial Pathology*, vol. 3, no. 2, pp. 65–67, 2012.

[15] R. Herrera-Goepfert, M. Lizano-Soberón, and M. Garcia-Perales, "Verruciform xanthoma of the esophagus," *Human Pathology*, vol. 34, no. 8, pp. 814–815, 2003.

[16] C.-H. Yu, T.-C. Tsai, J.-T. Wang et al., "Oral verruciform xanthoma: a clinicopathologic study of 15 cases," *Journal of the Formosan Medical Association*, vol. 106, no. 2, pp. 141–147, 2007.

[17] H. P. Philipsen, P. A. Reichart, T. Takata, and I. Ogawa, "Verruciform xanthoma: biological profile of 282 oral lesions based on a literature survey with nine new cases from Japan," *Oral Oncology*, vol. 39, no. 4, pp. 325–336, 2003.

[18] E. W. Odell and P. R. Morgan, Eds., *Biopsy Pathology of the Oral Tissue*, Chapman Hall, London, UK, 1st edition, 1998.

[19] S. Kimura, "Verruciform xanthoma of the scrotum," *Archives of Dermatology*, vol. 120, no. 10, pp. 1378–1379, 1984.

[20] K. A. Mostafa, T. Takata, I. Ogawa, N. Ijuhin, and H. Nikai, "Verruciform xanthoma of the oral mucosa: a clinicopathological study with immunohistochemical findings relating to pathogenesis," *Virchows Archiv*, vol. 423, no. 4, pp. 243–248, 1993.

[21] S. B. Connolly, E. J. Lewis, J. S. Lindholm, B. D. Zelickson, C. B. Zachary, and W. D. Tope, "Management of cutaneous verruciform xanthoma," *Journal of the American Academy of Dermatology*, vol. 42, no. 2, pp. 343–347, 2000.

# Prosthodontic Management of Xerostomic Patient: A Technical Modification

**Haraswarupa Gurkar, Omprakash Yadahally Venkatesh, Jagadeesh Mandya Somashekar, Muthuraj Hariharapura Lakshme Gowda, Madhavi Dwivedi, and Ishani Ningthoujam**

*Department of Prosthodontics, Farooqia Dental College and Hospital, Mysore 570021, India*

Correspondence should be addressed to Madhavi Dwivedi; madhavi.dwivedi1312@gmail.com

Academic Editor: Marco Antonio Compagnoni

Xerostomia is often a contributing factor in both minor and serious health problems. It can affect nutrition and dental as well as psychological health. Common problems faced by such patients are glossitis, mucositis, angular cheilitis, dysgeusia, and difficulty in chewing and swallowing. One of the major problems associated with xerostomic patients is the poor tolerance and retention of removable dental prostheses because of thin dry atrophic mucosa and lack of a saliva film. This paper describes a new technique of incorporating a salivary reservoir in the maxillary complete denture. The salivary reservoir fabricated by this technique provided good lubrication of the oral tissues and was easily cleansed by the wearer and was fabricated from routine denture materials.

## 1. Introduction

Saliva is a viscous, transparent liquid secreted by cells of the salivary glands. It plays a critical role in retention of dentures due to its lubricating function and, thus, dry mucosa often leads to compromise in the retention of prosthesis. Furthermore, salivary flow also facilitates the mastication and food bolus formation and its swallowing. It also aids in speech, mastication, or general oral health and function [1].

Xerostomia, a clinical condition caused by a decrease in the production of saliva, may present itself as a local symptom, as part of a systemic disease such as Sjogren's syndrome, diabetes, and alcoholism, or as a side effect of medications and other conditions such as menopause, following therapeutic radiation to the head and neck regions and vitamin deficiencies [2–6]. A temporary decrease could be from emotional reaction or sialolithiasis [1]. Edentulous patients suffering from xerostomia may complain not only of dry mouth, but also of difficulty in normal functions like eating, speaking, swallowing, and so forth and increased susceptibility to infections. Extreme discomfort in wearing dentures is a common complaint [2, 5].

Sugar-free gum or candies/lozenges may help to increase salivary output, and also drinking water on a regular basis [2–4, 6, 7]. Symptomatic relief can be provided by treatment with parasympathomimetics such as pilocarpine hydrochloride or neostigmine bromide [4, 6, 7]. Artificial saliva and salivary substitutes are other means of managing xerostomia. Artificial saliva acts by humidifying and lubricating the dehydrated oral mucosa. Saliva substitutes mainly consist of aqueous solutions containing the same mineral salts as those found in human saliva. To provide easier application of artificial saliva, an intraoral saliva reservoir in the hollowed lingual flange of a mandibular denture or palatal reservoir is also the technique of choice [6].

## 2. Case Report

A 65-year-old edentulous female patient reported to Department of Prosthodontics, Farooqia Dental College, having complaint of dryness of mouth and severe discomfort while speaking and eating. Intraoral examination revealed maxillary and mandibular edentulous residual ridges, severely resorbed mandibular ridges, areas of irritation associated with the maxillary denture, dry tongue, and minimal frothy saliva in the floor of the mouth (Figure 1). Patient's mouth was noted to be very dry with cracks at the corner of the mouth and lips. Medical history revealed that she was on medications for hypertension. The patient's general practitioner was also contacted and the medications were reduced or altered to

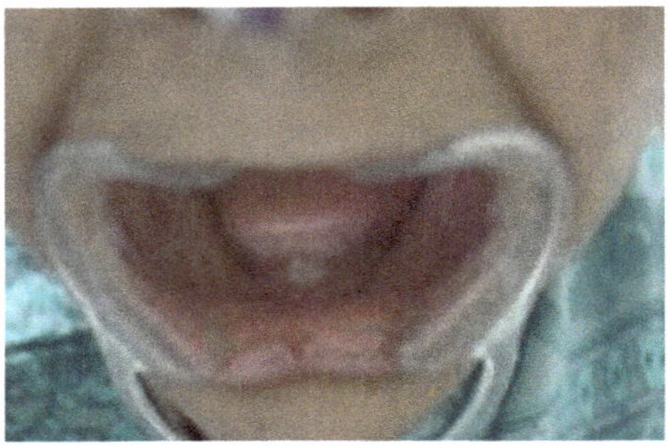

Figure 1

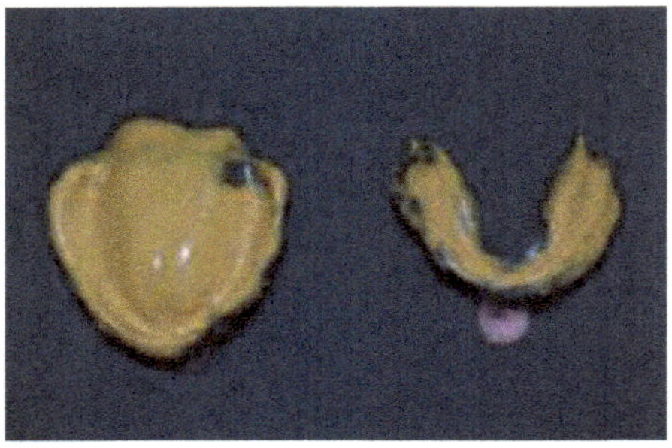

Figure 2

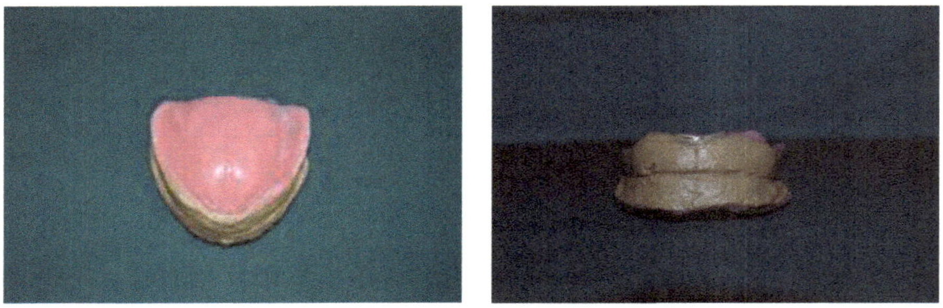

(a) (b)

Figure 3

reduce the xerostomia. She had been advised to use salivary substitute regularly and frequently drink water to overcome the dryness and discomfort.

## 3. Procedure

*3.1. Clinical Steps (Figures 2–5).* (1) Primary impression was made in irreversible hydrocolloid.

(2) Custom trays were fabricated, border moulding was done, and secondary impressions were made in light body elastomeric impression material (Aquasil Ultra LV Dentsply Caulk) (Figure 2).

(3) Occlusal rims were fabricated using impression compound (DPI Pinnacle) and jaw relation was obtained using closed mouth technique using temporary tissue liner material (Visco-gel Dentsply CE) on the tissue surface of the maxillary and mandibular temporary denture bases for their better stability (Figure 3).

(4) Impression compound occlusion rims were replaced with modeling wax (Hindustan Modelling Wax Number 2, Hyderabad, India) occlusion rims and tissue relining material with cold cure acrylic resin (DPI RR cold cure) (Figure 4).

(5) Teeth were arranged on occlusal rims and palatal surface of the maxillary denture base was covered by the wax to the thickness of 6 mm. Try-in was done using temporary tissue liner material on the polished surface and was allowed to stand in patient's mouth for 30 mins to allow recording the functional movements of tongue and to check for retention, stability, and speech (Figure 5).

*3.2. Laboratory Procedures (Figures 6–14).* (6) Vacuum formed thermoplastic sheet of 5 mm was heat pressed and cut 2-3 mm short of crest of maxillary ridge on palatal surface and posteriorly just anterior to vibrating line on the maxillary master cast to relieve posterior palatal seal and this sheet spacer was later used at the processing stage (Figure 6).

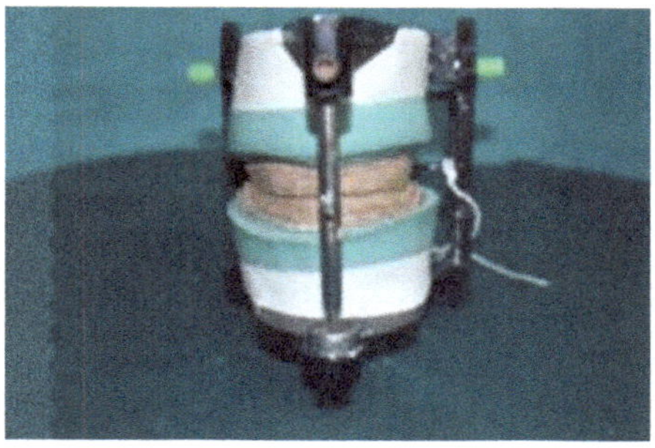

(a)

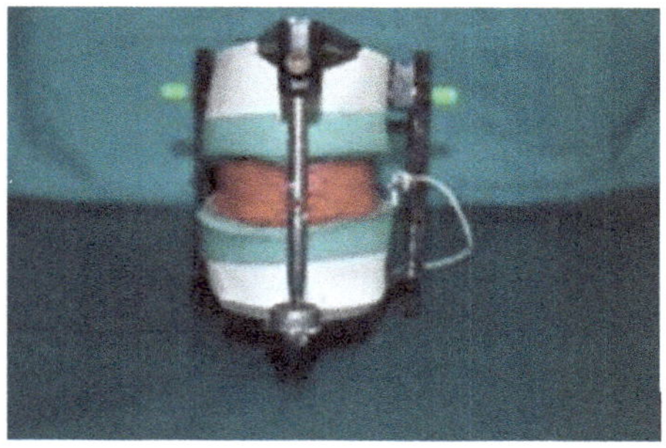

(b)

Figure 4

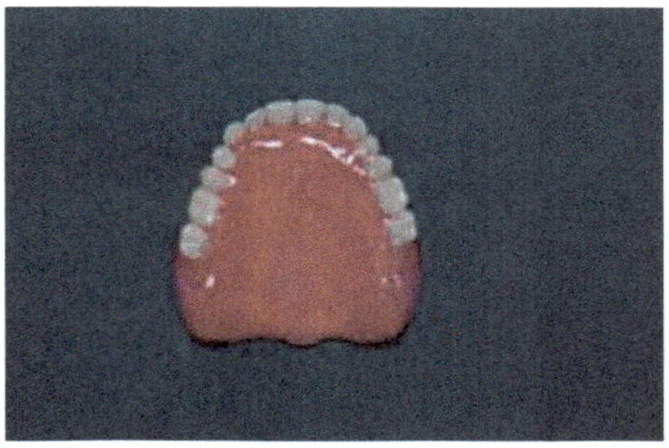

Figure 5

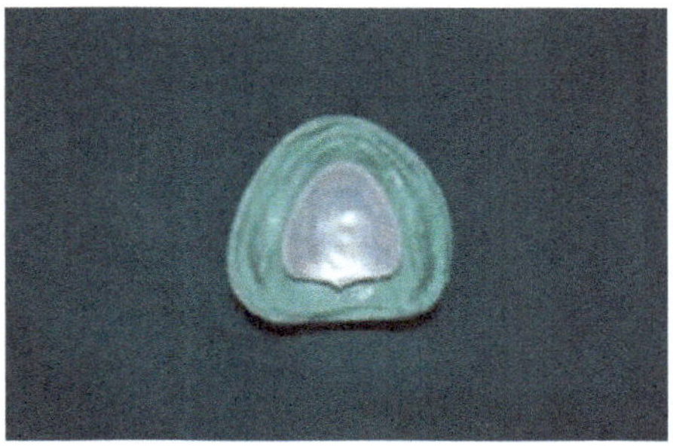

Figure 6

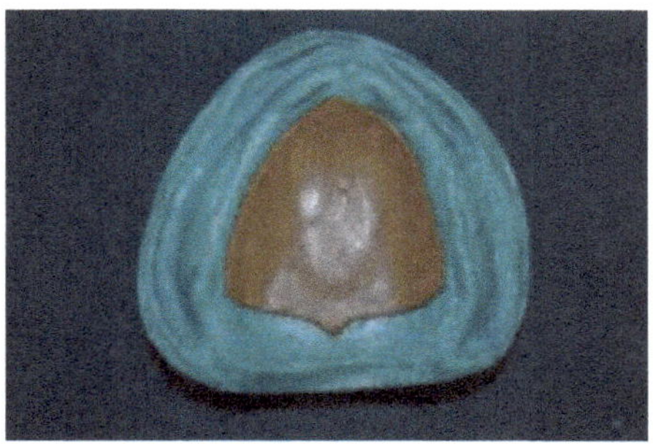

Figure 7

(7) Shellac base plate (Supernal Base plate, Lucknow, India) of 1 mm thickness was adapted over the maxillary cast and cut into the same size and shape as that of thermoplastic sheet for later use (Figure 7).

(8) Mandibular complete denture was processed in the conventional manner.

(9) For maxillary trial denture which has a thickness of 6 mm (step number (5)), flasking and dewaxing were done in conventional manner. Heat pressed thermoplastic sheet was placed over the cast. Heat cure acrylic resin (Acralyn-"H", Mumbai, India) was packed into the mould. Heat curing was done in conventional manner (Figure 8).

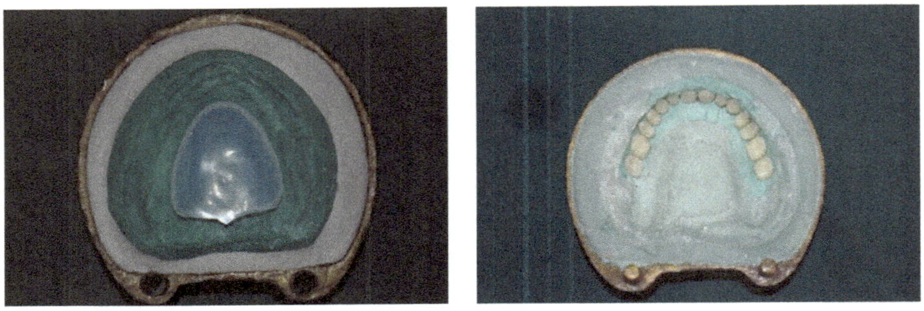

(a) (b)

Figure 8

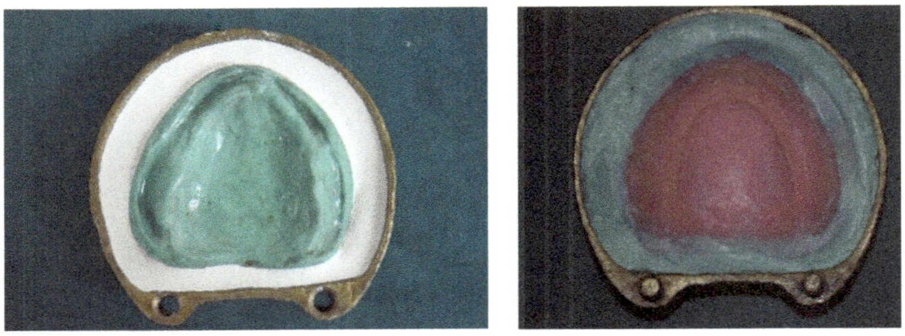

(a) (b)

Figure 9

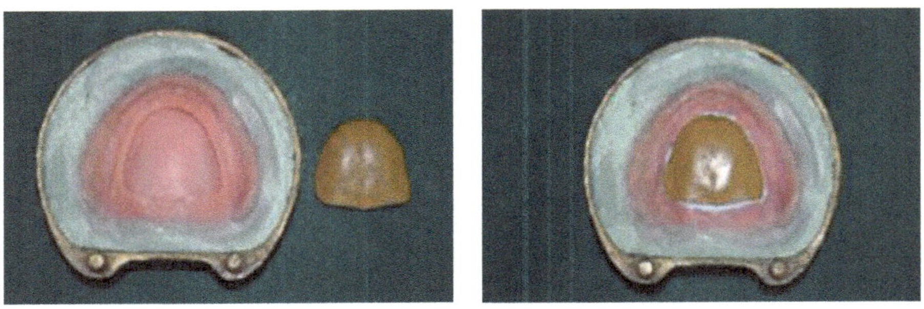

(a) (b)

Figure 10

(10) After heat curing was completed, flask was opened (Figure 9):

(a) Base part of flask-containing maxillary master cast (Figure 9(a)).

(b) Counterpart of the flask-containing teeth, polished surface of denture made of pink heat cure acrylic resin and tissue surface of the denture with space created by thermoplastic sheet of 5 mm (Figure 9(b)).

(11) Space of 5 mm created after retrieval of thermoplastic sheet was filled with the elastomeric putty material of thickness 4 mm (GC Flexceed) and closed with the shellac base plate lid of thickness 1 mm on the tissue surface of denture later to create space for clear heat cure acrylic resin (Acralyn-"H", Mumbai, India) and the base flask was closed with its counterpart (Figure 10).

(12) After the setting of putty material the base flask was opened and any excess putty and also shellac base plate lid (1 mm) were removed. It was again packed with clear heat cure acrylic resin to get the tissue surface of the denture and base flask was closed and it was heat cured again in the conventional manner.

(13) Both the dentures were then finished and polished. Now the processed maxillary denture has

(a) pink heat cure acrylic on the polished surface (1 mm);

(b) elastomeric putty material in-between (4 mm);

(c) clear heat cure acrylic on the tissue surface (1 mm).

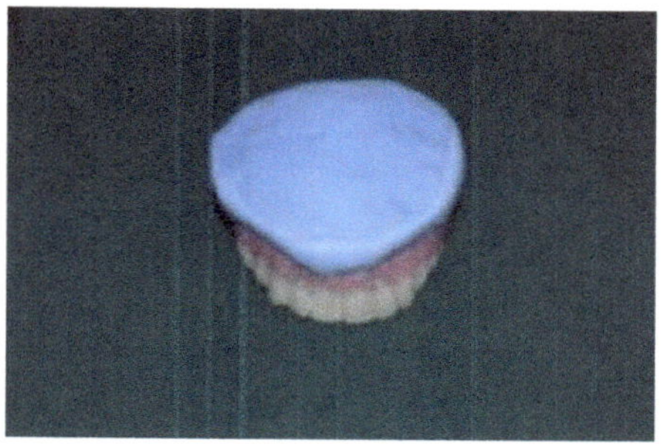

FIGURE 11

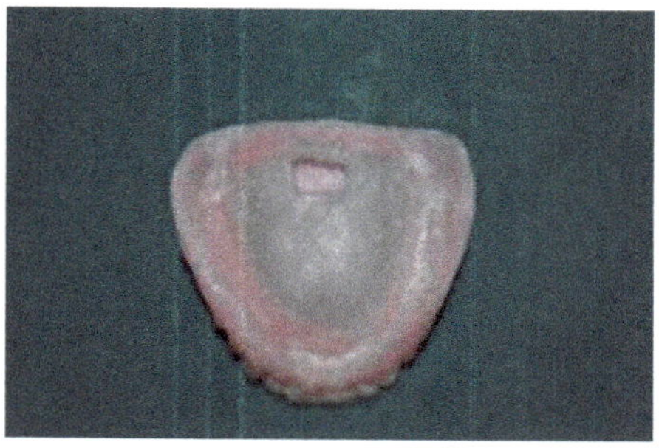

FIGURE 12

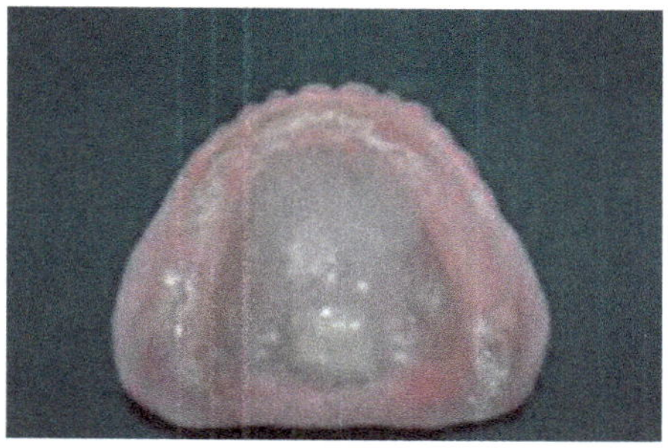

FIGURE 13

(14) Before removing putty spacer, an index impression of the tissue surface of denture was made using putty elastomeric impression material (Figure 11).

(15) The putty spacer was removed by creating a hole on the tissue surface of the denture as shown in Figure 12.

(16) After removal of putty spacer, the hole was closed using cold cure clear acrylic material (DPI-Heat Cure, Mumbai) using the putty index (Figure 13).

(17) Two holes were made: one bigger inlet hole at the tissue surface posteriorly and another smaller outlet hole on the polished surface on anterior palatal on mid-palatine raphae (Figure 14).

(18) Through the inlet hole artificial saliva was injected using 18 mm gauge needle and outlet was in the diameter of 26 mm gauge needle.

(19) The maxillary and mandibular dentures were checked in the patient's mouth for their retention, stability, occlusion, and border extensions and they were finally inserted and the patient was instructed for routine for denture and oral hygiene maintenance and recalled after one week (Figure 15). She was given instructions about how to fill the artificial salivary substitute through the inlet.

## 4. Discussion

Depending on the etiology of the xerostomia, various treatment aspects are available as mentioned above [4]. However 2 or 3 methods are employed to make the prosthesis successful. The goal in management of the xerostomia is to reduce the suffering from the disease and make wearing of dentures and performing normal oral functions comfortable for the patients. At the same time priority should be given to retention and stability of the dentures [4]. In order to enhance retention in xerostomic patients oral moisturizers, denture adhesives, denture reservoirs, soft liners, various denture bases, and various surface treatments are used in order to relieve them from the effects of xerostomia [7–9].

This case report describes the technique of fabrication of the maxillary denture with salivary reservoir. Xerostomic patients can benefit immensely from it as reservoir chamber

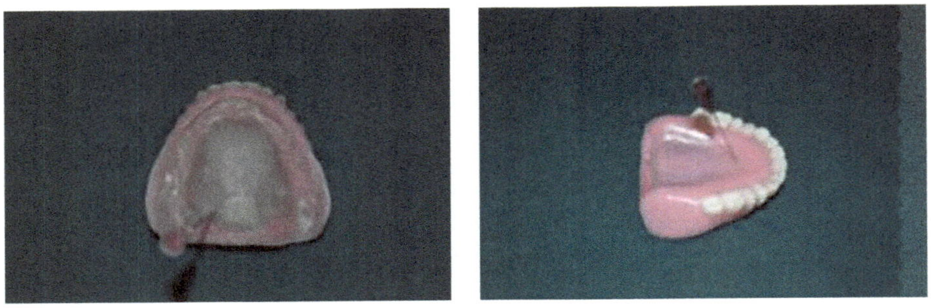

(a) (b)

FIGURE 14

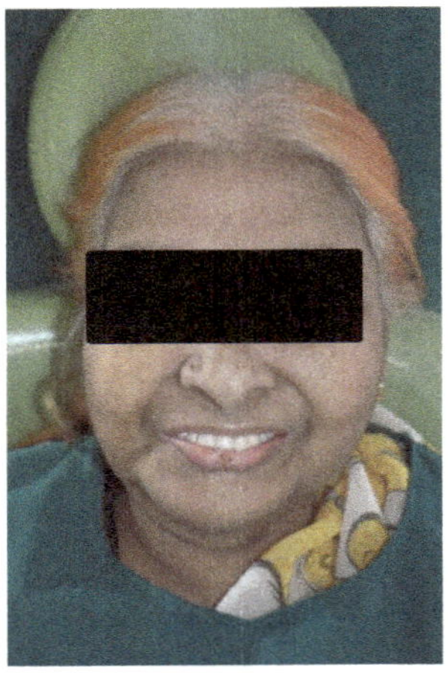

FIGURE 15

allows for more controlled flow of artificial saliva [3, 9]. The thickness of the palate was increased primarily in the palatal vault area with minimum increase at the periphery of the palate [4]. Volume of the reservoir was 4.5 mL with its working duration of 2 to 2.5 hours.

Its advantages are easy visibility of the level of salivary substitute in the chamber, easy accessibility to reservoir by the dentist [3], better retention and stability of the dentures, and functional impression of tongue on polished surface which makes room for tongue movements.

Limitations of this technique are that it requires bulky dentures, artificial saliva must be mechanically introduced into the dentures by the patient at regular intervals [5], and it requires additional laboratory steps [3]. The dentures and the reservoir require meticulous cleaning, and patients were instructed in the use of a disposable syringe for flushing with 2% sodium hypochlorite and refilling the chamber [4, 5]. Artificial saliva is contraindicated in conditions like asthma, iritis, and glaucoma as they cause tachycardia, bradycardia, sweating, and increased smooth muscle tone [8].

## 5. Conclusion

Prosthodontics management of xerostomic patient has been a challenging task for the dentist. But this case report provides various methods of treatment that cater to both the need of xerostomia and lack of retention due to resorbed ridges in completely edentulous patients. Since the quality and quantity of saliva have an important role in the success of complete dentures, the patients with hyposalivation need to be treated to prevent adverse effects on the oral mucosa [5, 6].

## Conflict of Interests

The authors declare that there is no conflict of interests regarding the publication of this paper.

## References

[1] S. Winkler, *Essentials of Complete Denture Prosthodontics*, Saunders Elsevier, Philadelphia, Pa, USA, 2nd edition, 2012.

[2] G. S. Chandu and M. N. Hombesh, "Management of xerostomia and hyposalivation in complete denture patients," *Indian Journal of Stomatology*, vol. 2, no. 4, pp. 263–266, 2011.

[3] L. S. Kaira, "Prosthodontic management of xerostomic patient with reservoir denture—a case report," *Journal of Dentofacial Sciences*, vol. 1, no. 1, pp. 37–41, 2012.

[4] S. R. Upadhyay, L. Kumar, and J. Rao, "Fabrication of a functional palatal saliva reservoir by using a resilient liner during processing of a complete denture," *Journal of Prosthetic Dentistry*, vol. 108, no. 5, pp. 332–335, 2012.

[5] S. B. Lagdive, R. B. Umbarkar, S. S. Lagdive, D. S. Gandhage, A. J. Bhandari, and S. A. Gangadhar, "Dentures as artificial saliva reservoirs in the irradiated edentulous cancer patient with xerostomia," *Indian Journal of Basic & Applied Medical Research*, vol. 1, no. 1, pp. 31–37, 2011.

[6] O. P. Singh, N. Rubina, N. Mittal, and R. Saini, "How to manage xerostomia in prosthodontics???" *Dental Journal of Advance Studies*, vol. 1, no. 3, pp. 144–151, 2013.

[7] V. Madhumathi, S. Sowmya, and R. Swamy, "Xerostomia and its dental implications: a review," *Journal of Oral Health & Community Dentistry*, vol. 7, no. 3, pp. 166–169, 2013.

[8] V. Murthy, V. Yuvraj, P. P. Nair, and S. Thomas, "Prosthodontic management of radiation induced xerostomic patient using flexible dentures," *BMJ Case Reports*, 2012.

[9] M. Rathee, P. Malik, and M. Bhoria, "Customized complete denture for xerostomic patients with resorbed ridge," *International Journal of Scientific Research*, vol. 3, no. 11, article 37, 2014.

# A Rare Case of an Artery Passing through the Median Perforating Canal of the Mandible

**Joe Iwanaga, Koichi Watanabe, Tsuyoshi Saga, Yoko Tabira, and Koh-ichi Yamaki**

*Department of Anatomy, Kurume University School of Medicine, Kurume, Fukuoka 830-0011, Japan*

Correspondence should be addressed to Joe Iwanaga; iwanaga_jyou@med.kurume-u.ac.jp

Academic Editor: Gilberto Sammartino

Along with the popularization of dental implant surgery, there has been considerable research on the lingual foramen using cone-beam computed tomography. Anatomical research has also revealed that the arteries entering the lingual foramina are branches of the submental and sublingual arteries. There have been no reports, however, of the submental or sublingual artery entering the mandible from the lingual foramen, perforating it, and then distributing to the inferior labial region. A 69-year-old man who donated his body to our department in 2015 was dissected. The mandible with overlying soft tissue of the mental region was resected and examined with microcomputed tomography, which showed that the canal perforated from the lingual foramen to the midline of the labial cortical plate. The canal was thus named the median perforating canal. To the best of our knowledge, there have been no other reports of a perforating artery of the mandible, so this case is thought to be rare. Hence, the existence of perforating arteries, such as in the present case, should be taken into consideration in preoperative diagnoses such as for dental implant surgery. Thus, the fusion of anatomical and radiological study is useful and necessary to understand surgical anatomy.

## 1. Introduction

The development of cone-beam computed tomography (CBCT) has contributed to finding many kinds of accessory foramina of the mandibular bone. The lingual foramen is well known as it enters branches of the submental or sublingual artery in the lingual cortical plate of the mandible [1]. Thus, a preoperative diagnosis of the anatomy for implant surgery in the incisive region is important to prevent accidental hemorrhage [2]. The morphology of the accessory foramina and canals could be clarified on CBCT images. The replacement site for the implant fixture should sometimes be modified to avoid injuring neurovascular bundles passing through those accessory foramina. The course of the artery outside the mandible, however, cannot be visualized by CBCT, and thoughtless handling in the soft tissue near the foramina has a risk of damaging arteries. Both the course of the artery before entering the mandible from the lingual foramen and the branches of the submental artery around the mental region have been studied in detail by gross anatomical dissection [1, 3]. Report of an artery perforating the mandible from the lingual to the labial cortical plate should be taken into consideration during surgical procedures.

Here we report a case of a perforating canal of the mandible, with an artery passing through the canal and distributing to the inferior labial region, which we confirmed anatomically and radiologically. This study was performed in keeping with the requirements of the Declaration of Helsinki (64th World Medical Assembly, Fortaleza, Brazil, October 2013).

## 2. Case Presentation

A 69-year-old Japanese man who died of cervical esophageal cancer donated his body to our medical school in 2015. An edentulous mandibular bone with the lateral area of overlying soft tissue was resected from his body and examined using microcomputed tomography ($\mu$CT) and anatomical dissection. The axial and sagittal images showed two small foramina and a canal connecting the two foramina near the inferior border of the mandible in the midline (Figures 1(a) and 1(b)). Three-dimensional reconstructed images showed

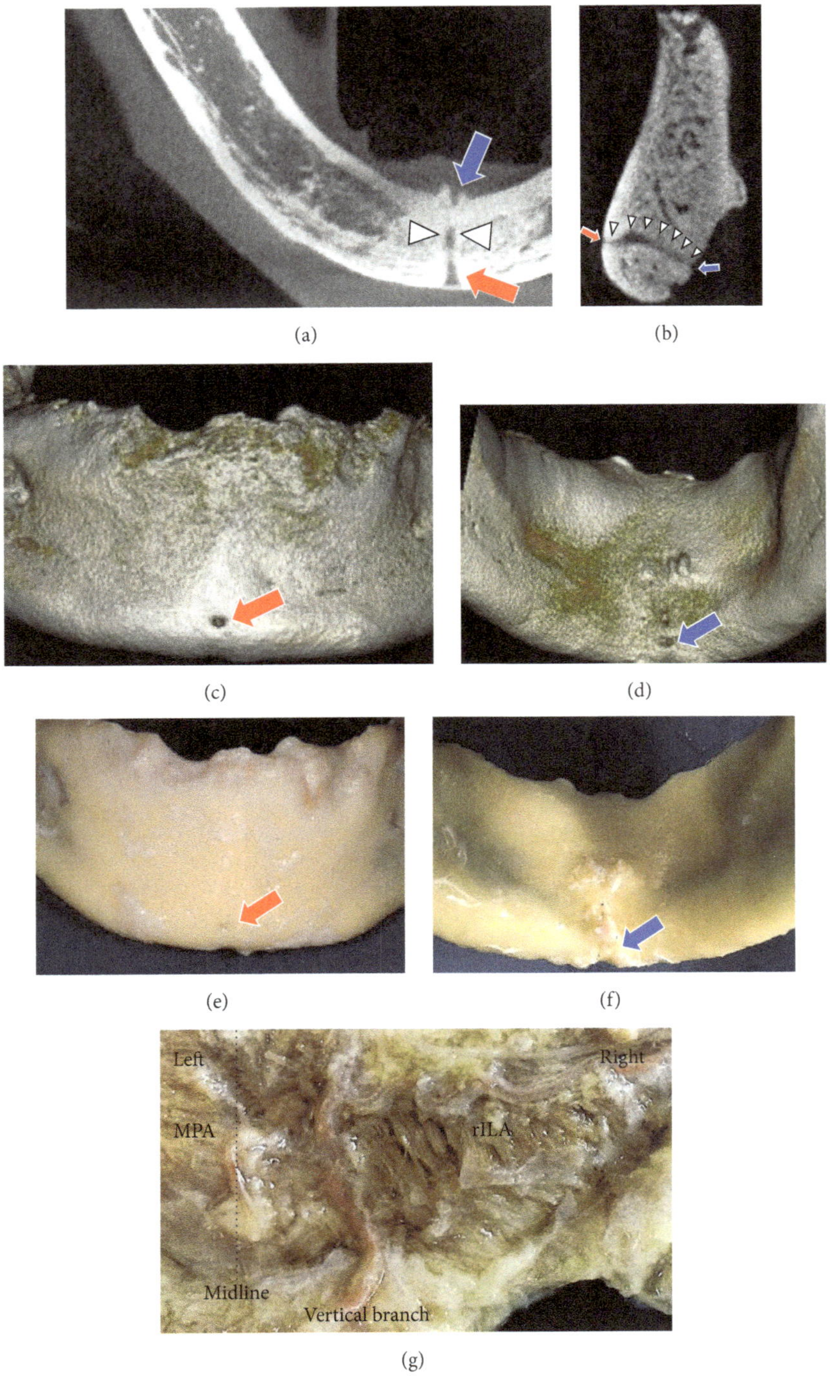


FIGURE 1: Axial (a) and sagittal (b) images of the mandible show two foramina located on the anterior (red arrow) and posterior (blue arrow) surfaces of the midline. A canal (white arrowheads), which has the continuity of those two foramina, was demonstrated. Three-dimensional computed tomography images of the mandible show anterior (c) and posterior (d) views of the mandible. After removing the overlying soft tissue, the mandible is seen in anterior (e) and posterior (f) views. The medial view of the dissected soft tissue after periosteal detachment shows the right ILA running horizontally and joining the vertical branch, which passes by the inferior border of the mandible (g). The median perforating artery (MPA) has no anastomosis with other branches. Red arrow, median labial foramen (MLaF); blue arrow, median lingual foramen (MLiF); rILA, right inferior labial artery.

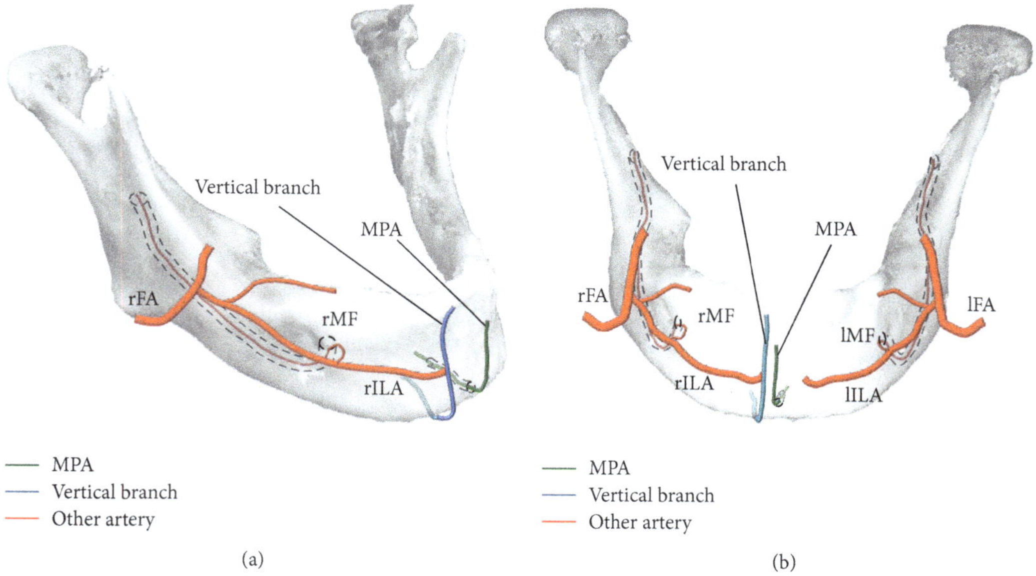


Figure 2: MPA (green line), vertical branch (blue line), and other arteries (red lines) are shown in lateral (a) and frontal (b) views. Both facial arteries branch off the inferior labial arteries (ILAs). Both ILAs anastomose with the mental arteries arising from the mental foramina. The right ILA anastomoses with the vertical branch coming from the inferior border of the mandible without perforating the mandible. The median perforating artery (MPA) comes from the posterior of the mandible and perforates the mandible. It then goes up to the inferior labial region. lFA, left facial artery; lILA, left inferior labial artery; lMF, left mental foramen; rFA, right facial artery; rILA, right inferior labial artery; rMF, right mental foramen.

that, in the frontal and posterior views, the labial and lingual accessory foramina were located near the inferior border of the mandible in the midline (Figures 1(c) and 1(d)).

The labial and lingual foramina were named the median labial foramen (MLaF) and the median lingual foramen (MLiF). The canal connecting the MLaF and MLiF was named the median perforating canal (MPC). The MPC was 9.2 mm long. The MLaF (1.1 × 1.2 mm) was located in the midline and 5.8 mm superior to the inferior border of the mandible. The MLiF (0.9 × 0.9 mm) was located in the midline and 3.6 mm superior to the inferior border of the mandible and inferior to the mental spine. Gross anatomical dissection was carried out to visualize the structure passing through the MPC. The overlying soft tissue was separated from the mandible (Figures 1(e) and 1(f)), and a structure was seen arising from the MLaF. Dissection revealed that only the artery passed through the MPC. It was named the median perforating artery (MPA). The MPA went up to and fed the medial inferior labial region. The vertical branch, which passed by the inferior border of the mandible, also went into the inferior labial region 3.0 mm to the right of the MPA and then anastomosed to the right inferior labial artery (rILA). It was difficult to dissect these thin arteries, so colored derivatives of contrast medium (Microfil red; Flow Tech, Hartford, CT, USA) were injected from both sides of the facial arteries (Figure 1(g)). The contrast medium revealed that the MPA had no anastomosis and directly fed the inferior labial region. The vertical branch went up and joined the rILA and fed the inferior labial region (Figures 2(a) and 2(b)).

In the present case, the mandible was resected from the head by cutting off the origin of the oral floor and tongue, which was on the medial side of the mandible. Hence, the origins of the MPA and the vertical branches were unknown, although they are thought to arise from the submental or sublingual artery.

## 3. Discussion

Bone morphology is easy to understand using CT images. Popularization of implant surgery has caused many more dentists to use CT, appreciating its high resolution that allowed us to visualize the accessory foramina. Cases of severe bleeding caused by injury to the lingual foramen have been reported. Wang et al. investigated the lingual and lateral lingual foramina to learn their epidemiology and morphology [4]. They researched the lingual foramen using CBCT, so the components of the neurovascular bundles were not seen. CBCT showed that 13.2% of the mandible had the lingual foramen in the midline which was >1 mm in diameter.

It is well known that the major nerve in the mental region is the mental nerve, which arises from the mental foramen. Iwanaga et al. [5] noted that the large accessory mental foramen, which was distant from the mental foramen, might contain an artery. Nakajima et al. [1] classified the artery that entered the median lingual foramen based on the patterns of the anastomosis of the sublingual and submental arteries. In the present case, the MPA entering the MLiF was thought to be a branch of the submental or sublingual artery. The artery perforated the mandibular bone and arose from the MLaF and then fed the inferior labial region without any anastomosis. Masui et al. also classified the course of the sublingual artery [6]. The artery passed by the inferior border of the mandible and in this case was thought to be the vertical labiomental artery proposed by Kawai [3]. Smartt Jr. et al. [7] stated that the blood supply to most of the postnatal developing mandible was via the inferior alveolar artery and the periosteal plexus provided by the terminal branches of the lingual and facial arteries. An anastomosis between the inferior *alveolar* artery branches and the submental artery has also been reported [8]. Many arteries fed the mandible during the development process, and the MPA was considered to be a remnant of the feeding artery of the mandible and its surrounding tissue. Embryologically, when both mandibles fused with the midline, it is possible that the bone formation around the MPA created the MPC.

The MPA matters clinically during dental implant surgery, and periosteal detachment of the mandible in the submandibular region must be corrected. CBCT makes it easy to diagnose those accessory foramina preoperatively. In plastic surgery, during a facelift or submental procedures, the submental artery is known to bleed. Hwang et al. explained that branches of the submental artery pass by the inferior border of the mandible, causing the submental artery to bleed [9]. When the submental region is touched during those procedures, variations in the vascular system and bone morphology should be taken into consideration.

This was a rare case of a perforating artery passing through the lingual foramen of the mandible. It is important to remember that findings from anatomical and radiological studies are useful clinically.

## Competing Interests

The authors declare that they have no conflict of interests.

## Acknowledgments

The authors thank all those who donate their bodies and tissues for the advancement of education and research.

## References

[1] K. Nakajima, A. Tagaya, M. Otonari-Yamamoto et al., "Composition of the blood supply in the sublingual and submandibular spaces and its relationship to the lateral lingual foramen of the mandible," *Oral Surgery, Oral Medicine, Oral Pathology and Oral Radiology*, vol. 117, no. 1, pp. e32–e38, 2014.

[2] Y. Katsumi, R. Tanaka, T. Hayashi, T. Koga, R. Takagi, and H. Ohshima, "Variation in arterial supply to the floor of the mouth and assessment of relative hemorrhage risk in implant surgery," *Clinical Oral Implants Research*, vol. 24, no. 4, pp. 434–440, 2013.

[3] K. Kawai, N. Imanishi, H. Nakajima, S. Aiso, M. Kakibuchi, and K. Hosokawa, "Arterial anatomy of the lower lip," *Scandinavian Journal of Plastic and Reconstructive Surgery and Hand Surgery*, vol. 38, no. 3, pp. 135–139, 2004.

[4] Y. M. Wang, Y. R. Ju, W. L. Pan, and C. P. Chan, "Evaluation of location and dimensions of mandibular lingual canals: a cone beam computed tomography study," *International Journal of Oral and Maxillofacial Surgery*, vol. 44, no. 9, pp. 1197–1203, 2015.

[5] J. Iwanaga, K. Watanabe, T. Saga et al., "Accessory mental foramina and nerves: application to periodontal, periapical and implant surgery," *Clinical Anatomy*, vol. 29, no. 4, pp. 493–501, 2016.

[6] T. Masui, S. Seki, K. Sumida, K. Yamashita, and S. Kitamura, "Gross anatomical classification of the courses of the human sublingual artery," *Anatomical Science International*, vol. 91, no. 1, pp. 97–105, 2016.

[7] J. M. Smartt Jr., D. W. Low, and S. P. Bartlett, "The pediatric mandible: I. A primer on growth and development," *Plastic and Reconstructive Surgery*, vol. 116, no. 1, pp. 14e–23e, 2005.

[8] T. Kawai, I. Sato, T. Yosue, H. Takamori, and M. Sunohara, "Anastomosis between the inferior alveolar artery branches and submental artery in human mandible," *Surgical and Radiologic Anatomy*, vol. 28, no. 3, pp. 308–310, 2006.

[9] K. Hwang, J. Y. Han, R. S. Chung, and I. H. Chung, "Submental perforating artery: a culprit of bleeding during facelift," *Journal of Craniofacial Surgery*, vol. 16, no. 1, pp. 3–5, 2005.

# Diagnosis and Surgical Management of Nonsyndromic Nine Supernumerary Teeth and Leong's Tubercle

**Christiane V. Cruz,[1] Andrea L. Soares,[2] David N. Braga,[3] and Marcelo C. Costa[1]**

[1] *Department of Pediatric Dentistry and Orthodontics, Federal University of Rio de Janeiro, Brazil*
[2] *Department of Oral Biology, Fluminense Federal University, Brazil*
[3] *Department of Maxillofacial Surgery, Federal University of Rio de Janeiro, Brazil*

Correspondence should be addressed to Marcelo C. Costa; odontopediatria@odonto.ufrj.br

Academic Editor: Hüsamettin Oktay

Nonsyndromic multiple supernumerary teeth (ST) and Leong's tubercle are a condition with a very low prevalence and a multidisciplinary approach is required to restore function and aesthetics. So, this case report aimed at presenting a rare case of nonsyndromic nine supernumerary teeth and Leong's tubercle in a pediatric patient, without any evident familial history, showing its diagnosis and surgical management.

## 1. Introduction

Supernumerary teeth (ST) are a numeric dental anomaly characterized by the formation of teeth in excess of the normal dental formula, occurring in both the primary and permanent dentition [1, 2]. The etiology of ST is still unknown. A number of theories have been postulated to try to explain their presence, including atavism (evolutionary throwback), tooth germ dichotomy, genetic and environmental factors, and hyperactivity of the dental lamina. However, all theories are hypothetical due to the inability to obtain sufficient embryologic material on their origin [3]. Their frequency ranges from 0.3% to 3.6% [4, 5] and they are two times more common in males than females [5, 6]. Multiple ST are usually associated with syndromes such as cleidocranial dysplasia and Gardner's syndrome [7]. However, multiple ST in nonsyndromic patients is a rare condition [8] and less than 1% of cases are reported [9, 10]. Nonetheless, teeth that remain unerupted may cause aesthetic and functional problems due to overretained primary teeth, delayed or ectopic eruption of permanent, displacement and rotation of adjacent teeth, crowding, development of diastema, crossbite [10, 11], eruption into the floor of the nasal cavity [12], and root resorption of adjacent teeth [10].

Accessory cusps are variations of tooth shape and their frequency varies depending on the type and the tooth affected. The most commonly reported accessory cusps are cusp of Carabelli of the molars that represents 68% [13], 8% for Leong's tubercle of premolars, and between 1% and 7.7% for the talons cusps of the incisors [14]. The clinical aspects include a cusp like accessory structure varying in size from a prominent cingulum to a marked projection affecting the enamel surface of the teeth [15]. Regarding clinical disturbances, it may cause occlusal interferences, esthetic disturbances, accidental cusp fracture leading to loss of pulp vitality, irritation of tongue during speech and mastication, nursing difficulties, caries, and displacement of the affected tooth [16].

The most reliable methods for the diagnosis of supernumerary teeth and accessories cusp are clinical and conventional radiographs (orthopantomogram, periapical and occlusal) and cone-beam computed tomography [7]. Early surgical intervention is the preferred method of treatment to prevent clinical problems and to minimize further complications. To the best of our knowledge, this is the first report that presents a case of multiple supernumerary teeth associated with accessory cusp. So, here we document a case of nine supernumerary teeth in a nonsyndromic pediatric

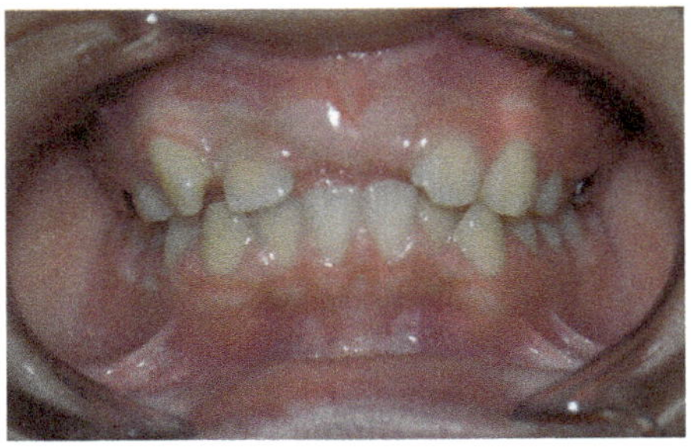

Figure 1: Frontal view showing the absence of the maxillary central incisors.

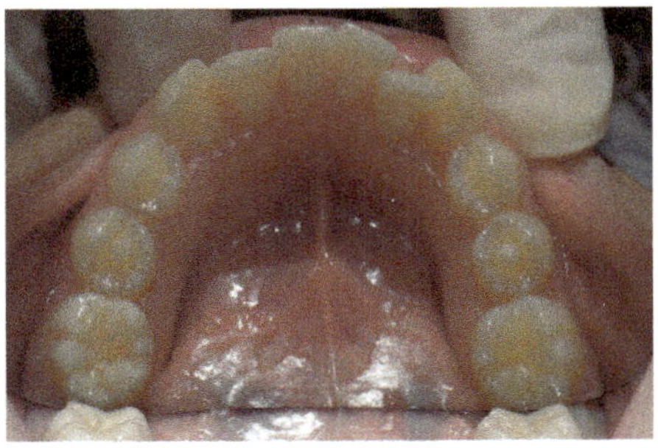

Figure 2: Occlusal view disclosing Leong's tubercle on the second mandibular premolars.

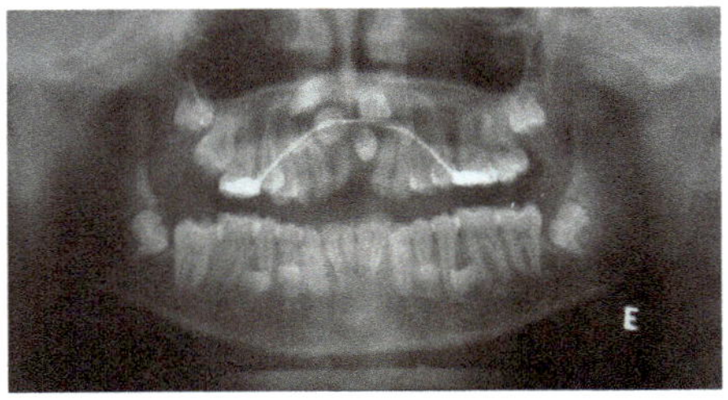



Figure 3: Orthopantomogram. Nine supernumerary teeth distributed in the maxillary and mandibular arches.

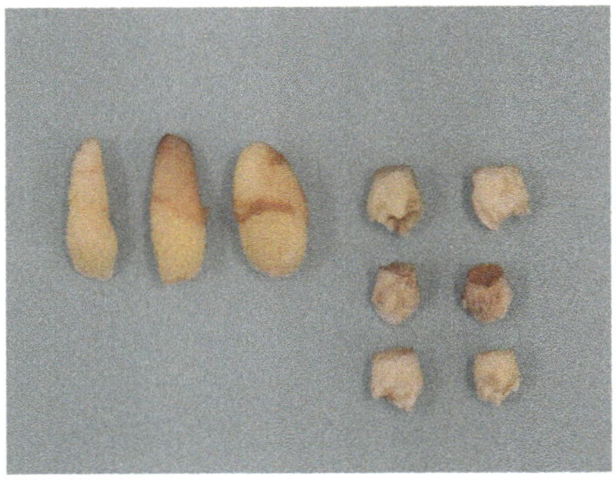

Figure 4: Nine supernumerary teeth.

patient and the presence of Leong's tubercle in the premolars usual dental formula, highlighting the diagnosis and surgical management using a multidisciplinary approach. This case report was performed according to The CARE guideline [17].

## 2. Case Report

A 10-year-old male, Caucasian patient was referred to the Continuing Education Clinical Program in Pediatric Dentistry at the Federal University of Rio de Janeiro due to the absence of teeth in the maxillary anterior region; this has influenced his social adjustment, impacting on his quality of life (Figure 1). The family's medical and dental history was noncontributory. General physical and extra oral examination did not show any abnormality. An intraoral examination revealed the presence of mixed dentition and the absence of the permanent maxillary central incisors. There was a wide anterior arch space, misalignment of permanent canines and mandibular incisors, and the lack of space for the alignment of the upper permanent incisors. Normal overjet and overbite were observed. The second usual premolars presented Leong's tubercle, which resulted in occlusal interference, performing a premature contact with their antagonists (Figure 2).

The analysis of the orthopantomogram and occlusal radiographs revealed the presence of nine impacted supernumerary teeth in the four quadrants, distributed as follows: in the maxilla there were one conical and two tuberculate mesiodens and two supplemental teeth in the posterior segment. In the mandible, there were four tuberculate teeth arranged in the premolar region, two in the right side and the other ones on the left side (Figure 3). The cone-beam computed tomography showed that the central incisors were arranged horizontally in the floor of the nasal cavity and presented a complete root development.

After a thorough diagnosis by the multidisciplinary team, pediatric dentistry, oral surgeon, and orthodontist, by analyzing the orthopantomogram and cone bean computed tomography as well as his systemic condition, the treatment plan was defined. The treatment of choice for Leong's tubercle was selective grinding. It was performed using a diamond stern conical drill under water to eliminate premature contact. The nine ST were extracted in a single surgical time under general anesthesia (Figure 4). The orthodontic traction of the superior central incisors was proposed aiming to their alignment in the upper arch. However, there was not enough space to carry out the tooth alignments in both the upper and lower arches. Thereby, we proposed the extraction of four premolars in order to obtain the correct alignment before the referred orthodontic traction, which could improve function and aesthetics. On the other hand, the prognosis of the orthodontic traction was questionable because of the risk of dental ankylosis due to the close contact with the buccal cortical bone. As a result, an additional treatment was proposed, implantology, and/or prosthetic restoration at the end of the growth spurt.

## 3. Discussion

It is essential not only to enumerate but also to identify the ST present clinically and radiographically before a definitive diagnosis and treatment plan can be formulated [9]. In this patient, the ST resulted in a wide anterior arch space because the unerupted mesiodens has caused a retardation or obstruction of eruption of the permanent central incisors which resulted in an aspect of dental absence in the anterior region, impacting the quality of life of the ST patient. The mesiodens in this patient has been probably originated from the permanent dentition tooth bud since in the primary dentition, supernumerary teeth occurred most often in the lateral incisor regions, as opposed to permanent supernumerary teeth, which prevailed in the central incisor regions [18]. Early diagnosis and extraction of mesiodens may prevent malocclusion and dental abnormalities such as delayed eruption, rotation of the permanent incisors and diastema [19, 20]. Teeth located in the nasal cavity are a rare phenomenon but a case has been previously reported in which mesiodens were left untreated and erupted in the nasal cavity [21]. In this patient, it is unlikely that the ST would erupt in the nasal cavity if they were left untreated because of their horizontal position. Nevertheless, it is worth noting that these teeth should be followed up in an attempt to decrease the risk of oral complications.

Classification of ST can be made on the basis of morphology and region [7]. Morphology variations include conical types (small peg-shaped or conical), tuberculate types (with more than one cusp or tubercle frequently described as barrel-shaped and may be invaginated), and supplemental teeth (refers to a duplication of teeth in the normal series). They can be found in almost any region of the dental arch but occur more frequently in the maxilla, especially in the anterior segment. ST may occur singularly or in multiple teeth and unilaterally or bilaterally [9]. Corroborating these findings, we found five ST in the maxilla, of which three were mesiodens (one conical and two tuberculate teeth) and two supplemental teeth which were located on either side of the posterior arch. In addition, we found four ST arranged in the posterior region of the jaw.

Thus in this patient, it was necessary to remove the ST under general anesthesia since the patient was not able to tolerate a long surgical procedure under local analgesia. Furthermore, when surgical removal is indicated, the advantage of avoiding the young children for local analgesia should be kept in mind where about 52% of the patients aged 5 to 10 years often require general anesthesia for removal of ST [22]. It has been advocated that a single surgical time could bring more benefits to the patient and his family has accorded to this decision. ST are associated with disturbances of tooth eruption, midline diastema, or development of a local malocclusion [15]. We decided not to use traction for the two permanent incisors at the same time because their position was unfavorable and the risk of ankylosis as well as their alignment will require the extraction of the first premolars; therefore, we chose conservative management. The right central incisor will undergo traction on a second time under local analgesia, and depending on the performance, the orthodontic plan can be followed up.

Accessory cusps are relatively rare anomalies. The size, shape, and location of these anomalies have wide variations. The central cusp on the occlusal surface of posterior teeth has also been given several descriptions such as supernumerary occlusal cusp, dens evaginatus, premolar odontome, occlusal tubercle, tuberculated premolar, Leong's tubercle, and Leong's premolar [22]. Patients with additional tooth projections should be placed under routine and periodic dental surveillance, which include monitoring of the degree of attrition and tooth vitality. Early diagnosis and management are important if complications are to be prevented. In this report, we performed the enamel grinding on the Leong's tubercle as an attempt to avoid occlusal disturbances such as functional crossbite, premature contact, and accidental cusp fracture to prevent disturbances in the pulp vitality.

Whenever the supernumerary teeth and accessory cusp are diagnosed, a decision with regard to the appropriate management should be made carefully. It is difficult to establish an ideal treatment for these cases. The clinical and radiographic exam is of vital importance to carry out a good treatment.

## 4. Conclusion

The approach to the patients with supernumerary teeth must be multidisciplinary. The management of the supernumerary teeth should form the part of a comprehensive treatment plan in cooperation with pediatric dentistry, oral surgeon, and orthodontists.

Leong's tubercle has to be evaluated in occlusal context and in cases of premature contact it has to be submitted into a selective grinding to avoid possible malocclusions and pulpal complications.

## Disclosure

This paper is a partial fulfillment of requirements for a Master's degree (Christiane V. Cruz) in the graduate faculty, Federal University of Rio de Janeiro, Brazil.

## Conflict of Interests

The authors declare that there is no conflict of interests regarding the publication of this paper.

## Acknowledgments

Support for this work was provided by CAPES (CVC fellowship), FAPERJ (M. C. Costa).

## References

[1] R. N. D'Souza and O. D. Klein, "Unraveling the molecular mechanisms that lead to supernumerary teeth in mice and men: current concepts and novel approaches," *Cells Tissues Organs*, vol. 186, no. 1, pp. 60–69, 2007.

[2] P. Srivatsan and N. Aravindha Babu, "Mesiodens with an unusual morphology and multiple impacted supernumerary teeth in a non-syndromic patient," *Indian Journal of Dental Research*, vol. 18, no. 3, pp. 138–140, 2007.

[3] F. N. Weber, "Supernumerary teeth," *Dental Clinics of North America*, vol. 1, pp. 509–517, 1964.

[4] E. Ferrés-Padró, J. Prats-Armengol, and E. Ferrés-Amat, "A descriptive study of 113 unerupted supernumerary teeth in 79

pediatric patients in Barcelona," *Medicina Oral, Patologia Oral y Cirugia Bucal*, vol. 14, no. 3, pp. E146–E152, 2009.

[5] U. Meriç, A. Brkic, N. Aksakalli, and V. Olgaç, "Supernumerary teeth associated with third molar impaction: a case report," *Acta Stomatologica Croatica*, vol. 2, pp. 123–127, 2010.

[6] A. Sharma, "Familial occurence of mesiodens—a case report," *Journal of the Indian Society of Pedodontics and Preventive Dentistry*, vol. 21, no. 2, pp. 84–85, 2003.

[7] M. T. Garvey, H. J. Barry, and M. Blake, "Supernumerary teeth overview of classification, diagnosis and management," *Journal of Canadian Dental Association*, vol. 65, no. 11, pp. 612–616, 1999.

[8] P. Batra, R. Duggal, and H. Parkash, "Non-syndromic multiple supernumerary teeth transmitted as an autosomal dominant trait," *Journal of Oral Pathology and Medicine*, vol. 34, no. 10, pp. 621–625, 2005.

[9] M. A. Scheiner and W. J. Sampson, "Supernumerary teeth: a review of the literature and four case reports," *Australian Dental Journal*, vol. 42, no. 3, pp. 160–165, 1997.

[10] L. D. Rajab and M. A. M. Hamdan, "Supernumerary teeth: review of the literature and a survey of 152 cases," *International Journal of Paediatric Dentistry*, vol. 12, no. 4, pp. 244–254, 2002.

[11] M. M. Gallas and A. García, "Retention of permanent incisors by mesiodens: a family affair," *British Dental Journal*, vol. 188, no. 2, pp. 63–64, 2000.

[12] N. M. King and A. M. P. Lee, "An intranasal tooth in a patient with a cleft lip and palate: report of case," *The Journal of the American Dental Association*, vol. 114, no. 4, pp. 475–478, 1987.

[13] K. Mavrodisz, N. Rózsa, M. Budai, A. Soós, I. Pap, and I. Tarján, "Prevalence of accessory tooth cusps in a contemporary and ancestral Hungarian population," *European Journal of Orthodontics*, vol. 29, no. 2, pp. 166–169, 2007.

[14] H. S. Chawla, A. Tewari, and N. S. Gopalakrishnan, "Talon cusp—a prevalence study," *Journal of the Indian Society of Pedodontics and Preventive Dentistry*, vol. 1, no. 1, pp. 28–34, 1983.

[15] Ö. Tulunoglu, D. U. Çankala, and R. C. Özdemir, "Talon's cusp: report of four unusual cases," *Journal of Indian Society of Pedodontics and Preventive Dentistry*, vol. 25, no. 1, pp. 52–55, 2007.

[16] F. N. Hattab, O. M. Yassin, and K. S. Al-Nimri, "Talon cusp in permanent dentition associated with other dental anomalies: review of literature and reports of seven cases," *Journal of Dentistry for Children*, vol. 63, no. 5, pp. 368–376, 1996.

[17] J. J. Gagnier, G. Kienle, D. G. Altman et al., "The CARE guidelines: consensus-based clinical case report guideline development," *Journal of Clinical Epidemiology*, vol. 67, no. 1, pp. 46–51, 2014.

[18] A. Diaz, J. Orozco, and M. Fonseca, "Multiple hyperodontia: report of a case with 17 supernumerary teeth with non-syndromic association," *Medicina Oral, Patologia Oral y Cirugia Bucal*, vol. 14, no. 5, pp. E229–E231, 2009.

[19] F. N. Hattab, O. M. Yassin, and M. A. Rawashdeh, "Supernumerary teeth: report of three cases and review of the literature," *ASDC Journal of Dentistry for Children*, vol. 61, no. 5-6, pp. 382–393, 1994.

[20] R. E. Primosch, "Anterior supernumerary teeth—assessment and surgical intervention in children," *Pediatric Dentistry*, vol. 3, no. 2, pp. 204–215, 1981.

[21] N. M. King and A. M. Lee, "An intranasal tooth in a patient with a cleft lip and palate: report of case," *The Journal of the American Dental Association*, vol. 114, no. 4, pp. 475–478, 1987.

[22] C. E. Jerome and R. J. Hanlon Jr., "Dental anatomical anomalies in Asians and Pacific Islanders," *Journal of the California Dental Association*, vol. 35, no. 9, pp. 631–636, 2007.

# Radix Entomolaris in Mandibular First Molars in Indian Population

**Kanika Attam, Ruchika Roongta Nawal, Shivani Utneja, and Sangeeta Talwar**

*Conservative Dentistry & Endodontics, Maulana Azad Institute of Dental Sciences, New Delhi 110002, India*

Correspondence should be addressed to Ruchika Roongta Nawal, ruchika.roongta@gmail.com

Academic Editors: D. Cogulu and C. Evans

*Purpose.* The aim of this paper is to present cases of mandibular first molars with an additional distolingual root and their management using appropriate instruments and techniques. *Basic Procedures and Main Findings.* Mandibular molars can sometimes present a variation called radix entomolaris, wherein the tooth has an extra root attached to its lingual aspect. This additional root may complicate the endodontic management of the tooth if it is misdiagnosed or maltreated. This paper reviews the prevalence of such cases in Indian population and reports the management of 6 such teeth. *Principal Conclusions.* (1) It is crucial to be familiar with variations in tooth/canal anatomy and characteristic features since such knowledge can aid location and negotiation of canals, as well as their subsequent management. (2) Accurate diagnosis and careful application of clinical endodontic skill can favorably alter the prognosis of mandibular molars with this root morphology.

## 1. Introduction

The primary aim of endodontic treatment is the elimination of bacteria from the infected root canal and the prevention of subsequent reinfection. This is mainly achieved by a thorough cleaning and shaping of the root canal, followed by a three-dimensional filling with a fluid tight seal. Establishing adequate access for cleaning and shaping is an integral part of this procedure. In order to achieve these endodontic goals, the clinician must have an in-depth knowledge of root canal anatomy and be aware of its anatomic diversities such as extra roots, extra canals, webs, fins, and isthmuses that may complicate the endodontic procedure. Several authors have reported about the morphology of the mandibular first molars [1–3]. These articles have shown that mandibular first molars usually have three or four canals. Along with the number of root canals, the number of roots may also vary. The majority of first and second mandibular molars are two rooted with two mesial and one distal canals [3, 4]. A major variant in this group is the mandibular first molar which has three roots. This has a frequency of less than 5% in white Caucasian (UK, Dutch, Finnish, German), African (Bantu Bushmen), Eurasian and Indian populations. In those with Mongoloid traits, such as the Chinese, Eskimos, and native American populations, it occurs with a frequency of 5 to more than 30% [5–8]. This third lingual root, first mentioned in the literature by Carabelli [9], is called the radix entomolaris (RE).

For successful endodontic treatment of all canals of the tooth careful radiographic diagnosis plays a pivotal role. Radiographs taken at different angulations reveal the basic information regarding the anatomy of a tooth and can thus help to detect any aberrant anatomy such as extra canals/roots [10]. However, a significant constraint in conventional radiography is that it produces a two-dimensional image of a three-dimensional object, resulting in the superimposition of the overlying structure. To achieve a more detailed understanding of the morphological structure of root canals and their interrelations, more advanced diagnostic tools are required.

Recently, cone-beam computed tomography (CBCT) has emerged as a useful tool to aid in the diagnosis of teeth with complex root anatomies [11, 12]. It is an imaging method employing tomography to generate a three-dimensional reconstruction of the entire tooth at different levels from a single imaging procedure. The advantages of CBCT imaging

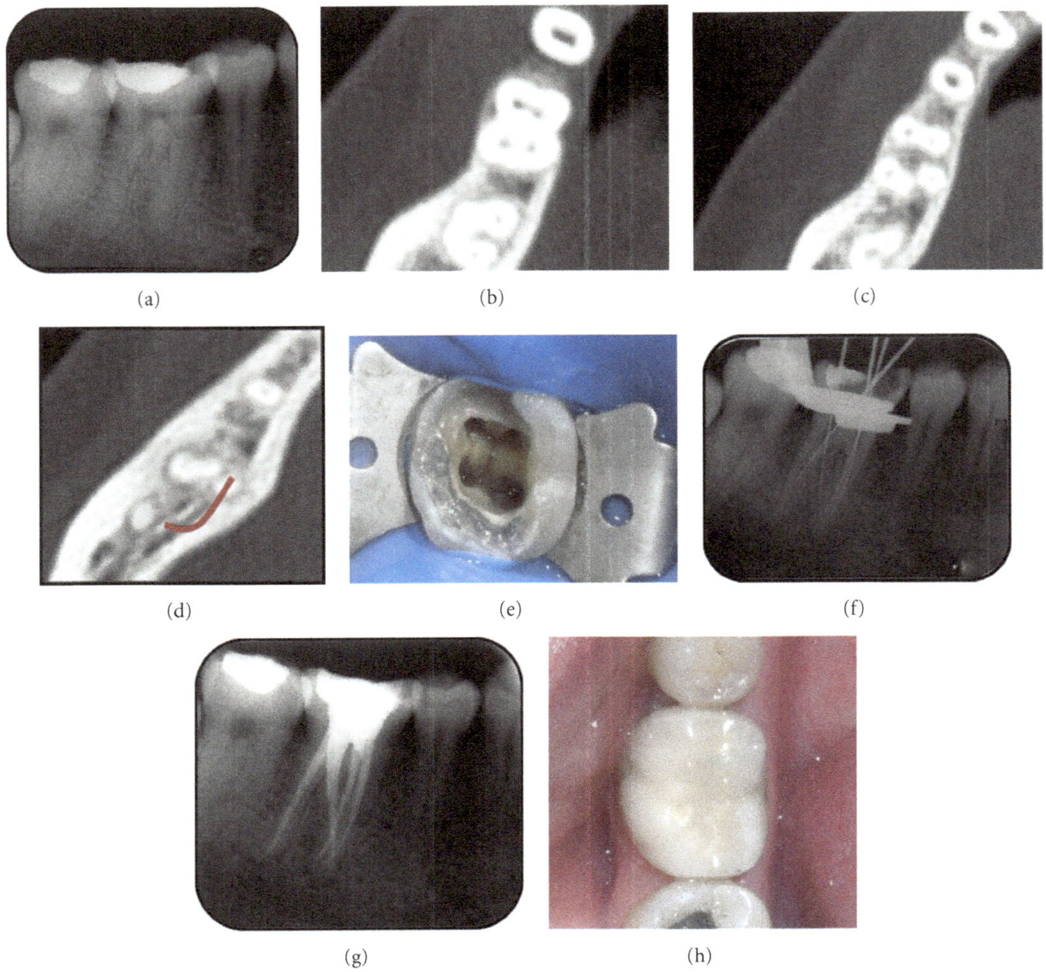


FIGURE 1: (a) Diagnostic radiograph, (b–d) computed tomographic scan in coronal, middle, and apical segments, respectively, (e) access cavity preparation, (f) working length determination, (g) post obturation, and (h) full coverage restoration.

are that it completely eliminates the superimposition of structural images outside the area of interest and provides a high-contrast resolution and data from a single computed tomography imaging process. Moreover, the images can be viewed in a coronal, sagittal, or even an oblique or curved image planes—a process referred to as multiplanar Reformation (MPR). In addition, CBCT data is amenable to reformation in a volume, rather than a slice, providing three-dimensional images in the axial, coronal, or sagittal planes [13].

RE has an occurrence of less than 5% in the Indian population, and such cases are rarely observed during routine endodontic procedures. We report on six such cases in this paper. RE was observed in the mandibular first molars of three patients being root canal treated. This anatomy was also present on three extracted mandibular teeth which were studied in detail to gain an understanding of their morphological characteristics. Knowledge of such variations can be beneficial in delivering treatment to patients presenting with related diversities in their root canal anatomy.

## 2. Case Reports

*Case 1.* A 22-year-old Indian female patient reported complaining of pain in a lower-right posterior tooth for a few days. The lower right first molar tooth had been restored with an amalgam restoration 10 years prior to this. Examination of the tooth revealed a large occlusal amalgam restoration with marginal ditching and tenderness to percussion. The mobility of the tooth was within physiologic limits and vitality testing revealed the tooth to be nonvital. The medical history of the patient was noncontributory. Radiographic examination (Figure 1(a)) revealed the restoration close to the distal pulp horn and periapical lamina dura widening. It also revealed the presence of an additional supernumerary root on distolingual side. In addition, a computed tomographic scan (Figures 1(b), 1(c), and 1(d)) of the lower jaw of the patient was available for surgical reasons. On evaluation, the scan illustrated the nature of origin and curvature of the extra root in a mesiobuccal direction as depicted by the arc (Figure 1(d)). The extra root originated from the distolingual part of the tooth and curved mesially.

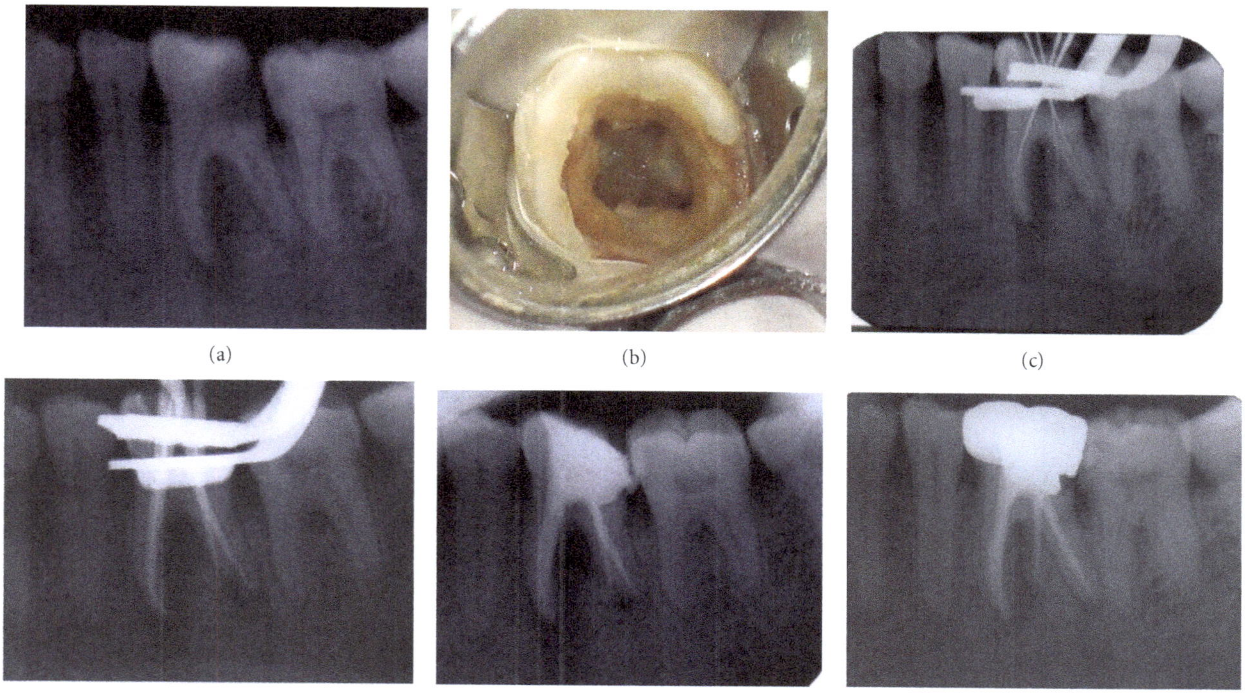

(a) (b) (c) (d) (e) (f)

FIGURE 2: (a) Diagnostic radiograph, (b) access cavity preparation, (c) working length determination, (d) master cone confirmation, (e) postobturation, and (f) eight-month followup.

A diagnosis was made as chronic apical periodontitis due to pulpal necrosis of the lower right first molar tooth. The pulp chamber was accessed and two mesial canal orifices and one distal canal orifice were located. In addition a dark line guided the operator towards an extra orifice located towards the distolingual part of the pulpal floor (Figure 1(e)). The root canal orifices were enlarged using gates glidden drills (Mani Inc., Kiyohara industrial park, Utsunomiya, Japan) to obtain a straight line access which modified the access shape to a more trapezoidal form. The root canals were explored with precurved K-file ISO number 15 (Dentsply Maillefer, Ballaigues, Switzerland), and radiographic length measurement was performed (Figure 1(f)). The root canals were instrumented using the ProTaper rotary files (Dentsply Maillefer, Ballaigues, Switzerland) in all the canals. During instrumentation adequate irrigation was performed using 1% sodium hypochlorite (I-Dent, Rohini, Delhi, India) and lubricated using Glyde (Dentsply Maillefer, Ballaigues, Switzerland). Obturation of the root canals was performed using AH plus sealer (Dentsply, Maillefer, Ballaigues, Switzerland) and corresponding ProTaper gutta percha points (Figure 1(g)). Postendodontic coronal restoration was done with full metal crown (Figure 1(h)).

*Case 2.* A 22-year-old Indian male patient reported to the Out Patient Department complaining of an inability to chew with lower left posterior tooth for the preceding few days. On clinical examination, the lower left first molar tooth had distoproximal caries and was tender to percussion. The periodontal status of the tooth was clinically normal, and the tooth had physiologic mobility.

Radiographic examination (Figure 2(a)) revealed periapical lesion in relation to both the mesial and distal roots of the tooth. It also revealed the presence of a supernumerary root in addition to a mesial and a distal root. The extra root originated from the distolingual part of the tooth and appeared to be relatively straight. As the tooth was unresponsive to electric pulp testing, it was diagnosed with pulpal necrosis and chronic apical periodontitis.

The pulp chamber was accessed, and two mesial canal orifices and one distal canal orifice were initially located. On further exploration, another orifice was located towards the distolingual part of the pulpal floor (Figure 2(b)). The root canals were explored with a K-file ISO number 15 and radiographic length measured (Figure 2(c)). Instrumentation was carried out using the ProTaper rotary files with intermittent irrigation using 1% sodium hypochlorite in all the canals. Master cone radiograph was obtained (Figure 2(d)). Obturation of the root canals was performed using the ProTaper gutta percha points and AH Plus sealer (Figure 2(e)). An eight-month follow-up radiograph of the patient illustrated resolving periapical radiolucency (Figure 2(f)).

*Case 3.* A 24-year-old female patient presented with pain in her lower right posterior region. The pain was continuous in nature and aggravated with hot food. On intraoral examination, an old leaking composite restoration was seen in the lower right first molar tooth. The tooth was hypersensitive to both hot and cold stimuli and was tender to percussion

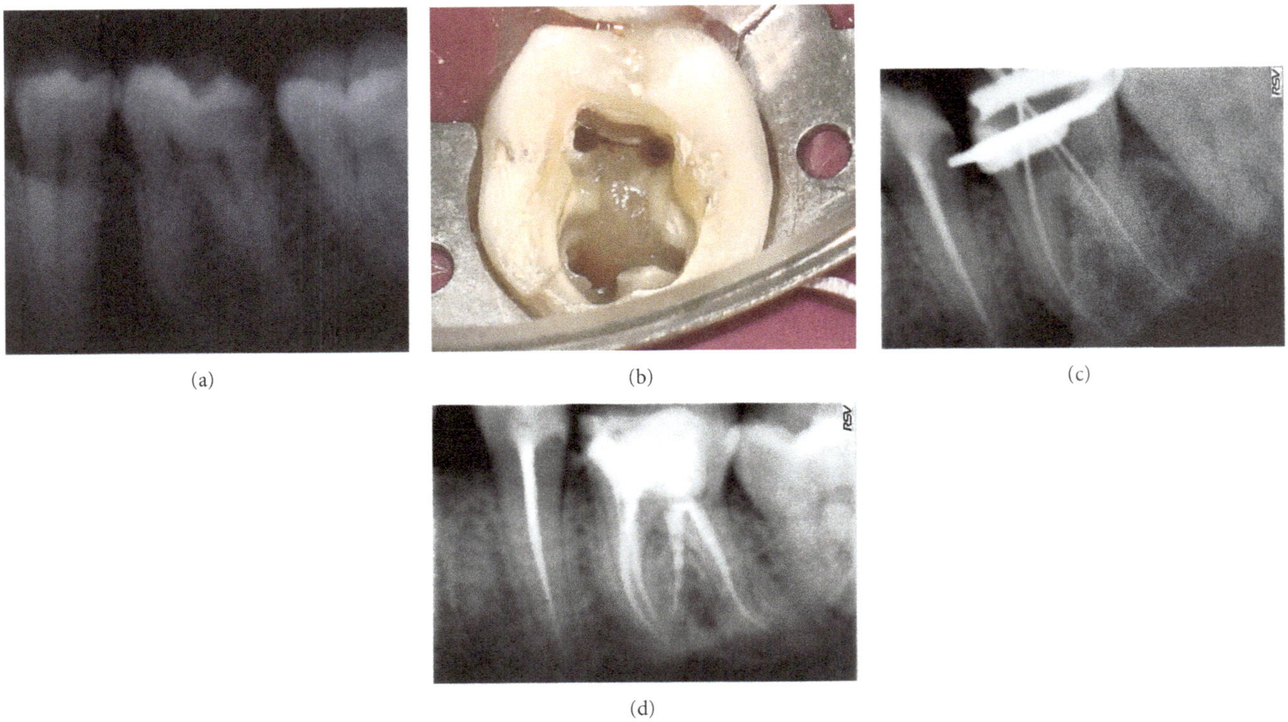


FIGURE 3: (a) Diagnostic radiograph, (b) access cavity preparation, (c) working length determination, and (d) postfilling.

although no pathologic mobility was observed. Radiographic assessment of the tooth revealed a large occlusal restoration close to the pulp of the tooth with an extra distal root. To confirm this observation, another radiograph at a horizontal angulation of 20 degrees was taken which clearly revealed the presence of an extra distal root that curved severely towards the mesial root (Figure 3(a)). No periapical changes could be seen thus a diagnosis of irreversible pulpitis was made, and root canal treatment was decided as the treatment option.

Upon access to the pulp chamber, the distal orifice was seen located eccentrically towards the buccal aspect of the tooth (Figure 3(b)). Following the laws of orifice location [14], another orifice was located on the distolingual side. The coronal shaping of all of the orifices was done using Gates Glidden drills (number 1–3). A number 10 K file was loose in all canals except in the disto-lingual canal where it stopped 3 mm short of the radiographic apex. Since there was a sharp apical curvature (Figure 3(c)) in the disto-lingual root, C+ files (Dentsply, Maillefer, Ballaigues, Switzerland) with batt tips (a unique feature of C+ files) were used to negotiate the canal. The canals were shaped from coronal to middle and apical to a ProTaper size F2 (Dentsply, Maillefer, Ballaigues, Switzerland) and obturated (Figure 3(d)) using the corresponding gutta percha cones.

## 3. Extracted Teeth

Three extracted teeth which exhibited RE morphology were also clinically and radiographically assessed. In all of the teeth, the extra root emerged from the lingual aspect of the tooth (Figures 4(a), 4(e), 4(i), 4(b), 4(f), and 4(j)) either attached to the distal root or midway between the mesial and the distal roots. After separating from the tooth, the root usually ran straight for the coronal part of its length and then in the middle or apical third, and it curved buccally and/or mesially. The third root was narrow and tapering towards the apex with a variable length. Thus care should be taken not to overprepare and shape such root canals to avoid any inadvertent perforation of the root (Figures 4(d), 4(h), and 4(l)).

Access opening was performed on all of the extracted molars (Figures 4(c), 4(g), and 4(k)). The location of the supplemental orifice was in a distal and/or lingual position, at times nearing the external enamel wall. To establish straight line access, it was required to have sufficient coronal enlargement using gates glidden drills.

## 4. Discussion

Anatomical variations are an acknowledged characteristic of mandibular permanent molars. Although a majority of the mandibular molars are two rooted with a mesial and distal root, an extra disto-lingual root may occasionally be encountered. Some authors consider a radix entomolaris as a genetic trait rather than a developmental anomaly [6, 15]. They have suggested that these "three-rooted molar" traits had a high degree of genetic penetration as reflected in the fact that pure Eskimo and Eskimo/Caucasian mixed-race individuals had a similar prevalence of the trait. While it may be a normal morphological variant in ethnic groups

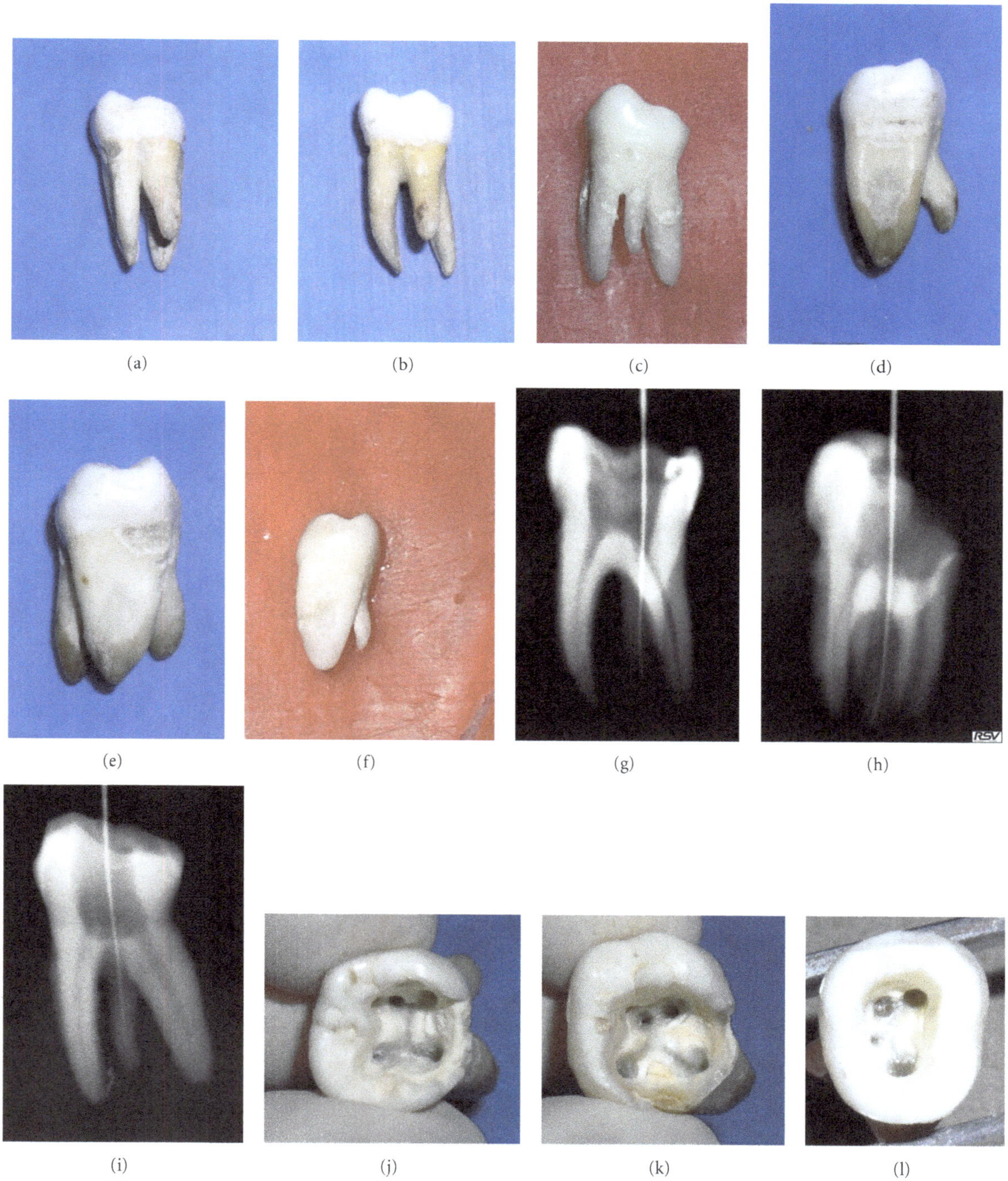


FIGURE 4: (a, e, and i) Lateral view of the extracted teeth, (b, f, and j) mesial view of the extracted teeth, (c, g, and k) access cavity preparation, and (d, h, and l) radiographic appearance.

of mongoloid origin (>30%), it has rather low prevalence (<5%) in other people such as the Indian population.

RE root is commonly found distolingually and ranges from being a short conical extension to a full-length root. The root may extend unilaterally or bilaterally [16] and may contain pulpal tissue even if it is short and conical in form [17]. RE can be classified into four different types depending on the location of its cervical part [18].

(i) Type A: the RE is located lingually to the distal root complex which has two cone-shaped macrostructures.

(ii) Type B: the RE is located lingually to the distal root complex which has one cone-shaped macrostructures.

(iii) Type C: the RE is located lingually to the mesial root complex.

(iv) Type AC: the RE is located lingually between the mesial and distal root complexes.

Each type has a subclassification to allow for the identification of separate or nonseparate RE.

An alternative classification of RE by De Moor et al. describes the curvature of the root or the root canal and is based on the work of Ribeiro et al. [10, 19].

(i) Type 1: a straight root or root canal.

(ii) Type 2: a curved coronal third which becomes straighter in the middle and apical third.

(iii) Type 3: an initial curve in the coronal third with a second buccally oriented curve which begins in the middle or apical third.

The infrequent occurrence of such an anomaly requires that the clinician be vigilant in diagnosis and management of the lower molar teeth. The clinical examination of the tooth can reveal a more bulbous outline of the crown, an extra cusp (tuberculum paramolare), or a more prominent occlusodistal or distolingual lobe. These in combination with a cervical prominence or convexity can indicate the presence of an additional root. Aids to clinical examination such as magnifying loupes, an intraoral camera, or a dental microscope may be useful in this respect. Radiographically a third root should normally be readily evident in about 90% of cases [20]. A careful inspection of the radiograph can sometimes reveal the presence of a "hidden" RE as indicated by an unclear view or outline of the distal root contour or the root canal. However, it may still be missed due to its slender dimensions occasionally. An additional exposure of the concerned tooth from different horizontal projections, the standard buccal-to-lingual projection, 20 degrees from the mesial and 20 degrees from the distal reveals all the basic information regarding the anatomy of the tooth [21, 22]. Cone-beam computed tomography has emerged as a useful tool to aid in diagnosis of complex root canal anatomy. In the first case report the CBCT images revealed the location and direction of the curvature. This was extremely beneficial during cleaning, shaping, and obturation of the type 3 curvature seen in this root.

Once a diagnosis is reached and an access cavity has to be prepared, care should be taken to establish a "straight-line" access. With the disto-lingually located orifice of the RE a modification of the classical triangular access cavity to a trapezoidal form is required to locate and access the root canal. The laws of orifice location [14] may aid in the location of extra orifices. However, care must be taken to avoid gouging or excessive removal of dentin as this may weaken the tooth structure.

Based on the literature, the majority of radices entomolaris are curved. In some cases there is an additional curve starting from the middle of the root or in the apical third. Hence using precurved files, to establish a smooth glide path to the apical segment and Nickel-Titanium rotary files for cleaning and shaping, is the desired option [23]. Adequate coronal enlargement avoids hindrances in the coronal segment of the canals and easy passage of the endodontic file to the apical segment. It would also allow root canal irrigants to pass on to the apical segment in larger volumes. Radiographs taken at different angulations/CBCT scan of the tooth should be studied carefully to estimate the root length and curvature. The root length in such cases can be confirmed with the help of electronic apex locators. Nonetheless, in spite of using the state-of-art gadgets endodontic mishaps may occur, and thus care has to be taken while negotiating and cleaning these curved canals.

## 5. Conclusion

Radix entomolaris has been reported to occur with a frequency of 0.2–32% in different populations. It is crucial to ascertain the exact nature/characteristic of the RE in terms of curvature and conformation to carry out a proper treatment. Therefore, such cases require judicial application of diagnostic tools and endodontic skills for their management. Careful interpretation of the radiograph, using different horizontal cone projections and advanced tools such as CBCT, may facilitate their recognition. Once diagnosed, management of the extra canal and root can be done using equipments such as magnification aids, orifice locators and flexible files.

## References

[1] A. E. Skidmore and A. M. Bjorndal, "Root canal morphology of the human mandibular first molar," *Oral Surgery, Oral Medicine, Oral Pathology*, vol. 32, no. 5, pp. 778–784, 1971.

[2] F. Pineda and Y. Kuttler, "Mesiodistal and buccolingual roentgenographic investigation of 7,275 root canals," *Oral Surgery, Oral Medicine, Oral Pathology*, vol. 33, no. 1, pp. 101–110, 1972.

[3] F. J. Vertucci, "Root canal anatomy of the human permanent teeth," *Oral Surgery Oral Medicine and Oral Pathology*, vol. 58, no. 5, pp. 589–599, 1984.

[4] B. C. W. Barker, K. C. Parsons, P. R. Mills, and G. L. Williams, "Anatomy of root canals. III. Permanent mandibular molars," *Australian Dental Journal*, vol. 19, no. 6, pp. 408–413, 1974.

[5] E. K. Tratman, "Three-rooted lower molars in man and their racial distribution," *British Dental Journal*, vol. 64, pp. 264–274, 1938.

[6] M. E. Curzon and J. A. Curzon, "Three-rooted mandibular molars in the Keewatin Eskimo," *Journal of the Canadian Dental Association*, vol. 37, no. 2, pp. 71–72, 1971.

[7] C. G. Turner, "Three-rooted mandibular first permanent molars and the question of American Indian origins," *American Journal of Physical Anthropology*, vol. 34, no. 2, pp. 229–241, 1971.

[8] S. C. Yew and K. Chan, "A retrospective study of endodontically treated mandibular first molars in a Chinese population," *Journal of Endodontics*, vol. 19, no. 9, pp. 471–473, 1993.

[9] G. Carabelli, *Systematisches Handbuch Der Zahnheilkunde*, Braumüller und Seidel, Vienna, Austria, 2 edition, 1844.

[10] R. J. G. De Moor, C. A. J. G. Deroose, and F. L. G. Calberson, "The radix entomolaris in mandibular first molars: an endodontic challenge," *International Endodontic Journal*, vol. 37, no. 11, pp. 789–799, 2004.

[11] V. Gopikrishna, J. Reuben, and D. Kandaswamy, "Endodontic management of a maxillary first molar with two palatal roots and a single fused buccal root diagnosed with spiral computed

tomography—a case report," *Oral Surgery, Oral Medicine, Oral Pathology, Oral Radiology and Endodontology*, vol. 105, no. 4, pp. e74–e78, 2008.

[12] V. Aggarwal, M. Singla, A. Logani, and N. Shah, "Endodontic management of a maxillary first molar with two palatal canals with the aid of spiral computed tomography: a case report," *Journal of Endodontics*, vol. 35, no. 1, pp. 137–139, 2009.

[13] Z. Kirzioglu, H. Karayilmaz, and B. Baykal, "Value of computed tomography (CT) in imaging the morbidity of submerged molars: a case report," *European Journal of Dentistry*, vol. 1, pp. 246–250, 2007.

[14] P. Krasner and H. J. Rankow, "Anatomy of the pulp-chamber floor," *Journal of Endodontics*, vol. 30, no. 1, pp. 5–16, 2004.

[15] R. T. Walker, "Root form and canal anatomy of mandibular second molars in a Southern Chinese population," *Endodontics & Dental Traumatology*, vol. 14, no. 7, pp. 325–329, 1988.

[16] W. Somogyi-Csizmazia and A. J. Simons, "Three-rooted mandibular first permanent molars in Alberta Indian children," *Journal of the Canadian Dental Association*, vol. 37, no. 3, pp. 105–106, 1971.

[17] P. A. Reichart and D. Metah, "Three-rooted permanent mandibular first molars in the Thai," *Community Dentistry and Oral Epidemiology*, vol. 9, no. 4, pp. 191–192, 1981.

[18] O. Carlsen and V. Alexandersen, "Radix entomolaris: identification and morphology," *Scandinavian Journal of Dental Research*, vol. 98, no. 5, pp. 363–373, 1990.

[19] F. C. Ribeiro and A. Consolaro, "Importancia clinica y antropologica de la raiz distolingual en los molares inferiores permamentes," *Endodoncia*, vol. 15, pp. 72–78, 1997.

[20] R. T. Walker and L. E. Quackenbush, "Three-rooted lower first permanent molars in Hong Kong Chinese," *British Dental Jornal*, vol. 159, no. 9, pp. 298–299, 1985.

[21] R. M. F. Klein, S. A. Blake, B. R. Nattress, and P. N. Hirschmann, "Evaluation of X-ray beam angulation for successful twin canal identification in mandibular incisors," *International Endodontic Journal*, vol. 30, no. 1, pp. 58–63, 1997.

[22] J. I. Ingle, G. S. Heithersay, and G. R. Hatwell, *Endodontic Diagnostic Procedures*, BC Decker, London, UK, 2002.

[23] F. L. Calberson, R. J. De Moor, and C. A. Deroose, "The radix entomolaris and paramolaris: clinical approach in endodontics," *Journal of Endodontics*, vol. 33, no. 1, pp. 58–63, 2007.

# 43

# Cracked Tooth: A Report of Two Cases and Role of Cone Beam Computed Tomography in Diagnosis

**Pishipati Vinayak Kalyan Chakravarthy,[1] Lahari Ajay Telang,[2] Jayashri Nerali,[3] and Ajay Telang[3]**

[1] *Department of Conservative Dentistry and Endodontics, Penang International Dental College, Level 18-21, NB Tower, 5050 Jalan Bagan Luar, 12000 Butterworth, Penang, Malaysia*
[2] *Department of Oral Medicine and Radiology, Penang International Dental College, 12000 Butterworth, Penang, Malaysia*
[3] *Department of Oral Pathology, Penang International Dental College, 12000 Butterworth, Penang, Malaysia*

Correspondence should be addressed to Pishipati Vinayak Kalyan Chakravarthy, kalyanendo@gmail.com

Academic Editors: S. S. De Rossi, L. Junquera, and P. Lopez Jornet

Cracked tooth is a distinct type of longitudinal tooth fracture which occurs very commonly and its diagnosis can be challenging. This type of fracture tends to grow and change over time. Clinical diagnosis is difficult because the signs and symptoms are variable or nonspecific and may even resemble post-treatment disease following root canal treatment or periodontal disease. This variety and unpredictability make the cracked tooth a challenging diagnostic entity. The use of cone beam computed tomography (CBCT) in diagnosis of complex endodontic cases has been well documented in the literature. In this paper we present two cases of cracked tooth and emphasise on the timely use of cone beam computed tomography as an aid in diagnosis and as a prognostic determinant.

## 1. Introduction

Longitudinal tooth fractures are characterized by an incomplete or complete fracture line that extends through the long axis of the tooth [1]. These linear fractures tend to grow and change over time [2]. They have been classified into 5 distinct groups, generally from least to most severe: craze lines; fractured cusp; cracked tooth; split tooth; vertical root fractures [3].

Cracked tooth is a distinct type of longitudinal fracture which may extend through either or both of the marginal ridges and through the proximal surface. The fracture may be restricted to the crown or may extend from crown to the proximal root for varying distances [3].

Cracked tooth is common and challenging [4]. It may be caused by excessive forces from mastication or occlusion, either large forces on a normal tooth or normal forces on a weakened tooth [1]. Complex restorative and endodontic treatments that remove dentin compromise the internal strength of the tooth making it susceptible to fracture [3]. The detection of non-displaced longitudinal fractures, such as a cracked tooth, is a significant challenge in clinical practice [4]. Clinical diagnosis is difficult because the signs and symptoms are variable or nonspecific and may even resemble post-treatment disease following root canal treatment or periodontal disease [5]. Radiographic signs are usually absent when the orientation of the X-ray beam is not parallel to the plane of the fracture making the diagnosis even more challenging [6]. Moreover superimposition of other structures further limits the sensitivity of radiographs for the detection of fractures.

Cracked tooth by itself is not a diagnosis, but is a finding. A cracked tooth can act as a pathway for bacteria that may induce pulpal and/or periapical inflammation or disease. The relationship between cracks in teeth and endodontic diagnosis depends upon the extent of the fracture. If the fracture is in or in close proximity to the pulp and allows bacterial byproducts or frank bacteria to communicate with the pulp, then inflammation and pulpal degeneration occurs. If the fracture is not in close proximity to the pulp and bacterial byproducts are neutralized in the dentinal tubules, then no pulpal inflammation or degeneration should be expected [7]. The prognosis of a tooth depends on extent of the fracture. The prognosis of cracked tooth that is not treated will progressively deteriorate and may evolve into a split tooth or result in severe periodontal defects [1]. Eventually the tooth may be lost. Therefore early diagnosis and treatment are essential in saving these teeth.

In this paper two case reports of cracked tooth which reported to the dental clinic of Penang International Dental College have been presented. The value of cone beam CT as a prognostic determinant has been highlighted.

## 2. Case Report 1

A female patient aged 49 years reported with pain on upper left second premolar, that is, 25, for the past two weeks. Pain was severe, throbbing in nature, and radiating towards the temporal region and the neck. It was aggravated on taking cold and hot drinks and relieved with pain killers (NSAIDs). No caries or fracture was detected nor was restoration present. The tooth was tender on percussion and no mobility was detected. Electric pulp test showed delayed response. Radiograph revealed no significant findings. Based on the history and clinical presentation it was diagnosed as apical periodontitis. Root canal treatment was performed with amalgam as post-endodontic restoration (Figure 1(c)). Thereafter, the patient failed to report for a crown restoration.

Fifteen months later, the patient returned with severe pain in the same tooth, that is, 25. Pain was radiating and aggravated on chewing and biting. Patient could recall episodes of dull aching pain even after the root canal therapy, for which she was taking pain killers for relief. Clinical examination revealed a fracture on the centre of occlusal surface running mesiodistally and over the marginal ridges onto the proximal surface (Figure 1(a)). A diffuse swelling was present on the buccal gingiva involving the marginal and attached gingiva (Figure 1(b)). Tooth was tender on percussion and exhibited grade II mobility. The fracture could not be separated by using wedging forces. Periodontal probing revealed deep isolated narrow pockets on both proximal sides. Radiograph did not reveal the fracture as it was mesiodistally oriented, but showed angular bone loss on both mesial and distal proximal aspects and generalised widening of periodontal ligament space (Figure 1(d)). Prognosis was considered poor and extraction was performed.

The fracture in this case was considered to be a cracked tooth as it originated on the occlusal surface and extended onto the proximal surface and then onto the root surface until the apical third on both mesial and distal surfaces (Figures 2(a) and 2(b)).

## 3. Case Report 2

A female patient aged 51 years reported with severe, throbbing pain in left upper first premolar, that is, 24, since three days. The pain was aggravated on chewing and lingered on for few hours after removal of stimulus. There was history of sensitivity to cold beverages. The patient could recall episodes of similar pain with the same tooth for the past two years which was only temporarily relieved with desensitising tooth paste.

On clinical examination, no caries was detected nor restoration was present but a very faint craze line could be seen on the distal marginal ridge extending onto the distal proximal surface of 24 (Figure 3(a)). The extent of the craze line could not be determined. The tooth was tender on percussion, it did not exhibit mobility, and the fracture could not be separated using wedging forces. Periodontal probing depths were normal. Electric pulp test revealed immediate response. Radiograph did not confirm the fracture line or reveal any significant findings (Figure 3(b)). The patient was given a choice of using cone beam computed tomography (CBCT) to determine the extent of fracture and the prognosis of the tooth. She was explained the benefits and also assured that radiation exposure would be kept as minimal as possible. An informed consent was obtained from the patient. Cone beam computed tomography (Vatech, PaX-Reve 3D plus, pulse type generator, $5 \times 5$ cm field of view (FOV) and 0.08 mm voxel size) was used to determine the relative depth of fracture apically and the proximity of fracture to the pulp (Figures 4(a) and 4(b)). The fracture line was found to extend mesiodistally involving lingual pulp horn and apically it did not extend below the level of alveolar bone. Prognosis was considered to be favourable. Root canal treatment followed by crown restoration was then decided as most appropriate treatment plan. The suspicion of fracture extending to deeper aspects of root, coupled with acute symptoms of pain in the patient prompted the usage of CBCT for a clearer diagnosis, prognosis, and treatment plan.

## 4. Discussion

Cracked tooth is a distinct type of longitudinal fracture of the tooth and studies have indicated increased incidence of cracked tooth [8, 9]. This type of fracture is not only associated with complex and long standing restorations but also with minimally restored teeth and teeth without any restorations as noticed in case report 2. The teeth usually involved are mandibular molars (restored and nonrestored) followed by maxillary premolars and then by maxillary first molars [1, 10, 11]. Cracks in teeth are almost invariably mesiodistal fractures [12] although mandibular molars may occasionally fracture toward the facial or lingual surface. Longitudinal fractures are common in root canal-treated teeth, because the strength of root canal treated tooth has already been compromised by caries, restorations, or overextended access preparations [13] making it vulnerable to fracture. Crown restorations given in posterior teeth after endodontic therapy provide bracing effect and prevent crack initiation and propagation. In case report 1, failure to deliver crown restoration after root canal therapy may have led to the propagation of crack over a period of time leading to devastating results and finally extraction of tooth.

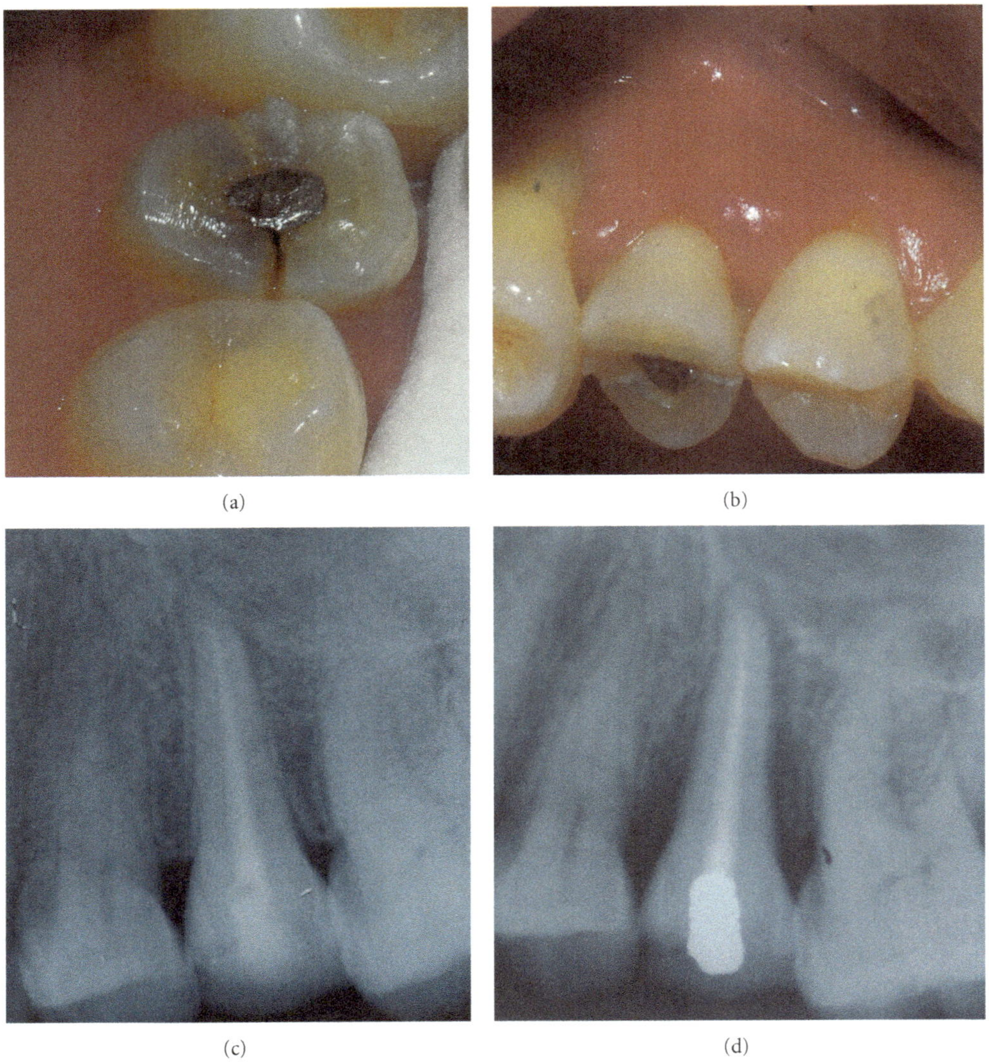

FIGURE 1: (a) Fracture extending mesiodistally on centre of occlusal surface and then onto proximal surface of 25. (b) Diffuse swelling of the buccal gingiva. (c) Post obturation intraoral periapical radiograph of 25. (d) Intraoral periapical radiograph taken after 15 months shows severe angular bone loss interproximally associated with propagation of fracture line.

Etiological factors of these fractures are repeated biting on hard substances [2], prominent masticatory muscles [14], parafunctional habits, deep class I and II restorations, thermal stresses created by difference of coefficient of thermal expansion of restoration and dentin [15, 16], retentive pin placement with twist drills [17], and endodontically treated teeth.

Cracked tooth is a fracture which usually begins on the occlusal surface and grows from this surface toward the cervical surface and down the root. In case report 1 the fracture was present on centre of occlusal surface and progressed until the junction of middle third and apical third of the root. The more centred the fracture on the occlusal surface, the more it has a tendency to extend deeper before it shears toward the root surface. The deeper the fracture extends on to the root surface, the poorer the prognosis [7]. This fracture is considered "greenstick" because it is incomplete (either to the mesial or distal surface) or does not extend to the facial or lingual root surface [8]. Wedging forces produce no separable segments. In contrast, a split tooth has a fracture which is complete and extends to a surface in all areas [14]. A split tooth is usually the end result of a cracked tooth.

Cracked tooth is not a diagnosis by itself, but a finding. The objective is to first detect and then determine the extent of the fracture. Useful aids in detection of cracked tooth are transillumination [8], careful visualisation after removal of restoration, selective biting on objects such as the Tooth Slooth or Fracfinder, dental operating microscopes, staining, and wedging forces [3].

The relationship between fractures in the teeth and endodontic diagnoses depends upon the extent of the fracture. A cracked tooth may present with a variety of symptoms ranging from pain on biting, sensitivity to thermal changes, and mild to very severe, spontaneous pain consistent with irreversible pulpitis, pulp necrosis, or apical periodontitis

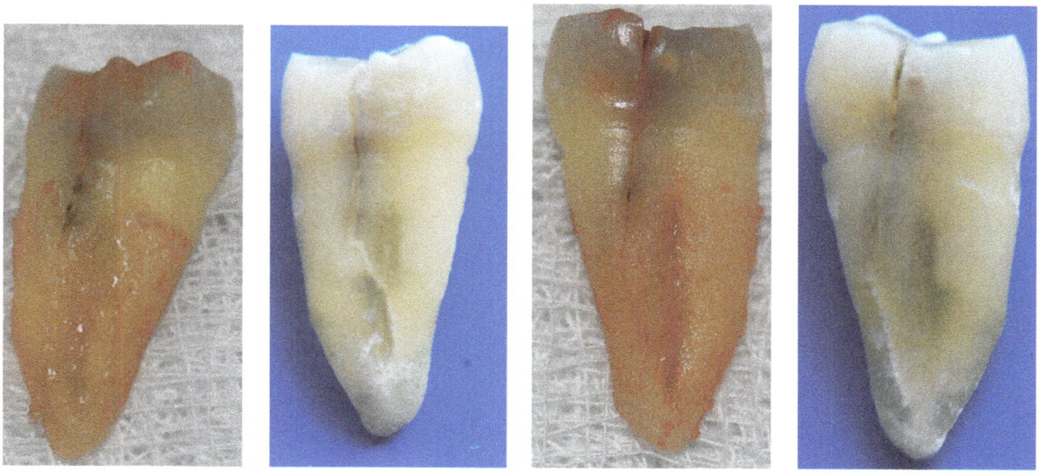

(a) (b)

FIGURE 2: (a) Fracture extending to junction of middle and apical third of root (mesial) of 25. (b) Fracture extending to apical third of root (distal) of 25.

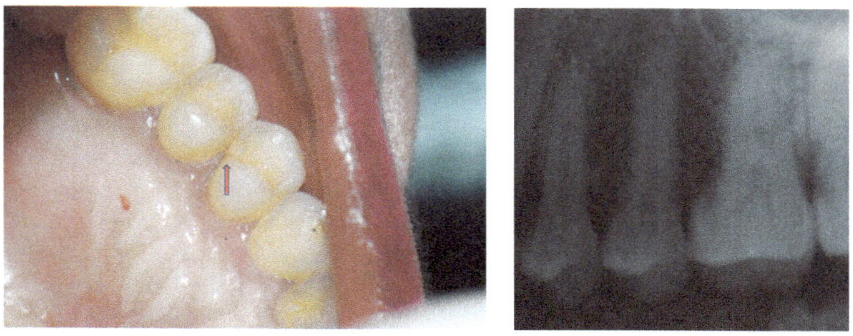

(a) (b)

FIGURE 3: (a) Faint fracture line can be detected on distal marginal ridge extending onto proximal surface of 24. (b) Intraoral periapical radiograph of 24 reveals no significant findings.

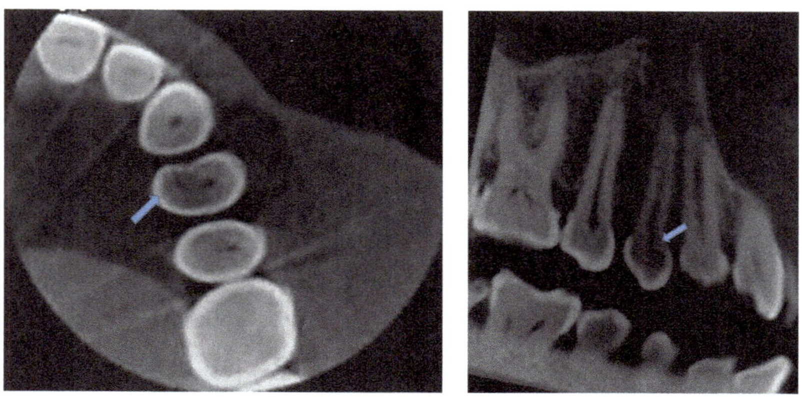

(a) (b)

FIGURE 4: (a) Axial view of CBCT reveals a fracture line extending mesiodistally involving lingual pulp horn. (b) Sagittal view of CBCT reveals a fracture line extending mesiodistally at the level of pulp horn.

[18]. Even an acute apical abscess, with or without swelling or a draining sinus tract, may be present if the pulp has undergone necrosis. Once the fracture has extended to and exposed the pulp, severe pulp and/or periapical pathosis may be present. This explains the variation in signs and symptoms and therefore the term "Cracked Tooth Syndrome" should not be used [7].

In a cracked tooth pulp and periapical tests also produce variable results. The pulp is usually responsive (vital) [14] but may be non-responsive (necrosis) as well. Directional percussion is also advocated. Percussion that separates the crack may cause pain due to stimulation of the periodontal ligament proprioceptors [7]. Periodontal probing is important and may disclose the approximate depth and severity of the fracture. However, subgingival fractures often do not create a probing defect. Therefore the absence of deep probing does not preclude a cracked tooth [19].

As the fracture in a cracked tooth is usually present in mesiodistal direction, it is not visible radiographically. Conventional dental radiography serves as an aid in assessing pulpal and periodontal compromise but gives little or no information on the direction and extent of the fracture. Depending on the extension towards the root and the relationship with the periodontium (below alveolar crest) the treatment is going to vary. If the fracture is limited to the crown surface, it can be restored. If a fracture extends below the alveolar crest, the prognosis is poor. Making the proper treatment decision is a challenge for the endodontist as there are limited noninvasive tools to assess the length of the fractures below the soft tissues and alveolar crest.

Newer methods of analysis, such as cone beam computed tomography (CBCT), are currently being studied in order to help identify longitudinal fractures in a nondestructive fashion [20]. The joint position statement by the American Association of Endodontists (AAE) and American Academy of Oral and Maxillofacial Radiology (AAOMR) regarding the use of CBCT in Endodontics states that "the patient's history and clinical examination must justify the use of CBCT by demonstrating that the benefits to the patient outweigh the potential risks [21]. Clinicians should use CBCT only when the need for imaging cannot be answered adequately by lower dose conventional dental radiography or alternate imaging modalities." Every effort should be made to reduce the effective radiation dose to the patient for endodontic-specific tasks. Using the smallest possible field of vision (FOV), the smallest voxel size, the lowest mA setting, and the shortest exposure time in conjunction with a pulsed exposure mode of acquisition is recommended [21].

In case report 2 we have used multi-slice view (thickness 1 mm, spacing 0.4 mm) of CBCT to detect the fracture at various planes and to determine the apical extent as well as proximity to the pulp and predict the prognosis. The volume of data acquired in a single scan allows visualizing a tooth from any coronal, sagittal, or axial view, and the ability to reslice the volume at any slice thickness. This volume of data can be manipulated repeatedly to gather large amount of information about the tooth and its periapical tissues.

Mora et al. [20] and Valizadeh et al. [22] in their in vitro study found local CT and CBCT, respectively, to be more efficient in detection of longitudinal tooth fractures compared to conventional dental radiographs.

Treatment of a cracked tooth depends on the nature (depth and location) of the fracture. If there are no symptoms of irreversible pulpitis, a crown may be placed. Some of these teeth may eventually manifest irreversible pulpitis or pulp necrosis [23]. In that case root canal treatment can be performed through the crown. After endodontic access, the pulp chamber floor is examined carefully; transillumination is a useful aid during this procedure. If the fracture extends through the chamber floor, further treatment is usually hopeless and extraction is preferred [24]. An exception is the maxillary molar, which may be hemisected along the fracture, saving half (or both halves) of the crown and supporting roots. If a partial fracture of the chamber floor is detected, the crown may be bound with an orthodontic band or temporary crown to protect the cusps until final restoration is performed [25]. This also helps to determine whether symptoms decrease during root canal treatment [26]. The rationale employed for treatment of cracked tooth is that if pain symptoms are not relieved, the prognosis is significantly poorer, and extraction may be necessary. The overall prognosis depends on the situation but is always questionable at best. The patient is informed about the possible outcomes and the unpredictability of the duration of treatment. The fracture may continue to grow and become a split tooth, with devastating consequences requiring tooth extraction or additional treatment. Tan et al. [19] studied a small number ($n = 50$) of root-filled cracked teeth with a diagnosis of irreversible pulpitis and determined a 2-year survival rate of 85.5%. Krell and Rivera [23] evaluated 127 patients with teeth diagnosed with reversible pulpitis that had a cracked tooth in which the treatment was placement of a crown restoration without performing root canal treatment. Twenty percent of these cases turned into irreversible pulpitis or necrosis within 6 months and required root canal treatment, but none of the other teeth required root canal treatment over the 6-year evaluation period. In case report 1 the failure to detect the crack and determine its severity, followed by failure to place a crown restoration after root canal treatment, may have led to crack propagation and poor prognosis of the tooth. In case report 2 early detection of extent and severity of the crack with the aid of CBCT helped in improving the overall prognosis of the tooth.

## 5. Conclusion

Early detection, diagnosis, and prompt treatment are the key to the successful management of a cracked tooth. Careful attention to signs and symptoms and using conventional techniques and advanced methods like CBCT along with timely treatment can limit the crack propagation. Assessment of the pattern or extent of fracture with the aid of CBCT can help the endodontist in making a decision about root canal treatment or extraction and reassuring the patient why root canal treatment or extraction is necessary for such a faint fracture line. It also helps in having reliable documentation and strong evidence for future reference. Nevertheless, the higher dose of radiation should be kept in mind and hence should be reserved for only challenging cases after thorough examination.

## References


[1] R. E. Walton, "Longitudinal tooth fractures," in *Torabinejad M. Principles and Practice of Endodontics*, R. E. Walton, Ed., pp. 499–519, WB Saunders Company, Philadelphia, Pa, USA, 3rd edition, 1995.

[2] E. M. Rivera and A. Williamson, "Diagnosis and treatment planning: cracked tooth," *Texas dental journal*, vol. 120, no. 3, pp. 278–283, 2003.

[3] E. M. Rivera and R. E. Walton, "Cracking the cracked tooth code: detection and treatment of various longitudinal tooth fractures," American Association of Endodontists Colleagues for Excellence, Newsletter, Summer 2008.

[4] J. D. Bader, J. A. Martin, and D. A. Shugars, "Preliminary estimates of the incidence and consequences of tooth fracture," *Journal of the American Dental Association*, vol. 126, no. 12, pp. 1650–1654, 1995.

[5] A. Schetritt and B. Steffensen, "Diagnosis and management of vertical root fractures," *Journal of Canadian Dental Association*, vol. 61, no. 7, pp. 607–613, 1995.

[6] A. Tamse, I. Zilburg, and J. Halpern, "Vertical root fractures in adjacent maxillary premolars: an endodontic-prosthetic perplexity," *International Endodontic Journal*, vol. 31, no. 2, pp. 127–132, 1998.

[7] E. M. Rivera and R. E. Walton, "Longitudinal tooth fractures: findings that contribute to complex endodontic diagnoses," *Endodontic Topics*, vol. 16, pp. 82–111, 2007.

[8] M. Abou-Rass, "Crack lines: the precursors of tooth fractures—their diagnosis and treatment," *Quintessence International*, vol. 14, no. 4, pp. 437–447, 1983.

[9] E. H. Ehrmann and M. J. Tyas, "Cracked tooth syndrome: diagnosis, treatment and correlation between symptoms and post-extraction findings," *Australian Dental Journal*, vol. 35, no. 2, pp. 105–112, 1990.

[10] M. K. Nair, U. D. P. Nair, H. G. Gröndahl, R. L. Webber, and J. A. Wallace, "Detection of artificially induced vertical radicular fractures using Tuned Aperture Computed Tomography," *European Journal of Oral Sciences*, vol. 109, no. 6, pp. 375–379, 2001.

[11] A. N. Van Daatselaar, S. M. Dunn, H. J. W. Spoelder et al., "Feasibility of local CT of dental tissues," *Dentomaxillofacial Radiology*, vol. 32, no. 3, pp. 173–180, 2003.

[12] F. S. Weine and J. A. Dewberry, "Cracked-tooth syndrome: vertical fractures of posterior teeth," in *Endodontic Therapy*, F. S. Weine, Ed., pp. 8–15, Mosby, St. Louis, Mo, USA, 3rd edition, 1982.

[13] W. S. Eakle, E. H. Maxwell, and B. V. Braly, "Fractures of posterior teeth in adults," *The Journal of the American Dental Association*, vol. 112, no. 2, pp. 215–218, 1986.

[14] C. E. Cameron, "The cracked tooth syndrome: additional findings," *The Journal of the American Dental Association*, vol. 93, no. 5, pp. 971–975, 1976.

[15] W. S. Brown, H. R. Jacobs, and R. E. Thompson, "Thermal fatigue in teeth," *Journal of Dental Research*, vol. 51, no. 2, pp. 461–467, 1972.

[16] W. S. Eakle, "Effect of thermal cycling on fracture strength and microleakage in teeth restored with a bonded composite resin," *Dental Materials*, vol. 2, no. 3, pp. 114–117, 1986.

[17] J. P. Standlee, E. W. Collard, and A. A. Caputo, "Dentinal defects caused by some twist drills and retentive pins," *The Journal of Prosthetic Dentistry*, vol. 24, no. 2, pp. 185–192, 1970.

[18] A. Brynjulfsen, I. Fristad, T. Grevstad, and I. Hals-Kvinnsland, "Incompletely fractured teeth associated with diffuse long-standing orofacial pain: diagnosis and treatment outcome," *International Endodontic Journal*, vol. 35, no. 5, pp. 461–466, 2002.

[19] L. Tan, N. N. Chen, C. Y. Poon, and H. B. Wong, "Survival of root filled cracked teeth in a tertiary institution," *International Endodontic Journal*, vol. 39, no. 11, pp. 886–889, 2006.

[20] M. A. Mora, A. Mol, D. A. Tyndall, and E. M. Rivera, "In vitro assessment of local computed tomography for the detection of longitudinal tooth fractures," *Oral Surgery, Oral Medicine, Oral Pathology, Oral Radiology and Endodontology*, vol. 103, no. 6, pp. 825–829, 2007.

[21] "AAE and AAOMR joint position statement. Use of cone-beam-computed tomography in endodontics," *Pennsylvania Dental Journal*, vol. 78, no. 1, pp. 37–39, 2011.

[22] S. Valizadeh, M. Khosravi, and Z. Azizi, "Diagnostic accuracy of conventional, digital andCone Beam CT in vertical root fracture detection," *Iranian Endodontic Journal*, vol. 6, no. 1, pp. 15–20, 2011.

[23] K. V. Krell and E. M. Rivera, "A six year evaluation of cracked teeth diagnosed with reversible pulpitis: treatment and prognosis," *Journal of Endodontics*, vol. 33, no. 12, pp. 1405–1407, 2007.

[24] J. C. Türp and J. P. Gobetti, "The cracked tooth syndrome: an elusive diagnosis," *Journal of the American Dental Association*, vol. 127, no. 10, pp. 1502–1507, 1996.

[25] E. S. Pane, J. E. A. Palamara, and H. H. Messer, "Stainless steel bands in endodontics: effects on cuspal flexure and fracture resistance," *International Endodontic Journal*, vol. 35, no. 5, pp. 467–471, 2002.

[26] P. O. Zimet and C. Endo, "Preservation of the roots—management and prevention protocols for cracked tooth syndrome," *Annals of the Royal Australasian College of Dental Surgeons*, vol. 15, pp. 319–324, 2000.

# Nasolabial Cyst Associated with Odontogenic Infection

**Eveline Claudia Martini,[1] Fabiana Madalozzo Coppla,[1]**
**Eduardo Bauml Campagnoli,[2] and Marcelo Carlos Bortoluzzi[2]**

[1]*Department of Dentistry, State University of Ponta Grossa, Rua Carlos Cavalcanti 4748, Bloco M, Uvaranas, 84030-900 Ponta Grossa, PR, Brazil*
[2]*Department of Stomatology, State University of Ponta Grossa, PR, Brazil*

Correspondence should be addressed to Eveline Claudia Martini; eve_fcs@hotmail.com

Academic Editor: Giuseppe Colella

The nasolabial cyst or Klestadt cyst is a relatively uncommon nonodontogenic cyst that develops in the nasal alar region; it has uncertain pathogenesis. This lesion has slow growth and variable dimensions and is characterized clinically by a floating tumefaction in the nasolabial fold area around the bridge of the nose, causing an elevation of the upper lip and relative facial asymmetry. Diagnosis is primarily made clinically; if necessary, this is complemented by imaging. This paper reports the case of a 39-year-old male patient who complained of pain in the right upper premolar region and poor aesthetics due to a firm tumor in the right wing of the nose. Initially, this was thought to be due to an odontogenic abscess; however, the differential diagnosis was that a nasolabial cyst was communicating with the apex of teeth 14 and 15. Surgical treatment was carried out, followed by histopathological examination and concomitant endodontic treatment of the teeth involved.

## 1. Introduction

Nasolabial cysts can be considered as lesions that are not odontogenic and that affect the soft tissues of the nasal vestibule, canine fossa, and upper lip. These effects are unilateral to the midline of the upper lip and the base alar [1–4]. Nasolabial cysts are relatively rare, representing 0.7% of cysts affecting the maxillofacial region [5, 6].

The nasolabial cyst was studied by Klestadt in 1953 [2], and the lesion was named in his honor. Other names used for this lesion since 1941 include *mucoid cyst*, *maxillary cyst*, *wind cyst*, *nasovestibular cyst*, *subalar cyst*, and *nasoglobular cyst*. Neville et al. [3] and Choi et al. suggested the term *nasoalveolar cyst*, defining it as a lesion located between the soft tissues of the upper lip and nasal vestibule.

The pathogenesis of this lesion is uncertain, and there are several theories for its origin. The most accepted current theory is that the cyst originates from epithelial remnants trapped along the fusion of the lateral nasal processes with the median and the jaw; other theories speculate that it is a fissure cyst or that it originates from the deposition of the nasolacrimal duct epithelium [7].

Clinically, a nasolabial cyst is characterized by an increase in the volume of the unilateral nasolabial area causing an elevation of the bridge of the nose and superior lip projection [8]; in some cases, nasal obstruction occurs [2]. It presents as a slow and asymptomatic growth except when associated with an infection [9]. A nasolabial cyst typically forms between the first and seventh decades of life and is more common in adults aged 40–50 years, females (3 : 1) [1], and dark-skinned people [10].

The diagnosis is usually based on clinical outcomes and can involve imaging tests like X-ray, computed tomography (CT), and magnetic resonance.

The treatment of nasolabial cysts can be accomplished with a fine aspiration needle or through incision and drainage, cystic enucleation for intraoral access, marsupialization, use of endoscopic [8, 11] or sclerosing agents [4], or intralesional injection.

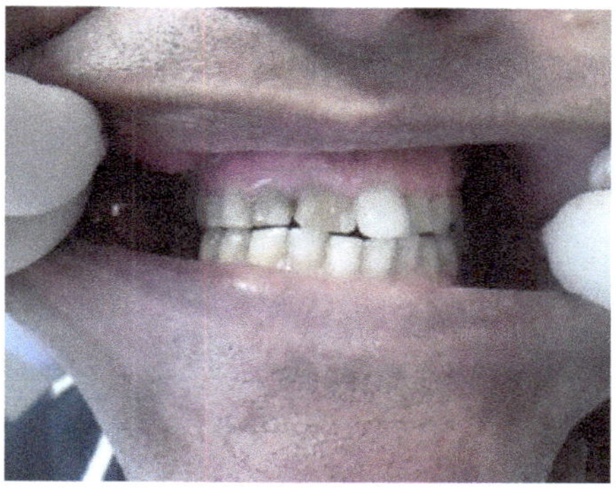

Figure 1: Initial dental appearance.

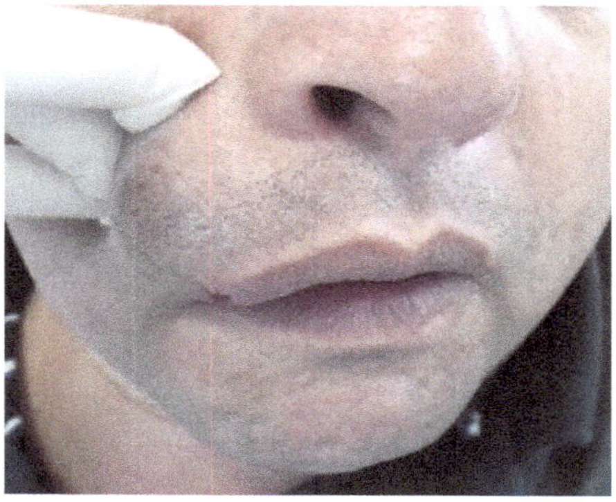

Figure 2: Initial view of the injury with external palpation of the face.

The aims of this paper are to present a case study of the treatment of a nasolabial cyst and discuss the diagnosis and characteristics of the lesion.

## 2. Case Report

The patient, a Caucasian, 39-year-old male, entered the emergency department at the State University of Ponta Grossa complaining of an increase in the size of the paranasal sinuses on the right side and of diffuse pain in the teeth in the same region; the patient also complained of poor aesthetics due to swelling for several months. During the intraoral clinical examination, palpation revealed an increased volume close to the bottom groove region (Figures 1, 2, and 3). Panoramic (Figure 4), periapical (Figure 5), and occlusal radiographs of the maxilla were requested. Relevant to the radiographic images, there was apical periodontitis in teeth 14 and 15 that was compatible with an abscess.

Bringing together the clinical characteristics with the radiographic images, a diagnosis of endodontic abscess was made, for which the emergency procedure involved opening and endodontic instrumentation in teeth 14 and 15 and prescriptions for diclofenac potassium (50 mg for 2 days) and amoxicillin (500 mg for 7 days). The aim was to reduce local swelling and other symptoms. Two days later, the patient returned to carry out an exchange of intracanal medication and receive endodontic reinstrumentation on both teeth.

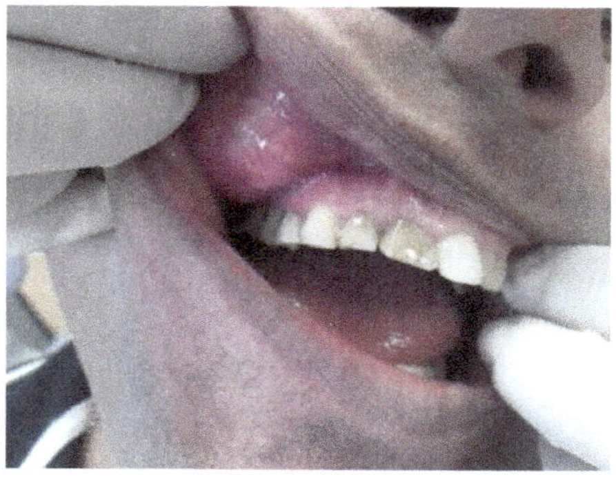

Figure 3: Initial view of the injury with internal palpation of the mucosa.

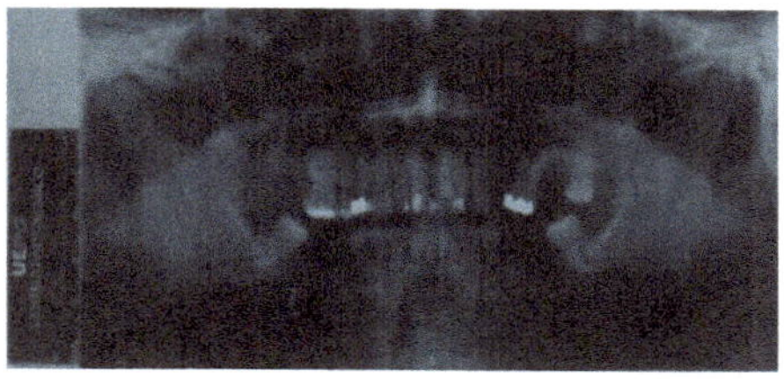

Figure 4: Panoramic radiograph of the patient.

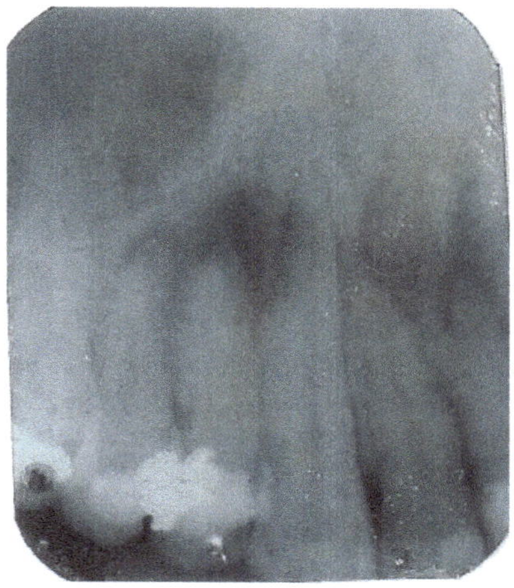

Figure 5: Periapical view of the right premolars. Extensive amalgam restorations on teeth 14 and 15 are observed; this location is close to the region of the apical periodontitis.

After 8 days, as no decrease in the lesion was observed and the patient complained of pain, another exchange of intracanal medication was carried out. The following were prescribed: amoxicillin (875 mg) and clavulanate potassium (125 mg) for 7 days and dipyrone sodium (500 mg) for 2 days.

After another 7 days, the patient returned with similar symptoms. Fistula tracking with gutta-percha points was then made, followed by radiographic examination, which confirmed that the periapical lesions in question actually came from teeth 14 and 15. The intracanal medication was switched again, and a pulp sensitivity test was conducted on all upper teeth; beyond those in question, teeth 21, 11, and 12

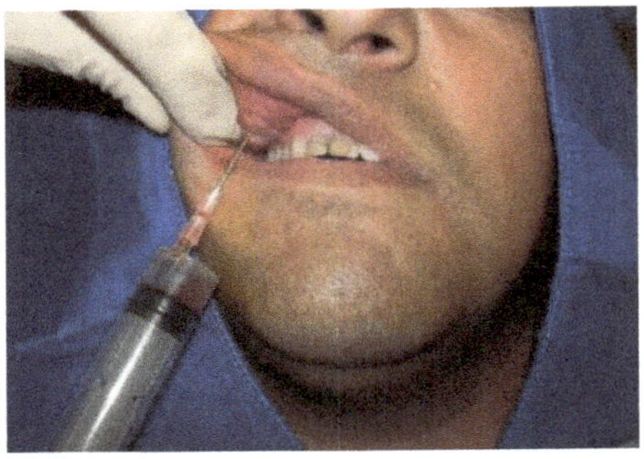

Figure 6: Aspiration of cystic content prior to surgery showed liquid with characteristics similar to that found in nasolabial cysts.

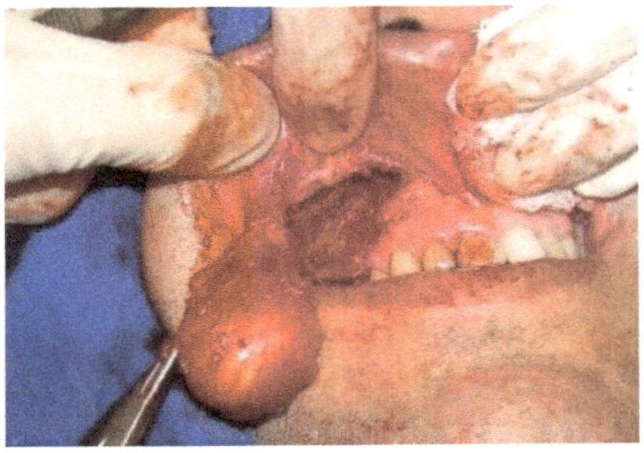

Figure 7: The view of the lesion; it was removed carefully because it was deeply embedded in tissues.

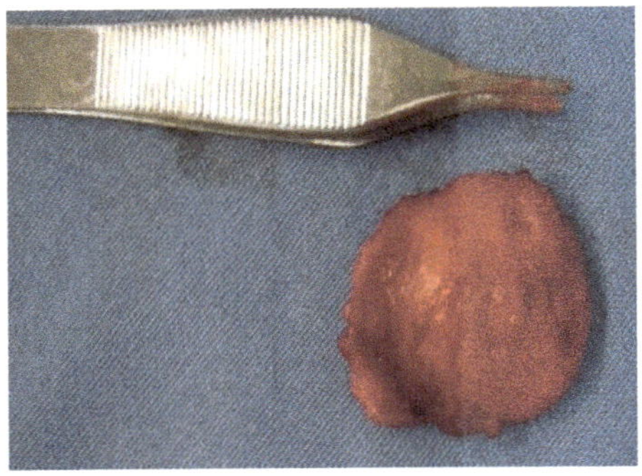

Figure 8: Appearance of the injury after complete removal.

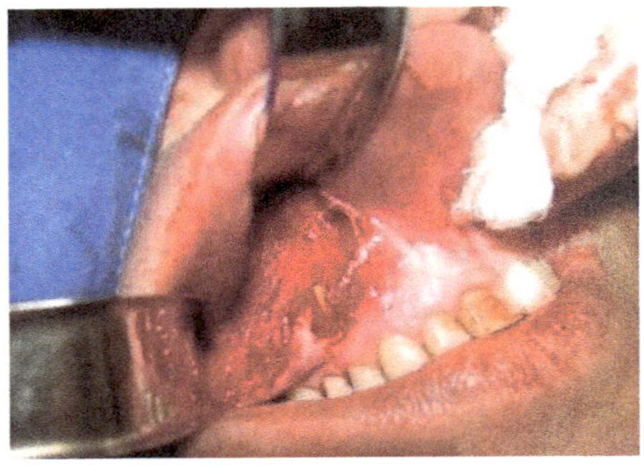

Figure 9: Note the close relationship of the lesion with the apex of premolars, which confirms the hypothesis of mutual periapical-cystic infection.

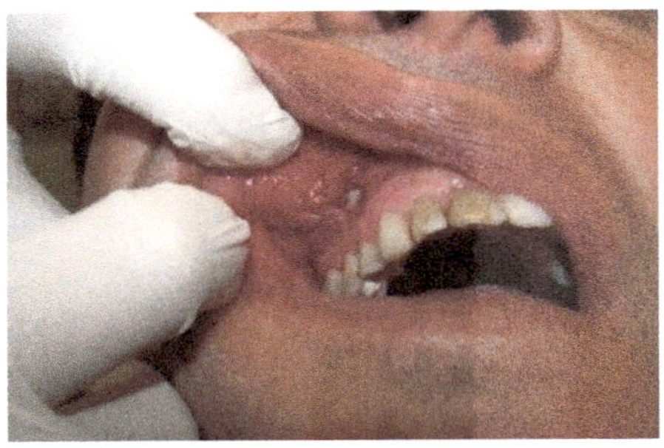

Figure 10: Appearance of the tissue after the end of the suture.

also did not respond to the test. These results were forwarded to endodontics, since besides the sensitivity test these teeth were seen to be darkened, which is compatible with pulp necrosis.

Because endodontic treatment has not shown the desired effect or remission of early symptoms, complete blood count and fasting glucose have been invited to check systemic condition and immune ability of the patient. Nothing abnormal in laboratory tests was observed; a diagnosis of nasolabial cyst in the right facial region with possible communication with the roots of the teeth 14 and 15 was raised. After 1 week, a further change to the intracanal medication was made due to a lack of remission in the initial symptoms.

Given that after this period the symptoms had not deteriorated, surgical treatment of the case was then proposed. This was initially performed using aseptic face PVPI to prepare the surgical field after local anesthesia of the infraorbital nerve and the cellular anterior nasopalatine region using three tubes of mepivacaine (2%) and epinephrine (1:100,000). First, the cystic lesion contents were aspirated (Figure 6), followed by an excisional biopsy (Figure 7). The surgery had no complications.

We found in the swelling an oval, whitish, noninfiltrating lesion (Figure 8); it had a smooth surface with defined borders, and it was hardened, sessile, and approximately 5 cm in diameter. After removal of the lesion, attention was drawn to the root of tooth 14, which had communication with the location of the cyst, confirming that there was a contamination relationship between the nasolabial cyst and the apical periodontitis, explaining why the endodontic treatment had not had the desired effect (Figure 10). The suture was performed (Figure 9) with Vicryl polyglycolic acid yarn (Janssen Pharmaceutica Ethicon Inc., New Brunswick, New Jersey, EUA).

The lesion was properly stored and sent to clinical pathology for analysis, and the patient received a prescription for anti-inflammatory postoperative medication (600 mg ibuprofen for 3 days). The outer immediate postoperative appearance of the patient may be observed in Figure 11; this appearance was satisfactory, as the main complaint was the increase in the volume of the face region, and this was removed during the surgical procedure.

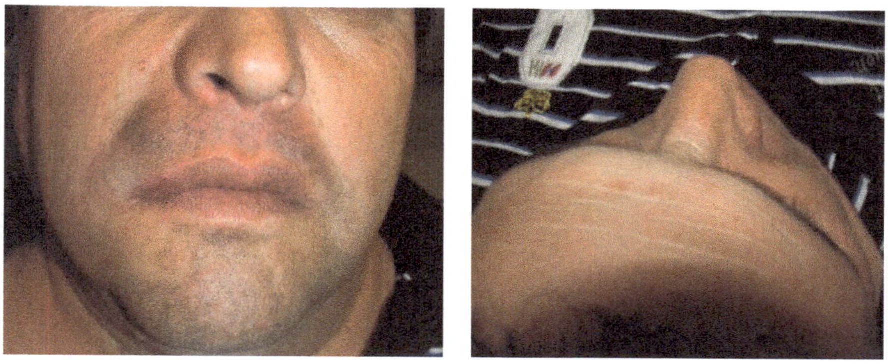

(a) (b)

FIGURE 11: (a) and (b) Front and top facial views in the immediate postoperative period.

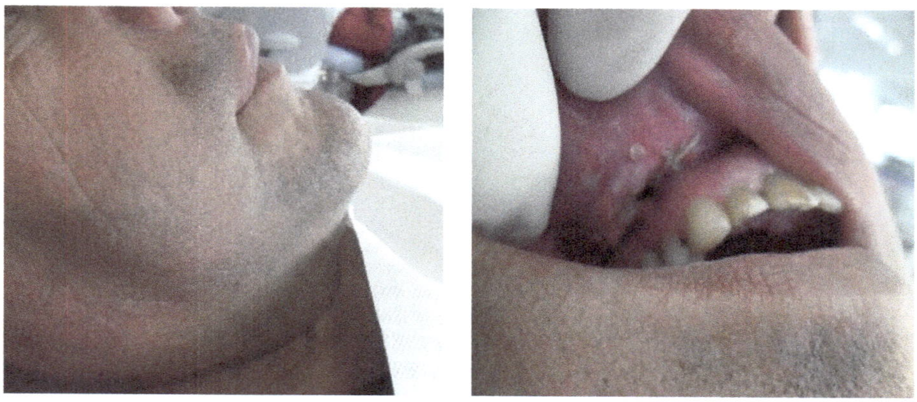

(a) (b)

FIGURE 12: (a) and (b) Appearance of the face and the patient's mucosa in the postoperative period (after 7 days).

The clinical pathology analysis showed that the specimen consisted of a fibrous cyst wall with a light-coated cylindrical pseudostratified epithelium enclosing mucous-secreting goblet cells and inflammatory cells (due to the constant cystic contamination), which were seen communicating with the periapical region of the right premolars, as previously described. After examination, the diagnosis of a nasolabial cyst was confirmed.

Postoperative controls were made at 7 days (Figure 12), 15 days (Figure 14), and 1 month to evaluate possible volume increase and symptom recurrence in the region, including site pain, paresthesia, or any other signs of neurological changes in the region. At the first postoperative visit, paresthesia of the nasolabial and labial region was observed; these sites were listed for laser therapy sessions (Figure 13) aimed at recovering sensitivity in the region. The patient has conducted 2 sessions of laser therapy; after the second one, the patient reported that he was beginning to feel the surgical site.

## 3. Discussion

This case report illustrates the most common features found in patients affected by nasolabial cysts, which corroborates previous studies [4, 6, 7, 12]. Some common clinical signs observed here, such as the deletion of the nasolabial folds and the elevation of the nasal wings, could have led to the final diagnosis upon first contact with the patient; however, the story reported by the patient made it difficult to diagnose an injury that did not involve bone tissue. This difficulty can lead to a demand for various professionals to ensure the complete resolution of the case [10].

The patient reported growth of the injury within a few months, along with painful symptoms, unlike what is commonly found [2, 6, 8], and he was complaining about poor aesthetics due to bulging in the region. This differed from the literature [6], in which some patients reported development of this lesion over a period of 3 to 5 years and did not seek treatment due to its slow, asymptomatic growth and the absence of pain and discomfort. In other cases [13], there was a sudden growth of the lesion after 1 year, and in one case, after a period of only 2 months, the lesion became excessive.

Regarding the preference for race, the present case also differs from the literature, as dark-skinned people have shown the highest number of occurrences with respect to age and gender [12, 14]. In this case, the lesion was diagnosed unilaterally after a thorough evaluation of the opposite side

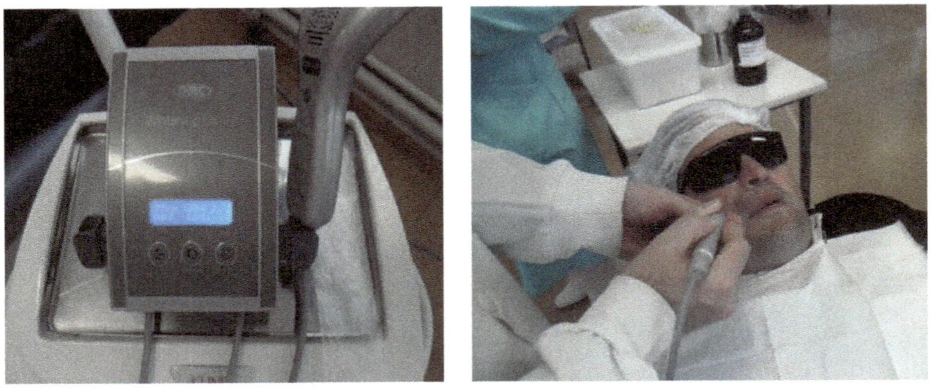

(a) (b)

FIGURE 13: (a) and (b) Equipment of laser therapy and procedure performed in the region of the surgery 7 days after the chirurgic procedure.

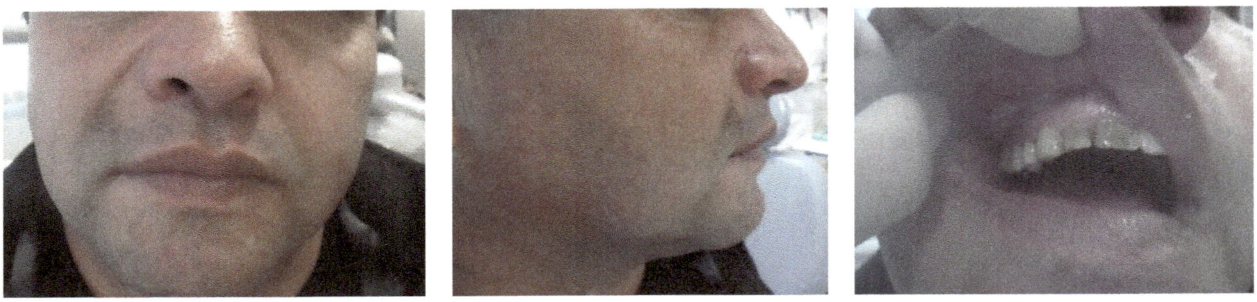

(a) (b) (c)

FIGURE 14: (a, b, and c) View of the patient's frontal and lateral face and mucosa 15 days after the operation.

and a pulpal vitality test of the teeth in quadrant 2. There are few cases of bilateral nasolabial cysts in the literature.

The diagnosis of nasolabial cysts is almost exclusively clinical, in which bidigital palpation of the region is essential and should be careful [2, 6, 12]. What hinders the process is that it is a relatively rare lesion and that the differential diagnosis can include many other conditions affecting the anterior maxillary region, including odontogenic cysts, periapical granulomas, and abscesses. The pulp vitality test of the adjacent teeth is essential for a proper diagnosis, and it must first be carried out, as if it is not apical periodontitis, the teeth in question will show positive results for vitality in the presence of nasolabial cyst. This feature made it difficult to diagnose this case, as the clinical characteristics of the patient matched with apical periodontitis and the teeth in question responded negatively to the pulp vitality test.

Dermal and epidermal cysts should also be considered in the differential diagnosis, although these are associated with the yellowing of the overlying mucosa; in cases of nasolabial cysts, they hold to your labial mucosa with normal color or bluish color, due to the presence of local vascularization and depending on their size [7, 12, 15]. In addition, epidermoid cysts are usually diagnosed in childhood, while nasolabial cysts are more common in adult patients [12], as was noted in this case.

El-Din and el-Hamd [6] reported that complications of the injury, when occurring, generally cause nasal obstruction and appearance of cosmetic redness on the patient's face. According to Nixdorf et al. [13], patients only seek therapy when there is deformity, nasal obstruction, or an infection caused by the lesion [5, 9, 15]. However, this patient sought treatment because he thought the injury was of dental origin, as there was a communication of the nasolabial cyst with the root tips of teeth 14 and 15.

Regarding treatment of the injury, most studies have reported enucleation as the treatment of choice for nasolabialis [2, 4, 5, 8, 10, 12] and cysts, as they are composed entirely of soft tissue, which does not respond well to marsupialization. Alternative methods of treatment have been suggested, including aspiration, cauterization, injection of sclerosing agents, and incision with drainage. However, these methods are associated with higher rates of relapse [3, 11, 12, 15]. Therefore, in view of the ease of surgical resection and its curative potential, we believe this procedure should be the treatment of choice in most cases. For this patient, despite the size of the lesion, we chose to perform surgical removal after a histological study of the region.

As for the cyst aspiration procedure, which aims to assess the possible presence of cholesterol crystals, remove odontogenic injuries, and enable injection of radiopaque

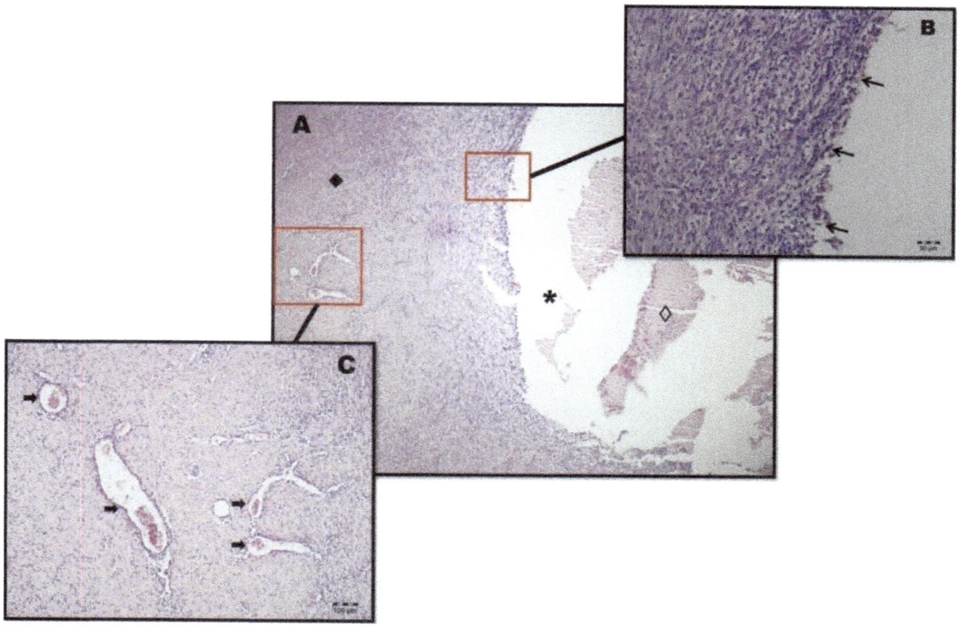


FIGURE 15: (A) View of the cystic nature of the lesion; the cystic cavity (*) had the presence of necrotic material (◊), and the cystic capsule was found to be quite thick (◆) (HE, 40x). (B) View of the destruction of the epithelial lining demarcating the cystic cavity (arrows) and the presence of intense inflammation associated with granulation tissue (HE 200x) due to recurrent episodes of infection associated with cystic tooth infection. (C) View of the cystic capsule, which has been collagenized and cellularized and shows several blood vessels that are dilated and have an accumulation of erythrocytes inside (arrows) but no atypical cells (HE, 100x).

solution, this method was contraindicated by some authors because it may increase the risk of lesion recurrence [12–14, 16], especially when it is chosen as the only form of treatment. In this case, this was only an auxiliary part of the diagnosis; therefore it could be used.

In our patient, the histopathology was not entirely consistent with what we usually see in the histology of nasolabial cysts (Figure 15); due to a process of chronic recurrent inflammation, the cyst eventually lost some of its epithelial characteristics. However, we did observe characteristics of a cystic lesion with chronic inflammation signals, a fibrous capsule, bright and smooth inner surface, and dyed yellow seromucous content; therefore, through the combination of histological findings and clinical features found in the lesion the diagnosis of a nasolabial cyst was confirmed.

## 4. Conclusion

This paper presented clinical characteristics and histological findings consistent with a nasolabial cyst despite the framework that was initially described as being only of dental origin. This soft tissue injury should always be considered in the differential diagnosis when there is swelling in the soft tissue of the nasal alar region. The treatment in this case covers endodontic conduct in conjunction with surgical excision of the lesion; the treatment was conservative, as this type of lesion is a rare recurrence.

## Conflict of Interests

The authors declare that there is no conflict of interests regarding the publication of this paper.

## References

[1] A. P. Sumer, P. Celenk, M. Sumer, N. T. Telcioglu, and O. Gunhan, "Nasolabial cyst: case report with CT and MRI findings," *Oral Surgery, Oral Medicine, Oral Pathology, Oral Radiology and Endodontology*, vol. 109, no. 2, pp. e92–e94, 2010.

[2] C. Sahin, "Nasolabial cyst," *Case Reports in Medicine*, vol. 2009, Article ID 586201, 2 pages, 2009.

[3] B. W. Neville, D. D. Damm, C. M. Allen, and J. E. Bouquot, *Patologia Oral e Maxilofacial*, Guanabara Koogan, Rio de Janeiro, Brazil, 2009.

[4] J. H. Choi, J. H. Cho, H. J. Kang, S. W. Chae, S. H. Lee, and S. J. Hwang, "Nasolabial cyst: a retrospective analysis of 18 cases," *Ear, Nose & Throat Journal*, vol. 81, no. 2, pp. 94–96, 2002.

[5] W.-C. Chao, C.-C. Huang, P.-H. Chang, Y.-L. Chen, C.-W. Chen, and T.-J. Lee, "Management of nasolabial cysts by transnasal endoscopic marsupialization," *Archives of Otolaryngology—Head and Neck Surgery*, vol. 135, no. 9, pp. 932–935, 2009.

[6] K. El-Din and A. A. el-Hamd, "Nasolabial cyst: a report of eight cases and a review of the literature," *The Journal of Laryngology & Otology*, vol. 113, no. 8, pp. 747–749, 1999.

[7] R. S. L. Tiago, M. S. Maia, G. M. S. Do Nascimento, J. P. Correa, and D. C. Salgado, "Nasolabial cyst: diagnostic and therapeutical aspects," *Brazilian Journal of Otorhinolaryngology*, vol. 74, no. 1, pp. 39–43, 2008.

[8] C.-Y. Su, C.-Y. Chien, and C.-F. Hwang, "A new transnasal approach to endoscopic marsupialization of the nasolabial cyst," *Laryngoscope*, vol. 109, no. 7 I, pp. 1116–1118, 1999.

[9] S. Özer, C. Cabbarzade, and O. Öğretmenoğlu, "A new transnasal approach to nasolabial cyst: endoscopic excision of nasolabial cyst," *Journal of Craniofacial Surgery*, vol. 24, no. 5, pp. 1748–1749, 2013.

[10] C. H. Bettoni, F. Jaerger, R. L. Alvarenga, and F. O. Rezende, "Cisto nasolabial: revisão da literatura e relato de caso clínico," in *Revista Portuguesa de Estomatologia, Medicina Dentária e Cirurgia Maxilofacial*, vol. 52, pp. 157–160, 2011.

[11] C.-N. Chen, C.-Y. Su, H.-C. Lin, and C.-F. Hwang, "Microdebrider-assisted endoscopic marsupialization for the nasolabial cyst: comparisons between sublabial and transnasal approaches," *American Journal of Rhinology and Allergy*, vol. 23, no. 2, pp. 232–236, 2009.

[12] H.-W. Yuen, C.-Y. L. Julian, and C.-L. Y. Samuel, "Nasolabial cysts: clinical features, diagnosis, and treatment," *British Journal of Oral and Maxillofacial Surgery*, vol. 45, no. 4, pp. 293–297, 2007.

[13] D. R. Nixdorf, E. Peters, and K. E. Lung, "Clinical presentation and differential diagnosis of nasolabial cyst," *Journal of the Canadian Dental Association*, vol. 69, no. 3, pp. 146–149, 2003.

[14] T. Hillman, E. B. Galloway, and L. P. Johnson, "Pathology quiz case 1: nasoalveolar cyst," *Archives of Otolaryngology—Head & Neck Surgery*, vol. 128, no. 4, pp. 452–455, 2002.

[15] D. B. Kuriloff, "The nasolabial cyst-nasal hamartoma," *Otolaryngology—Head and Neck Surgery*, vol. 96, no. 3, pp. 268–272, 1987.

[16] M. A. Cohen and Y. Hertzanu, "Huge grow potential of nasolabial cyst," *Oral Surgery, Oral Medicine, Oral Pathology*, vol. 59, no. 5, pp. 441–445, 1985.

# 45

# Different Occlusal Schemes in a Persistent Protruding Complete Denture Wearer

**Carolina Mayumi Iegami, Danilo de Melo Lopes, Atlas Edson Moleros Nakamae, Priscila Nakasone Uehara, and Regina Tamaki**

*Department of Prosthodontics, School of Dentistry, University of Sao Paulo, Avenida Professor Lineu Prestes, 2227 Cidade Universitaria, 05508-000 Sao Paulo, SP, Brazil*

Correspondence should be addressed to Regina Tamaki; retamaki@usp.br

Academic Editor: Asja Celebić

Different types of artificial teeth and occlusal designs can be used in complete dentures. Bilateral balanced occlusion, lingualized occlusion, canine guidance, and monoplane are the main occlusal designs; however there is no agreement on which tooth arrangement is ideal for achieving success in complete dentures. This report presents an alternative for persistent involuntary protruding complete denture wearers through the use of artificial teeth with higher cusps. Due to an old and worn pair of complete dentures, the patient had the habit of protruding. New dentures were made with Biotone artificial teeth and in the trial session, the patient would still protrude. A new set was made with Premium artificial teeth, which present higher cusps. With these dentures, the involuntary protrusion did not occur. From the delivery to the follow-up sessions, the patient stopped protruding.

## 1. Introduction

Despite the efforts to reduce tooth loss in the world, edentulism prevails in most countries, presenting higher rates, especially in countries where poverty exists [1]. In these countries, complete dentures are the primary choice of the edentulous patients for cost reasons and most patients, while satisfied, do not replace their dentures in the recommended period.

Long-time use of the same pair of complete dentures might lead to aesthetics impairment, loss of vertical dimension, and reduction of masticatory efficiency [2, 3]. Since complete dentures are mucosa-supported, they require stability on the support area to function properly. Therefore, occlusion is a key component for denture stability [4]. Although complete dentures have been used in prosthodontics for over a hundred years, there is no consensus on which tooth arrangement is ideal for achieving success in complete dentures [5, 6]. Among the various commercial brands available, posterior teeth can present different morphology, being anatomical or monoplane. Anatomical posterior teeth are similar to the natural posterior teeth and can present different cusp angles and cusp heights, improving masticatory efficiency [5]. Bilateral balanced occlusion provides comfort for the patient, protects the tissues, and improves retention [7]. Canine-guided occlusion presents good retention and masticatory performance levels [5]. Lingualized balanced occlusion also provides comfort, retention and is the occlusion choice for patients with residual ridge resorption [8, 9]. Monoplane posterior teeth are flat and were developed to minimize horizontal forces and improve stability [10].

According to Hanau, artificial dental cusps height may vary according to the inclination of the condylar guidance. The higher the inclination of the condylar guidance is, the higher the artificial teeth cusps can be [11]. Height of cusps also improves esthetics and may please the patient, since they are similar to natural teeth [12, 13]. Therefore, despite the little options available in the market, some patients need teeth with different cusps heights, according to their condylar guidance inclination.

In theory, teeth with higher cusps should allow better comminution of food, since their smaller area of contact with

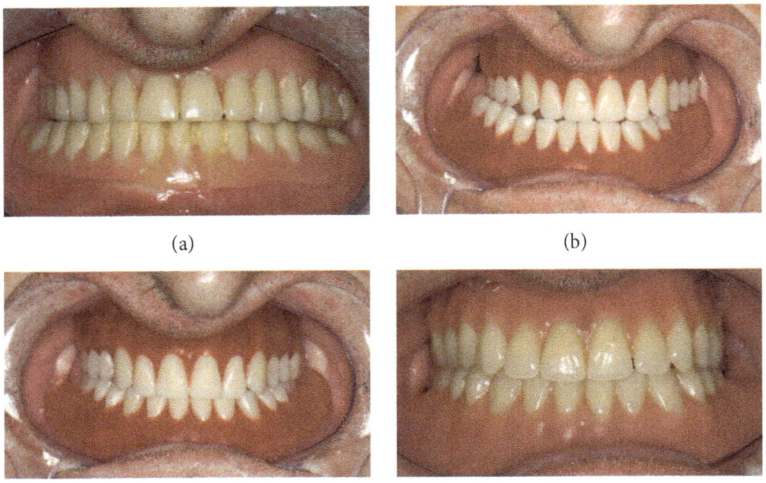

(a) (b)

(c) (d)

Figure 1: (a) Old complete dentures. (b) Repetitive movement with Biotone artificial teeth. (c) Trial complete dentures with Biotone artificial teeth. (d) Complete dentures with Premium artificial teeth.

the food promotes greater penetrating power into the food bolus; however, it has not yet been proven [4].

This clinical report displays how the application of different posterior teeth cusps heights can influence the excursive movements of the patient.

## 2. Case Presentation

This study was submitted to the University of Sao Paulo, School of Dentistry Ethics Committee under the protocol 90/2010 and approved FR330287.

A 59-year-old man, complete denture wearer for over 10 years, presented severe occlusal wear in the premolar and molar areas, vertical dimension was reduced, and the denture bases were ill adapted. Due to the posterior teeth wear, the patient was able to generate excursive movements freely (Figure 1(a)).

Given that the patient's complaint was that the dentures were old and teeth were abraded, new complete dentures were suggested as treatment.

Preliminary maxillary and mandibular impressions were made with modeling plastic impression compound (Godibar Placas; Lysanda Produtos Odontologicos Ltda, Brazil). Custom trays (JET; Artigos Odontologicos Classico Ltda, Brazil) were fabricated by taking reference of anatomical landmarks present in the diagnostic casts. Then, final casts were made with an impression with custom trays and a zinc-enolic paste (Pasta Lysanda; Lysanda Produtos Odontologicos Ltda, Brazil). Maxillary and mandibular wax rims were made with trial denture bases according to the esthetics requirements and vertical dimension was reestablished. Horizontal maxillomandibular record presented to be difficult as a result of the previous reduced vertical dimension and the posterior teeth wear.

Among the available techniques for the horizontal maxillomandibular record, the Paterson technique was chosen. In this technique, a mixture of carborundum and plaster is used to individualize the plane of occlusion and to promote neuromuscular disarrangement, allowing the horizontal maxillomandibular record.

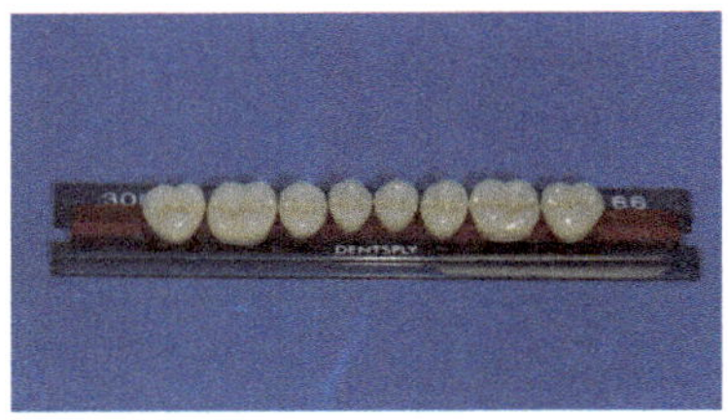

Figure 2: Biotone artificial teeth.

Occlusal rims were mounted in an articulator (Articulador A7 Plus; Bio-Art Equipamentos Odontológicos Ltda, Brazil) with a facebow transfer and occlusal rims were fixed with metal staples.

Teeth chosen for the complete dentures were the Biotone (BT) (Dentsply International, Pennsylvania, USA) and the chosen occlusal scheme was the bilateral balanced occlusion. In the trial session, an unstable mandibular position was observed. The patient protruded repetitively, promoting the movement of the artificial teeth (Figures 1(b) and 1(c)).

A second pair of complete dentures was made with Premium (PT) (Heraeus Kulzer GmbH/Hanau, Germany) artificial teeth, which have posterior teeth with higher cusps (2.39 mm) than BT (1.67 mm), resembling more natural teeth cusps (Figures 2 and 3) [4]. Different from the BT teeth trial, in the PT trial, the patient did not perform protrusion movements.

The patient received both pairs and wore the complete dentures for two months each. While the patient was wearing the BT dentures, the involuntary protrusion movements remained. However, with the PT dentures, from the delivery

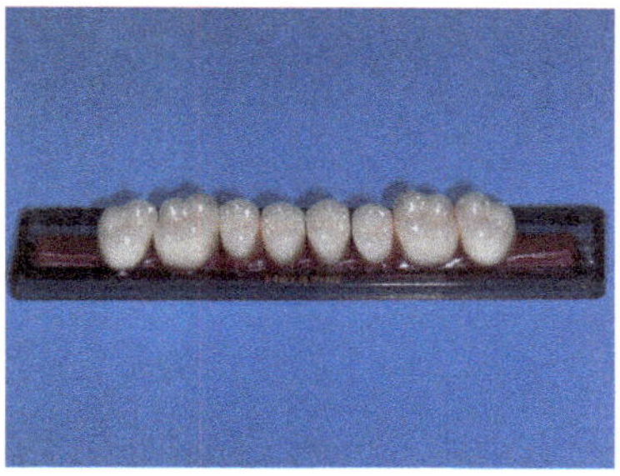

FIGURE 3: Premium artificial teeth.

session through the follow-up sessions, the maxillomandibular relation remained stable in maximal intercuspal position without traumatizing the mucosa. Harmonious occlusion and articulation were achieved without denture base dislodging during excursive movements (Figure 1(d)). According to the patient, masticatory function and retention were similar between BT and PT. Weekly follow-up sessions occurred up to 2 months. After that period, monthly follow-up sessions were set up to 1 year.

## 3. Discussion

Since the patient's old dentures were severely abraded, not only was vertical dimension decreased, but also masticatory efficiency was reduced. Mandibular displacement and alteration of the pathways that drive mastication and fatigue of the masticatory muscles are also consequences of abrasion of the artificial teeth [14, 15], which might have led to the involuntary movements of the mandible.

Both BT and PT complete dentures presented the same vertical dimension. Yet, the increase of vertical dimension itself was not sufficient to stop the involuntary protrusion movements that occurred with the old dentures and persisted with BT dentures. According to Hanau, cusp height or inclination is related to the inclination of the condylar guidance and influences the balanced occlusion of complete dentures [11]. If complete dentures are not balanced, the bases could shift during the eccentric movements and result in uneven force distribution and injure the mucosa. The selection of anatomical higher cusps artificial teeth in PT denture, closer to the patient's condylar guidance, combined with the bilateral balanced occlusion, provided a satisfactory result, since they helped the patient to maintain maximal intercuspal position and stopped the involuntary mandible movements.

Although higher cusp artificial teeth were beneficial in this case, the use of these teeth might change the direction of forces applied, as well as generating stress of greater magnitude [16]. The higher the cusps are, the more instable the prosthesis becomes, because the horizontal forces are maximized. When the residual ridge is extremely resorbed, horizontal forces tend to dislodge the denture more easily, which is negative for the patient.

Esthetics was also improved, since the higher cusps teeth were more similar to the natural teeth than the lower cusps teeth. However, this condition was only achieved due to the correct horizontal maxillomandibular record and to an accurate occlusal adjustment.

Furthermore, the chosen occlusal scheme contributed to the stability and function of the complete dentures. A lingualized balanced or a monoplane occlusion other than bilaterally balanced occlusion would not stop the patient from protruding. Selecting an occlusal scheme with higher cusps provided mandibular stability for the patient.

## 4. Conclusion

The complete dentures with higher cusps reestablished the patient's vertical dimension and masticatory function and prevented the protruding involuntary movement.

## Competing Interests

The authors declare that they have no competing interests.

## References

[1] G. E. Carlsson and R. Omar, "The future of complete dentures in oral rehabilitation. A critical review," *Journal of Oral Rehabilitation*, vol. 37, no. 2, pp. 143–156, 2010.

[2] K. A. Mays, "Reestablishing occlusal vertical dimension using a diagnostic treatment prosthesis in the edentulous patient: a clinical report," *Journal of Prosthodontics*, vol. 12, no. 1, pp. 30–36, 2003.

[3] R. Matsuda, Y. Yoneyama, M. Morokuma, and C. Ohkubo, "The influence of vertical dimension of occlusion changes on the electroencephalograms of complete denture wearers," *Journal of Prosthodontic Research*, vol. 58, no. 2, pp. 121–126, 2014.

[4] W. F. Barbosa, C. M. Iegami, P. N. Uehara, R. J. Furuyama, and R. Tamaki, "In vivo comparison of the masticatory efficiency of artificial teeth with two different cusp heights in complete dentures: a preliminary study," *Journal of Prosthodontics*, 2015.

[5] K. Zhao, Q.-Q. Mai, X.-D. Wang, W. Yang, and L. Zhao, "Occlusal designs on masticatory ability and patient satisfaction with complete denture: a systematic review," *Journal of Dentistry*, vol. 41, no. 11, pp. 1036–1042, 2013.

[6] S. Kimoto, A. Gunji, A. Yamakawa et al., "Prospective clinical trial comparing lingualized occlusion to bilateral balanced occlusion in complete dentures: a pilot study," *International Journal of Prosthodontics*, vol. 19, no. 1, pp. 103–109, 2006.

[7] I. Peroz, A. Leuenberg, I. Haustein, and K.-P. Lange, "Comparison between balanced occlusion and canine guidance in complete denture wearers—a clinical, randomized trial," *Quintessence International*, vol. 34, no. 8, pp. 607–612, 2003.

[8] Y. Matsumaru, "Influence of mandibular residual ridge resorption on objective masticatory measures of lingualized and fully bilateral balanced denture articulation," *Journal of Prosthodontic Research*, vol. 54, no. 3, pp. 112–118, 2010.

[9] M. Shirani, R. Mosharraf, and M. Shirany, "Comparisons of patient satisfaction levels with complete dentures of different occlusions: a randomized clinical trial," *Journal of Prosthodontics*, vol. 23, no. 4, pp. 259–266, 2014.

[10] J. Abduo, "Occlusal schemes for complete dentures: a systematic review," *The International Journal of Prosthodontics*, vol. 26, no. 1, pp. 26–33, 2013.

[11] R. Hanau, "Articulation defined, analyzed, and formulated," *Journal of the American Dental Association*, vol. 13, pp. 1694–1709, 1926.

[12] J. Lamoureux, R. Taché, and P. De Grandmont, "Patient evaluation of treatment success as related to denture tooth type," *International Journal of Prosthodontics*, vol. 12, no. 3, pp. 272–278, 1999.

[13] B. R. Lang, "Complete denture occlusion," *Dental Clinics of North America*, vol. 48, no. 3, pp. 641–665, 2004.

[14] S. Hirano, K. B. May, W. C. Wagner, and C. H. Hacker, "In vitro wear of resin denture teeth," *The Journal of Prosthetic Dentistry*, vol. 79, no. 2, pp. 152–155, 1998.

[15] A. Ekfeldt and S. Karlsson, "Changes of masticatory movement characteristics after prosthodontic rehabilitation of individuals with extensive tooth wear," *International Journal of Prosthodontics*, vol. 9, no. 6, pp. 539–546, 1996.

[16] N. Mankani, R. Chowdhary, and S. Mahoorkar, "Comparison of stress dissipation pattern underneath complete denture with various posterior teeth form: an in vitro study," *Journal of Indian Prosthodontist Society*, vol. 13, no. 3, pp. 212–219, 2013.

# 46

# Gingival Recession: Review and Strategies in Treatment of Recession

**Koppolu Pradeep,[1] Palaparthy Rajababu,[2] Durvasula Satyanarayana,[2] and Vidya Sagar[2]**

*[1] Department of Periodontics, Sri Sai College of Dental Surgery, Vikarabad, Andhra Pradesh, India*
*[2] Department of Periodontics, Kamineni Institute of Dental Sciences, Narketpally, Andhra Pradesh, India*

Correspondence should be addressed to Koppolu Pradeep, drpradeepk08@gmail.com

Academic Editors: N. Brezniak and A. Markopoulos

One of the most common esthetic concerns associated with the periodontal tissues is gingival recession. Gingival recession is the exposure of root surfaces due to apical migration of the gingival tissue margins; gingival margin migrates apical to the cementoenamel junction. Although it rarely results in tooth loss, marginal tissue recession is associated with thermal and tactile sensitivity, esthetic complaints, and a tendency toward root caries. This paper reviews etiology, consequences, and the available surgical procedures for the coverage of exposed root surfaces, including three case reports.

## 1. Introduction

Gingival recession is a problem affecting almost all middle and older aged to some degree. Gingival recession is the apical migration of gingival margin to the cementoenamel junction (CEJ). The distance between the CEJ and gingival margin gives the level of recession. Gingival recession can be caused by periodontal disease, accumulations, inflammation, improper flossing, aggressive tooth brushing, incorrect occlusal relationships, and dominant roots. These can appear as localized or generalized gingival recession. Recession can occur with or without loss of attached tissue. Gingival recession may effect in accentuated sensitivity because of the exposed dentin, it can be assessed by an appearance of a long clinical tooth and varied proportion of the teeth when compared with adjacent teeth.

## 2. Prevalence

According to the US National Survey, 88% of seniors (age 65 and over) and 50% of adults (18 to 64) present recession in one or more sites; progressive increase in frequency and extent of recession is observed with increase in age [1].

In the youngest age cohort (30 to 39 years), the prevalence of recession was 37.8% and the extent averaged 8.6% teeth. In contrast, the oldest cohort, aged 80 to 90 years, had a prevalence of 90.4% (more than twice as high) and the extent averaged 56.3% teeth (more than six times as large) [2].

Gingival recession is associated with the presence of supragingival and subgingival calculus and showed that the lingual surfaces of the lower anterior teeth were most frequently affected in 20–34 year age group in Tanzanian adult population [3].

## 3. Etiology

*3.1. Calculus.* Association between gingival recession with supragingival and subgingival calculus can be noted because of inadequate access to prophylactic dental care [3].

*3.2. Tooth Brushing.* Khocht et al. showed that use of hard tooth brush was associated with recession [4].

*3.3. High Frenal Attachment.* This may impede plaque removal by causing pull on the marginal gingival [5].

*3.4. Position of the Tooth.* Tooth which erupts close to mucogingival line may show localised gingival recession as there may be very little or no keratinized tissue [6].

*3.5. Tooth Movement by Orthodontic Forces.* The movement of tooth such as excessive proclination of incisors and expansion of the arch expansion are associated with greater risk of gingival recession [7].

*3.6. Improperly Designed Partial Dentures.* The partial dentures which have been maintained or designed which cause the gingival trauma and aid in the plaque retention have the tendency to cause gingival recession [8].

*3.7. Smoking.* The people who smoke have more gingival recession than nonsmokers.

The recession sites were found on the buccal surfaces of maxillary molars, premolars, and mandibular central incisors [9].

*3.8. Restorations.* Subgingival restoration margins increase the plaque accumulation, gingival inflammation, and alveolar bone loss [10].

*3.9. Chemicals.* Topical cocaine application causes gingival ulcerations and erosions [11].

## 4. Consequences

*4.1. Aesthetics.* The appearance of tooth becomes unattractive [12].

*4.2. Gingival Bleeding and Plaque Retention.* The recession may be a site clinically which offers plaque retention.

*4.3. Hypersensitivity.* Recession will uncover the cervical dentine. Hypersensitivity is usually of a sharp and short duration often associated with cold stimulus. The mechanism of hypersensitivity that is accepted is the hydrodynamic theory of pain, which states that the movement of dental fluid in the dentinal tubules triggers sensory nerve fibers in the inner dentine and dentinopulpal junction [13].

*4.4. Caries.* There may be a risk of the development of root caries as root surfaces are exposed to oral environment and aid in the withholding of plaque. Patients on periodontal maintenance with an average of 64.7 exposed root surfaces per patient; the mean number of caries lesions which were detected were 4.3 in a prevalence study [14].

## 5. Treatment

*5.1. Restorations, Crowns, and Veneers.* Crowns may be placed to widen the clinical crown which may camouflage the exposed root surface

*5.2. Construction of Gingival Mask.* Patients who have several teeth with recession may have unaesthetic appearance because of black triangles. In these cases, where surgical procedure is not appropriate, silicone flexible gingival veneer or mask may be used.

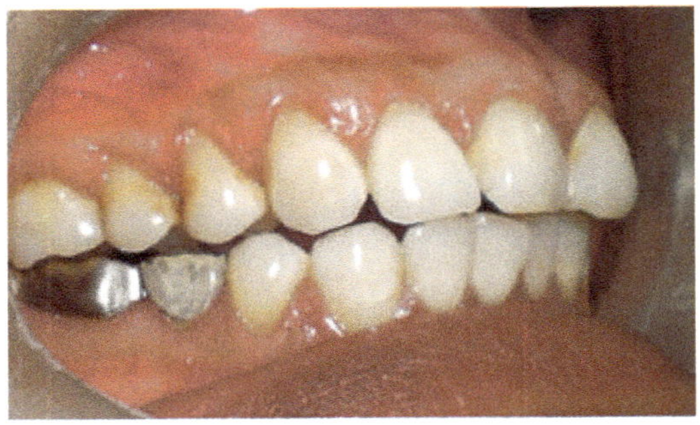

FIGURE 1: Facial view of gingival recession on 1st premolar and canine. The patient complained of root sensitivity in addition to the unaesthetic appearance when smiling.

*5.3. Root Conditioning.* Application of tetracycline HCL or citric acid to root surface before placement of soft tissue graft.

*5.4. Frenectomy.* When the recession is caused by frenal pull in those cases, frenectomy is advised. If appropriate hygiene aids do not enable the patient to maintain the area plaque free, then frenectomy is advised to give ease to entrance to the site [15].

*5.5. Surgical Root Coverage Techniques*

(i) Free epithelialised gingival graft [16].

(ii) Subepithelial connective tissue graft [17].

(iii) Semilunar flap [18].

(iv) Coronally advanced flap [19].

(v) Guided tissue regeneration [GTR] [20].

## 6. Case Report 1

A 43-year-old female patient complained of hypersensitivity inspite of using anti-hypersensitivity paste since 2 months and was also concerned about the esthetics. Patient had gingival recession on the maxillary left canine and first premolar at the first examination (Figure 1). The recession measured 2 mm on the canine and 3 mm on the first premolar, respectively. The clinical attachment loss was 4 mm from the CEJ for the canine and 5 mm for the first premolar, respectively. Oral prophylaxis has been done and oral hygiene instructions were given so as to achieve satisfactory plaque control prior to periodontal surgery. After reevaluation, a Semilunar incision and intracrevicular incisions have been given using Tarnow technique 22 (Figure 2). The roots were planed with hand curettes to remove the flecks of the calculus and to obtain smooth surfaces and then treated with tetracycline for 3 minutes (using a burnishing technique) (Figure 3). The root surfaces were then rinsed with saline. The flap was positioned as coronally as possible. The postoperative healing after 2 months revealed an increase of 2 mm and root coverage was achieved (Figure 5).

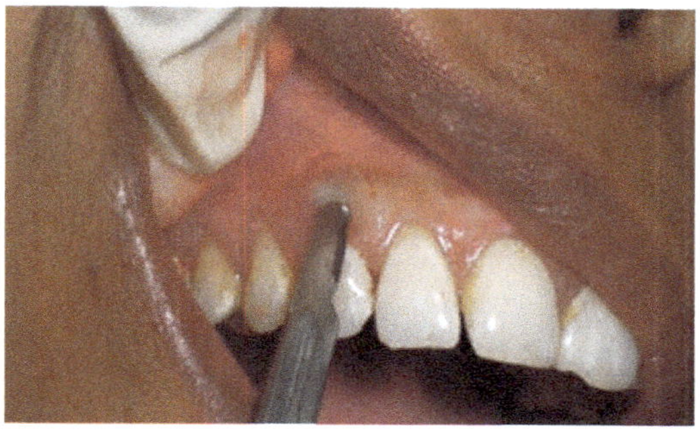

FIGURE 2: Semilunar incision placed apically.

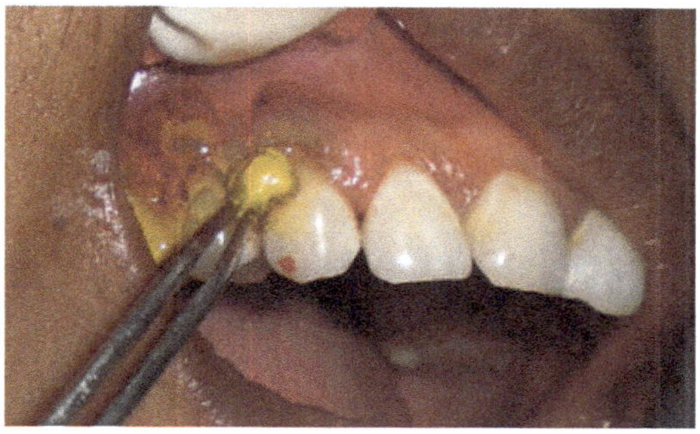

FIGURE 3: Root conditioning with tetracycline.

## 7. Case 2

A 31-year-old female patient complained of a black triangle in the upper front teeth region since 6 months and was concerned about the esthetics and whistling sound while speaking (Figure 6).

The interdental papilla between maxillary right central and lateral incisor was blunt (Figure 6). Oral prophylaxis has been done and oral hygiene instructions were given so as to achieve satisfactory plaque control prior to surgery. An intrasulcular incision is made at the tooth surfaces facing the interdental area to be reconstructed (Figure 7), consequently an incision is placed across the facial aspect of the interdental area and an envelope-type, split-thickness flap is elevated; simultaneously, a semilunar incision was given apical to the mucogingival junction and the flap was coronally displaced using Langers technique. A connective tissue graft is harvested from palate (Figure 8) and placed under the flap in interdental area (Figure 9) and sutured back (Figure 10). In Figure 11 postoperative healing after 6 months revealed the excellent closure of black triangle between the left upper central and lateral incisors.

## 8. Case 3

A 25-year-old female patient complained of hypersensitivity in the lower front teeth region since 2 months and was concerned about the esthetics. Patient had gingival recession on the mandibular right central incisor at the first examination (Figure 12). The clinical attachment loss was 5 mm

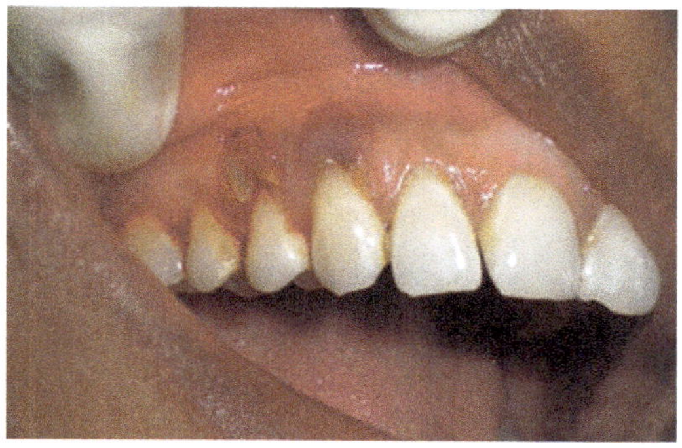

FIGURE 4: Repositioning of the flap coronally.

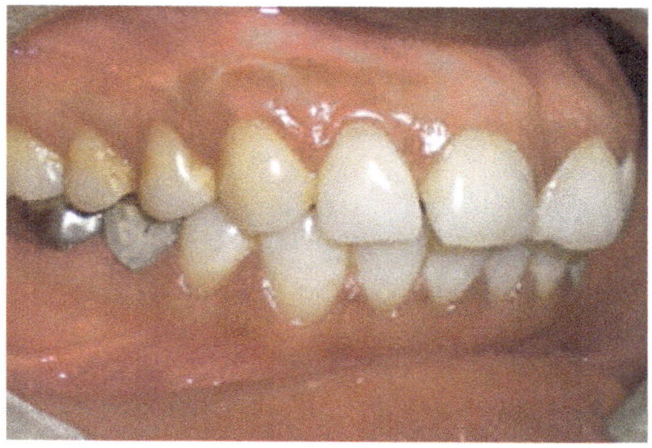

FIGURE 5: One -year postoperative view. Complete root coverage is observed.

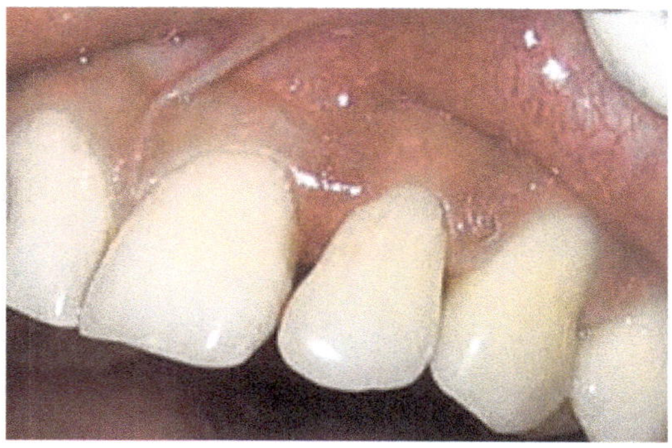

FIGURE 6: Blunting of interdental papilla between central and lateral incisor.

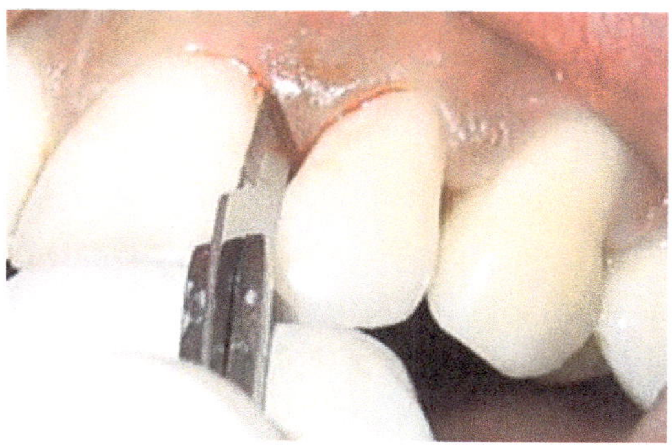

FIGURE 7: Intrasulcular incision.

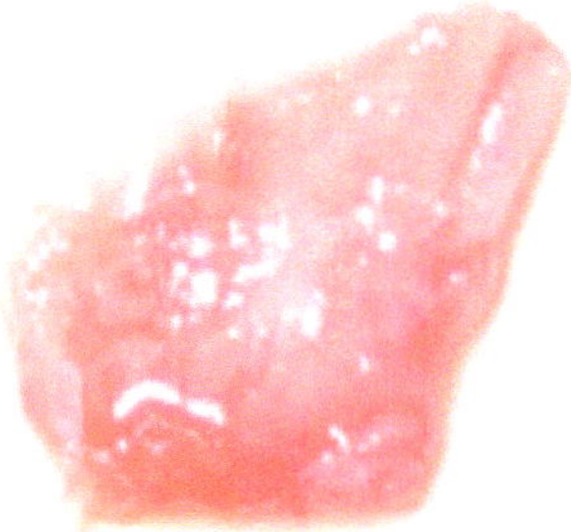

Figure 8: Connective tissue graft taken from palate.

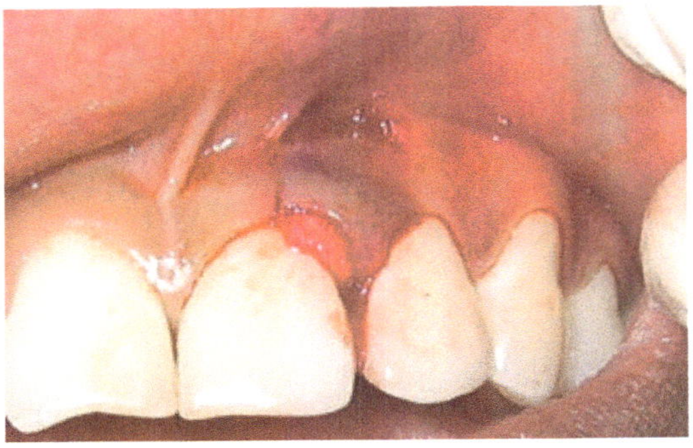

Figure 9: Graft placement under the flap.

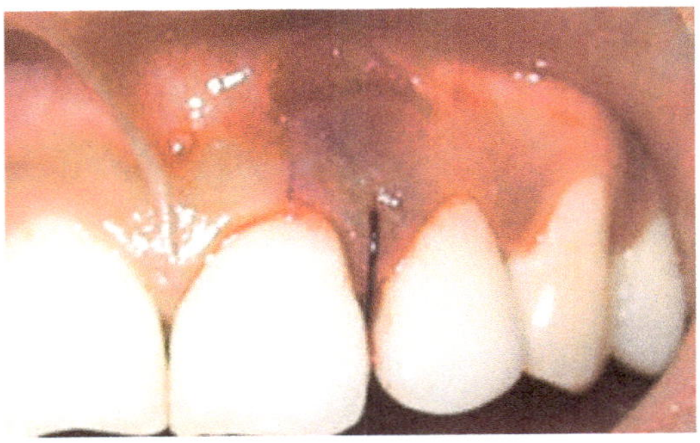

Figure 10: Placement of suture.

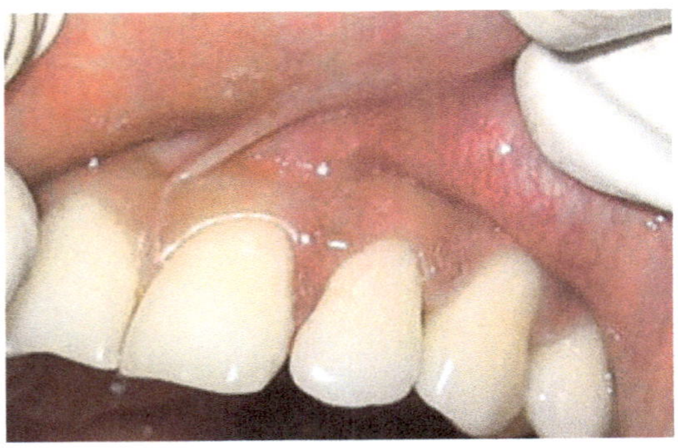

Figure 11: Closure of interdental papilla 6 months postoperatively.

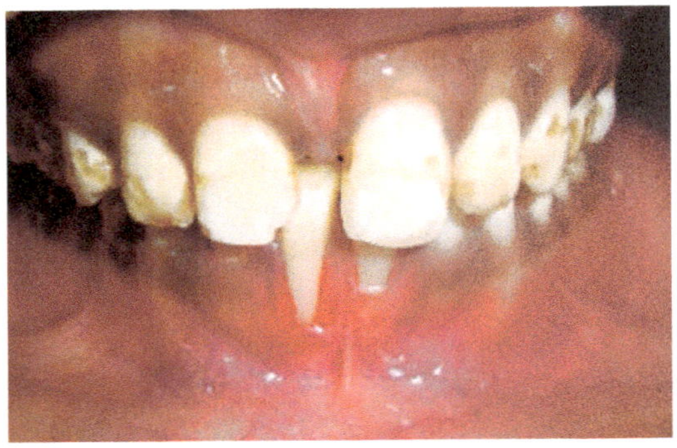

Figure 12: Recession of right central incisor.

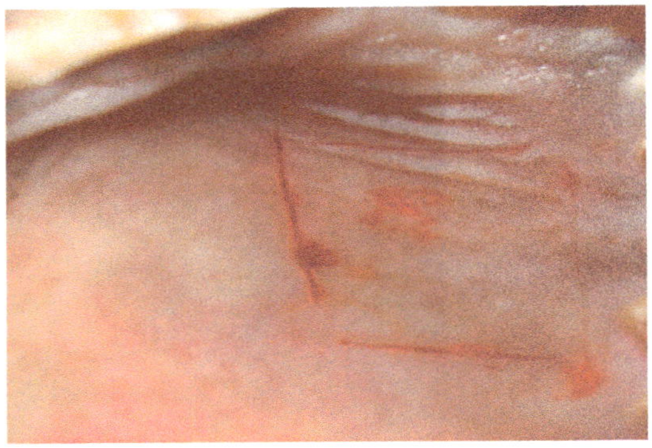

Figure 13: Incisions given for the removal of graft.

from the CEJ. Oral prophylaxis has been done and oral hygiene instructions were given so as to achieve satisfactory plaque control prior to periodontal surgery. The root surface was gently scaled and planed; instrumentation was done by utilizing manual and power driven scalers and curets. The shape of the root was not altered. The root surface was then treated with a tetracycline 500 mg by attempting to burnish, with small cotton pledgets. The donor tissue was removed from the palate and trimmed to a thickness of 2 to 3 mm (Figure 15). Within minutes of removal, the donor tissue was placed at the recipient site. Vertical stabilizing sutures (4–0 silk) were used to secure the graft (Figure 16). Postoperative healing after 6 months reveal excellent healing of the site and complete coverage of recession was achieved (Figure 17).

## 9. Discussion

The main goal of periodontal therapy is to improve periodontal health and thereby to maintain a patient's functional dentition right through his/her life. However, aesthetics symbolize an inseparable part of today's oral therapy, and numerous procedures have been proposed to preserve or enhance patient aesthetics. This treatment has principally been justified by the patient's wish to advance the aesthetic appearance when there is an exposed root.

Etiology and the contributing factors are chief when deciding on appropriate treatment procedures for patients with localized gingival recession. In the cases presented,

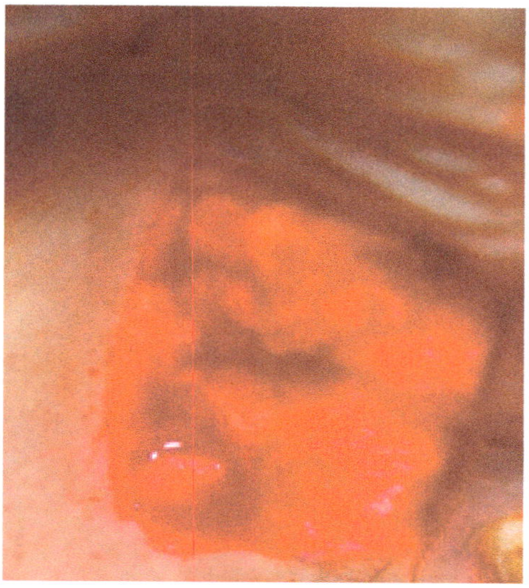

FIGURE 14: View of the palate after removal of the graft.

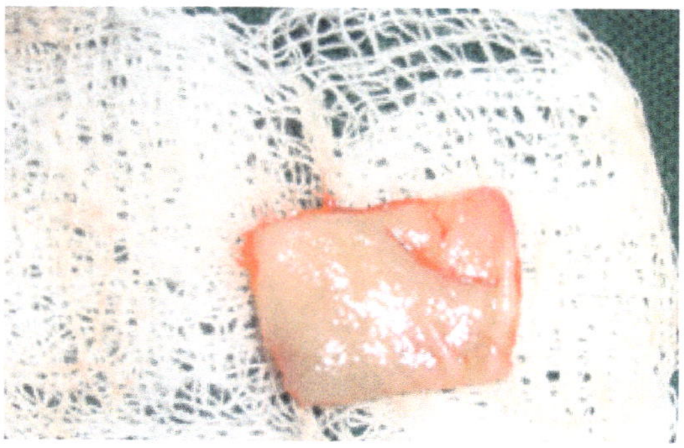

FIGURE 15: The donor tissue.

the etiologies of the gingival recession were scarce vestibular depth and inadequate width of keratinized gingiva. If malposition of teeth is supposed to be the etiology for recession, then orthodontic treatment needs to be given a thought with or without periodontal therapy. Due to the existence of multiple mucogingival problems, it was decided to use a free gingival graft to accomplish root coverage and to form functional attached gingiva. The band of keratinized tissue was determined to be adequate in all cases. The color match and the tissue contour were satisfactory to the patients in all cases mentioned above. In some cases the color match and tissue contour match were good enough to make it complex to determine the position of the original defect.

The outcome of the current cases confirm aesthetics as the primary indication for root coverage. A recent survey showing that aesthetic concern was the foremost indication for root coverage procedures [21]. Indications other than aesthetic, root sensitivity were low and were grouped in the other category, accounting for 1.84% of the indications.

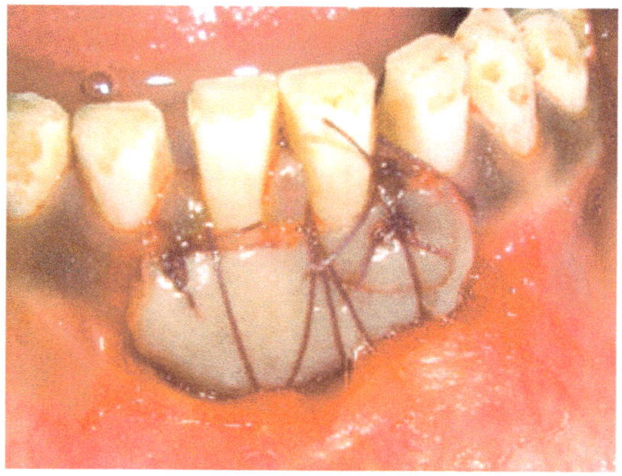

FIGURE 16: Suturing.

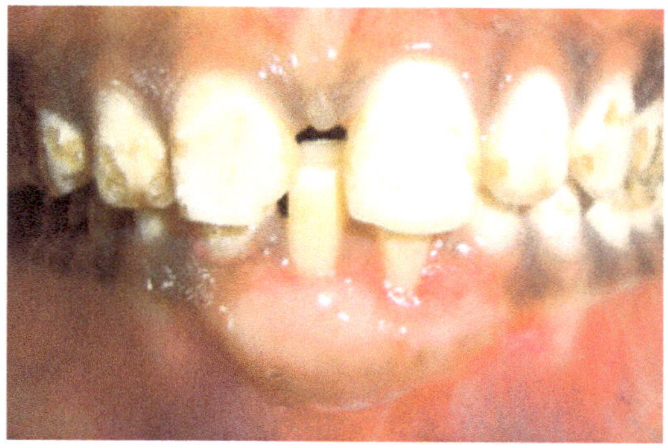

FIGURE 17: Six months postoperative healing.

## 10. Conclusion

Gingival recession is one of the main esthetic complaints of patients. This also exposes patients to sensitivity and greater risk for root caries. Mucogingival surgery endeavors' to reestablish the periodontium to a healthy circumstance Periodontal plastic surgery strives to restore the periodontium to a healthy, efficient, and aesthetic state. For coverage of exposed roots, there is a vast range of mucogingival grafting procedures available in the present epoch. These procedures are quite predictable and produce satisfactory solutions to the problems presented by gingival recessions. Choice of appropriate procedure and surgical technique will recommend successful and exceedingly predictable results in the management of gingival recession .

*Key Finding(s).* The present paper suggests that the selection of suitable procedure and specific and meticulous surgical technique will provide successful and exceedingly predictable results in the management of gingival recession.

## References

[1] A. J. Miller, J. A. Brunelle, J. P. Carlos, L. J. Brown, and H. Löe, *Oral Health of United States Adults. The National Survey of Oral Health in U.S. Employed Adults and Seniors: 1985-1986*, NIH publication no. 87-2868.

[2] J. M. Albandar and A. Kingman, "Gingival recession, Gingival bleeding, and dental calculus in adults 30 years of age and older in the United States, 1988–1994," *Journal of Periodontology*, vol. 70, no. 1, pp. 30–43, 1999.

[3] W. H. Van Palenstein Helderman, B. S. Lembariti, G. A. Van Der Weijden, and M. A. Van't Hof, "Gingival recession and its association with calculus in subjects deprived of prophylactic dental care," *Journal of Clinical Periodontology*, vol. 25, no. 2, pp. 106–111, 1998.

[4] A. Khocht, G. Simon, P. Person, and J. L. Denepitiya, "Gingival recession in relation to history of hard toothbrush use," *Journal of Periodontology*, vol. 64, no. 9, pp. 900–905, 1993.

[5] J. R. Trott and B. Love, "An analysis of localized gingival recession in 766 Winnipeg High School students," *The Dental Practitioner and Dental Record*, vol. 16, no. 6, pp. 209–213, 1966.

[6] B. U. Zachrisson, "Orthodontics and periodontics," in *Clinical Periodontology and Implant Dentistry*, J. Lindhe, Ed., pp. 741–793, Munksgaard, Copenhagen, Denmark, 3rd edition, 1998.

[7] J. Årtun and O. Krogstad, "Periodontal status of mandibular incisors following excessive proclination A study in adults with surgically treated mandibular prognathism," *American Journal of Orthodontics and Dentofacial Orthopedics*, vol. 91, no. 3, pp. 225–232, 1987.

[8] P. S. Wright and P. H. Hellyer, "Gingival recession related to removable partial dentures in older patients," *The Journal of Prosthetic Dentistry*, vol. 74, no. 6, pp. 602–607, 1995.

[9] J. C. Gunsolley, S. M. Quinn, J. Tew, C. M. Gooss, C. N. Brooks, and H. A. Schenkein, "The effect of smoking on individuals with minimal periodontal destruction," *Journal of Periodontology*, vol. 69, no. 2, pp. 165–170, 1998.

[10] S. Parma-Benfenati, P. A. Fugazzato, and M. P. Ruben, "He effect of restorative margins on post—surgical development and nature of periodontium," *The International Journal of Periodontics & Restorative Dentistry*, vol. 5, pp. 31–51, 1985.

[11] A. M. Quart, C. Butkus Small, and R. S. Klein, "The cocaine connection. Users imperil their gingiva," *The Journal of the American Dental Association*, vol. 122, no. 1, pp. 85–87, 1991.

[12] P. R. Greene, "The flexible gingival mask: an aesthetic solution in periodontal practice," *British Dental Journal*, vol. 184, no. 11, pp. 536–540, 1998.

[13] M. Brannstrom and A. Astrom, "The hydrodynamics of the dentine; its possible relationship to dentinal pain," *International Dental Journal*, vol. 22, no. 2, pp. 219–227, 1972.

[14] J. Reiker, U. Van Der Velden, D. S. Barendregt, and B. G. Loos, "A cross-sectional study into the prevalence of root caries in periodontal maintenance patients," *Journal of Clinical Periodontology*, vol. 26, no. 1, pp. 26–32, 1999.

[15] J. L. Wennström, "Mucogingival therapy," *Annals of Periodontology*, vol. 1, no. 1, pp. 671–701, 1996.

[16] H. C. Sullivan and J. H. Atkins, "Free autogenous gingival grafts. I. Principles of successful grafting," *Periodontics*, vol. 6, no. 3, pp. 121–129, 1968.

[17] B. Langer and L. Langer, "Subepithelial connective tissue graft technique for root coverage," *Journal of Periodontology*, vol. 56, no. 12, pp. 715–720, 1985.

[18] D. P. Tarnow, "Semilunar coronally repositioned flap," *Journal of Clinical Periodontology*, vol. 13, no. 3, pp. 182–185, 1986.

[19] C. F. Sumner III, "Surgical repair of recession on the maxillary cuspid: incisally repositioning the gingival tissues," *Journal of Periodontology*, vol. 40, no. 2, pp. 119–121, 1969.

[20] G. Pini Prato, C. Tinti, G. Vincenzi, C. Magnani, P. Cortellini, and C. Clauser, "Guided tissue regeneration versus mucogingival surgery in the treatment of human buccal gingival recession," *Journal of Periodontology*, vol. 63, no. 11, pp. 919–928, 1992.

[21] C. A. Zaher, J. Hachem, M. A. Puhan, and A. Mombelli, "Interest in periodontology and preferences for treatment of localized gingival recessions: a survey among Swiss dentists," *Journal of Clinical Periodontology*, vol. 32, no. 4, pp. 375–382, 2005.

# Permissions

All chapters in this book were first published in CRID, by Hindawi Publishing Corporation; hereby published with permission under the Creative Commons Attribution License or equivalent. Every chapter published in this book has been scrutinized by our experts. Their significance has been extensively debated. The topics covered herein carry significant findings which will fuel the growth of the discipline. They may even be implemented as practical applications or may be referred to as a beginning point for another development.

The contributors of this book come from diverse backgrounds, making this book a truly international effort. This book will bring forth new frontiers with its revolutionizing research information and detailed analysis of the nascent developments around the world.

We would like to thank all the contributing authors for lending their expertise to make the book truly unique. They have played a crucial role in the development of this book. Without their invaluable contributions this book wouldn't have been possible. They have made vital efforts to compile up to date information on the varied aspects of this subject to make this book a valuable addition to the collection of many professionals and students.

This book was conceptualized with the vision of imparting up-to-date information and advanced data in this field. To ensure the same, a matchless editorial board was set up. Every individual on the board went through rigorous rounds of assessment to prove their worth. After which they invested a large part of their time researching and compiling the most relevant data for our readers.

The editorial board has been involved in producing this book since its inception. They have spent rigorous hours researching and exploring the diverse topics which have resulted in the successful publishing of this book. They have passed on their knowledge of decades through this book. To expedite this challenging task, the publisher supported the team at every step. A small team of assistant editors was also appointed to further simplify the editing procedure and attain best results for the readers.

Apart from the editorial board, the designing team has also invested a significant amount of their time in understanding the subject and creating the most relevant covers. They scrutinized every image to scout for the most suitable representation of the subject and create an appropriate cover for the book.

The publishing team has been an ardent support to the editorial, designing and production team. Their endless efforts to recruit the best for this project, has resulted in the accomplishment of this book. They are a veteran in the field of academics and their pool of knowledge is as vast as their experience in printing. Their expertise and guidance has proved useful at every step. Their uncompromising quality standards have made this book an exceptional effort. Their encouragement from time to time has been an inspiration for everyone.

The publisher and the editorial board hope that this book will prove to be a valuable piece of knowledge for researchers, students, practitioners and scholars across the globe.

# List of Contributors

**Anoop Jain and Shivakumar Puranik**
Department of Prosthodontics, HKE'S S N Institute of Dental Sciences & Research, Gulbarga, Karnataka 585105, India

**M. S. Jagadeesh**
Department of Prosthodontics, Farooqia Dental College and Hospital, Mysore, Karnataka 570015, India

**Puttaraj Kattimani**
Department of Prosthodontics, Pandit Deendayal Upadhyay Dental CollegeHospital&Research Centre, Solapur,Maharastra 413255, India

**Savita Akki**
Department of Prosthodontics, SB Patil Dental College & Hospital, Bidar, Karnataka 585401, India

**Pawan Kumar**
Department of Prosthodontics, Al-Badar Dental College & Hospital, Gulbarga, Karnataka 585105, India

**Vijaya laxmi'**
Department of Prosthodontics, G. Pulla Reddy Dental College, Andhra Pradesh 518002, India

**Massimo Amato**
Department ofMedicine and Surgery, University of Salerno, Fisciano, 84084 Salerno, Italy

**Vincenzo Bruno, Giuseppe Pantaleo, Gianrico Spagnuolo and Gilberto Sammartino**
Department of Neurosciences, Reproductive and Odontostomatological Sciences, University of Naples Federico II, 80131 Naples, Italy

**Antonio Cerutti**
School of Dentistry, University of Brescia, 25121 Brescia, Italy

**S. Padmashree, Chaitra H. Ramprakash and Rema Jayalekshmy**
Department of Oral Medicine & Radiology, Vydehi Institute of Dental Sciences and Research Centre, No. 82, EPIP Area, Whitefield, Bangalore 560 066, India

**Konstantinos X. Michalakis**
Division of Graduate and Postgraduate Prosthodontics, Tufts University School of Dental Medicine, Boston, MA 02111, USA
Department of Prosthodontics, Division of Removable Prosthodontics, Faculty of Dentistry, Aristotle University School of Health Sciences, 54124 Thessaloniki, Greece
Private Practice Limited to Prosthodontics, 54622 Thessaloniki, Greece

**Hiroshi Hirayama**
Division of Graduate and Postgraduate Prosthodontics, Tufts University School of Dental Medicine, Boston, MA 02111, USA

**Pasquale Lino Calvani**
Division of Graduate and Postgraduate Prosthodontics, Tufts University School of Dental Medicine, Boston, MA 02111, USA
Private Practice Limited to Prosthodontics, 00198 Rome, Italy

**Argiris L. Pissiotis**
Department of Prosthodontics, Division of Removable Prosthodontics, Faculty of Dentistry, Aristotle University School of Health Sciences, 54124 Thessaloniki, Greece
Private Practice Limited to Prosthodontics, 54622 Thessaloniki, Greece

**Christos D. R. Kalpidis**
Private Practice Limited to Periodontics, 54623 Thessaloniki, Greece

**Yvone Kirmanidou**
Private Practice, 54622Thessaloniki, Greece

**Ishani Karhade and Meenal N. Gulve**
Usha Kiran Bunglow, Anand Nagar, Behind Muktidham, Opp Maharshi Hospital, Nashik Road, Nashik, Maharashtra 422101, India

**Prashanthi Chippagiri**
Department of Oral Medicine and Radiology, MS Ramaiah Dental College and Hospital, Bangalore, Karnataka 560010, India

**Spoorthi Banavar Ravi**
Department of Oral Pathology, MS Ramaiah Dental College and Hospital, Bangalore, India

**Neha Patwa**
Department of Dentistry, Indiragandhi District Hospital, Mandsaur, Madhya Pradesh 458001, India

**Tupili Muralikrishna, Butchibabu Kalakonda and Pradeep Koppolu**
Department of Periodontics, Sri Sai College of Dental Surgery, Kothrepally, Vikarabad, Andhra Pradesh 501101, India

**Sumanth Gunupati**
Department of Periodontics, Narayana Dental College and Hospital, Chinthareddypalem, Nellore, Andhra Pradesh 524003, India

**Gaurav Sharma**
Department of Oral Medicine and Radiology, Sudha Rustagi College of Dental Sciences and Research, Faridabad, Haryana 121002, India

**Amritpreet Nagra**
Ahead Academy, Rajinder Nagar, New Delhi 11060, India

**Gurkeerat Singh and Vishal Bhardwaj**
Department of Orthodontics, Sudha Rustagi College of Dental Sciences and Research, Faridabad, Haryana 121002, India

**Archna Nagpal**
Department of Oral Medicine and Radiology, PDM Dental College and Research Institute, Bahadurgarh, Haryana 124507, India

**Atul Soin**
Department of Prosthodontics, Kalka Dental College, Meerut 250006, India

**Nedim Özer and Serdar Yilmaz**
Department of Oral and Maxillofacial Surgery, Faculty of Dentistry, Istanbul Medipol University, Turkey

**Fulya Üçem, Alp SaruhanoLlu and HakkJ Tanyeri**
Department of Oral and Maxillofacial Surgery, Faculty of Dentistry, Istanbul University, Istanbul, Turkey

**Manasa Anand Meundi**
Department of Oral Medicine, Diagnosis and Radiology, Dayananda Sagar College of Dental Sciences, Shavige Malleshwara Hills, Kumaraswamy Layout, Bangalore 560078, India

**Gopakumar R. Nair**
Department of Oral Medicine, Diagnosis and Radiology, New Horizon Dental College & Research institute, Sakri, Bilaspur 495001, India

**Prathima Sreenivasan**
Department of Oral Medicine, Diagnosis and Radiology, Kannur Dental College, Anjarakkandy post, Kannur 670612, India

**A. C. Raj**
Department of Oral Medicine, Diagnosis and Radiology, KVG Dental College and Hospital, Vidhyanagar post, Kurunjibagh, Sullia 574327, India

**Saad Al-Almaie**
KFMMC, Dental Department, P.O. Box 946, Dhahran 31932, Saudi Arabia

**Renata Reis dos Santos**
Universidade Estadual Paulista, UNESP Arac¸atuba Dental School, Preventive and Social Dentistry, Rua José Bonifácio 1193, Vila Mendonça, Araçatuba16015-050, SP, Brazil

**Artênio José Isper Garbin**
Universidade Estadual Paulista, UNESP Arac¸atuba Dental School, Post-Graduation Program, Rua José Bonifácio 1193, Vila Mendonça, Araçatuba 16018-050, SP, Brazil

**Cléa Adas Saliba Garbin**
Universidade Estadual Paulista, UNESP Araçatuba Dental School, Orthodontics and Preventive and Social Dentistry, Rua José Bonifácio, 1193, Vila Mendonça, Araçatuba-16015-050, SP, Brazil

**Santosh Hunasg and Anila Koneru**
Department of Oral and Maxillofacial Pathology, Navodaya Dental College and Hospital, Raichur, Karnataka 584103, India

**Dinesh Singh Chauhan and Yadavalli Guruprasad**
Department of Oral and Maxillofacial Surgery, AME's Dental College, Raichur, Karnataka 584103, India

**Suryakant C. Deogade, Sneha S. Mantri and Pushkar Gupta**
Department of Prosthodontics, Hitkarini Dental College & Hospital, Jabalpur, Madhya Pradesh 482001, India

**Dinesh Naitam and Ashish Dewangan**
Department of Prosthodontics, Rungta College of Dental Sciences & Research, Bhilai, Chhattisgarh 490024, India

**Gunjan Dube**
Department ofOral Surgery,Hitkarini Dental College&Hospital, Jabalpur, Madhya Pradesh 482001, India

**Fahad F. Alsulaimani and Ahmed R. Afify**
Orthodontic Division, Department of Preventive Dental Sciences, Faculty of Dentistry, King Abdul-Aziz University, Jeddah, Saudi Arabia

**Maisa O. Al-Sebaei**
2Oral andMaxillofacial SurgeryDepartment, Faculty ofDentistry, King Abdul-AzizUniversity, Jeddah, Saudi Arabia

**G. Siva Prasad Reddy, Shravan Kumar Regonda and Harish Kumar TVS**
Department of Oral and Maxillofacial Surgery, Panineeya Institute of Dental Sciences, Road No. 5, Kamala Nagar, Dilsukhnagar, Hyderabad, Andhra Pradesh 500060, India

**B. Surya Kumar**
Department of Dental Surgery, Mediciti Hospital, Near Secretariate, Hyderabad, India

**RadhikaMuppa**
Department of Pedodontics, Panineeya Institute of Dental Sciences, Hyderabad, India

**Kaustubh Suresh Thakare, M. L. Bhongade, Pretti Charde, Priyanka Jaiswal, B. K. Somnath and Sunil Pendor**
Department of Periodontology & Implantology, Sharad Pawar Dental College and Hospital,Wardha, Maharashtra 442001, India

**Shweta Kale**
Department of Prosthodontics, Sharad Pawar Dental College and Hospital,Wardha, Maharastra 442001, India

**Mahesh Jayachandran and Rethi Mahesh**
Noorul Islam College of Dental Sciences, Aralammoodu PO,Thiruvananthapuram, Kerala 695123, India

**Shalini Kapoor**
SGT Dental College, Hospital & Research Institute, Gurgaon, Delhi, India

**Mohammad Hoseini, SeyedMorteza Saadat Mostafavi and Navid Rezaei**
Department of Orthodontics and Dentofacial Orthopedics, School of Dentistry, Shahid Sadoughi University of Medical Sciences, Daheye Fajr BLV, Imam Avenue, Yazd 89195/165, Iran

**Ehsan Javadzadeh Boluri**
School of Dentistry, Shahid Sadoughi University of Medical Sciences, Daheye Fajr BLV, Imam Avenue, Yazd 89195/165, Iran

**Sabrina Araújo Pinho Costa,Mário César Pereira Brinhole, Rogério Almeida da Silva, Daniel Hacomar dos Santos, and Mayko Naruhito Tanabe**
Department of Oral andMaxillofacial Surgery, Vila Penteado General Hospital, Avenue Ministro Petrônio Portela, 1642, Freguesia do Ó, 02802-120 Saõ Paulo, SP, Brazil

**Meenakshi Bhasin**
Department of Oral Medicine, Mansarovar Dental College, Bhopal, Madhya Pradesh 462042, India
Department ofOralMedicine & Radiology, 153 AdarshNagar,Narmada Road, Jabalpur, Madhya Pradesh 482002, India

**Vinny Bhasin**
Department of Orthodontia, Mansarovar Dental College, Bhopal, Madhya Pradesh 462042, India

**Abhilasha Bhasin**
Department of Prosthodontics, Hithkarni Dental College, Jabalpur, Madhya Pradesh 482002, India

**Mahnaz Hatami**
Department of Prosthodontics, School of Dentistry, Shahid Sadoughi University of Medical Sciences, Yazd, Iran

**Hamid Badrian**
Dental Implant Research Center, School of Dentistry, Isfahan, Iran

**Siamak Samanipoor**
Department of Endodontics, School of Dentistry, Shahid Bahonar University of Medical Sciences, Kerman, Iran

**Marcelo Coelho Goiato**
Faculty of Dentistry of Araçatuba, University of the State of São Paulo, Jose Bonifacio 1193, 16015-050 Araçatuba, SP, Brazil

**Satish G. Patil, Aaisha Siddiqua, Udupi Krishna Joshi, and AnandMangalgi**
Department of Oral and Maxillofacial Surgery, S. Nijalingappa Institute of Dental Sciences and Research, Gulbarga, Karnataka 585105, India

**Pallavi K. Deshmukh**
Department of Oral Medicine and Radiology, S. Nijalingappa Institute of Dental Sciences and Research, Gulbarga, Karnataka 585105, India

**Bindu S. Patil**
Department of Periodontics, S. Nijalingappa Institute of Dental Sciences and Research, Gulbarga, Karnataka 585105, India

**Flávia SayuriMatsuo and Paulo Rogério de Faria**
Department of Morphology, Laboratory of Histology, Institute of Biomedical Science, Federal University of Uberlândia, Avenue Pará 1720, Block 2B, Room 2B-256, 38405-320 Uberlândia, Minas Gerais, Brazil

**Alceu Luiz Camargo Villela Berbert and Sônia Antunes de Oliveira Mantese**
Department of Dermatology, School of Medicine, Federal University of Uberlândia, Avenue Pará 1720, Block 2U, Room23, 38405-302 Uberlândia, Minas Gerais, Brazil

**AdrianoMota Loyola and Sérgio Vitorino Cardoso**
Department of Oral Pathology, School of Dentistry, Federal University of Uberlândia, Avenue Pará 1720,UniversityHospital, Room 2K07, 38405-302 Uberlândia, Minas Gerais, Brazil

**Butchibabu Kalakonda, Koppolu Pradeep, AshankMishra, Krishnanjaneya Reddy, Tupili Muralikrishna, Vijaya Lakshmi and Radhika Challa**
Department of Periodontics, Sri Sai College of Dental Surgery, Vikarabad 501101, India

**Poulami Majumder and Subrata Kumar Dey**
Department of Biotechnology, Centre for Genetic Studies, School of Biotechnology and Biological Sciences, West BengalUniversity of Technology, BF-142, Sector I, Salt Lake City, Kolkata, West Bengal 700064, India

**Vineet Nair and Malancha Mukherjee**
Department of Periodontics&Oral Implantology,Dr. R. AhmedDental College & Hospital, Kolkata, West Bengal 700014, India

**Sujoy Ghosh**
Department of Zoology, University of Calcutta, 35 Ballygunge Circular Road, Kolkata,West Bengal 700019, India

**Shailesh Menat and Kaushal Goyal**
Department of Oral and Maxillofacial Surgery, Narsinhbhai Patel Dental College and Hospital, Visnagar, Gujarat 384315, India

**Shylaja MD**
Department of Oral Pathology and Microbiology, Narsinhbhai Patel Dental College and Hospital, Visnagar, Gujarat 384315, India

**Kailash Attur**
Department of Conservative and Endodontics, Narsinhbhai Patel Dental College and Hospital, Visnagar, Gujarat 384315, India

**Mostafa Ibrahim Mostafa and Mennat Allah IsmailMehrez**
Department of Oro-Dental Genetics, National Research Centre, 33 Tahrir Street, Dokki, Cairo 12311, Egypt

**Nehad Samir Taha**
Oral Histopathology Department, Misr International University (MIU), Cairo, Egypt

**Umberto Romeo,Marco Lollobrigida, Gaspare Palaia, Domenica Laurito, Riccardo Cugnetto and Alberto De Biase**
Division of Oral Surgery, Department of Oral and Maxillofacial Sciences, Sapienza University of Rome, Via Caserta 6, 00161 Rome, Italy

**Mamta Kaushik and NehaMehra**
Department of Conservative Dentistry and Endodontics, Army College of Dental Sciences, Jai Jawahar Nagar, Secunderabad, Andhra Pradesh 500094, India

**Nádia Carolina Teixeira Marques, Carla Vecchione Gurgel, Ana Paula Fernandes and Maria Aparecida AndradeMoreira Machado**
Department of Pediatric Dentistry, Orthodontics and Public Health, Bauru School of Dentistry, University of São Paulo, Al. Octávio Pinheiro Brisolla 9-75, 17012-901, Bauru-SP 73, Brazil

**Marta Cunha Lima**
Matrix Dynamics Group, Faculty of Dentistry, University of Toronto, Toronto, ON, Canada

**Simone Soares**
Department of Prosthetic Dentistry, Bauru School of Dentistry, University of São Paulo, São Paulo, Bauru, Brazil
Hospital for the Rehabilitation of Craniofacial Anomalies, University of São Paulo, São Paulo, SP, Brazil

**Thais Marchini Oliveira**
Department of Pediatric Dentistry, Orthodontics and Public Health, Bauru School of Dentistry, University of São Paulo, Al. Octávio Pinheiro Brisolla 9-75, 17012-901, Bauru-SP 73, Brazil
Hospital for the Rehabilitation of Craniofacial Anomalies, University of São Paulo, São Paulo, SP, Brazil

**Andreas Thor**
Department of Plastic & Oral and Maxillofacial Surgery, Institute of Surgical Sciences, Uppsala University, 751 85 Uppsala, Sweden

**Naresh Shetty**
Department of Oral & Maxillofacial Surgery, Faculty of Dentistry, Melaka Manipal Medical College, 75150 Melaka, Malaysia

**Rajanikanth K.Malaviya**
Department of Oral & Maxillofacial Surgery, Sharad Pawar Dental College, Wardha 442005, India

**M. K. Gupta**
Department of Oral & Maxillofacial Surgery, Peoples Dental Academy, Bhopal 462010, India

**OrlandoMotohiro Tanaka**
Graduate Dentistry Program in Orthodontics, Pontifícia Universidade Católica do Paraná, Rua Imaculada Conceição 1155, 80215-901 Curitiba, PR, Brazil
Postdoctoral Fellowship at The Center for Advanced Dental Education, Saint Louis University, St. Louis, MO, USA

**Isabelle Adad Fornazari**
Dentistry, Pontifícia Universidade Católica do Paraná, Curitiba, PR, Brazil

**Ariane Ximenes Graciano Parra and Bruno Borges de Castilhos**
Orthodontics, Pontif´ıcia Universidade Católica do Paraná, Curitiba, PR, Brazil

**Ademir Franco**
Department of Oral Health Sciences, Forensic Dentistry, KU Leuven and Dentistry, University Hospitals Leuven, Leuven, Belgium
Stomatology, Pontif´ıcia Universidade Católica do Paraná, Curitiba, PR, Brazil

**SepidehMokhtari and Ali Lotfi**
Department of Oral and Maxillofacial Pathology, Dental School of Shahid Beheshti University of Medical Sciences, Tehran 4739, Iran

**SaeedehMokhtari**
Department of of Pediatric Dentistry, Dental School of Shahid Beheshti University of Medical Sciences, Tehran 4739, Iran

**K. Pavan Kumar, Surya Kumari Nujella, S. Sujatha Gopal and K. Karthik Roy**
Conservative Dentistry & Endodontics, MNR Dental College and Hospital, Sangareddy, Telangana 522094, India

**Parth Purwar**
Department of Periodontology, Faculty of Dental Sciences, King George's Medical University, Lucknow, Uttar Pradesh, India
Ankur Diagnostic Center, Lakhimpur Road, Gola Gokaran Nath, Kheri, Uttar Pradesh 262802, India

**Abhishek Gupta**
Department of Community Medicine, Hind Institute of Medical Sciences, Barabanki, Uttar Pradesh, India

**Rajiv Ratan Singh Yadav**
Emergency Medicine, Dr. Ram Manohar Lohia Institute of Medical Sciences, Uttar Pradesh, India

**Utkarsh Bansal**
Department of Paediatrics, Hind Institute of Medical Sciences, Barabanki, Uttar Pradesh, India

**Akshay Shetty**
Department of Oral and Maxillofacial Surgery, Sri Rajiv Gandhi College of Dental Sciences and Hospital, Cholanagar, RT Nagar, Bangalore 560032, India

**Kourosh Nakhaei, Maryam Mohseni and Iman Mohebatzadeh**
Sri Rajiv Gandhi College of Dental Sciences andHospital, Cholanagar, RTNagar, Bangalore 560032, India

**Yogesh Lakkashetty**
Department of Oral and Maxillofacial Pathology, Sri Rajiv Gandhi College of Dental Sciences and Hospital, Cholanagar, RT Nagar, Bangalore 560032, India

**Haraswarupa Gurkar, Omprakash Yadahally Venkatesh, JagadeeshMandya Somashekar, Muthuraj Hariharapura Lakshme Gowda, Madhavi Dwivedi and Ishani Ningthoujam**
Department of Prosthodontics, Farooqia Dental College and Hospital, Mysore 570021, India

**Joe Iwanaga, Koichi Watanabe, Tsuyoshi Saga, Yoko Tabira and Koh-ichi Yamaki**
Department of Anatomy, Kurume University School of Medicine, Kurume, Fukuoka 830-0011, Japan

**Christiane V. Cruz and Marcelo C. Costa**
Department of Pediatric Dentistry and Orthodontics, Federal University of Rio de Janeiro, Brazil

**Andrea L. Soares**
Department of Oral Biology, Fluminense Federal University, Brazil

**David N. Braga**
Department of Maxillofacial Surgery, Federal University of Rio de Janeiro, Brazil

**Kanika Attam, Ruchika Roongta Nawal, Shivani Utneja and Sangeeta Talwar**
Conservative Dentistry & Endodontics, Maulana Azad Institute of Dental Sciences, New Delhi 110002, India

**Pishipati Vinayak Kalyan Chakravarthy**
Department of Conservative Dentistry and Endodontics, Penang International Dental College, Level 18-21, NB Tower, 5050 Jalan Bagan Luar, 12000 Butterworth, Penang, Malaysia

**Lahari Ajay Telang**
Department of Oral Medicine and Radiology, Penang International Dental College, 12000 Butterworth, Penang, Malaysia

**Jayashri Nerali and Ajay Telang**
Department of Oral Pathology, Penang International Dental College, 12000 Butterworth, Penang, Malaysia

**Eveline Claudia Martini and FabianaMadalozzo Coppla**
Department of Dentistry, State University of Ponta Grossa, Rua Carlos Cavalcanti 4748, Bloco M, Uvaranas, 84030-900 Ponta Grossa, PR, Brazil

**Eduardo Bauml Campagnoli and Marcelo Carlos Bortoluzzi**
Department of Stomatology, State University of Ponta Grossa, PR, Brazil

**Carolina Mayumi Iegami, Danilo deMelo Lopes, Atlas EdsonMoleros Nakamae, Priscila Nakasone Uehara and Regina Tamaki**
Department of Prosthodontics, School of Dentistry, University of Sao Paulo, Avenida Professor Lineu Prestes, 2227 Cidade Universitaria, 05508-000 Sao Paulo, SP, Brazil

**Koppolu Pradeep**
Department of Periodontics, Sri Sai College of Dental Surgery, Vikarabad, Andhra Pradesh, India

**Palaparthy Rajababu, Durvasula Satyanarayana and Vidya Sagar**
Department of Periodontics, Kamineni Institute of Dental Sciences, Narketpally, Andhra Pradesh, India

# Index

## P



## R



## S



## T



## U



## X